ANNALS OF THE NEW YORK ACADEMY OF SCIENCES

Volume 1084

DIABETES MELLITUS AND ITS COMPLICATIONS

Molecular Mechanisms, Epidemiology, and Clinical Medicine

Edited by Ernest Adeghate, Hussein Saadi, Abdu Adem, and Enyioma Obineche

Published by Blackwell Publishing on behalf of the New York Academy of Sciences
Boston, Massachusetts
2006

Library of Congress Cataloging-in-Publication Data

International Conference on Recent Advances in Diabetes Mellitus and its Complications (2006 : Al Ain, United Arab Emirates)
Diabetes mellitus and its complications : molecular mechanisms, epidemiology, and clinical medicine / edited by Ernest Adeghate... [et al.].
p. ; cm. – (Annals of the New York Academy of Sciences, ISSN 0077-8923 ; v. 1086) Includes bibliographical references.
Includes bibliographical references.
ISBN-13: 978-1-57331-635-4 (paper : alk. paper)
ISBN-10: 1-57331-635-0 (paper : alk. paper)
1. Diabetes–Complications–Congresses. I. Adeghate, Ernest. II. New York Academy of Sciences. III. Title. IV. Series.
[DNLM: 1. Diabetes Mellitus–Congresses. 2. Diabetes Complications–Congresses.
W1 AN626YL v.1086 2006 / WK 810 I5913d 2006]

RC660.D5344 2006
616.4'62–dc22

2006032968

The *Annals of the New York Academy of Sciences* (ISSN: 0077-8923 [print]; ISSN: 1749-6632 [online]) is published 28 times a year on behalf of the New York Academy of Sciences by Blackwell Publishing, with offices located at 350 Main Street, Malden, Massachusetts 02148 USA, PO Box 1354, Garsington Road, Oxford OX4 2DQ UK, and PO Box 378 Carlton South, 3053 Victoria Australia.

Information for subscribers: Subscription prices for 2006 are: Premium Institutional: $3850.00 (US) and £2139.00 (Europe and Rest of World).
Customers in the UK should add VAT at 5%. Customers in the EU should also add VAT at 5% or provide a VAT registration number or evidence of entitlement to exemption. Customers in Canada should add 7% GST or provide evidence of entitlement to exemption. The Premium Institutional price also includes online access to full-text articles from 1997 to present, where available. For other pricing options or more information about online access to Blackwell Publishing journals, including access information and terms and conditions, please visit www.blackwellpublishing.com/nyas.

Membership information: Members may order copies of the *Annals* volumes directly from the Academy by visiting www.nyas.org/annals, emailing membership@nyas.org, faxing 212-888-2894, or calling 800-843-6927 (US only), or +1 212 838 0230, ext. 345 (International). For more information on becoming a member of the New York Academy of Sciences, please visit www.nyas.org/membership.

Journal Customer Services: For ordering information, claims, and any inquiry concerning your institutional subscription, please contact your nearest office:
UK: Email: customerservices@blackwellpublishing.com; Tel: +44 (0) 1865 778315; Fax +44 (0) 1865 471775
US: Email: customerservices@blackwellpublishing.com; Tel: +1 781 388 8599 or 1 800 835 6770 (Toll free in the USA); Fax: +1 781 388 8232
Asia: Email: customerservices@blackwellpublishing.com; Tel: +65 6511 8000; Fax: +61 3 8359 1120
Members: Claims and inquiries on member orders should be directed to the Academy at email: membership@nyas.org or Tel: +1 212 838 0230 (International) or 800-843-6927 (US only).

Printed in the USA.
Printed on acid-free paper.

Mailing: The *Annals of the New York Academy of Sciences* are mailed Standard Rate. **Postmaster:** Send all address changes to *Annals of the New York Academy of Sciences*, Blackwell Publishing, Inc., Journals Subscription Department, 350 Main Street, Malden, MA 01248-5020. Mailing to rest of world by DHL Smart and Global Mail.

Annals are available to subscribers online at the New York Academy of Sciences and also at Blackwell Synergy. Visit www.annalsnyas.org or www.blackwell-synergy.com to search the articles and register for table of contents e-mail alerts. Access to full text and PDF downloads of *Annals* articles are available to nonmembers and subscribers on a pay-per-view basis at www.annalsnyas.org.

The paper used in this publication meets the minimum requirements of the National Standard for Information Sciences Permanence of Paper for Printed Library Materials, ANSI Z39.48_1984.

ISSN: 0077-8923 (print); 1749-6632 (online)
ISBN-10: 1-57331-635-0 (paper); ISBN-13: 978-1-57331-635-4 (paper)

A catalogue record for this title is available from the British Library.

Digitization of the *Annals of the New York Academy of Sciences*

An agreement has recently been reached between Blackwell Publishing and the New York Academy of Sciences to digitize the entire run of the *Annals of the New York Academy of Sciences* back to volume one.

The back files, which have been defined as all of those issues published before 1997, will be sold to libraries as part of Blackwell Publishing's Legacy Sales Program and hosted on the Blackwell Synergy website.

Copyright of all material will remain with the rights holder. Contributors: Please contact Blackwell Publishing if you do not wish an article or picture from the *Annals of the New York Academy of Sciences* to be included in this digitization project.

ANNALS OF THE NEW YORK ACADEMY OF SCIENCES

Volume 1084
November 2006

DIABETES MELLITUS AND ITS COMPLICATIONS

Molecular Mechanisms, Epidemiology, and Clinical Medicine

Editors
ERNEST ADEGHATE, HUSSEIN SAADI, ABDU ADEM, AND ENYIOMA OBINECHE

This volume is the result of a conference entitled **International Conference on Recent Advances in Diabetes Mellitus and Its Complications,** held on March 6–9, 2006 in Al Ain, United Arab Emirates.

CONTENTS

Preface. *By* ERNEST ADEGHATE, HUSSEIN SAADI, ABDU ADEM, AND ENYIOMA OBINECHE xiii

Part I. Epidemiology of Diabetes Mellitus

An Update on the Etiology and Epidemiology of Diabetes Mellitus. *By* ERNEST ADEGHATE, PETER SCHATTNER, AND EARL DUNN 1

Part II. Metabolic Syndrome

Inflammation in Metabolic Syndrome and Type 2 Diabetes: Impact of Dietary Glucose. *By* KERSTIN KEMPF, BETTINA ROSE, CHRISTIAN HERDER, URSULA KLEOPHAS, STEPHAN MARTIN, AND HUBERT KOLB 30

Part III. Immunology of Diabetes, the Pancreas, and Transplantation

Functional Capacity of Macrophages Determines the Induction of Type 1 Diabetes. *By* EPK MENSAH-BROWN, A. SHAHIN, KHATIJA PAREKH, A. AL HAKIM, M. AL SHAMISI, D.K. HSU, AND M.L. LUKIC 49

Effect of Insulin on Acetylcholine-Evoked Amylase Release and Calcium Mobilization in Streptozotocin-Induced Diabetic Rat Pancreatic Acinar Cells. *By* REKHA PATEL, JOSÉ A. PARIENTE, MARIA A. MARTINEZ, GINÉS M. SALIDO, AND JAIPAUL SINGH 58

Mechanism of Exocrine Pancreatic Insufficiency in Streptozotocin-Induced Type 1 Diabetes Mellitus. *By* REKHA PATEL, AMIL SHERVINGTON, JOSE A. PARIENTE, MARIA A. MARTINEZ-BURGOS, GINES M. SALIDO, ERNEST ADEGHATE, AND JAIPAUL SINGH 71

Inflammatory Process in Type 2 Diabetes: The Role of Cytokines. *By* KRYSTALLENIA ALEXANDRAKI, CHRISTINA PIPERI, CHRISTOS KALOFOUTIS, JAIPAUL SINGH, ANTONIS ALAVERAS, AND ANASTASIOS KALOFOUTIS 89

Part IV. Gestational Diabetes

Beneficial Effect of Supplemental Lipoic Acid on Diabetes-Induced Pregnancy Loss in the Mouse. *By* RENGASAMY PADMANABHAN, SHAFIULLAH MOHAMED, AND SARABJIT SINGH 118

Audit of Pregnancies Complicated by Diabetes from One Center Five Years Apart with Selective versus Universal Screening. *By* M. EZIMOKHAI, ANNIE JOSEPH, AND P. BRADLEY-WATSON 132

Part V. Cardiovascular Complications of Diabetes

Blockade of the Renin–Angiotensin System Attenuates Sarcolemma and Sarcoplasmic Reticulum Remodeling in Chronic Diabetes. *By* XUELIANG LIU, HIDEAKI SUZUKI, RAJAT SETHI, PARAMJIT S. TAPPIA, NOBUAKIRA TAKEDA, AND NARANJAN S. DHALLA 141

Effects of Brain Natriuretic Peptide on Contraction and Intracellular Ca^{2+} in Ventricular Myocytes from the Streptozotocin-Induced Diabetic Rat. *By* FRANK C. HOWARTH, NOURA AL SHAMSI, MARYAM AL QAYDI, MARIAM AL MAZROUEI, ANWAR QURESHI, S.I. CHANDRANATH, ELSADIG KAZZAM, AND ABDU ADEM 155

Differences in Expression of Cardiovascular Risk Factors among Type 2 Diabetes Mellitus Patients of Different Age. *By* CHRISTOS KALOFOUTIS, CHRISTINA PIPERI, AIKATERINI ZISAKI, JAIPAUL SINGH, FRED HARRIS, DAVID PHOENIX, ANTONIS ALAVERAS, AND ANASTASIOS KALOFOUTIS 166

Effect of Streptozotocin-Induced Type 1 Diabetes Mellitus on Contraction, Calcium Transient, and Cation Contents in the Isolated Rat Heart. *By* JAIPAUL SINGH, APURVA CHONKAR, NICHOLAS BRACKEN, ERNEST ADEGHATE, ZAY LATT, AND MUNIR HUSSAIN 178

Predicting the Development of Macrovascular Disease in People with Type 1 Diabetes: A 9-Year Follow-up Study. *By* LATIKA SIBAL, HUONG NAI LAW, JANICE GEBBIE, UMESH K. DASHORA, SHARAD C. AGARWAL, AND PHILIP HOME 191

Effects of Streptozotocin-Induced Diabetes on Contraction and Calcium Transport in Rat Ventricular Cardiomyocytes. *By* NICHOLAS BRACKEN, FRANK C. HOWARTH, AND JAIPAUL SINGH 208

Part VI. Diabetic Nephropathy

Alterations in Atrial Natriuretic Peptide and Its Receptor Levels in Long-Term, Streptozotocin-Induced, Diabetes in Rats. *By* ENYIOMA OBINECHE, IRWIN CHANDRANATH, ERNEST ADEGHATE, SHEELA BENEDICT, MOHAMED FAHIM, AND ABDU ADEM 223

Part VII. Genetics

Diabetic Neuropathy Differs in Type 1 and Type 2 Diabetes. *By* ANDERS A.F. SIMA AND HIDEKI KAMIYA 235

Treatment of Diabetic Polyneuropathy: Update 2006. *By* DAN ZIEGLER 250

The Effect of Streptozotocin-Induced Diabetes on the Rat Seminal Vesicle: A Possible Pathophysiological Basis for Disorders of Ejaculation. *By* J.F.B. MORRISON, S. DHANASEKARAN, RAJAN SHEEN, C.M. FRAMPTON, AND ERIC MENSAH-BROWN 267

Changes of the Different Neuropeptide-Containing Nerve Fibers and Immunocells in the Diabetic Rat's Alimentary Tract. *By* ERZSÉBET FEHÉR, BAYARCHIMEG BATBAYAR, ÁGOTA VÉR, AND TIVADAR ZELLES 280

Pattern of Distribution of Calcitonin Gene–Related Peptide in the Dorsal Root Ganglion of Animal Models of Diabetes Mellitus. *By* ERNEST ADEGHATE, HAMEED RASHED, SATYAN RAJBANDARI, AND JAIPAUL SINGH 296

Cardiovascular Risk Factors Predicting the Development of Distal Symmetrical Polyneuropathy in People with Type 1 Diabetes: A 9-Year Follow-up Study. *By* LATIKA SIBAL, HUONG NAI LAW, JANICE GEBBIE, AND PHILIP HOME 304

Part VIII. Diabetes Education/Screening/Community Health

Audit of a Diabetes Clinic at Tawam Hospital, United Arab Emirates, 2004–2005. *By* B. AFANDI, S. AHMAD, H. SAADI, S. ELKHUMAIDI, M.A. KARKOUKLI, B. KELLY, H. ASSAF, AND D. MATEAR 319

A Controlled Study of Psychosocial Factors in Young People with Diabetes in the United Arab Emirates. *By* VALSAMMA EAPEN, ABDEL AZIM MABROUK, SUFIAN SABRI, AND SALEM BIN-OTHMAN 325

Diabetic Patients: Psychological Aspects. *By* FATEMEH ADILI, BAGHER LARIJANI, AND MOHAMMADREZA HAGHIGHATPANAH 329

Effect of Psychological Intervention on Exercise Adherence in Type 2 Diabetic Subjects. *By* ROBERT MARTINUS, ROD CORBAN, HENNING WACKERHAGE, STEVE ATKINS, AND JAIPAUL SINGH 350

Part IX. Nutrition

The Effect of a Fat-Enriched Diet on the Pattern of Distribution of Pancreatic Islet Cells in the C57BL/6J Mice. *By* ERNEST ADEGHATE, FRANK CHRISTOPHER HOWARTH, HAMEED RASHED, TARIQ SAEED, AND AMSTRONG GBEWONYO 361

Effect of Vitamin C on Liver and Kidney Functions in Normal and Diabetic Rats. *By* MARIAM AL SHAMSI, AMR AMIN, AND ERNEST ADEGHATE 371

The Protective Effect of *Tribulus terrestris* in Diabetes. *By* AMR AMIN, MOHAMED LOTFY, MOHAMED SHAFIULLAH, AND ERNEST ADEGHATE 391

Effect of High-Calorie Diet on the Prevalence of Diabetes Mellitus in the One-Humped Camel (*Camelus dromedarius*). *By* M. AL HAJ ALI, FRED NYBERG, S.I. CHANDRANATH, A.S. PONERY, A. ADEM, AND E. ADEGHATE 402

Vitamin E Ameliorates Some Biochemical Parameters in Normal and Diabetic Rats. *By* MARIAM AL SHAMSI, AMR AMIN, AND ERNEST ADEGHATE 411

Vitamin E Decreases the Hyperglucagonemia of Diabetic Rats. *By* MARIAM AL SHAMSI, AMR AMIN, AND ERNEST ADEGHATE 432

Part X. The Neuromuscular System and Diabetes

Contraction and Cation Contents of Skeletal Soleus and EDL Muscles in Age-Matched Control and Diabetic Rats. *By* APURVA CHONKAR, RICHARD HOPKIN, ERNEST ADEGHATE, AND JAIPAUL SINGH 442

Part XI. Molecular Genetics of Diabetes

Calpains and Their Multiple Roles in Diabetes Mellitus. *By* FREDERICK HARRIS, SUMAN BISWAS, JAIPAUL SINGH, SARAH DENNISON, AND DAVID A. PHOENIX 452

Lipid Peroxidation and Serum Antioxidant Enzymes in Patients with Type 2 Diabetes Mellitus. *By* FEROZA N. AHMED, FARZANA N. NAQVI, AND FAKHRA SHAFIQ 481

Signaling Proteins Associated with Diabetic-Induced Exocrine Pancreatic Insufficiency in Rats. *By* REKHA PATEL, PHILIP ATHERTON, HENNING WACKERHAGE, AND JAIPAUL SINGH 490

Part XII. Miscellaneous

Effects of Streptozotocin-Induced Type 1 Diabetes Mellitus on Total Protein Concentrations and Cation Contents in the Isolated Pancreas, Parotid, Submandibular, and Lacrimal Glands of Rats. *By* NAVIN R. CHANGRANI, APURVA CHONKAR, ERNEST ADEGHATE, AND JAIPAUL SINGH 503

Mucormycosis Mimicks Sinusitis in a Diabetic Adult. *By* GYÖRGY SZALAI, VERONIKA FELLEGI, ZSUZSANNA SZABÓ, AND LAJOS CSOKONAI VITÉZ 520

Index of Contributors 531

Financial assistance was received from:

- Faculty of Medicine & Health Sciences, UAE University
- Sheikh Hamdan Bin Rashid Al Maktoum Award for Medical Sciences
- Department of Health & Medical Services, Dubai
- Etihad Airways
- Merck
- Aventis
- Servier
- Life Scan (Johnson & Johnson)
- Roche Diagnostics

Preface

ERNEST ADEGHATE,[a] HUSSEIN SAADI,[b] ABDU ADEM,[c]
AND ENYIOMA OBINECHE[b]

[a]*Department of Anatomy,* [b]*Department of Internal Medicine,* [c]*Department of Pharmacology, Faculty of Medicine and Health Sciences, UAE University, Al Ain, United Arab Emirates*

This volume of the *Annals of New York Academy of Sciences* is based on the proceedings of the International Conference on Recent Advances in Diabetes Mellitus and its Complications, held in Al Ain, United Arab Emirates, from March 6–9, 2006. The meeting was organized by the Diabetes and Cardiovascular Research Group, Faculty of Medicine and Health Sciences, UAE University, United Arab Emirates under the patronage of His Excellency Sheikh Nahayan Mabarak Al-Nahayan, Minister of Higher Education and Scientific Research and Chancellor of UAE University.

The meeting was convened because diabetes has become a major global health problem.[1,2] According to the projections of Zimmet *et al.*,[1] the total number of people with diabetes mellitus worldwide will reach 220 million in the year 2010 and 300 million in 2025, compared to the current estimate of around 160 million. Diabetes mellitus is also becoming a major challenge in the Middle East, where prevalence estimates have ranged from 13% to 40% of the adult population.[3]

The main objectives of the conference were threefold: (1) to present recent advances in the area of diabetes mellitus and its complications, from molecular to clinical medicine spanning several areas, including epidemiology, diagnosis, complications, prevention, treatment, pancreatic β cell function, metabolic syndrome, glucose and lipid metabolism, and drug targets; (2) to facilitate exchange of information and collaboration among investigators from different specialty areas of diabetes; and (3) to emphasize the role of diabetes education in the prevention and management of diabetes mellitus. This was achieved through the teaching of healthcare professionals involved in the care of diabetic patients. The meeting was attended by more than 600 delegates from 35 countries.

The meeting covered a wide variety of the most current issues related to diabetes mellitus; these are reflected in this volume. Contributions include both basic and clinical research on diabetes mellitus. Topics covered in this

Address for correspondence: Ernest Adeghate, M.D., M.F.M., Ph.D., Department of Anatomy, Faculty of Medicine and Health Sciences, UAE University, P.O. Box 17666, Al Ain, United Arab Emirates. Voice: +971-3-7137496; fax: +971-3-7672033.
e-mail: eadeghate@uaeu.ac.ae

Ann. N.Y. Acad. Sci. 1084: xiii–xiv (2006). © 2006 New York Academy of Sciences.
doi: 10.1196/annals.1372.035

volume include epidemiology of diabetes mellitus; metabolic syndrome; the immunology of diabetes, the pancreas and pancreatic transplantation; gestational diabetes; cardiovascular complications of diabetes mellitus; diabetic nephropathy; diabetic neuropathy; diabetes education/screening/community health; nutrition and diabetes mellitus; the neuromuscular system and diabetes mellitus; and the molecular genetics of diabetes mellitus.

Supported grants came from the Faculty of Medicine and Health Sciences, UAE University, Al Ain and from several government and/or nonprofit institutions, including the Department of Health and Medical Services, Dubai; the Sheikh Hamdan Bin Rashid Al Maktoum Award for Medical Sciences; and other companies (listed separately). We are grateful for the help of many of our colleagues at the UAE University and to members of the Emirates Diabetes Society, as well as to all of the outstanding authors who have contributed to this volume.

Working with the editorial department of the *Annals of the New York Academy of Sciences*, especially Linda Mehta, Hilary Burdge, and Ralph Brown; and with Julia Keller and Carol DiPalermo (Blackwell Publishing) has been a pleasant and rewarding experience. We trust that this volume will be useful to all of those who wish to know and learn more about the basic and clinical aspects of diabetes mellitus and its complications.

REFERENCES

1. Zimmet, P., K.G. Alberti & J. Shaw. 2001. Global and societal implications of the diabetes epidemic. Nature **414:** 782–787.
2. Adeghate, E. 2001. Diabetes mellitus—multifactorial in aetiology and global in prevalence. Arch. Physiol. Biochem. **109:** 197–199.
3. Malik, M., A. Bakir., B.A. Saab. & H. King. 2005. Glucose intolerance and associated factors in the multi-ethnic population of the United Arab Emirates: results of a national survey. Diabetes Res. Clin. Pract. **69:** 188–195.

An Update on the Etiology and Epidemiology of Diabetes Mellitus

ERNEST ADEGHATE,[a] PETER SCHATTNER,[b] AND EARL DUNN[c]

[a]*Department of Human Anatomy, Faculty of Medicine and Health Sciences, UAE University, Al Ain, United Arab Emirates*

[b]*Department of Community Medicine and General Practice, Monash University, East Bentleigh, Victoria, Australia 3165*

[c]*Department of Family Medicine, Faculty of Medicine and Health Sciences, UAE University, Al Ain, United Arab Emirates*

ABSTRACT: **Diabetes mellitus is one of the most common endocrine disorders affecting almost 6% of the world's population. The number of diabetic patients will reach 300 million in 2025 (International Diabetes Federation, 2001). More than 97% of these patients will have type II diabetes. The projected increase in the number of diabetic patients will strain the capabilities of healthcare providers the world over. Thus it is of paramount importance to revisit the causes and epidemiology of diabetes mellitus. Diabetes mellitus is caused by both environmental and genetic factors. The environmental factors that may lead to the development of diabetes mellitus include physical inactivity, drugs and toxic agents, obesity, viral infection, and location. While type I diabetes is not a genetically predestined disease, an increased susceptibility can be inherited. Genetic susceptibility plays a crucial role in the etiology and manifestation of type II diabetes, with concordance in monozygotic twins approaching 100%. Genetic factors may have to be modified by environmental factors for diabetes mellitus to become overt. An individual with a susceptible gene may become diabetic if environmental factors modify the expression of these genes. Since there is an increase in the trend at which diabetes prevail, it is evident that environmental factors are playing a more increasing role in the cause of diabetes mellitus. The incidence of type I diabetes ranged from 1.9 to 7.0/100,000/yr in Africa, 0.13 to 10/100,000/yr in Asia, ∼4.4/100,000/yr in Australasia, 3.4 to 36/100,000/yr in Europe, 2.62 to 20.18/100,000/yr in the Middle East, 7.61 to 25.7/100,000/yr in North America, and 1.27 to 18/100,000/yr in South America. The epidemiology of type II diabetes is equally bleak. The prevalence of type II diabetes ranged from 0.3 to 17.9% in Africa, 1.2 to 14.6% in Asia, 0.7 to**

Address for correspondence: Ernest Adeghate, M.D., M.F.M., Ph.D., Department of Anatomy, Faculty of Medicine and Health Sciences, UAE University, P. O. Box 17666, Al Ain, United Arab Emirates. Voice: 971-3-7137496; fax: 971-3-7672033.
e-mail: eadeghate@uaeu.ac.ae

Ann. N.Y. Acad. Sci. 1084: 1–29 (2006).
doi: 10.1196/annals.1372.029

11.6% in Europe, 4.6 to 40% in the Middle East, 6.69 to 28.2% in North America, and 2.01 to 17.4% in South America.

KEYWORDS: diabetes; etiology; epidemiology; environmental; genetic factors; populations

INTRODUCTION

Diabetes mellitus is one of the most common endocrine disorders affecting almost 6% of the world's population. The prevalence of this chronic metabolic disease is on the increase.[1] According to the projections of Amos *et al.*,[2] the total number of people with diabetes mellitus all over the world will reach 221 million in the year 2010 in contrast to the 124 million estimated for 1997. According to other estimates, this number of diabetic patients is estimated to reach 300 million in 2025.[3] This chronic metabolic disorder affects the metabolism of carbohydrates, protein, fat, water, and electrolytes, leading to structural changes in tissues of many organ systems in the body, especially those of the vascular system. The symptoms of diabetes mellitus are well known. They include weight loss, thirst, and sweet-smelling urine. These symptoms were well known to the ancient Greek, Roman, and Egyptian physicians.[4]

ETIOLOGY OF DIABETES MELLITUS

The causes of diabetes mellitus are incompletely understood. It has now been widely accepted that the cause of diabetes mellitus is multifactorial and that both genetic and environmental factors play a contributing role.

GENETIC FACTORS AND DIABETES MELLITUS

Familial Aggregation of Diabetes

The ancient Hindu physicians had long recognized that diabetes can be passed from generation to generation.[4] The frequency of diabetic patients with positive family history ranges from 25 to 50%.[5] In order to determine whether diabetes mellitus is truly familial, Pincus and White[6] examined the prevalence of the disease among relatives of diabetic patients. The prevalence among close relatives (parents, siblings) of patients suffering from diabetes was as high as 10–30% when measured with more sensitive markers, such as oral, intravenous, and cortisone-induced glucose tolerance test. This is very high compared to the 1–6% observed in similar relatives of nondiabetic patients. Thus, the prevalence of both clinical and impaired glucose tolerance is significantly higher among the close relatives of diabetics than among similar relatives of nondiabetics.[6,7]

Genetics of Type I Diabetes

Although type I diabetes is not a genetically predestined disease, an increased susceptibility can be inherited. For example, the identical twins of a patient with type I diabetes have about 30–50% concordance rate for the disease. Other evidence of genetic involvement in the etiology of type I diabetes is that 95% of type I diabetes patients carry HLA-DR3, HLA-DR4, or both.[8] The relative risk of type I diabetes conferred by DR3 is 7 times, by DR4 9 times and by both DR3 and DR4 is more than 14 times that of normal. Type I diabetes is linked to the HLA complex at chromosome 6.[7] Homozygosity of the short (class I) allele is found in about 80% of subjects suffering from diabetes as against 40% of controls.[8] The precise nature of the genetic determinants of diabetes mellitus also remained elusive for many years despite the fact that twin studies showed that a major component of the familial association in diabetes was due to genetic factors.[9] Investigators have been confronted with several obstacles in their attempt to decipher the exact role of genetic factors in the etiology of diabetes mellitus. These obstacles include the modification of the expression of the diabetic genotype by environmental factors and the variability in the age of onset of diabetes.[5–7]

Genetics of Type II Diabetes

The majority (~97%) of diabetic patients have type II diabetes. The prevalence of this disease is on the increase.[3] The association of genetic factors with type II diabetes mellitus is well documented in many parts of the world. Genetic susceptibility plays a crucial role in the etiology and manifestation of the disease, with concordance in monozygotic twins approaching 100%.[8] Physiological variability in glucose metabolism has been suggested for many years. For example, the maximum plasma insulin response to oral glucose load found in nondiabetic Ravajos and Pima Indians was over three times as great as that observed in Western Europeans.[10] In addition, the insulin output of maturity-onset diabetic American Indians was different from than of maturity-onset diabetic Europeans.[5]

Comparison of the phenotypic characteristics of the disease has also given more information on the nature of the genetic factors in this disease. For example studies on Asian Indians with type II diabetes showed that they are more insulin resistant than are Caucasians with type II diabetes, even when the degree of obesity is comparable.[11] This suggests that there may be distinct subtypes of type II diabetes in different ethnic groups depending on the phenotype of the diabetes gene. Intrapopulation studies have also shown that there may be an important but delicate phenotypic difference in glucose metabolism even in nondiabetic subjects in a given population. Several studies on populations have demonstrated physiological variability in insulin action and secretion even in nondiabetics.[12] For example, in a population of Swedish male nondiabetics, the subjects were found to be either low or high insulin responders, a difference that was attributed in part to physical fitness.[13]

In Australian Aborigines, major differences in insulin response have been reported for populations living in the desert and in the coastal regions.[14] All of these examples suggest physiological differences in glucose metabolism, which may in turn be due to genetic differences even within a single population. More recent data[15] suggests that loci on chromosomes 2 (NIDDM1) and 15 may interact to increase susceptibility to diabetes in Mexican Americans.

Genes Associated with Diabetes Mellitus

Many genes have been shown to be associated with type II diabetes. These genes include Gc genotype gene located on chromosome 4, HLA gene on chromosome 6, lipoprotein antigen gene on chromosome 6, insulin gene polymorphism on chromosome 11, apo-lipoprotein genes on chromosomes 2 and 11, glucose transporter genes on chromosomes 1 and 12, haptoglobulin gene on chromosome 16, and insulin receptor gene on chromosome 19.[16] These genes have been shown to be present in different populations and may be analogous to the different phenotypes of diabetes observed between and within populations. More recent studies on a population-based study in Denmark[17] on the heritability of type II diabetes mellitus suggest that even though genetic factors may be important in the development of abnormal glucose tolerance, nongenetic factors possibly have a predominant role in controlling whether a genetically predisposed individual progresses to overt type II diabetes.

In summary, it is clear that genetic factors do have a role in the etiopathogenesis of diabetes mellitus. This genetic factor may have to be modified by environmental factors for diabetes mellitus to become overt. An individual with a susceptible gene may become diabetic if environmental factors modify the expression of these genes.

ENVIRONMENTAL AND ETHNIC FACTORS AND DIABETES MELLITUS

Environmental and Ethnic Factors and Type I Diabetes

Environmental factors have been implicated in the pathogenesis and outcome of both type I and type II diabetes. There is a major ethnic and geographical difference in the prevalence and incidence of type I diabetes.[18] The highest reported cases of type I diabetes are in the Nordic countries, with the highest incidence in Finland (35/100,000/year) of the population in children aged 0–14 years. The lowest incidence is seen in Asia (0.5–1.3/100,000/year). Low rates are also reported in Africa and Latin America.[19] These significant differences between the incidence of type I diabetes are possibly due to variations in genetic and environmental factors.[20,21]

Many reports have shown significant variability in the prevalence and clinical features of diabetes mellitus.[22] This variability among ethnic groups may be secondary to both genetic and environmental modifying factors. It may also indicate the presence of genetic differences between various ethnic groups. It appears that there is a correlation of overnutrition and the prevalence of diabetes. In certain populations, such as the Kurdish and Yemenite Jews in Israel, the prevalence of diabetes has markedly increased following their migration to Israel with subsequent alterations in their diet.[23] Environmental factors thus have a role in ethnic differences in the prevalence of diabetes mellitus. However, there are clear differences in the clinical phenotype of diabetes between different ethnic groups,[22] which are indicative of a genetic role.

The annual rate of incidence of childhood type I diabetes in France, between 1988 and 1995, was comparable to that observed in the Nordic countries. In spite of the similarity in the annual rate of incidence of childhood type I diabetes, the overall incidence of type I diabetes in childhood is still smaller in France. This shows that environmental factors play a major role in the pathogenesis of type I diabetes.[24]

Gender Differences

In a study of subjects aged 15–29 years, Bruno *et al.*[25] observed a significantly higher incidence of type I diabetes in males compared to females. This may be due to the influence of sex hormones or differential exposure to environmental contaminants. In contrast to this finding, many investigators did not observe any sex difference in the incidence of type I diabetes in the provinces of Rzeszow in Poland,[26] Edmonton in Canada,[27] and Abruzzo in Italy.[28]

Ethnicity

Some reports have shown that physical environmental factors are not the only issues that contribute to the development of diabetes mellitus. In a study of the incidence of diabetes mellitus in a region in Chile between 1983 and 1993, there was a significant difference between the incidence of type I diabetes in native Chileans (0.42/100,000) compared to Caucasian Chileans (1.58/100,000).[29]

Location

Location has also been implicated in the development of diabetes mellitus. In a study comparing the incidence of childhood-onset type I diabetes in black

African heritage populations in the Caribbean, significant differences were noted in the incidence of type I diabetes. Incidence of type I diabetes was highest (2.57/100,000) in the Barbados and lowest (0.09/100,000) in St. Croix.[30] There was no difference between the incidence of type I diabetes in the rural and urban populations.[26]

Seasonal Variation

Most investigators agree that the incidence of type I diabetes is highest in the autumn and winter[7,31] when compared to the incidence in other seasons.

Nutritional Factors

Nutrition given during the neonatal period and early infancy, such as the consumption of cow's milk protein in early life, may increase susceptibility to type I diabetes mellitus.[32,33] In addition to these studies, Verge and associates[34] showed that there is an increased risk of type I diabetes in children with early dietary exposure to cow's milk containing feed, short duration of exclusive breast feeding, and high intake of cow's milk protein in recent diet.

Toxic Agents

In children there is epidemiological evidence that high intake of nitrites and *N*-nitroso compounds increases the risk of type I diabetes.[35]

Viruses and Infection

Viruses have long been implicated in the pathogenesis of type I diabetes. This suspicion is based on the comparable seasonal incidence of the type I diabetes in both hemispheres, anecdotal associations, and analysis of viral antibody titres at diagnosis. IgM antibodies against Coxsackie B4 have been reported in 20–30% of new cases of type I diabetes.[36] High incidence of diabetes is also associated with congenital rubella.[37] For example, 20% of children with congenital rubella develop type I diabetes.[38] Increased risk of type I diabetes was also reported in children with recent infection.[34]

Immunological Aspects

There is ample evidence suggesting that autoimmune processes are involved in the etiology of type I diabetes. Autoimmune diseases, such as Addison's disease, pernicious anemia, and autoimmune thyroid disease, are more common in type I diabetes patients and their relatives[5] than in the normal population. More than 70% of the newly diagnosed type I diabetes patients have islet cell antibodies. Islet cell antibodies may appear in circulation months or even years before the actual onset of diabetes.[39] These antibodies react with pancreatic islet cells and can be detected by immunofluorescence. Increased T lymphocyte levels are also observed in these patients. In addition to increased T lymphocyte levels, there is increase in insulin autoantibodies and anti-GAD antibodies in diabetes mellitus.[40,41]

ENVIRONMENTAL AND ETHNIC FACTORS AND TYPE II DIABETES

Ethnicity

It appears that environment is not the only factor that influence the development of diabetes, ethnicity may also play a role on whether a subject is likely to be diabetic or not. For example the prevalence of type II diabetes is much higher (8.9%) in South African Indians when compared to South African blacks (4.2%). Differences in the prevalence of type II diabetes among people of different ethnic origins were also reported in Asia. The overall prevalence of type II diabetes in Aborigines and Malays living in the same community was 4.4% and 11.3%, respectively. Again, this shows that ethnicity may, in addition to other factors, contribute to an increase in the prevalence of diabetes mellitus.[42] Pregnancy has been shown to be associated with a decreased glucose tolerance caused by insulin resistance especially in late gestation. In some of these women, glucose intolerance is increased by a defect in β cell function and diabetes mellitus occurs.[43]

Some reports in literature have described a significant difference in the ethnic distribution of gestational diabetes.[44] The fact that type II diabetes is extremely high (>50%) in the Pima Indians of Arizona[6,45] and the urbanized Pacific Islanders of Nauru[46] and Fiji[47] suggests a genetic (ethnic) role in the etiology of diabetes mellitus.

Gender Differences

Reports exist in the literature, which show that the prevalence of type II diabetes is more common in females than in males. This has been demonstrated in a selected African[48] population. In contrast to these findings, Lerman *et al.*[49] reported that type II diabetes is more prevalent in men (16.7%) than in females (9.5%) in Mexican populations of all age groups.

Location (Urban vs. Rural)

Several studies on the prevalence of diabetes have demonstrated the importance of residence on the prevalence of diabetes mellitus. In a recent study performed in Saudi Arabia, Al-Nuaim[50] showed that age-adjusted prevalence of diabetes mellitus was significantly higher in the urban population (males 12%, females 14%) compared to rural (males 7%, females 7.7%) population. In the UAE, El Mugamer and associates[51] reported a similar finding. In Asia, the difference in the prevalence of type II diabetes between rural and urban population was also observed. In a study of the prevalence of diabetes mellitus in adult Malays living in rural and urban centres, a striking significant difference in prevalence of type II diabetes between the two groups were observed. The prevalence of type II diabetes was 2.8% in a traditional village compared to 8.2% in the urban.[42] This pattern of prevalence of diabetes in rural–urban areas is also true for South America.[49] In spite of the fact that majority of the published papers reported a higher prevalence of type II diabetes in urban subjects, Elbagir *et al.*[52] did not find any difference in the prevalence of type II diabetes between urban and rural populations in Sudan. The role of geographical difference in the development of type II diabetes is supported by the fact that Japanese living in Brazil have higher prevalence of type II diabetes compared to those in Japan.[53] Similarly, Japanese Americans living in Hawaii and Los Angeles have a higher prevalence of type II diabetes than native Japanese.[54] Since Japanese Americans are genetically indistinguishable from native Japanese, environmental factors like location can be ascribed to the etiology of type II diabetes.

The difference between the prevalence of diabetes in the urban and rural setting may be due to two reasons. Namely, people in the urban setting may be more affluent and eat more junk food in contrast to people in the rural setting. Second, people in the rural setting are more lilkely to be involved in more physical activity compared to their urban counterparts, thereby reducing the likelihood of developing type II diabetes.

Physical Inactivity

It has been shown that regular physical activity increases insulin sensitivity and glucose tolerance.[55] Moreover, it has been recently shown that physical activity reduces the risk of type II diabetes.[56] In a recent study performed on an African American population in the United States, it was observed that the prevalence of diabetes increases with the degree of inactivity and obesity.[7,54,56] The potentially important role of physical activity in development of type II diabetes was reported by Pereira and associates[57] on the multiethnic population of Mauritius.

Body Weight and Fat Distribution

Obesity has been implicated as a risk factor for type II diabetes.[58–60] Body mass index is directly associated with increased risk of type II diabetes in many ethnic groups.[7] The extent of intra-abdominal rather than subcutaneous fat is important in the development of diabetes mellitus.[61–63] Some investigators have reported a strong correlation between obesity and type II diabetes. In a study of the pattern of diabetes mellitus in 3229 patients, it was shown that 57.7% of the diabetic women were obese and 30.2% were overweight.[64]

Nutritional Factors and Obesity

Obesity is present in about 80% of type II diabetes patients. There is a strong association of obesity and type II diabetes.[61,62,65] The introduction of energy-rich food, rich in saturated fats, refined and simple sugars, and deficient in complex carbohydrates (fibers) may contribute to the development of obesity and type II diabetes. In a recent study on the prevalence of diabetes in Mexicans, it was shown that higher fat, low carbohydrate, and low fiber diets is associated with a higher prevalence of diabetes.[49]

Severe and Prolonged Stress

Severe and prolonged stress associated with today's modern life may also be associated with glucose intolerance and may hence increase the risk of diabetes.[66] The development of diabetes after severe and prolonged stress may be caused by the activation of the adrenal hormones, notably the glucocorticoids that have been noted to cause glucose intolerance.

Drugs

Drugs like corticosteroids and some oral contraceptive steroids may cause glucose intolerance and type II diabetes in susceptible individuals.[67] The role of other drugs like diuretics and β-adrenoceptor blocking agents in the etiology of glucose intolerance and type II diabetes is, however, questionable.

Abnormal Insulin Secretion and Action

Most patients with type II diabetes have reduced insulin secretion relative to the plasma blood glucose levels. This is accompanied by progressive β cell loss although not to the extent seen in type I diabetes. Islet amyloid is a characteristic feature of the pancreas of type II diabetes patients. Amyloid (derived from islet amyloid polypeptide [IAPP]) deposits in the endocrine pancreas may act as a passenger to the pathogenesis of diabetes.[68]

EPIDEMIOLOGY OF TYPE I DIABETES

The incidence rate of type I diabetes varies with age and rarely occurs before the first 6 months of age[69] with the exception of a very few cases recorded in a large registry in Great Britain.[70] The incidence of type I diabetes begins sharply to rise at about 9 months of age, continues to rise until age 12–14 years, and then declines.[71] A similar pattern is seen in many other countries irrespective of whether the overall incidence of type I diabetes is low or high.[72] Available data in the United States of America suggest that there is a temporal increase in the incidence of type I diabetes over the last 50 years from about 5% in 1940 to 20% in 1980.[73] Data from other countries are comparable with that from the United States.[72]

Many studies have been performed on the incidence rate of diabetes in various parts of the world to allow for examination of the geographical pattern of type I diabetes. The incidence of type I diabetes is lowest in Japan, the Caribbean, and southern Europe while the highest incidence rates are in the Scandinavian countries,[74] particularly in Finland, and in Sardinia in Italy.[7] The incidence rate of type I diabetes in the white population of the United States is higher than those recorded for countries of northern Europe but significantly lower than those in Sweden and Finland. The incidence of type I diabetes in African Americans was lower than in white Americans.[75] Accumulated data on the incidence of type I diabetes during the last 20 years show that type I diabetes occurs in most racial and ethnic groups but the risk is highest among white population.[74] While these differences among races may be determined in part by genes, the variation within the white population is almost as large as that observed among all races. All of these examples support the role of genetic and environmental factors in the etiology of diabetes. A more recent study shows that climate has a role in the etiology of type I diabetes.[76] The continued increase in the incidence of type I diabetes in many parts of the world would suggest that the role of environmental factors in the etiology of diabetes mellitus is extremely important (TABLE 1).

REGIONAL DISTRIBUTION OF TYPE I DIABETES

Africa

The incidence and prevalence of type I diabetes mellitus in Africa has not been widely reported compared to other regions of the world. There is increasing incidence and prevalence of type I diabetes among the African population. The incidence of type I diabetes varies from 1.9/100,000/year in Mauritius[77] to 7.0/100,000/year in Bengazzi, Libya.[78] A relatively high incidence was recorded in Beja, Monastir, and Gafsa regions of Tunisia.[79] There is a nonsignificant increase in the incidence of type 1 diabetes in Africa.[80] The incidence of type I diabetes is less than that recorded in Asia, Australia, Europe, Middle East, and North and South America. The reason for the low incidence of type I diabetes may be due to several reasons, namely, it is truly low because people are relatively poor and do not have access to abundant food and luxurious modes of transportation. Hence, people are more physically active. The disparity may also be due to different time points at which the studies were performed. It may also be due to the fact that not enough studies were performed on the incidence of type I diabetes in this continent (TABLE 1).

Asia

This region holds a large and significant part of the world population. Therefore the impact of the disease in this part of the world is significant. Studies performed on the prevalence of diabetes in this region are relatively more compared to that performed in Africa. The reported incidence of type I diabetes in Asia ranged from 0.13 to 1.61/100,000/yr in China[81] to 10.5/100,000/yr in India.[82] The incidence reported in Singapore (2.46/100,000/yr),[83] Japan (2.1–3.5/100,000/yr),[84] Pakistan (1.0/100,000/yr),[85] and Thailand (0.3–1.65/100,000/yr)[86,87] lies between these two incidence rates. Like in other parts of the world, the incidence of type I diabetes is also increasing in Asia.[87] This may be due to the introduction of more sensitive investigative procedures, less of physical activity and inappropriate, nutrition (TABLE 1).

Australasia

The incidence rate of type I diabetes reported for Australia was 4.4/100,000/yr)[88] and the prevalence rate given for New Zealand[89] was 227/100,000. However, it has been reported that these rates continue to rise due to factors mentioned in the section for Asia. The development of new diagnostic methods in medicine and in technology at large may also identify cases that were undetected by older methods in the past. This may contribute to the increase in the number of new cases that we observe worldwide today. (TABLE 1)

Europe

The largest and most comprehensive studies performed on the incidence of type I diabetes were performed in Europe. These studies covered most of

TABLE 1. Incidence of type I diabetes in some countries

Continent	Country	Location or ethnicity	Period	Age group (years)	Incidence/ 100,000/ year	Author(s)
Africa	Mauritius		1986–1990	0–19	1.9	Tuomilehto *et al.* (77)
	Libya	Bengazzi	1981–1990	0–14	7.0	Kadiki and Moawad (78)
	Tunisia	Beja, Monastir, and Gafsa	1990	0–14	6.76	Ben Khalifa *et al.* (79)
	Libya	Bengazzi	1991–2000	0–14	7.8	Kadiki and Roaeid (80)
Asia	China	All regions	1991	0–14	0.13–1.61	Yang *et al.* (81)
	India	Madras	1991–1994	0–14	10.5	Ramachadran *et al.* (82)
	Singapore		1992–1994	0–12	2.46	Lee *et al.* (83)
	Japan		1986–1990	0–14	2.1–3.5	Kida *et al.* (84)
	Pakistan	Karachi	1989–1993	0–14	1.02	Staines *et al.* (85)
	Thailand	North East	1991–1995	0–15	0.3	Panamonta *et al.* (86)
	Thailand	Bangkok	1991–1995	0–15	1.65	Tuchinda *et al.* (87)
Australasia	Australia	New South Wales	1990–1996	0–14	4.4	Craig *et al.* (88)
	New Zealand	Canterbury	2001	0–24	227/100,000 (prevalence)	Wu *et al.* (89)
Europe	Finland	Finland	1990–1994	0–14	36.5	Karvonen *et al.* (90)
	Sweden		1978–1997	0–14	21.1–31.9	Dahlquist and Mustonen (91)
	Denmark		1989–1993	0–14	17.4	Svendsen *et al.* (92)
	Italy	Sardinia	1989–1992	0–14	34.4	Muntoni *et al.* (93)
		Liguria	1989–1998	0–14	12.56	Cotellessa *et al.* (94)
	UK	Scotland	1981–1993	10–14	31.9	Rangasami *et al.* (95)
		Northern Ireland	1989–2003	0–14	24.7	Cardwell *et al.* (96)
	The Netherlands		1988–1990	0–20	13.2	Ruwaard *et al.* (97)
			1996–1999	0–14	18.6	van Wouwe *et al.* (98)
	Germany		1987–1993	0–14	11.6	Neu *et al.* (99)
	Germany		1988–1995	0–14	14.2	Rosenbauer *et al.* (100)

Continued

TABLE 1. Continued

Continent	Country	Location or ethnicity	Period	Age group (years)	Incidence/ 100,000/ year	Author(s)
	Spain	Navarre	1975–1991	0–16	13.7	Chueca *et al.* (101)
		Caceres	1988–1999	0–14	16.8	Lora-Gomez *et al.* (102)
	Hungary	Hungary	1987–1997	0–14	10.7	Gyurus *et al.* (103)
	Cyprus	Nicosia	1990–1994	0–14	10.5	Skordis and Hadjiloizou (104)
	Czech Republic		1990–1997	0–14	10. 1	Cinek *et al.* (105)
	Poland		1998	0–29	9.9	Kretowski *et al.* (106)
	France		1988–1995	0–20	9.28	Levy-Marchal (24)
	Slovakia		1985–1992	0–14	8.92	Michalkova *et al.* (107)
	Lithuania		1991–2000	0–39	8.2	Pundziute-Lycka *et al.* (108)
	Slovenia	Slovenia	1988–1995	0–14	8.0	Battelino and Krzisnik (109)
	Russia	Siberia (Novosibirsk)	1983–1989	10–14	4.7	Podar *et al.* (110)
	Belarus	Gomel	1976–1999	0–14	4.6	Martinucci *et al.* (111)
Middle East	Kuwait		1992–1993	0–14	15.4	Shaltout *et al.* (112)
			1995–1999	0–14	20.18	Abdul-Rasoul *et al.* (113)
	Saudi Arabia	Eastern Province	1986–1997	0–14	12.3	Kulaylat and Narchi (114)
	Jordan	Amman	1992–1996	0–14	3.6	Ajlouni *et al.* (115)
	Oman	Muscat	1993–1994	0–14	2.62	Soliman *et al.* (116)
North America	Canada	Edmonton	1990–1995	0–14	25.7	Toth *et al.* (27)
	USA	Hawaii	1980–1990	0–14	7.61	Patrick *et al.* (117)
	USA	Philadelphia	1993	0–14	13.4	Lipman (118)
South America	Puerto Rico		1985–1994	0–14	18.0	Frazer de Llado *et al.* (119)
	Brazil	Passo Fundo	1996	0–14	12	Lisboa *et al.* (120)
	Bahamas	Africans	2005	0–14	10.1	Peter *et al.* (121)
	West Indies	Barbados	1982–1991	0–14	5.0	Jordan *et al.* (122)
	Chile	IX region	1980–1993	0–14	1. 27	Larenas *et al.* (29)

the European countries, including new independent states like Lithuania. The highest incidence rate so far was reported in Finland, with 36.5/100,000/yr.[90] Sweden (21.1-31.9/100,000/yr)[91] and Denmark (17.4/1000,000/yr)[92] which are located in the same geographical area (Scandinavia) as Finland have also reported high incidence rate of type I diabetes. In addition to the high incidence rate reported in the Scandinavian countries, some areas in Southern Europe, such as Sardinia (34.4/100,000/yr)[93] and Liguria (12.56/100,000/yr)[94] in Italy, and Scotland (31.9/100,000/yr)[95] and Northern Ireland (24.7/100,000/yr)[96] in the UK have reported very high incidence rates. The incidence of type I diabetes in The Netherlands ranges between 13.2/100,000/yr[97] and 18.6/100,000/yr.[98] The incidence rate of type I diabetes is also on the rise in Germany (11.6/100,000/yr),[99] 14.6/1000,000/yr,[100] and Spain with a reported incidence rate of between 13.7/100,000/yr[101] and 16.8/100,000/yr.[102] Moderate rate of incidence of type I diabetes were observed in Hungary (10.7/100,000/yr),[103] Cyprus (10.5/100,000/yr),[104] Czech Republic (10.1/100,000/yr),[105] Poland (9.9/100,000/yr),[106] France, (9.28/100,000/yr),[24] Slovakia (8.92/100,000/yr),[107] Lithuania (8.2/100,000/yr),[108] and Slovenia (8.0/100,000/yr).[109] European countries with low incidence rate of diabetes include Russia (4.7/100,000/yr)[110] and Belarus (4.6/100,000/yr).[111] It is not clear why the incidence of type I diabetes is very high in the Scandinavian countries and in some areas of southern Europe. The reason may be a combination of lifestyle, environmental, and genetic factors (TABLE 1).

Middle East

The Middle East is seeing an explosion in the incidence and prevalence of diabetes mellitus. The highest reported incidence of type I diabetes was in Kuwait. The incidence of type I diabetes rose from 15.4/100,000/yr[112] in 1993 to 20.18/100,000/yr in 1999.[113] High incidence of type I diabetes was also recorded in Saudi Arabia (12.3/100,000/yr).[114] Jordan (3.6/100,000/yr)[115] and Oman (2.62./100,000/yr)[116] have relatively low incidence rates of type I diabetes (TABLE 1).

North America

The incidence rate of type I diabetes in North America is comparable to that of Europe and somehow follow the same pattern. Incidence rates are higher in the northern colder countries, such as Canada (25.7/100,000/yr),[27] and relatively lower in the United States. The incidence rate varies from 7.61/100,000/yr in Hawaii[117] to 13.4/100,000/yr in Philadelphia.[118] However, there are regional variations. The comparable incidence rates of North America and Europe points to a possible interplay of genetic, environmental, and lifestyle factors in the etiology of type I diabetes (TABLE 1).

South America

Some of the countries in South America have the lowest incidence rates of type I diabetes. The incidence of type I diabetes is highest in Puerto Rico (18/100,000/yr).[119] It is noteworthy that Puerto Rico is part of the United States, where lifestyle is similar to that of mainland United States. Brazil (12.0/100,000/yr)[120] and the Bahamas (10.1/100,000/yr)[121] have relatively high incidence rates of type I diabetes. The incidence of type I diabetes is low in the West Indies (5.0/100,000/yr)[122] and in Chile (1.27/100,000/yr).[29]

EPIDEMIOLOGY OF TYPE II DIABETES

The overall prevalence of type II diabetes in U.S. population aged 20–74 years was 6.6% in 1980, corresponding to more than 8 million people. Diagnosed diabetes mellitus accounted for one-half of these cases. The prevalence of type II diabetes was slightly higher in women than in men, except for the age group 65–74 years. The prevalence of type II diabetes among blacks was higher than among whites at all ages and for both sexes.[123]

The prevalence in Hispanic minorities (Cubans in Florida and Mexican Americans in the border states) was even higher,[124] but did not approach that of Pima Indians of Arizona.[125] The prevalence of type II diabetes in the European population is relatively low compared with the prevalence recorded for these American populations. In European populations, the prevalence of type II diabetes is less than half of the prevalence observed in American populations.[126] The prevalence of type II diabetes in Saudi Arabia is similar to that obtained in U.S. populations, while in Central Asia the prevalence among men aged 50 years and over is similar to that in European men.[127] The above data and those in TABLE 2 are comparable to that obtained by King and Rewers.[46] TABLE 2 shows a more recent data on the prevalence of type II diabetes in many countries.

The substantial difference in the occurrence of diabetes among white populations, particularly between those in Europe and North America, points to an environmental component in the development of diabetes mellitus in white populations. In addition, type II diabetes is more prevalent in Chinese living outside Asia than those in China. For example, the prevalence of type II diabetes among Chinese living in the island of Mauritius is more than 20.8%, more than the value obtained for native Chinese.[60]

REGIONAL DISTRIBUTION OF TYPE II DIABETES

Africa

In recent years the continent of Africa has seen tremendous increases in the prevalence rate of type II diabetes. This is most likely due to changes

TABLE 2. Prevalence of type II diabetes in some countries

Continent	Country	Location or ethnicity	Period	Age group (years)	% Prevalence	Author(s)
Africa	Mauritius		1998	Adult	17.9	Soderberg *et al.* (128)
	South Africa	Blacks	1994	Adults	4.2	Omar *et al.* (129)
		Indians	1994	Adult	9.8	Omar *et al.* (129)
	Algeria	Setif Wilaya	2001	30–64	8.3	Malek *et al.* (130)
	Sudan	(North)	1998	>25	8.3	Elbagir *et al.* (131)
	Nigeria	Ibadan	1997	Adult	2.8	Owoaje *et al.* (132)
	Mauritania		1996	30–64	2.61	Ducorps *et al.* (48)
	Sierra Leone	Bo	1997	Adult	2.4	Ceesay *et al.* (133)
	Gambia		1997	>15	0.3	van de Sande *et al.* (134)
Asia	Nepal	Bhadrakali, Kotyang	2003	>20	2.5 rural 14.6 urban	Singh and Bhattarai (135)
			1999	Adult	6.3	Karki *et al.* (143)
	India	Madras	1994–1995		11.6	Ramachandran *et al.* (136)
		Shimla	1997	>40	4.86	Dhadwal *et al.* (145)
	Japan		1959–1992	>40	4–11	Kuzuya (137)
	Taiwan		1996		9.2	Chang *et al.* (138)
	Singapore		1998	18–69	9.0	Lee (139)
	Bangladesh	Dhaka	2004	≥20	8.1	Hussain *et al.* (140)
		Khagrachari	2004	20–70	6.4	Abu Sayeed *et al.* (142)
	Korea		2001	Adult	7.6	Kim *et al.* (141)
	Malaysia		1993	Adult	2.8 (rural)	Ali *et al.* (42)
			1993	Adult	8.2 (urban)	Ali *et al.* (42)
	Indonesia		2000	>15	1.2–2.3	Sutanegara and Budhiarta (144)
Australasia	Tonga		2002	Adult	15.1	Colagiuri *et al.* (146)
	Australia		1985	Adult	2.5	Glatthaar *et al.* (147)
	Papua N. Guinea		1996	Adult	0.001	Fujimoto (148)
	New Zealand		2002	Adolesc.	11	Hotu *et al.* (149)

Continued

TABLE 2 Continued

Continent	Country	Location or ethnicity	Period	Age group (years)	% Prevalence	Author(s)
Europe	Turkey	Adana	2003	20–79	11.6	Gokcel *et al.* (150)
	Spain	Asturias	2002	30–75	9.9	Botas Cervero *et al.* (151)
	Italy		2004	35–74	7.2	Pilotto *et al.* (152)
			1995	>44	8.5	Garancini *et al.* (153)
	France		1998	All	2.3	Detournay *et al.* (154)
			2001	35–64	5.1	Gourdy *et al.* (155)
	Russia	Moscow	1993	>75	4.43	Kuraeva *et al.* (156)
	Sweden	Laxa	1972–1987	35–79	4.3	Andersson *et al.* (157)
			2005	64	4.7–14.4	Brohall *et al.* (161)
	The Netherlands		2001	30–74	2.7–3.2	Baan and Feskens (158)
	Poland	Szczecin	2005	3–95	3.56	Fabian *et al.* (159)
	UK	Poole	1983–1996	Adult	2.13	Gatling *et al.* (160)
	Denmark		2003	30–60	0.7–9.7	Glumer *et al.* (162)
Middle East	UAE	Multi ethnic	1999–2000	Adult	13–40	Malik *et al.* (163)
	Kuwait		1995	>20	14.8	Abdella *et al.* (164)
	Saudi Arabia		1997	>15	7–7.5 (rural) 12–14 (urban)	Al-Nuaim (50)
	Palestine		2000	30–65	9.8	Husseini *et al.* (165)
	Yemen		2004	25–65	4.6	Al-Habori *et al.* (166)
North America	USA	American Indian (Apache)	1989	>35	9.8	Carter *et al.* (167)
		American Indian (Zuni)	1989	>35	28.2	Carter *et al.* (167)
		African American	1998	>20	11.4	Herman *et al.* (168)
	Canada	Manitoba	1986–1991	>25	6.69	Blanchard *et al.* (169)
South America	Brazil	Multicenter	1992	Adult	2.7–17.4	Malerbi and Franco (170)
		Japanese Brazil	1996	Adults	12.8–16.2	Franco (53)
		Sao Palo	2003	30–69	12.1	Torquato *et al.* (171)
	Chile	Mapuches	2001	>20	3.2	Perez-Bravo *et al.* (172)
		Aboriginal (Mapuche)	2004	>20	8.2	Carrasco *et al.* (173)
	Mexico	Mexico City	1997	>20	2.01	Castro-Sanchez *et al.* (174)

in lifestyle. The highest recorded prevalence of type II diabetes was found in the multiethnic Mauritian population, with a startling figure of 17.9%,[128] followed by South African Indians (9.8%).[129] North African countries of Algeria (8.3%)[130] and Sudan (8.3%)[131] also recorded high prevalence of diabetes. West African countries such as Nigeria (2.8%),[132] Mauritania (2.61%),[48] Sierra Leone (2.4%),[133] and Gambia (0.3%)[134] have low prevalence of type II diabetes. The prevalence of type II diabetes has continued to rise in some African countries[128] (TABLE 2).

Asia

A large majority of the people live in the Asian continent. The highest prevalence of type II diabetes was recorded in Nepalese living in Bhadrakali (14.6%).[135] High prevalence of type II diabetes was also reported in Indians living in Madras (11.6%)[136] and in some Japanese populations (4–11%).[137] High prevalence was also reported in Taiwan (9.2%),[138] Singapore (9.0%),[139] urban regions of Malaysia (8.2%),[42] and in Bangladesh (8.1%).[140] A medium prevalence was observed in South Korea (7.6%),[141] rural areas of Bangladesh (6.4),[142] and Nepal (6.3%).[143] The lowest reported prevalence (1.2–2.3%)[144] of type II diabetes was in Indonesia. Again, there are regional variations within a given country.[136,145] The differences in the prevalence of type II diabetes is particularly high between the urban and rural regions of Nepal and Malaysia[42,135] (TABLE 2).

Australasia

The highest recorded prevalence of type II diabetes was in Tonga (15.1%),[146] part of the Micronesia, a region well known for its high prevalence of type II diabetes. Prevalence is small in Australia (2.5%)[147] and very low in Papua New Guinea (0.001%).[148] However, the prevalence of type II diabetes is increasing in adolescents of New Zealand (11.0%).[149]

Europe

The Adana region of Turkey has one of the highest prevalence (11.6%)[150] of type II diabetes in Europe. Other areas with high prevalence in Europe include the Asturias region of Spain (9.9%)[151] and Italy (7.2–8.5%).[152,153] Most of the European countries, including France (2.3–5.1%),[154,155] Russia (4.43%),[156] Sweden (4.3%),[157] The Netherlands (2.7–3.2%),[158] Poland (3.56%),[159] and the UK (2.13%)[160] have a relatively low prevalence of type II diabetes. There are variations between age groups. For example, in a study performed on 64-year old subjects in Sweden, the prevalence of type II diabetes in the group ranged between 4.7 and 14.4%.[161] A high variation of between 0.7 and 9.7% was observed in a Danish population aged 30–60 years of age.[162]

The Middle East

The Middle East has seen a large increase in the prevalence of type II diabetes in the last decade. The prevalence of type II diabetes is particularly high in the UAE, where it ranged between 13 and 40%.[163] There is variation between rural and urban setting, age groups, and different nationalities living in the UAE. High prevalence of type II diabetes is also seen in Kuwait (14.8%)[164] and in Saudi Arabia (12–14%).[50] Relatively high prevalence was also seen in Palestine (9.8%).[165] Yemen recorded a small prevalence (4.6%)[166] of type II diabetes compared to other Middle Eastern countries.

North America

The prevalence of type II diabetes is significantly high among American Indians (9.8–28.2%)[167] and, to some extent, in the African American population (11.4%).[168] The prevalence of type II diabetes is relatively low (6.69%)[169] in the Manitoba region of Canada compared to the United States.

South America

The prevalence of type II diabetes varies between different regions and countries in South America. The highest prevalence of type II diabetes in South America is recorded in Brazil (2.7–17.4%).[170] It is particularly high in urban areas such as Sao Paulo (12.1%)[171] and in Japanese Brazilians (12.8–16.2%).[53] The prevalence of type II diabetes has continued to rise among the Aboriginal (Mapuche) population of Chile. In 2001 the prevalence of type was 3.2%.[172] By 2004 it has risen to 8.2%.[173] The prevalence of type II diabetes in Mexico (2.01%)[175] is among the lowest in Central/South America (TABLE 2).

CONCLUSIONS

The number of diabetic patients will continue to increase in all regions of the world. Although a steady increase in the incidence of type I diabetes has been reported, most of the diabetic patients the world over will be suffering from type II diabetes. The projected increase in the number of diabetic patients will cause a big burden for the healthcare systems. Diabetes mellitus is caused by an interplay of genetic and environmental factors. Many environmental factors (physical inactivity, drugs and toxic agents, obesity, viral infection, and location) contribute to the development of diabetes. While type I diabetes is not a genetically predestined disease, an increased susceptibility can be inherited. Genetic susceptibility plays an important role in the etiology and manifestation of type II diabetes, with concordance in monozygotic twins approaching 100%. Genetic factors may have to be influenced by environmental factors for diabetes mellitus to become overt.

REFERENCES

1. Townsend, T. 2000. A decade of diabetes research and development. Int. J. Diabetes Metab. **8:** 88–92.
2. Amos, A.F., D.J. McCarty & P. Zimmet. 1997. The rising global burden of diabetes and its complications: estimates and projections to the year 2010. Diabetes Med. **14:** S1–S85.
3. Zimmet, P. 2003. The burden of type 2 diabetes: are we doing enough? Diabetes Metab. **29**(Suppl 6): 59–518.
4. Frank, L.L. 1957. Diabetes mellitus in the texts of old Hindu medicine (Charaka, Susruta, Vagbhata). Am. J. Gastroenterol. **27:** 76–95.
5. Vadheim, C.M., D.L. Rimoin & J.I. Rotter. 1991. Diabetes mellitus. *In* Principles and Practice of Medical Genetics. A.E.H. Emery, & D.L. Rimoin, Eds.: 1521–1558. Churchill Livingstone. Edinburgh.
6. Pincus, G., P. White. 1933. On the inheritance of diabetes mellitus. I. Analysis of 675 family histories. Am. J. Med. Sci. **186:** 1–14.
7. Trevisan, R., M. Vedovato & A. Tiengo. 1998. The epidemiology of diabetes mellitus. Nephrol. Dial. Transplant **13:** 2–5.
8. Kumar, P.J. & M.L. Clark. 1999. Diabetes mellitus and other disorders of metabolism. *In* Clinical Medicine, 4th ed. P.J. Kumar & M.L. Clark, Eds.: 959–1005. Sounders, London.
9. Rotter, J.I., D.I. Rimoin & I.M. Samloff. 1978. Genetic heterogeneity in diabetes mellitus and peptic ulcer. *In* Genetic Epidemiology. N.E. Morton & C.S. Chung, Eds.: 381–414. Academic Press. New York.
10. Rimoin, D.L. 1969. Ethnic variability in glucose tolerance and insulin secretion. Arch. Intern. Med. **124:** 695–700.
11. Sharp, P.S., V. Mohan, J.C. Levy, *et al.* 1987. Insulin resistance in patients of Asian and European origin with non-insulin dependent diabetes. Horm. Metab. Res. **19:** 84–85.
12. Raeven, G.M. 1990. Non-insulin dependent diabetes (NIDDM): speculations on aetiology. *In* Diabetic Annual 5. K.G.M.M. Alberti & L.P. Krall Eds.: 51–71. Elsevier. Amsterdam.
13. Berntorp, K., F. Lindgarde & J. Malmquist. 1984. High and low insulin responders: relations to oral glucose tolerance, insulin secretion and physical fitness. Acta Med. Scand. **216:** 111–117.
14. O'Dea, K., K. Traianedes, J.L. Hooper & R.G. Larkins. 1988. Impaired glucose tolerance, hyperinsulinaemia, and hypertriglyceridaemia in Australian Aborigines from the desert. Diabetes Care **11:** 23–29.

15. COX, N.J., D.L. NICOLAE, P. CONCANNON, *et al.* 1999. Loci on chromosomes 2 (NIDDM1) and 15 interact to increase susceptibility to diabetes in Mexicans Americans. Nat. Genet. **21:** 213–215.
16. BELL, G.I. 1991. Molecular defects of diabetes mellitus. Diabetes **40:** 413–422.
17. POULSEN, P., K. OHM KYVIK & H. BECK-NIELSEN. 1999. Heritability of Type II (non-insulin dependent) diabetes mellitus and abnormal glucose tolerance–a population-based twin study. Diabetologia **42:** 139–145.
18. KARVONEN, M., J. TUOMILEHTO, I. LIBMAN & R.E. LAPORTE. 1993. Review of the recent epidemiological data on the worldwide incidence of Type I (insulin dependent) diabetes mellitus. Diabetologia **36:** 883–892.
19. REWERS, M., R.E. LAPORTE, H. KING & J. TUOMILEHTO. 1988. Trends in the prevalence and incidence of diabetes: insulin-dependent diabetes mellitus in childhood. World Health Stat. Q. **41:** 179–189.
20. LAPORTE, R.E., N. TAJIMA, H.K. AKERBLOM, *et al.* 1985. Geographical differences in the risk of insulin dependent diabetes mellitus: the importance of registries. Diabetes Care **8:** 101–107.
21. Anonymous. 1992. Childhood diabetes, epidemics, and epidemiology: an approach for controlling diabetes. World Health Organization DIAMOND Project Group on Epidemics. Am. J. Epidemiol. **135:** 803–816.
22. WEST, K.M. 1978. Epidemiology of Diabetes and Its Vascular Lesions. Elsevier. New York.
23. COHEN, A.M. & L. MAROM. 1993. Diabetes and accompanying obesity, hypertension and ECG abnormalities in Yemenite Jews 40 years after immigration to Israel. Diabetes Res. **23:** 65–74.
24. LEVY-MARCHAL, C. 1998. Evolution of the incidence of IDDM in childhood in France. Rev. Epidemiol. Sante Publique **46:** 157–163.
25. BRUNO, G., F. MERLETTI, A. VUOLO, *et al.* 1993. Sex differences in incidence of IDDM in age-group 15–29 yr. Higher risk in males in province of Turin, Italy. Diabetes Care **16:** 133–136.
26. GRZYWA, M.A. & A.K. SOBEL. 1995. Incidence of IDDM in the province of Rzeszow, Poland, 0–29 year old age-group, 1980–1992. Diabetes Care **18:** 542–544.
27. TOTH, E., K.C. LEE, R.M. COUCH & L.F. MARTIN. 1997. High incidence of IDDM over 6 years in Edmonton, Alberta, Canada. Diabetes Care **20:** 311–313.
28. ALTOBELLI, E., F. CHIARELLI, M. VALENTI, *et al.* 1998. Incidence of insulin-dependent diabetes mellitus (0–14) in the Abruzzo Region, Italy, 1990-1995: results from a population register. J. Pediatr. Endocrinol. Metabol. **11:** 555–562.
29. LARENAS, G., A. MONTECINOS, M. MANOSALVA, *et al.* 1996. Incidence of insulin-dependent diabetes mellitus in the IX region of Chile: ethnic differences. Diabetes Res. Clin. Pract. **34:** S147–S151.
30. TULL, E.S., O.W. JORDAN, L. SIMON, *et al.* 1997. Incidence of childhood-onset IDDM in black African-heritage populations in the Caribbean. The Caribbean African Heritage IDDM Study (CAHIS) Group. Diabetes Care **20:** 309–310.
31. SOLTESZ, G., L. MADACSY, D. BEKEFI & I. DANKO. 1990. Rising incidence of type 1 diabetes in Hungarian children (1978–1987). Hungarian Childhood Diabetes Epidemiology Group. Diabet. Med. **7:** 111–114.
32. BORCH-JOHNSEN, K., G. JONER, T. MANDRUP-POULSEN, *et al.* 1984. Relationship between breast feeding and incidence rates of insulin dependent diabetes mellitus. A hypothesis. Lancet **8411:** 1083–1086.

33. VIRTANEN, S.M., L. RASANEN, A. ARO, *et al.* 1991. Childhood diabetes in Finland Study Group. Infant feeding in children <7 years of age with newly diagnosed IDDM. Diabetes Care **14:** 415–417.
34. VERGE, C.F., N.J. HOWARD, L. IRWIG, *et al.* 1994. Environmental factors in childhood IDDM. A population-based case-control study. Diabetes Care **17:** 1381–1389.
35. VIRTANEN, S.M. & A. ARO. 1994. Dietary factors in the aetiology of diabetes. Ann. Med. **26:** 469–478.
36. ROIVAINEN, M., M. KNIP, H. HYOTY, *et al.* 1998. Several different enterovirus serotypes can be associated with prediabetic autoimmune episodes and onset of overt IDDM. Childhood Diabetes in Finland (DiMe) Study Group. J. Med. Virol. **56:** 74–78.
37. SYLLABA, J. 1994. New findings in type I diabetes. Cas Lek Cesk **133:** 37–40.
38. WHO STUDY GROUP. 1994. Prevention of Diabetes Mellitus. WHO Technical Report Series 844, 18–21. World Health Organisation. Geneva.
39. POZZILLI, P., N. VISALLI, R. BUZZETTI, *et al.* 1998. Metabolic and immune parameters at clinical onset of insulin-dependent diabetes: a population-based study. IMDIAB Study Group on Immunotherapy. Diabetes Metab. **47:** 1205–1210.
40. ZIMMET, P.Z., R.B. ELLIOTT, I.R. MACKAY, *et al.* 1994. Autoantibodies to glutamic acid decarboxylase and insulin in islet cell antibody positive pre-symptomatic type 1 diabetes mellitus: frequency and segregation by age and gender. Diabet. Med. **11:** 866–871.
41. PARDINI, V.C., D.M. MOURAO, P.D. NASCIMENTO, *et al.* 1999. Frequency of islet cell autoantibodies (IA-2 and GAD) in young Brazilian type 1 diabetes patients. Braz. J. Med. Biol. Res. **32:** 1195–1198.
42. ALI, O., T.T. TAN, O. SAKINAH, *et al.* 1993. Prevalence of NIDDM and impaired glucose tolerance in aborigines and Malays in Malaysia and their relationship to sociodemographic, health, and nutritional factors. Diabetes Care **16:** 68–75.
43. GERONOOZ, I., A.J. SCHEEN & J.M. FOIDART. 1999. Gestational diabetes: definition, screening and management. Rev. Med. Liege **54:** 429–433.
44. HUGHES, P.F., M. AGARWAL, P. NEWMAN & J. MORRISON. 1995. Screening for gestational diabetes in a multi-ethnic population. Diabetes Res. Clin. Pract. **28:** 73–78.
45. PETTITT, D.J., W.C. KNOWLER, H.R. BAIRD & P.H. BENNETT. 1980. Gestational diabetes: infant and maternal complications of pregnancy in relation to third-trimester glucose tolerance in the Pima Indians. Diabetes Care **3:** 458–564.
46. KING, H. & M. REWERS. 1993. Global estimates for prevalence of diabetes mellitus and impaired glucose tolerance in adults. WHO Ad Hoc Diabetes Reporting Group. Diabetes Care **16:** 157–177.
47. HOSKINS, P.L., D.J. HANDELSMAN, T. HANNELLY, *et al.* 1987. Diabetes in the Melanesian and Indian peoples of Fiji: a study of risk factors. Diabetes Res. Clin. Pract. **3:** 269–276.
48. DUCORPS, M., S. BALEYNAUD, H. MAYAUDON, *et al.* 1996. Prevalence survey of diabetes in Mauritania. Diabetes Care **19:** 761–763.
49. LERMAN, I.G., A.R. VILLA, C.L. MARTINEZ, *et al.* 1998. The prevalence of diabetes and associated coronary risk factors in urban and rural older Mexicans. J. Am. Geriatric Soc. **46:** 1387–1395.
50. AL-NUAIM, A.R. 1997. Prevalence of glucose intolerance in urban and rural communities in Saudi Arabia. Diabet. Med. **14:** 595–602.

51. EL MUGAMER, I.T., A.S. ALI ZAYAT, M.M. HOSSAIN & R.N. PUGH. 1995. Diabetes, obesity and hypertension in urban and rural people of Bedouin origin in the United Arab Emirates. J. Trop. Med. Hyg. **98:** 407–415.
52. ELBAGIR, M.N., M.A. ELTOM, E.M. ELMAHADI, *et al.* 1998. A high prevalence of diabetes mellitus and impaired glucose tolerance in the Danagla community in northern Sudan. Diabet. Med. **15:** 164–169.
53. FRANCO, L.J. 1996. Diabetes in Japanese-Brazilians: influence of the cultural process. Diabetes Res. Clin. Pract. **34:** S51–S57.
54. HARA, H., G. EGUSA & M. YAMAKIDO. 1996. Incidence of non-insulin-dependent diabetes mellitus and its risk factors in Japanese-Americans living in Hawaii and Los Angeles. Diabet. Med. **13:** S133–S142.
55. KRISKA, A.M., M.A. PEREIRA, R.L. HANSON, *et al.* 2001. Association of physical activity and serum insulin concentrations in two populations at high risk for type 2 diabetes but differing by BMI. Diabetes Care **24:** 1175–1180.
56. HELMRICH, S.P., D.R. RAGLAND, R.W. LEUNG & R.S. PAFFENBARGER JR. 1991. Physical activity and reduced occurrence of non-insulin-dependent diabetes mellitus. N. Engl. J. Med. **325:** 147–152.
57. PEREIRA, M.A., A.M. KRISKA, M.L. JOSWIAK, *et al.* 1995. Physical inactivity and glucose intolerance in the multiethnic island of Mauritius. Med. Sci. Sports Exerc. **27:** 1626–1634.
58. HAFFNER, S.M., M.P. STERN, H.P. HAZUDA, *et al.* 1986. Role of obesity and fat distribution in non-insulin dependent diabetes mellitus in Mexican Americans and non-Hispanic whites. Diabetes Care **9:** 153–161.
59. OHLSON, L.O., B. LARSSON, P. BJORNTORP, *et al.* 1988. Risk factors for Type II (non-insulin dependent) diabetes mellitus. Thirteen and one-half years of follow up of the participants in a study of Swedish men born in 1913. Diabetologia **31:** 798–805.
60. DOWSE, G.K., H. GAREEBOO, P.Z. ZIMMET, *et al.* 1990. High prevalence of NIDDM and impaired glucose tolerance in Indian, Creole, and Chinese Mauritians. Mauritius Non-communicable Disease Study Group. Diabetes **39:** 390–396.
61. KISSEBAH, A.H., N. VYDELINGUM, R. MURRAY, *et al.* 1982. Relation of body fat distribution to metabolic complications of obesity. J. Clin. Endocrinol. Metab. **54:** 254–260.
62. BRAY, G.A. 1987. Overweight is risking fate. Definition, classification, prevalence, and risks. Ann. N.Y. Acad. Sci. **499:** 14–28.
63. KISSEBAH, A.H. & A.N. PEIRIS. 1989. Biology of regional body fat distribution: relationship to non-insulin-dependent diabetes mellitus. Diabetes Metab. Rev. **5:** 83–109.
64. ABDELLA, N.A., M.M. KHOGALI, A.D. SALMAN, *et al.* 1995. Pattern of non-insulin dependent diabetes mellitus in Kuwait. Diabetes Res. Clin. Pract. **29:** 129–136.
65. JAMES, W.P. 1998. What are the health risks? The medical consequences of obesity and its health risks. Exp. Clin. Endocrinol. Diabetes **106:** 1–6.
66. HUANG, Z., V. CABANELA & T. HOWELL. 1997. Stress, bottle feeding, and diabetes. Lancet **350:** 889.
67. NATIONAL DIABETES DATA GROUP. 1979. Classification and diagnosis of diabetes mellitus and other categories of glucose intolerance. Diabetes **28:** 1039–1057.
68. FERRANNINI, E. 1998. Insulin resistance versus insulin deficiency in non-insulin-dependent diabetes mellitus: problems and prospects. Endocr. Rev. **19:** 477–490.

69. MELTON, L.J. III, P.J. PALUMBO & C.P. CHU. 1983. Incidence of diabetes mellitus by clinical type. Diabetes Care **6:** 75–86.
70. GAMBLE, D.R. 1980. The epidemiology of insulin-dependent diabetes mellitus with special reference to the relationship of virus infection to its aetiology. Epidemiol. Rev. **2:** 49–70.
71. CHRISTAU, B., H. KROMANN, M. CHRISTY, *et al.* 1979. Incidence of insulin-dependent diabetes mellitus (0–29 years at onset) in Denmark. Acta Med. Scand. **624:** 54–60.
72. SEARCH for Diabetes in Youth Study Group; A.D. LIESE, R.B. D'AGOSTINO, JR., R.F. HAMMAN, *et al.* 2006. The burden of diabetes mellitus among US youth: prevalence estimates from the SEARCH for Diabetes in Youth Study. Pediatrics **118:** 1510–1518.
73. KROLESWKI, A.S., J.H. WARRAM, L.I. RAND & C.R. KAHN. 1987. Epidemiological approach to the aetiology of Type I diabetes mellitus and its complications. N. Engl. J. Med. **317:** 1390–1398.
74. PATRICK, S.L., C.S. MOY & R.E. LAPORTE. 1989. The world of insulin-dependent diabetes mellitus: what international epidemiological studies reveal about the aetiology and natural history of IDDM. Diabetes Metab. Rev. **5:** 571–578.
75. DIABETES EPIDEMIOLOGY RESEARCH INTERNATIONAL GROUP. 1988. Geographic patterns of childhood insulin-dependent diabetes mellitus. Diabetes **37:** 1113–1119.
76. YANG, Z., X. LONG, J. SHEN, *et al.* 2005. Epidemics of type 1 diabetes in China. Pediatr. Diabetes **6:** 122–128.
77. TUOMILEHTO, J., J. DABEE, M. KARVONEN, *et al.* 1993. Incidence of IDDM in Mauritian children and adolescents from 1986 to 1990. Diabetes Care **16:** 1588–1591.
78. KADIKI, O.A. & S.E. MOAWAD. 1993. Incidence and prevalence of type 1 diabetes in children and adolescents in Benghazi, Libya. Diabet. Med. **10:** 866–869.
79. BEN KHALIFA, F., A. MEKAOUAR, S. TAKTAK, *et al.* 1997. A five-year study of the incidence of insulin-dependent diabetes mellitus in young Tunisians (preliminary results). Diabetes Metab. **23:** 395–400.
80. KADIKI, O.A. & R.B. ROAEID. 2002. Incidence of type 1 diabetes in children (0–14 years) in Benghazi, Libya (1991–2000). Diabetes Metab. **28:** 463–467.
81. YANG, Z., K. WANG, T. LI, *et al.* 1998. Childhood diabetes in China. Enormous variation by place and ethnic group. Diabetes Care **21:** 525–529.
82. RAMACHANDRAN, A., C. SNEHALATHA & C.V. KRISHNASWAMY. 1996. Incidence of IDDM in children in urban population in southern India. Madras IDDM Registry Group Madras, South India. Diabetes Res. Clin. Pract. **34:** 79–82.
83. LEE, W.W., B.C. OOI, A.C. THAI, *et al.* 1998. The incidence of IDDM in Singapore children. Singapore Med. J. **39:** 359–362.
84. KIDA, K., G. MIMURA, T. ITO, *et al.* 2000. Incidence of Type 1 diabetes mellitus in children aged 0–14 in Japan, 1986–1990, including an analysis for seasonality of onset and month of birth: JDS study. The Data Committee for Childhood Diabetes of the Japan Diabetes Society (JDS). Diabet. Med. **17:** 59–63.
85. STAINES, A., S. HANIF, S. AHMED, *et al.* 1997. Incidence of insulin dependent diabetes mellitus in Karachi, Pakistan. Arch. Dis. Child **76:** 121–123.
86. PANAMONTA, O., M. LAOPAIBOON & C. TUCHINDA. 2000. Incidence of childhood type 1 (insulin dependent) diabetes mellitus in northeastern Thailand. J. Med. Assoc. Thai. **83:** 821–824.

87. Tuchinda, C., S. Likitmaskul, K. Unachak, *et al.* 2002. The epidemiology of type I diabetes in Thai children. J. Med. Assoc. Thai. **85:** 648–652.
88. Craig, M.E., N.J. Howard, M. Silink & A. Chan. 2000. The rising incidence of childhood type 1 diabetes in New South Wales, Australia. J. Pediatr. Endocrinol. Metab. **13:** 363–372.
89. Wu, D., D. Kendall, H. Lunt, *et al.* 2005. Prevalence of tye 1 diabetes in new Zealanders aged 0–24 years. NZ. Med. J. **118:** U1557.
90. Karvonen, M., M. Viik-Kajander, E. Moltchanova, *et al.* 2000. Incidence of childhood type 1 diabetes worldwide. Diabetes Mondiale (DiaMond) Project Group. Diabetes Care **23:** 1516–1526.
91. Dahlquist, G. & L. Mustonen. 2000. Analysis of 20 years of prospective registration of childhood onset diabetes time trends and birth cohort effects. Swedish Childhood Diabetes StudyGroup. Acta Paediatr. **89:** 1231–1237.
92. Svendsen, A.J., J.C. Kreutzfeld, E.B. Lund, *et al.* 1997. Incidence of juvenile-onset diabetes in Denmark. A prospective registration in the counties of Fyn, Ribe, Sonderjylland and Vejle. Laeger **159:** 1257–1260.
93. Muntoni, S., L. Stabilini, M. Stabilini, *et al.* 1995. Steadily high IDDM incidence over 4 years in Sardinia. Diabetes Care **18:** 1600–1601.
94. Cotellessa, M., P. Barbieri, M. Mazzella, *et al.* 2003. High incidence of childhood type 1 diabetes in Liguria, Italy, from 1989 to 1998. Diabetes Care **26:** 1786–1789.
95. Rangasami, J.J., D.C. Greenwood, B. McSporran, *et al.* 1997. Rising incidence of type 1 diabetes in Scottish children, 1984-93. The Scottish Study Group for the Care of Young Diabetics. Arch. Dis. Child **77:** 210–213.
96. Cardwell, C.R., D.J. Carson & C.C. Patterson. 2006. Higher incidence of childhood-onset type 1 diabetes mellitus in remote areas: a UK regional small-area analysis. Diabetologia **49:** 2074–2077.
97. Ruwaard, D., R.A. Hirasing, H.M. Reeser, *et al.* 1994. Increasing incidence of type I diabetes in the Netherlands. The second nationwide study among children under 20 years of age. Diabetes Care **17:** 599–601.
98. van Wouwe, J.P., G.F. Mattiazzo, N. el Mokadem, *et al.* 2004. The incidence and initial symptoms of diabetes mellitus type 1 in 0–14-year-olds in the Netherlands, 1996–1999. Ned. Tijdschr. Geneeskd. **148:** 1824–1829.
99. Neu, A., M. Kehrer, R. Hub & M.B. Ranke. 1997. Incidence of IDDM in German children aged 0–14 years. A 6-year population-based study (1987–1993). Diabetes Care **20:** 530–533.
100. Rosenbauer, J., A. Icks & G. Giani. 2002. Incidence and prevalence of childhood type 1 diabetes mellitus in Germany—model-based national estimates. J. Pediatr. Endocrinol. Metab. **15:** 1497–1504.
101. Chueca, M., M. Oyarzabal, F. Reparaz, *et al.* 1997. Incidence of type I diabetes mellitus in Navarre, Spain (1975–91). Acta Paediatr. **86:** 632–637.
102. Lora-Gomez, R.E., F.M. Morales-Perez, F.J. Arroyo-Diez & J. Barquero-Romero. 2005. Incidence of Type 1 diabetes in children in Caceres, Spain, during 1988–1999. Diabetes Res. Clin. Pract. **69:** 169–174.
103. Gyurus, E., B. Gyork, A. Green, *et al.* 1999. Incidence of type 1 childhood diabetes in Hungary (1978–1997). Hungarian Committee on the Epidemiology of Childhood Diabetes. Orv. Hetil. **140:** 1107–1111.
104. Skordis, N. & S. Hadjiloizou. 1997. Incidence of insulin dependent diabetes mellitus in Greek Cypriot children and adolescents, 1990–1994. J. Pediatr. Endocrinol. Metab. **10:** 203–207.

105. CINEK, O., V. LANSKA, S. KOLOUSKOVA, *et al.* 2000. Type 1 diabetes mellitus in Czech children diagnosed in 1990–1997: a significant increase in incidence and male predominance in the age group 0–4 years. Collaborators of the Czech Childhood Diabetes Registry. Diabet. Med. **17:** 64–69.
106. KRETOWSKI, A., I. KOWALSKA, J. PECZYNSKA, *et al.* 1999. Epidemiology of diabetes type 1 in the 0 to 29 year-old age group in Northeastern Poland, 1994–1998—prospective observations. Pol. Arch. Med. Wewn. **101:** 509–515.
107. MICHALKOVA, D.M., J. CERNAY, A. DANKOVA, *et al.* 1995. Incidence and prevalence of childhood diabetes in Slovakia (1985–1992). Slovak Childhood Diabetes Epidemiology Study Group. Diabetes Care **18:** 315–320.
108. PUNDZIUTE-LYCKA, A., B. URBONAITE, R. OSTRAUSKAS, *et al.* 2003. Incidence of type 1 diabetes in Lithuanians aged 0–39 years varies by the urban-rural setting, and the time change differs for men and women during 1991–2000. Diabetes Care **26:** 671–676.
109. BATTELINO, T. & C. KRZISNIK. 1998. Incidence of type 1 diabetes mellitus in children in Slovenia during the years 1988–1995. Acta Diabetol **35:** 112–114.
110. PODAR, T., R.E. LAPORTE, J. TUOMILEHTO & E. SHUBNIKOV. 1993. Risk of childhood type 1 diabetes for Russians in Estonia and Siberia. Int. J. Epidemiol. **22:** 262–267.
111. MARTINUCCI, M.E., G. CURRADI, A. FASULO, *et al.* 2002. Incidence of childhood type 1 diabetes mellitus in Gomel, Belarus. J. Pediatr. Endocrinol. Metab. **15:** 53–57.
112. SHALTOUT, A.A., M.A. QABAZARD, N.A. ABDELLA, *et al.* 1995. High incidence of childhood-onset IDDM in Kuwait. Kuwait Study Group of Diabetes in Childhood. Diabetes Care **18:** 923–927.
113. ABDUL-RASOUL, M., H. AL-QATTAN, A. AL-HAJ, *et al.* 2002. Incidence and seasonal variation of Type 1 diabetes in children in Farwania area, Kuwait (1995–1999). Diabetes Res. Clin. Pract. **56:** 153–157.
114. KULAYLAT, N.A. & H. NARCHI. 2000. A twelve-year study of the incidence of childhood type 1 diabetes mellitus in the Eastern Province of Saudi Arabia. J. Pediatr. Endocrinol. Metab. **13:** 135–140.
115. AJLOUNI, K., Y. QUSOUS, A.K. KHAWALDEH, *et al.* 1999. Incidence of insulin-dependent diabetes mellitus in Jordanian children aged 0–14 y during 1992–1996. Acta Paediatr. **88:** 11–13.
116. SOLIMAN, A.T., I.S. AL-SALMI & M.G. ASFOUR. 1996. Epidemiology of childhood insulin-dependent diabetes mellitus in the Sultanate of Oman. Diabet. Med. **13:** 582–586.
117. PATRICK, S.L., J.K. KADOHIRO, S.H. WAXMAN, *et al.* 1997. IDDM incidence in a multiracial population. The Hawaii IDDM Registry, 1980–1990. Diabetes Care **20:** 983–987.
118. LIPMAN, T.H. 1993. The epidemiology of type I diabetes in children 0–14 yr of age in Philadelphia. Diabetes Care **16:** 922–925.
119. FRAZER DE LLADO, T.E., L. GONZALEZ DE PIJEM & B. HAWK. 1998. Incidence of IDDM in children living in Puerto Rico. Puerto Rican IDDM Coalition. Diabetes Care **21:** 744–746.
120. LISBOA, H.R., R. GRAEBIN, L. BUTZKE & C.S. RODRIGUES. 1998. Incidence of type 1 diabetes mellitus in Passo Fundo, RS, Brazil. Braz. J. Med. Biol. Res. **31:** 1553–1556.
121. PETER, S.A., R. JOHNSON, C. TAYLOR, *et al.* 2005. The incidence and prevalence of type I diabetes mellitus. J. Natl. Med. Assoc. **97:** 250–252.

122. JORDAN, O.W., R.B. LIPTON, E. STUPNICKA, *et al.* 1994. Incidence of type I diabetes in people under 30 years of age in Barbados, West Indies, 1982–1991. Diabetes Care **17:** 428–431.
123. WARRAM, J.H., S.S. RICH & A.S. KROLESWKI. 1994. Epidemiology and Genetics of diabetes mellitus. *In* Joslin's Diabetes Mellitus, 13th ed. C.R., Kahn & G., Weir, Eds.: 210–215. Lea and Febiger. Philadelphia.
124. FLEGAL, K.M., T.M. EZZATI, M.I. HARRIS, *et al.* 1991. Prevalence of diabetes in Mexican Americans, Cubans, and Puerto Ricans from the Hispanic Health and Nutrition Examination Survey, 1982–1984. Diabetes Care **14:** 628–638.
125. KNOWLER, W.C., D.J. PETTITT, M.F. SAAD & P.H. BENNETT. 1990. Diabetes mellitus in the Pima Indians: incidence, risk factors and pathogenesis. Diabetes Metab. Rev. **6:** 1–27.
126. TUOMILEHTO, J., H.J. KORHONEN, L. KARTOVAARA, *et al.* 1991. Prevalence of diabetes mellitus and impaired glucose tolerance in the middle-aged population of three areas in Finland. Int. J. Epidemiol. **20:** 1010–1017.
127. BACCHUS, R.A., J.L. BELL, M. MADKOUR & B. KILSHAW. 1982. The prevalence of diabetes mellitus in male Saudi Arabs. Diabetologia **23:** 330–332.
128. SODERBERG, S., P. ZIMMET, J. TUOMILEHTO, *et al.* 2005. Increasing prevalence of Type 2 diabetes mellitus in all ethnic groups in Mauritius. Diabet. Med. **22:** 61–68.
129. OMAR, M.A., M.A. SEEDAT, A.A. MOTALA, *et al.* 1993. The prevalence of diabetes mellitus and impaired glucose tolerance in a group of urban South African blacks. S. Afr. Med. J. **83:** 641–643.
130. MALEK, R., F. BELATECHE, S. LAOUAMRI, *et al.* 2001. Prevalence of type 2 diabetes mellitus and glucose intolerance in the Setif area (Algeria). Diabetes Metab. **27:** 164–171.
131. ELBAGIR, M.N., M.A. ELTOM, E.M. ELMAHADI, *et al.* 1996. A population-based study of the prevalence of diabetes mellitus and impaired glucose tolerance in adults in northern Sudan. Diabetes Care **19:** 1126–1128.
132. OWOAJE, E.E., C.N. ROTIMI, J.S. KAUFMAN, *et al.* 1997. Prevalence of adult diabetes in Ibadan, Nigeria. East. Afr. Med. J. **74:** 299–302.
133. CEESAY, M.M., M.W. MORGAN, M.O. KAMANDA, *et al.* 1997. Prevalence of diabetes in rural and urban populations in southern Sierra Leone: a preliminary survey. Trop. Med. Int. Health **2:** 272–277.
134. VAN DE SANDE, M.A., R. BAILEY, H. FAAL, *et al.* 1997. Nation-wide prevalence study of hypertension and related non-communicable diseases in the Gambia. Trop. Med. Int. Health **2:** 1039–1048.
135. SINGH, D.L. & M.D. BHATTARAI. 2003. High prevalence of diabetes and impaired fasting glycaemia in urban Nepal. Diabet. Med. **20:** 170–171.
136. RAMACHANDRAN, A., C. SNEHALATHA, E. LATHA, *et al.* 1997. Rising prevalence of NIDDM in an urban population in India. Diabetologia **40:** 232–237.
137. KUZUYA, T. 1994. Prevalence of diabetes mellitus in Japan compiled from literature. Diabetes Res. Clin. Pract. **24:** S15–S21.
138. CHANG, C., F. LU, Y.C. YANG, *et al.* 2000. Epidemiologic study of type 2 diabetes in Taiwan. Diabetes Res. Clin. Pract. **50:** S49–S59.
139. LEE, W.R. 2000. The changing demography of diabetes mellitus in Singapore. Diabetes Res. Clin. Pract. **50:** S35–S39.
140. HUSSAIN, A., M. RAHIM, A.K. AZAD KHAN, *et al.* 2005. Type 2 diabetes in rural and urban population: diverse prevalence and associated risk factors in Bangladesh. Diabet. Med. **22:** 931–936.

141. KIM, S.M., J.S. LEE, J. LEE, *et al.* 2006. Prevalence of diabetes and impaired fasting glucose in Korea: Korean National Health and Nutrition Survey 2001. Diabetes Care **29:** 226–231.
142. ABU SAYEED, M., H. MAHTAB, P. AKTER KHANAM, *et al.* 2004. Diabetes and impaired fasting glycemia in the tribes of Khagrachari hill tracts of Bangladesh. Diabetes Care **27:** 1054–1059.
143. KARKI, P., N. BARAL, M. LAMSAL, *et al.* 2000. Prevalence of non-insulin dependent diabetes mellitus in urban areas of eastern Nepal: a hospital based study. Southeast Asian J. Trop. Med. Public Health **31:** 163–166.
144. SUTANEGARA, D. & A.A. BUDHIARTA. 2000. The epidemiology and management of diabetes mellitus in Indonesia. Diabetes Res. Clin. Pract. **50:** S9–S16.
145. DHADWAL, D., S.K. AHLUWALIA, D.J. DAS GUPTA, *et al.* 1997. Prevalence of NIDDM in the general population (>40 years) in Shimla. Indian J. Med. Sci. **51:** 459–464.
146. COLAGIURI, S., R. COLAGIURI, S. NA'ATI, *et al.* 2002. The prevalence of diabetes in the kingdom of Tonga. Diabetes Care **25:** 1378–1383.
147. GLATTHAAR, C., T.A. WELBORN, N.S. STENHOUSE & P. GARCIA-WEBB. 1985. Diabetes and impaired glucose tolerance. A prevalence estimate based on the Busselton 1981 survey. Med. J. Aust. **143:** 436–440.
148. FUJIMOTO, W.Y. 1996. Overview of non-insulin-dependent diabetes mellitus (NIDDM) in different population groups. Diabet. Med. **13:** S7–S10.
149. HOTU, S., B. CARTER, P.D. WATSON, *et al.* 2004. Increasing prevalence of type 2 diabetes in adolescents. J. Paediatr. Child Health. **40:** 201–204.
150. GOKCEL, A., A.K. OZSAHIN, N. SEZGIN, *et al.* 2003. High prevalence of diabetes in Adana, a southern province of Turkey. Diabetes Care **26:** 3031–3034.
151. BOTAS CERVERO, P., E. DELGADO ALVAREZ, G. CASTANO FERNANDEZ, *et al.* 2002. Prevalence of diabetes mellitus and glucose intolerance in the population aged 30 to 75 years in Asturias. Rev. Clin. Esp. **202:** 421–429.
152. PILOTTO, L., A. GAGGIOLI, C. LO NOCE, *et al.* & GRUPPO DI RICERCA DELL'OSSERVATORIO EPIDEMIOLOGICO CARDIOVASCOLARE. 2004. Diabetes in Italy: a public health problem. Ital. Heart J. Suppl. **5:** 480–486.
153. GARANCINI, M.P., G. CALORI, G. RUOTOLO, *et al.* 1995. Prevalence of NIDDM and impaired glucose tolerance in Italy: an OGTT-based population study. Diabetologia **38:** 306–313.
154. DETOURNAY, B., F. VAUZELLE-KERVROEDAN, M.A. CHARLES, *et al.* 1999. Epidemiology, management and costs of type 2 diabetes in France in 1998. Diabetes Metab. **25:** 356–365.
155. GOURDY, P., J.B. RUIDAVETS, J. FERRIERES, *et al.* & MONICA STUDY. 2001. Prevalence of type 2 diabetes and impaired fasting glucose in the middle-aged population of three French regions - The MONICA study 1995–1997. Diabetes Metab. **27:** 347–358.
156. KURAEVA, T.L., A.S. SERGEEV, N.B. LEBEDEV, *et al.* 1993. Diabetes mellitus incidence and its prevalence in Moscow. Probl. Endokrinol. (Mosk.) **39:** 4–7.
157. ANDERSSON, D.K., K. SVARDSUDD & G. TIBBLIN. 1991. Prevalence and incidence of diabetes in a Swedish community 1972–1987. Diabet. Med. **8:** 428–434.
158. BAAN, C.A. & E.J. FESKENS. 2001. Disease burden of diabetes mellitus type II in the Netherlands: incidence, prevalence and mortality. Ned. Tijdschr. Geneeskd. **145:** 1681–1685.

159. FABIAN, W., L. MAJKOWSKA, A. STEFANSKI & P. MOLEDA. 2005. Prevalence of diabetes, antidiabetic treatment and chronic diabetic complications reported by general practitioners. Przegl. Lek. **62:** 201–205.
160. GATLING, W., S. BUDD, D. WALTERS, *et al.* 1998. Evidence of an increasing prevalence of diagnosed diabetes mellitus in the Poole area from 1983 to 1996. Diabet. Med. **15:** 1015–1021.
161. BROHALL, G., C.J. BEHRE, J. HULTHE, *et al.* 2006. Prevalence of diabetes and impaired glucose tolerance in 64-year-old Swedish women: experiences of using repeated oral glucose tolerance tests. Diabetes Care **29:** 363–367.
162. GLUMER, C., T. JORGENSEN, K. BORCH-JOHNSEN, & INTER99 STUDY. 2003. Prevalences of diabetes and impaired glucose regulation in a Danish population: the Inter99 study. Diabetes Care **26:** 2335–2340.
163. MALIK, M., A. BAKIR, B.A. SAAB & H. KING. 2005. Glucose intolerance and associated factors in the multi-ethnic population of the United Arab Emirates: results of a national survey. Diabetes Res. Clin. Pract. **69:** 188–195.
164. ABDELLA, N., M. AL AROUJ, A. AL NAKHI, *et al.* 1998. Non-insulin-dependent diabetes in Kuwait: prevalence rates and associated risk factors. Diabetes Res. Clin. Pract. **42:** 187–196.
165. HUSSEINI, A., H. ABDUL-RAHIM, F. AWARTANI, *et al.* 2000. Type 2 diabetes mellitus, impaired glucose tolerance and associated factors in a rural Palestinian village. Diabet. Med. **17:** 746–748.
166. AL-HABORI, M., M. AL-MAMARI & A. AL-MEERI. 2004. Type II diabetes mellitus and impaired glucose tolerance in Yemen: prevalence, associated metabolic changes and risk factors. Diabetes Res. Clin. Pract. **65:** 275–281.
167. CARTER, J., R. HOROWITZ, R. WILSON, *et al.* 1989. Tribal differences in diabetes: prevalence among American Indians in New Mexico. Public Health Rep. **104:** 665–669.
168. HERMAN, W.H., T.J. THOMPSON, W. VISSCHER, *et al.* 1998. Diabetes mellitus and its complications in an African-American Community: project DIRECT. J. Natl. Med. Assoc. **90:** 147–156.
169. BLANCHARD, J.F., H. DEAN, K. ANDERSON, *et al.* 1997. Incidence and prevalence of diabetes in children aged 0–14 years in Manitoba, Canada, 1985–1993. Diabetes Care **20:** 512–515.
170. MALERBI, D.A. & L.J. FRANCO. 1992. Multicenter study of the prevalence of diabetes mellitus and impaired glucose tolerance in the urban Brazilian population aged 30–69 yr. The Brazilian Co-operative Group on the Study of Diabetes Prevalence. Diabetes Care **15:** 1509–1516.
171. TORQUATO, M.T., R.M. MONTENEGRO JUNIOR, L.A. VIANA, *et al.* 2003. Prevalence of diabetes mellitus and impaired glucose tolerance in the urban population aged 30–69 years in Ribeirao Preto (Sao Paulo), Brazil. Sao Paulo Med. J. **121:** 224–230.
172. PEREZ-BRAVO, F., E. CARRASCO, J.L. SANTOS, *et al.* 2001. Prevalence of type 2 diabetes and obesity in rural Mapuche population from Chile. Nutrition **17:** 236–238.
173. CARRASCO, E.P., F.B. PEREZ, B.B. ANGEL, *et al.* 2004. Prevalence of type 2 diabetes and obesity in two Chilean aboriginal populations living in urban zones. Rev. Med. Chil. **132:** 1189–1197.
174. CASTRO-SANCHEZ, H. & J. ESCOBEDO-DE LA PENA. 1997. Prevalence of non insulin dependent diabetes mellitus and associated risk factors in the Mazatec population of the State of Oaxaca, Mexico (Spanish). Gac. Med. Ex. **133:** 527–534.

Inflammation in Metabolic Syndrome and Type 2 Diabetes

Impact of Dietary Glucose

KERSTIN KEMPF, BETTINA ROSE, CHRISTIAN HERDER, URSULA KLEOPHAS, STEPHAN MARTIN, AND HUBERT KOLB

German Diabetes Clinic, German Diabetes Center, Leibniz Institute at Heinrich-Heine-University Düsseldorf, 40225 Düsseldorf, Germany

ABSTRACT: Chronic overnutrition combined with a lack of exercise is the main cause for the rapidly increasing prevalence of overweight and obesity. It seems accepted that *adipositis* (macrophage infiltration and inflammation of adipose tissue in obesity) and systemic low grade inflammation affect the pathogenesis of the metabolic syndrome or type 2 diabetes mellitus (T2DM). Therefore, modern weight reduction programs additionally focus on strategies to attenuate the inflammation state. Exercise is one major factor, which contributes to the reduction of both the incidence of T2DM and inflammation, and the immunomodulatory effects of exercise are supported by similarly beneficial effects of dietary changes. In this context, glucose is the most extensively studied nutrient and current investigations focus on postprandial glucose-induced inflammation, one possible reason why hyperglycemia is detrimental. Indeed, glucose may modulate the mRNA expression and serum concentrations of immune parameters but these alterations rapidly normalize in normoglycemic subjects. In case of an impaired metabolic state, however, postprandial hyperglycemia increases magnitude and duration of systemic inflammatory responses, which probably promotes the development of T2DM and of cardiovascular disease.

KEYWORDS: type 2 diabetes; obesity; inflammation; lifestyle; exercise; nutrition; glucose

INTRODUCTION

Any generalized and simplified scheme of the natural course of type 2 diabetes mellitus (T2DM) has to acknowledge several key stages on the way to overt clinical disease. The first stage appears to be during fetal development by

Address for correspondence: Dr. Kerstin Kempf, German Diabetes Clinic, German Diabetes Center, Leibniz Institute at Heinrich-Heine-University Düsseldorf, Auf'm Hennekamp 65, 40225 Düsseldorf, Germany. Voice: +49-211-3382-647; fax: +49-211-3382-653.
e-mail: kerstin.kempf@ddz.uni-duesseldorf.de

Ann. N.Y. Acad. Sci. 1084: 30–48 (2006).
doi: 10.1196/annals.1372.012

priming of gene expression through DNA methylation and other mechanisms, and also by the metabolic intrauterine environment that affects the relative beta cell mass at birth or birth weight.[1,2] Fetal priming appears to affect later inflammation status, as judged from the negative association of birth weight and systemic interleukin-6 (IL-6) levels of monozygotic twins later in life.[3]

Because of genetic predisposition, fetal priming, and lifestyle, insulin resistance evolves at some (unknown) time after birth, without requiring prior obesity.[4,5] In addition, loss of pulsatile insulin secretion and increased circulating proinsulin levels are noted.[6–8] Obesity often develops as an additional risk factor,[9,10] accompanied by macrophage infiltration and inflammation of obese adipose tissue, "adipositis."[11,12] Even clear symptoms of metabolic disturbances, such as impaired glucose tolerance (IGT) may precede overt disease by many years.

Beta cells initially compensate for insulin resistance by expanding cell numbers and insulin output. IGT and subsequent T2DM will develop in those individuals whose islets have deficient mechanisms of coping with the extra stress.[13–18] Hence, overt T2DM results from the failure of beta cells to compensate for increased demands due to insulin resistance (summarized in FIG. 1).

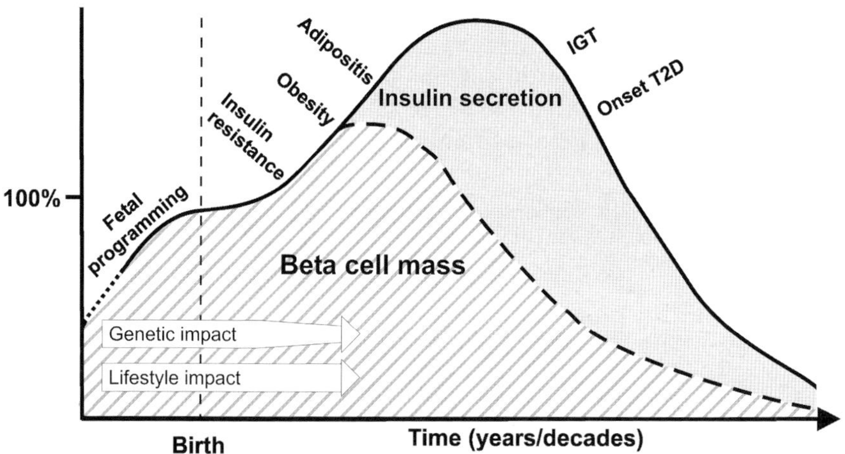

FIGURE 1. Natural course of type 2 diabetes, a generalized and simplified scheme. Programming of metabolic regulation and gene expression occurs *in utero*. Insulin resistance with or without obesity develops in childhood, adolescence, or early adulthood and is compensated by increased beta cell mass and insulin secretion. Probably in response to obesity/fat cell stress macrophages invade fat tissue and give rise to local inflammation ("adipositis"). The failure of islets to compensate for increased insulin demand is primarily caused by beta cell death. This leads to IGT and eventually to overt T2DM. Evidence of systemic low grade inflammation and of oxidative stress/mitochondrial dysfunction is noted from early on.

LOW GRADE INFLAMMATION

At which stage of disease development does low grade inflammation become visible? Early observations of the presence of subclinical systemic inflammation were done only after diagnosis of diabetes.[19–24] To date, virtually all systemic indicators of inflammation have been found abnormal in patients with T2DM. These include acute-phase proteins, cytokines, chemokines, and mediators associated with endothelial activation[25–27] (see also Ref. 28 for a comprehensive review). It is important to note that the degree of immune activation is far below that seen in acute infections. Prospective studies have demonstrated the presences of low grade inflammation years to decades before diagnosis of metabolic syndrome (MetS) or T2DM. These subtle changes include increased leukocyte counts and elevated concentrations of circulating immune mediators.[25,28–31]

Another argument in favor of a pathogenetic role of low grade inflammation is the association of several immune gene alleles with risk of T2DM. Associations of gene polymorphisms with insulin resistance, MetS, or T2DM have been reported for the HLA locus, for tumor necrosis factor-α (TNF-α), TNF-β, TNF-α receptor 80, IL-6, IL-6 receptor-α, C-reactive protein (CRP), transforming growth factor-β (TGF-β), monocyte chemoattractant protein-1 (MCP-1), plasminogen activator inhibitor-1 (PAI-1), CD14, or BPI (bactericidal/permeability-increasing protein).[28,32–36] Although many of these associations still await confirmation in large population-based studies, it is of relevance that the alleles in question usually have an impact on immune reactivity and hence contribute to the genetic control of inflammation.

Further support in favor of a contribution of immune gene products to disease development comes from animal studies. In fact, most of the genes reported associated with human T2DM do modulate the risk of developing insulin resistance, obesity, and diabetes also in animals, after appropriate genetic modification.[37–43]

IMMUNE INTERVENTION

The infusion of the cytokines TNF-α or IL-6 significantly reduces insulin sensitivity in animals.[44–48] In humans, there is only limited experience. Exogenous TNF-α was observed to cause insulin resistance while infusions of IL-6 showed little effects.[49] Additional insight comes from immunomodulatory intervention. In animals, the neutralization of TNF-α by injected monoclonal antibody improved insulin sensitivity while this was not observed in humans.[50–53] Therapeutic studies with high-dose aspirin in T2DM patients support a role of inflammation. Such treatment caused a decrease of systemic CRP levels and concomitantly a 25% reduction in fasting blood glucose and an even larger decrease of serum triglyceride levels.[54]

Taken together, arguments in favor of a causal role of the immune system in the pathogenesis of the MetS or T2DM are (*a*) the systemic low grade inflammation seen years prior to clinical symptoms, (*b*) the association of disease risk with immune gene alleles, (*c*) the causal role of immune gene products in animal models, (*d*) the observation that infused cytokines cause insulin resistance, and (*e*) the amelioration of insulin resistance by anti-cytokine or anti-inflammatory treatment (summarized in FIG. 2).

PATHOGENESIS: IMPACT OF LIFESTYLE FACTORS VIA THE IMMUNE SYSTEM?—EXERCISE

If the proinflammatory status is influenced by environmental factors and if inflammation plays an important role in the development of T2DM as suggested by the interaction of "Western" lifestyle, "adipositis" and increasing T2DM prevalence, any therapeutic approach to protect against T2DM would have to include effective anti-inflammatory mechanisms. Recent studies emphasized the value of exercise in reducing both the incidence of T2DM and inflammation. The efficacy of exercise and diet-based intervention to delay or prevent the progression to T2DM in individuals at high risk (IGT and/or overweight) was clearly demonstrated in the Finnish Diabetes Prevention Study,[55] the Diabetes Prevention Program in the USA,[56] the Da Qing IGT and Diabetes

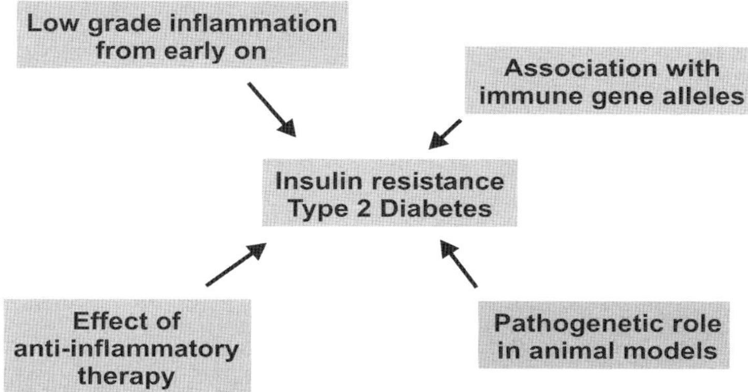

FIGURE 2. Arguments in favor of immune mediators as pathogenic factors in the development of insulin resistance and type 2 diabetes. Immunological changes in blood suggesting systemic low grade inflammation are seen years to decades before overt clinical symptoms. Immune gene polymorphisms are associated with disease risk. Immune gene alleles cause insulin resistance and diabetes in animal models. Infused cytokines may cause insulin resistance and anti-inflammatory therapy by pharmacological and nonpharmacological means ameliorates insulin resistance.

Study in China,[57] the Indian Diabetes Prevention Programme,[58] and other randomized controlled trials[59] with relative risk reductions up to 58%. The relative importance of exercise in most of these studies has not been investigated, but data from the Finnish and Chinese studies indicate a diet-independent beneficial effect of physical activity.[57,60]

The mechanisms of these interactions are currently analyzed on the cellular and systemic level. Exercise and weight loss may have direct anti-inflammatory effects on the innate immune system and on adipose tissue, but several studies also indicate that skeletal muscle is an important tissue in this context. Skeletal muscle expresses a range of immune mediators including TNF-α, IL-6, and IL-18 with potentially important differences between muscle fiber types.[61] Strenuous exercise results in substantial upregulation of IL-6 (but not TNF-α) in muscle and sequential upregulation of anti-inflammatory cytokines including IL-10 and IL-1 receptor antagonist (IL-1ra).[62] This cascade has been postulated to link the skeletal muscle with liver, adipose tissue, immune cells, and the brain and thereby mediate long-term metabolic and immunological health benefits.[63] Further research can be expected to lead to a better understanding of these mechanisms and of the (at a first glance) paradoxical observation that acute (short-term) exercise training results in *upregulation* of IL-6 and other immune mediators, whereas the aforementioned and other intervention studies as well as population-based cohorts clearly show significantly *lower* systemic levels of inflammatory markers (including IL-6) and reduced T2DM incidence associated with regular exercise and higher cardiorespiratory fitness.[64–66] From the clinician's point of view, it is interesting that the IL-6 response of skeletal muscle to exercise appears to be preserved during aging,[67] which is in line with the observation that lifestyle modification is equally effective in attenuating systemic inflammation and reducing the incidence of T2DM across a wide age range.[56,66]

It can be assumed that the immunomodulatory effects of exercise were complemented by similarly beneficial effects of changes in dietary habits on low grade inflammation and T2DM development in the aforementioned large diabetes prevention studies.[55–58] The impact of diet on inflammation and T2DM has been investigated by many groups and will be discussed in more detail in the following sections with a specific focus on glucose as most extensively studied nutrient.

PATHOGENESIS: IMPACT OF LIFESTYLE FACTORS VIA IMMUNE SYSTEM?—DIET

Diet Modulates Low Grade Inflammation (Long-Term Effects)

Chronic overnutrition combined with a lack of exercise is the main cause for the rapid increase of overweight and obesity in industrialized countries. The increase of adipose tissue mass is associated with significant invasion of immune cells (i.e., macrophages)[11,12,68] and secretion of proinflammatory immune mediators (i.e., adipokines, cytokines, chemokines, adhesion molecules, and acute-phase proteins) that mediate not only local "adipositis," but also a systemic low grade inflammation. Associated with significant risk factors for cardiometabolic diseases (e.g., insulin resistance, dyslipidemia, hypertension, and low grade inflammation), obesity has become a major public health problem with major implications for morbidity, mortality, and socioeconomic cost.

Various dietary strategies have been tested to reduce weight and the associated risk for T2DM and cardiovascular disease (CVD). The Women's Health Initiative Dietary Modification Trial including 48,835 postmenopausal women demonstrated that reduced intake of total fat combined with increased intake of vegetables and fruits (4.9 versus 3.8 servings/day) achieved only modest improvements of CVD risk factors after 8 years and did not significantly effect on incidence of coronary heart disease, stroke, or CVD. A trend was observed toward a reduced risk among those with >6.5 servings of vegetables and fruits per day.[69] This is in line with a meta-analysis based on nine independent cohorts and 257,551 individuals, which demonstrated that increased fruit and vegetable intake (>5 versus 3–5 servings/day) was clearly associated with a reduced risk of stroke.[70] While increased consumption of fruits and vegetables is favorable, the effect of low-carbohydrate diets is discussed. A meta-analysis of five trials including 447 individuals after 6 months showed that the weight loss of individuals assigned to low carbohydrate was higher than in individuals randomized to low-fat diets but this difference was no longer obvious after 12 months. The change of triglycerides and high-density lipoprotein (HDL) cholesterol levels was more favorable after the low-carbohydrate diet, while improvement of total and low-density lipoprotein (LDL) cholesterol values was stronger in individuals assigned to low-fat diets.[71] On the other hand, low-carbohydrate diets have been reported to be effective in T2DM, not only by reducing weight but also by improving CVD risk factors like dyslipidemia, blood pressure, postprandial glycemia, and insulin secretion.[72] Controlled clinical trials, such as the Kumamoto Study[73] and UKPDS[74] have established that therapies directed at achieving normal glycemia are effective in reducing the development and delaying the progression of long-term diabetic complications. Therefore, the key question is: Why is hyperglycemia so detrimental?

Short-Term Effects of Diet: Glucose

In nondiabetic individuals, fasting plasma glucose concentrations generally range from 70 to 110 mg/dL. Glucose concentrations begin to rise ~10 min after the start of a meal as a result of the absorption of dietary carbohydrates and peak after ~60 min, rarely exceed 140 mg/dL, and return due to insulin action to preprandial levels within 2–3 h. In T2DM patients, peak insulin levels are delayed and the magnitude and duration of postprandial glucose peaks are higher.[75]

There is evidence that obesity and persistent elevated blood glucose levels promote oxidative stress and it was shown that caloric restriction in obese subjects for a brief period of 4 weeks leads to a significant reduction in oxidative stress.[76] Moreover, it has been speculated that under certain conditions an increase in blood glucose is associated with an acute inflammatory response, and that glucose intake induces oxidative stress and inflammation at the cellular and molecular level. We could show that factors of the MetS could "prime" leukocytes to upregulate proinflammatory cytokines in response to oral glucose challenge (Kempf *et al.*, unpublished data). We analyzed TNF-α and IL-6 expression in peripheral blood leukocytes from normal glucose tolerant (NGT) subjects with ($n = 39$) and without MetS ($n = 35$) before and 2 h after an oral glucose tolerance test (OGTT). Glucose significantly increased mean expression of both proinflammatory cytokines only in the MetS group (FIG. 3). Our results are supported by other studies demonstrating that *in vitro* cultivation of monocytes in high-glucose medium increased the expression and secretion of IL-6 and TNF-α.[77,78] *In vivo*, oral glucose challenges (75 g glucose) or glucose clamps increased plasma levels of adhesion molecules (intercellular adhesion molecule-1 [ICAM-1], vascular cell adhesion molecule-1 [VCAM-1], and E-selectin), cytokines (IL-6, TNF-α, IL-18), chemokines (IL-8), or reactive oxygen species in NGT subjects[79] and patients with IGT or T2DM. Nevertheless, in NGT subjects plasma levels normalized within 2–3 h, while in obese, IGT, or T2DM subjects glucose-induced inflammation was stronger or lasted longer.[80–83] Similarly, an increase of IL-6 was only seen during hyperglycemic clamp and hyperinsulinemic euglycemic clamp but not during normoglycemic clamps[84] and a high-carbohydrate meal had no obvious impact on inflammation parameters in NGT subjects but more pronounced effects in T2DM patients[85,86] Nevertheless, published results are conflicting and even anti-inflammatory effects of glucose have been reported. It was shown that during an OGTT white blood count[87] and plasma concentrations of adhesion molecules fell promptly in NGT and T2DM subjects[88] and even after a carbohydrate-rich meal serum IL-6 and TNF-α decreased after 1 h or 4–6 h, respectively, in T2DM patients.[89] In sum, it can be stated that although the net effect of glucose on serum concentrations of inflammation parameters is controversial, we and others saw only marginal effects when comparing changes of inflammation parameters before and 2 h after an oral glucose challenge in metabolic healthy subjects.

To examine if the described changes in systemic immune marker levels depend on the time point of blood withdrawal, we took blood from NGT subjects ($n = 10$; 5 men and 5 women; mean age 37.3 ± 11.3 years, mean BMI 24.7 ± 2.3 kg/m^2) every 30 min until 4 h after glucose load using a permanent venous catheter. Glucose ingestion led to a marked increase of serum levels of IL-6 ($P < 0.01$ for 180 and 240 min) and a slight decrease of systemic IL-8 ($P < 0.05$ for 60 to 240 min), IL-18 ($P < 0.01$ for 60 to 240 min), MCP-1 ($P < 0.05$ for 90

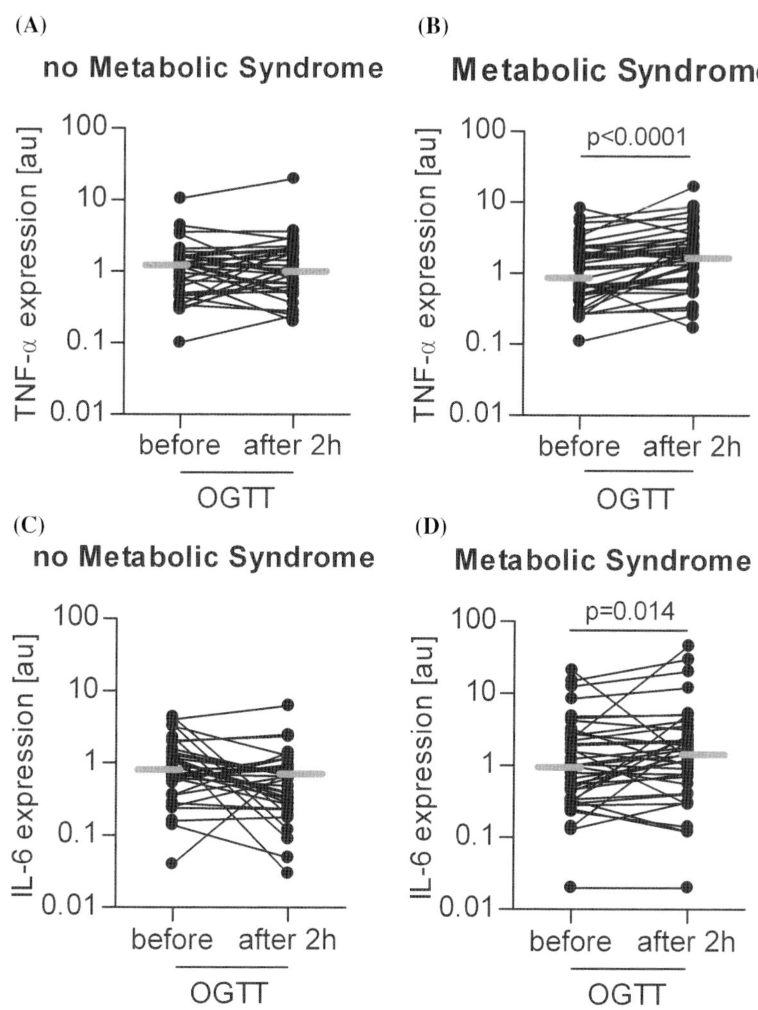

FIGURE 3. Glucose-induced expression of proinflammatory genes in peripheral leukocytes. Blood was drawn from NGT subjects by direct venipuncture before and 2 h after an OGTT and gene expression was analyzed using quantitative RT-PCR. For individuals without ($n = 35$) or with MetS ($n = 39$) arbitrary units (au) of (**A, B**) TNF-α and (**C, D**) IL-6 expression are shown. Differences were determined by Wilcoxon signed rank test, and medians are marked by *horizontal gray lines* (modified after Kempf *et al.*, unpublished data).

to 240 min), and interferon gamma-inducible protein (IP)-10 levels ($P < 0.01$ for 240 min), whereas no difference was found for TNF-α (FIG. 4). Interestingly, almost no difference between ingestion of 75 g glucose in 300 mL water, water alone, and fasting state was observed. These effects might be explained

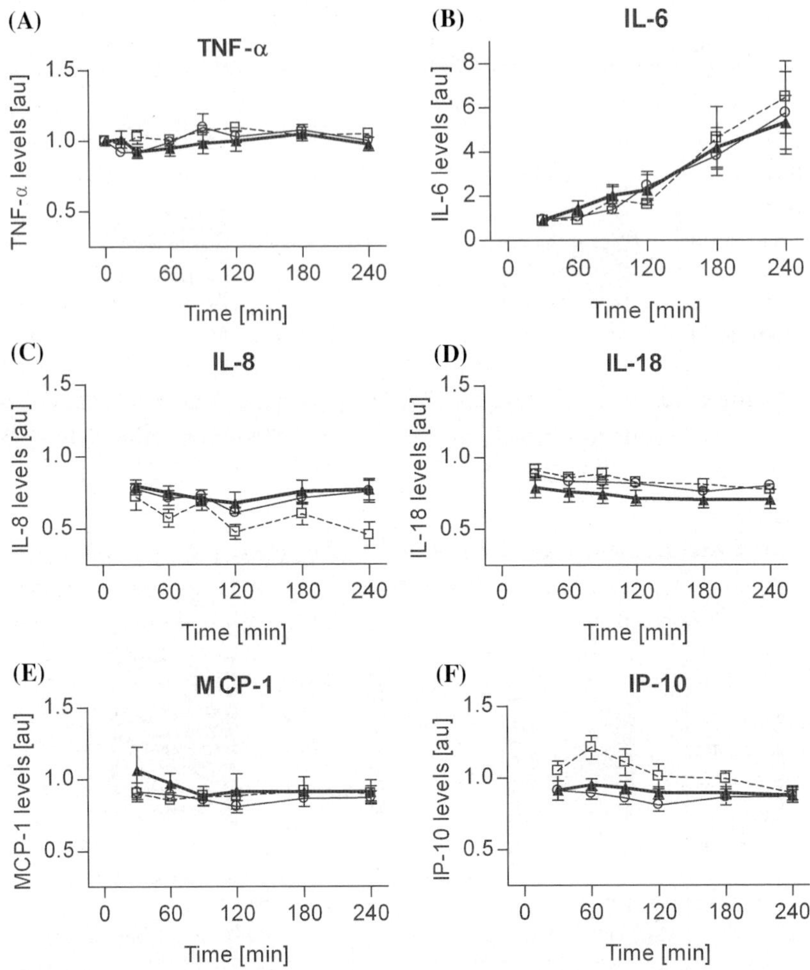

FIGURE 4. Glucose-mediated systemic cytokine levels in NGT subjects. Protein levels of (**A**) TNF-α, (**B**) IL-6, (**C**) IL-8, (**D**) IL-18, (**E**) MCP-1, and (**F**) IP-10 were analyzed in sera from NGT subjects after a 75 g oral glucose challenge (▲; $n = 10$), 300 mL water (o; $n = 10$), or in fasting state (□; $n = 9$). Blood was drawn every 30 min using an i.v. cannula. Data are shown as mean ± SEM.

by a study that showed that endothelial activation due to the placement of a permanent catheter in a forearm vein for more than 3 h leads to a local tissue production of IL-6.[90] Thus, serum analyses of blood that was drawn using a permanent catheter might represent local cytokine production and not systemic concentrations of circulating immune mediators and therefore show the limitations of this method. To deal with this problem, we additionally analyzed the expression of cytokine/chemokine genes in peripheral leukocytes. The analysis showed a transient increase of TNF-α and IL-18 expression peaking at 90 min ($P < 0.01$ for TNF-α $P < 0.05$ for IL-18), while no significant change was seen in IL-6, IL-8, MCP-1, and IP-10 expression (FIG. 5). Different gene expression responses after glucose ingestion compared to fasting state have been observed in our study for TNF-α, IL-6, and IL-8, with glucose inducing a higher or faster expression response. So far technical problems in isolating blood cell RNA prevented intensive gene expression analyses because of gene expression stimulation during blood withdrawal or RNA degradation.[91–94] Novel lysis and stabilization solutions allow gene expression analyses of peripheral blood cells without gene induction or RNA degradation. Alterations in gene expression are visible much faster than *de novo* protein synthesis and better reflect glucose-mediated effects on circulating leukocytes and systemic inflammation because circulating proteins do not originate only from circulating immune cells but may also be secreted from various other tissues (e.g., adipose tissue, muscle tissue, endothelial cells). Therefore, gene expression analysis can now be used as new and specific tool for the analysis of glucose-mediated changes of the activation state of peripheral blood leukocytes.

Interestingly, for most immune mediators investigated here only little differences were seen after ingestion of 75 g glucose in 300 mL water or water alone, whereas for some parameters the effects of complete fasting were different. This implicates that other mechanisms than glucose challenge must contribute to expression changes of inflammatory genes in peripheral blood cells. Only few data are available in the literature showing the effect of an oral glucose challenge in comparison to water uptake. A cross-over study with 10 NGT subjects showed that there was no significant difference in plasma antioxidants or oxidative stress comparing glucose or water ingestion[95] and although only glucose infusion led to an increase of neutrophils and IL-8 in 8 NGT subjects, a gradual increase of leukocytes and IL-6 could be seen in response to both, glucose and water.[96] Our data confirm these observations regarding a glucose- or water-mediated increase of leukocyte levels ($P < 0.01$ for glucose; $P < 0.001$ for water), but also extend previous studies by demonstrating that leukocyte counts under complete fasting conditions do not differ significantly from the other two experimental settings. The analysis of leukocyte subpopulations led to similar results. We found a transient decrease of lymphocytes ($P < 0.05$) and an increase of neutrophils ($P < 0.05$) not only after ingestion of glucose or water, but also in the fasting state (FIG. 6). This suggests that published studies regarding glucose-mediated effects in NGT subjects without water and fasting control are not suitable to describe glucose-induced alterations.

One might speculate that neuronal effects due to stomach filling or diurnal rhythms of cytokine secretion[96] contribute to immune mediator alterations but another possible explanation might be differences in the amount and migration potential of leukocytes. In malnutrition, one of the earliest changes in immune function is leukopenia due to simultaneous decrease in granulocyte, lymphocyte, and monocyte counts.[97] The mechanism of leukopenia during

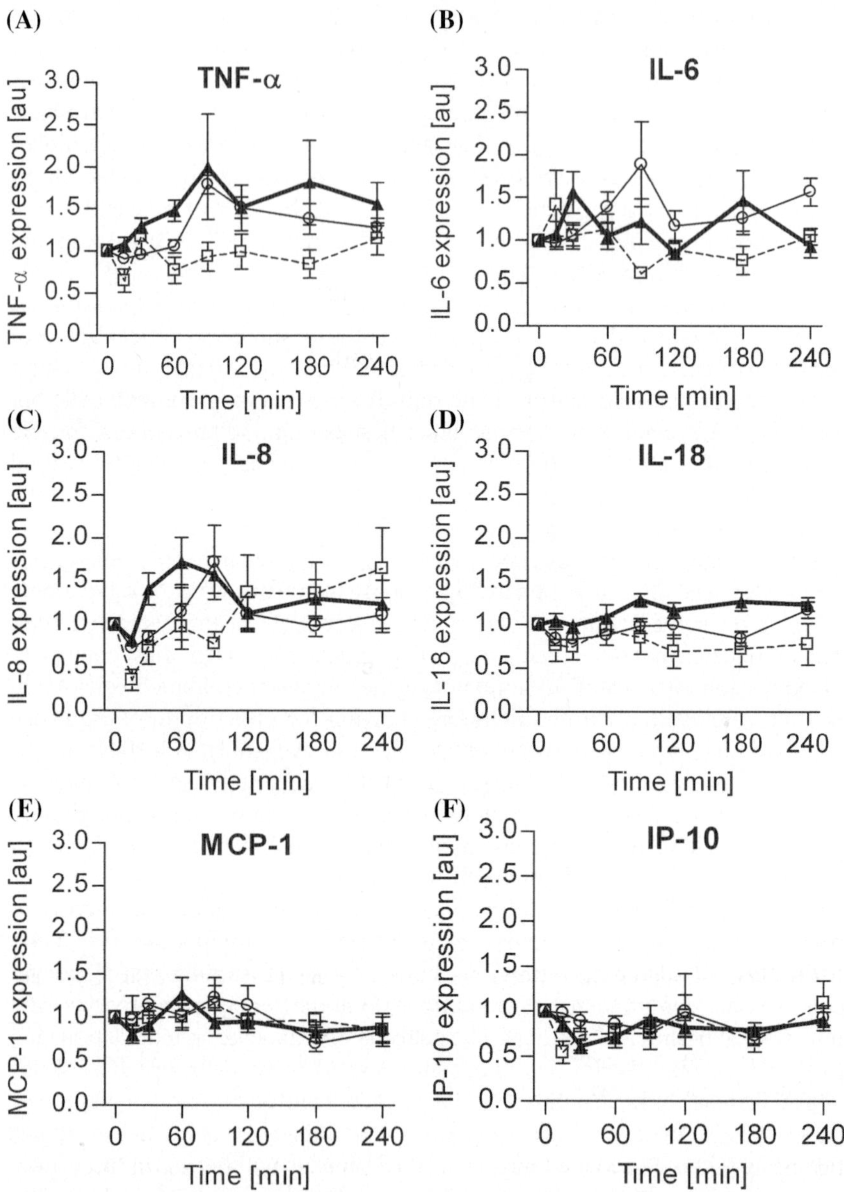

FIGURE 5. Glucose-mediated gene expression in peripheral leukocytes from NGT subjects. Gene expression of (**A**) TNF-α, (**B**) IL-6, (**C**) IL-8, (**D**) IL-18, (**E**) MCP-1, and (**F**) IP-10 was analyzed in peripheral blood leukocytes from NGT subjects after a 75 g oral glucose challenge (▲; n = 10), 300 mL water (o; n = 10), or in fasting state (□; n = 6). Blood was drawn every 30 min using an i.v. cannula. Data are shown as mean ± SEM.

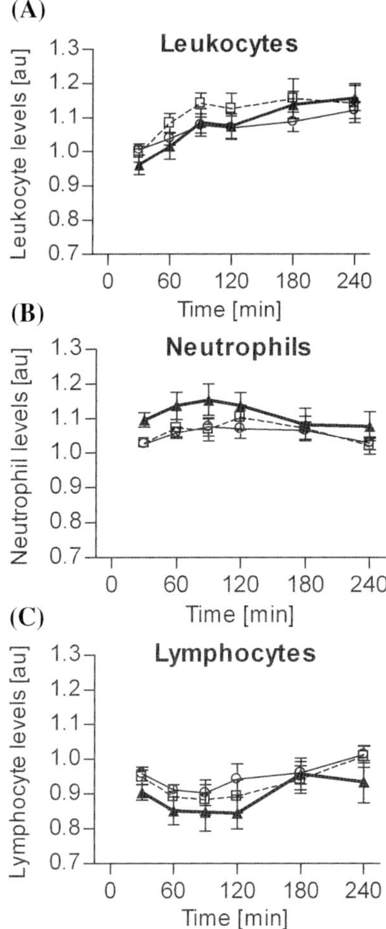

FIGURE 6. Glucose-mediated count of leukocytes and subpopulations from NGT subjects. (**A**) Leukocyte count, (**B**) proportion of neutrophil granulocytes, and (**C**) lymphocytes were analyzed in NGT subjects after a 75 g oral glucose challenge (▲; $n = 10$), 300 mL water (o; $n = 10$), or in fasting state (□; $n = 6$). Blood was drawn every 30 min using an i.v. cannula. Data are shown as mean ± SEM.

fasting is still unknown but mouse models showed that fasting induced neutrophils recruitment in the liver, while immunodeficient mice failed to show this response but instead became hypoglycemic.[98] The nutritional state also has a significant effect on leukocyte counts in humans and the migratory response of leukocyte subpopulations to nutritional fluctuations was impaired in elderly.[99] Such effects should be taken into account when studies are initiated to clarify the immunomodulatory properties of glucose and other nutrients.

In conclusion, an increase in blood glucose in the postprandial phase is a typical event for both normoglycemic and diabetic subjects, but in case of an impaired metabolic state, persistent postprandial hyperglycemia might affect magnitude and duration of glucose and immune parameter peaks, which both increase the risk for the development of T2DM and CVD.

REFERENCES

1. Bhargava, S.K., H.S. Sachdev, C.H. Fall, *et al.* 2004. Relation of serial changes in childhood body-mass index to impaired glucose tolerance in young adulthood. N. Engl. J. Med. **350:** 865–875.
2. Gluckman, P.D. & M.A. Hanson. 2004. Living with the past: evolution, development, and patterns of disease. Science **305:** 1733–1736.
3. Grunnet, L., P. Poulsen, B.K. Pedersen, *et al.* 2004. Interleukin 6 (IL-6), tumor necrosis factor-α (TNF-α) and soluble TNF receptor 1 (sTNFR1) in healthy twins—aetiology and relation to *in vivo* insulin action. Diabetologia **47:** (Suppl1): A226–A227.
4. Goldstein, B.J. 2003. Insulin resistance: from benign to type 2 diabetes mellitus. Rev. Cardiovasc. Med. **4**(Suppl 6): S3–S10.
5. Petersen, K.F., S. Dufour, D. Befroy, *et al.* 2004. Impaired mitochondrial activity in the insulin-resistant offspring of patients with type 2 diabetes. N. Engl. J. Med. **350:** 664–671.
6. Porksen, N. 2002. Early changes in beta-cell function and insulin pulsatility as predictors for type 2 diabetes. Diabetes Nutr. Metab. **15:** 9–14.
7. Zethelius, B., L. Byberg, C.N. Hales, *et al.* 2003. Proinsulin and acute insulin response independently predict type 2 diabetes mellitus in men—report from 27 years of follow-up study. Diabetologia **46:** 20–26.
8. Srinivasan, S.R., A. Elkasabani, E.R. Dalferes Jr., *et al.* 1998. Characteristics of young offspring of type 2 diabetic parents in a biracial (black-white) community-based sample: the Bogalusa Heart Study. Metabolism **47:** 998–1004.
9. Srinivasan, S.R., L. Myers & G.S. Berenson. 2002. Predictability of childhood adiposity and insulin for developing insulin resistance syndrome (syndrome X) in young adulthood: the Bogalusa Heart Study. Diabetes **51:** 204–209.
10. Srinivasan, S.R., M.G. Frontini & G.S. Berenson. 2003. Longitudinal changes in risk variables of insulin resistance syndrome from childhood to young adulthood in offspring of parents with type 2 diabetes: the Bogalusa Heart Study. Metabolism **52:** 443–450.
11. Xu, H., G.T. Barnes, Q. Yang, *et al.* 2003. Chronic inflammation in fat plays a crucial role in the development of obesity-related insulin resistance. J. Clin. Invest. **112:** 1821–1830.
12. Weisberg, S.P., D. McCann, M. Desai, *et al.* 2003. Obesity is associated with macrophage accumulation in adipose tissue. J. Clin. Invest **112:** 1796–1808.
13. Rosmond, R., M. Chagnon, C. Bouchard, *et al.* 2003. Increased abdominal obesity, insulin and glucose levels in nondiabetic subjects with a T29C polymorphism of the transforming growth factor-beta1 gene. Horm. Res. **59:** 191–194.

14. BUTLER, A.E., J. JANSON, S. BONNER-WEIR, *et al.* 2003. Beta-cell deficit and increased beta-cell apoptosis in humans with type 2 diabetes. Diabetes **52:** 102–110.
15. GOLDSTEIN, B.J. 2002. Insulin resistance as the core defect in type 2 diabetes mellitus. Am. J. Cardiol. **90:** 3G–10G.
16. LINGOHR, M.K., R. BUETTNER & C.J. RHODES. 2002. Pancreatic beta-cell growth and survival—a role in obesity-linked type 2 diabetes? Trends Mol. Med. **8:** 375–384.
17. SESTI, G. 2002. Apoptosis in the beta cells: cause or consequence of insulin secretion defect in diabetes? Ann. Med. **34:** 444–450.
18. GODSLAND, I.F., J.A. JEFFS & D.G. JOHNSTON. 2004. Loss of beta cell function as fasting glucose increases in the non-diabetic range. Diabetologia **47:** 1157–1166.
19. WINZLER, R.J. 1960. Glycoproteins. *In* The Plasma Proteins. F.W. Putnam, Ed.: 309. London Academic Press, New York.
20. COGAN, D.G., L. MEROLA & P.R. LAIBSON. 1961. Blood viscosity, serum hexosamine and diabetic retinopathy. Diabetes **10:** 393–395.
21. BERGSTRAND, C.G., P. FURST, Y. LARSSON, *et al.* 1962. Serum haptoglobin in juvenile diabetes. Scand. J. Clin. Lab. Invest **14:** 629–632.
22. GANROT, P.O., K. GYDELL & H. EKELUND. 1967. Serum concentration of alpha-2-macroglobulin, haptoglobin and alpha-1-antitrypsin in diabetes mellitus. Acta Endocrinol. (Copenh.) **55:** 537–544.
23. CLEVE, H., K. ALEXANDER, H.J. MITZKAT, *et al.* 1968. Serum glycoproteins in diabetes mellitus; quantitative immunological determination of acid alpha 1-glycoprotein, Gc, alpha 2-macroglobulin and hemopexin in diabetics with and without angiopathy. Diabetologia **4:** 48–55.
24. MCMILLAN, D.E. 1970. Changes in serum proteins and protein-bound carbohydrates in diabetes mellitus. Diabetologia **6:** 597–604.
25. PICKUP, J.C. 2004. Inflammation and activated innate immunity in the pathogenesis of type 2 diabetes. Diabetes Care **27:** 813–823.
26. HERDER, C., B. HAASTERT, S. MULLER-SCHOLZE, *et al.* 2005. Association of systemic chemokine concentrations with impaired glucose tolerance and type 2 diabetes: results from the Cooperative Health Research in the region of Augsburg Survey S4 (KORA S4). Diabetes **54:** S11–S17.
27. HERDER, C., H. KOLB, W. KOENIG, *et al.* 2006. Association of systemic concentrations of macrophage migration inhibitory factor with impaired glucose tolerance and type 2 diabetes: results from the Cooperative Health Research in the region of Augsburg, Survey 4 (KORA S4). Diabetes Care **29:** 368–371.
28. KOLB, H. & T. MANDRUP-POULSEN. 2005. An immune origin of type 2 diabetes? Diabetologia **48:** 1038–1050.
29. THORAND, B., H. KOLB, J. BAUMERT, *et al.* 2005. Elevated levels of interleukin-18 predict the development of type 2 diabetes: results from the MONICA/KORA Augsburg Study, 1984–2002. Diabetes **54:** 2932–2938.
30. THORAND, B., J. BAUMERT, L. CHAMBLESS, *et al.* 2006. Elevated markers of endothelial dysfunction predict type 2 diabetes mellitus in middle-aged men and women from the general population. Arterioscler. Thromb. Vasc. Biol. **26:** 398–405.
31. HERDER, C., J. BAUMERT, B. THORAND, *et al.* 2006. Chemokines as risk factors for type 2 diabetes—results from the MONIKA/KORA Augsburg Study, 1984–2002. Diabetologia **29:** 1626–1631.

32. FERNANDEZ-REAL, J.M. 2006. Genetic predispositions to low-grade inflammation and type 2 diabetes. Diabetes Technol. Ther. **8:** 55–66.
33. SIMEONI, E., M.M. HOFFMANN, B.R. WINKELMANN, *et al.* 2004. Association between the A-2518G polymorphism in the monocyte chemoattractant protein-1 gene and insulin resistance and type 2 diabetes mellitus. Diabetologia **47:** 1574–1580.
34. HAMID, Y.H., S.A. URHAMMER, C. GLUMER, *et al.* 2005. The common T60N polymorphism of the lymphotoxin-alpha gene is associated with type 2 diabetes and other phenotypes of the metabolic syndrome. Diabetologia **48:** 445–451.
35. SHIN, H.D., K.S. PARK, B.L. PARK, *et al.* 2006. Common promoter polymorphism in monocyte differentiation antigen CD14 is associated with serum triglyceride levels and body mass index in non-diabetic individuals. Diabet. Med. **23:** 72–76.
36. GUBERN, C., A. LOPEZ-BERMEJO, J. BIARNES, *et al.* 2006. Natural antibiotics and insulin sensitivity: the role of bactericidal/permeability-increasing protein. Diabetes **55:** 216–224.
37. UYSAL, K.T., S.M. WIESBROCK, M.W. MARINO, *et al.* 1997. Protection from obesity-induced insulin resistance in mice lacking TNF-alpha function. Nature **389:** 610–614.
38. DONG, Z.M., J.C. GUTIERREZ-RAMOS, A. COXON, *et al.* 1997. A new class of obesity genes encodes leukocyte adhesion receptors. Proc. Natl. Acad. Sci. USA **94:** 7526–7530.
39. WALLENIUS, V., K. WALLENIUS, B. AHREN, *et al.* 2002. Interleukin-6-deficient mice develop mature-onset obesity. Nat. Med. **8:** 75–79.
40. SCHAFER, K., K. FUJISAWA, S. KONSTANTINIDES, *et al.* 2001. Disruption of the plasminogen activator inhibitor 1 gene reduces the adiposity and improves the metabolic profile of genetically obese and diabetic ob/ob mice. FASEB J. **15:** 1840–1842.
41. MA, L.J., S.L. MAO, K.L. TAYLOR, *et al.* 2004. Prevention of obesity and insulin resistance in mice lacking plasminogen activator inhibitor 1. Diabetes **53:** 336–346.
42. LIJNEN, H.R., E. MAQUOI, P. MORANGE, *et al.* 2003. Nutritionally induced obesity is attenuated in transgenic mice overexpressing plasminogen activator inhibitor-1. Arterioscler. Thromb. Vasc. Biol. **23:** 78–84.
43. PERREAULT, M. & A. MARETTE. 2001. Targeted disruption of inducible nitric oxide synthase protects against obesity-linked insulin resistance in muscle. Nat. Med. **7:** 1138–1143.
44. LANG, C.H., C. DOBRESCU & G.J. BAGBY. 1992. Tumor necrosis factor impairs insulin action on peripheral glucose disposal and hepatic glucose output. Endocrinology **130:** 43–52.
45. LING, P.R., B.R. BISTRIAN, B. MENDEZ, *et al.* 1994. Effects of systemic infusions of endotoxin, tumor necrosis factor, and interleukin-1 on glucose metabolism in the rat: relationship to endogenous glucose production and peripheral tissue glucose uptake. Metabolism **43:** 279–284.
46. SENN, J.J., P.J. KLOVER, I.A. NOWAK, *et al.* 2003. Suppressor of cytokine signaling-3 (SOCS-3), a potential mediator of interleukin-6-dependent insulin resistance in hepatocytes. J. Biol. Chem. **278:** 13740–13746.
47. KLOVER, P.J., T.A. ZIMMERS, L.G. KONIARIS, *et al.* 2003. Chronic exposure to interleukin-6 causes hepatic insulin resistance in mice. Diabetes **52:** 2784–2789.

48. Kim, H.J., T. Higashimori, S.Y. Park, *et al.* 2004. Differential effects of interleukin-6 and -10 on skeletal muscle and liver insulin action *in vivo*. Diabetes **53:** 1060–1067.
49. Krogh-Madsen, R., P. Plomgaard, K. Moller, *et al.* 2006. Influence of TNF-alpha and IL-6 infusions on insulin sensitivity and expression of IL-18 in human. Am. J. Physiol. Endocrinol. Metab **291:** E108–E114.
50. Hotamisligil, G.S., N.S. Shargill & B.M. Spiegelman. 1993. Adipose expression of tumor necrosis factor-alpha: direct role in obesity-linked insulin resistance. Science **259:** 87–91.
51. Paquot, N., M.J. Castillo, P.J. Lefebvre, *et al.* 2000. No increased insulin sensitivity after a single intravenous administration of a recombinant human tumor necrosis factor receptor: Fc fusion protein in obese insulin-resistant patients. J. Clin. Endocrinol. Metab **85:** 1316–1319.
52. Di Rocco, P., M. Manco, G. Rosa, *et al.* 2004. Lowered tumor necrosis factor receptors, but not increased insulin sensitivity, with infliximab. Obes. Res. **12:** 734–739.
53. Ofei, F., S. Hurel, J. Newkirk, *et al.* 1996. Effects of an engineered human anti-TNF-alpha antibody (CDP571) on insulin sensitivity and glycemic control in patients with NIDDM. Diabetes **45:** 881–885.
54. Shoelson, S.E., J. Lee & M. Yuan. 2003. Inflammation and the IKK beta/I kappa B/NF-kappa B axis in obesity and diet-induced insulin resistance. Int. J. Obes. Relat. Metab. Disord. **27**(Suppl 3): S49–S52.
55. Tuomilehto, J., J. Lindstrom, J.G. Eriksson, *et al.* 2001. Prevention of type 2 diabetes mellitus by changes in lifestyle among subjects with impaired glucose tolerance. N. Engl. J. Med. **344:** 1343–1350.
56. Knowler, W.C., E. Barrett-Connor, S.E. Fowler, *et al.* 2002. Reduction in the incidence of type 2 diabetes with lifestyle intervention or metformin. N. Engl. J. Med. **346:** 393–403.
57. Pan, X.R., G.W. Li, Y.H. Hu, *et al.* 1997. Effects of diet and exercise in preventing NIDDM in people with impaired glucose tolerance. The Da Qing IGT and Diabetes Study. Diabetes Care **20:** 537–544.
58. Ramachandran, A., C. Snehalatha, S. Mary, *et al.* 2006. The Indian Diabetes Prevention Programme shows that lifestyle modification and metformin prevent type 2 diabetes in Asian Indian subjects with impaired glucose tolerance (IDPP-1). Diabetologia **49:** 289–297.
59. Yamaoka, K. & T. Tango. 2005. Efficacy of lifestyle education to prevent type 2 diabetes: a meta-analysis of randomized controlled trials. Diabetes Care **28:** 2780–2786.
60. Laaksonen, D.E., J. Lindstrom, T.A. Lakka, *et al.* 2005. Physical activity in the prevention of type 2 diabetes: the Finnish Diabetes Prevention Study. Diabetes **54:** 158–165.
61. Plomgaard, P., M. Penkowa & B.K. Pedersen. 2005. Fiber type specific expression of TNF-alpha, IL-6 and IL-18 in human skeletal muscles. Exerc. Immunol. Rev. **11:** 53–63.
62. Petersen, A.M. & B.K. Pedersen. 2005. The anti-inflammatory effect of exercise. J. Appl. Physiol. **98:** 1154–1162.
63. Pedersen, B.K. & M. Febbraio. 2005. Muscle-derived interleukin-6—a possible link between skeletal muscle, adipose tissue, liver, and brain. Brain Behav. Immun. **19:** 371–376.

64. HAFFNER, S., M. TEMPROSA, J. CRANDALL, *et al.* 2005. Intensive lifestyle intervention or metformin on inflammation and coagulation in participants with impaired glucose tolerance. Diabetes **54:** 1566–1572.
65. VALLE, T., S. MULLER, J. LINDSTROEM, *et al.* 2003. Changes in C-reactive protein and interleukin-6 correlate with a change in glucose in women but not in men with impaired glucose tolerance in the Finnish Diabetes Prevention Study. Diabetes **52:**(Suppl 1): A231.
66. NICKLAS, B.J., T. YOU & M. PAHOR. 2005. Behavioural treatments for chronic systemic inflammation: effects of dietary weight loss and exercise training. CMAJ **172:** 1199–1209.
67. PEDERSEN, M., A. STEENSBERG, C. KELLER, *et al.* 2004. Does the aging skeletal muscle maintain its endocrine function? Exerc. Immunol. Rev. **10:** 42–55.
68. CURAT, C.A., A. MIRANVILLE, C. SENGENES, *et al.* 2004. From blood monocytes to adipose tissue-resident macrophages: induction of diapedesis by human mature adipocytes. Diabetes **53:** 1285–1292.
69. HOWARD, B.V., L. VAN HORN, J. HSIA, *et al.* 2006. Low-fat dietary pattern and risk of cardiovascular disease: the Women's Health Initiative Randomized Controlled Dietary Modification Trial. JAMA **295:** 655–666.
70. HE, F.J., C.A. NOWSON & G.A. MACGREGOR. 2006. Fruit and vegetable consumption and stroke: meta-analysis of cohort studies. Lancet **367:** 320–326.
71. NORDMANN, A.J., A. NORDMANN, M. BRIEL, *et al.* 2006. Effects of low-carbohydrate vs low-fat diets on weight loss and cardiovascular risk factors: a meta-analysis of randomized controlled trials. Arch. Intern. Med. **166:** 285–293.
72. ARORA, S.K. & S.I. MCFARLANE. 2005. The case for low carbohydrate diets in diabetes management. Nutr. Metab. (Lond.) **2:** 16
73. OHKUBO, Y., H. KISHIKAWA, E. ARAKI, *et al.* 1995. Intensive insulin therapy prevents the progression of diabetic microvascular complications in Japanese patients with non-insulin-dependent diabetes mellitus: a randomized prospective 6-year study. Diabetes Res. Clin. Pract. **28:** 103–117.
74. UK Prospective Diabetes Study (UKPDS) Group. 1998. Intensive blood-glucose control with sulphonylureas or insulin compared with conventional treatment and risk of complications in patients with type 2 diabetes (UKPDS 33). Lancet **352:** 837–853.
75. American Diabetes Association Diabetes Care. 2001. Postprandial blood glucose. **24:** 775–778.
76. DANDONA, P., P. MOHANTY, H. GHANIM, *et al.* 2001. The suppressive effect of dietary restriction and weight loss in the obese on the generation of reactive oxygen species by leukocytes, lipid peroxidation, and protein carbonylation. J. Clin. Endocrinol. Metab **86:** 355–362.
77. MOROHOSHI, M., K. FUJISAWA, I. UCHIMURA, *et al.* 1995. The effect of glucose and advanced glycosylation end products on IL-6 production by human monocytes. Ann. N. Y. Acad. Sci. **748:** 562–570.
78. MOROHOSHI, M., K. FUJISAWA, I. UCHIMURA, *et al.* 1996. Glucose-dependent interleukin 6 and tumor necrosis factor production by human peripheral blood monocytes *in vitro*. Diabetes **45:** 954–959.
79. MOHANTY, P., W. HAMOUDA, R. GARG, *et al.* 2000. Glucose challenge stimulates reactive oxygen species (ROS) generation by leucocytes. J. Clin. Endocrinol. Metab **85:** 2970–2973.

80. CERIELLO, A., L. QUAGLIARO, L. PICONI, *et al.* 2004. Effect of postprandial hypertriglyceridemia and hyperglycemia on circulating adhesion molecules and oxidative stress generation and the possible role of simvastatin treatment. Diabetes **53:** 701–710.
81. ESPOSITO, K., F. NAPPO, R. MARFELLA, *et al.* 2002. Inflammatory cytokine concentrations are acutely increased by hyperglycemia in humans: role of oxidative stress. Circulation **106:** 2067–2072.
82. STRACZKOWSKI, M., S. DZIENIS-STRACZKOWSKA, A. STEPIEN, *et al.* 2002. Plasma interleukin-8 concentrations are increased in obese subjects and related to fat mass and tumor necrosis factor-alpha system J. Clin. Endocrinol. Metab. **87:** 4602–4606.
83. STRACZKOWSKI, M., I. KOWALSKA, A. NIKOLAJUK, *et al.* 2003. Plasma interleukin 8 concentrations in obese subjects with impaired glucose tolerance. Cardiovasc. Diabetol. **2:** 5.
84. KROGH-MADSEN, R., K. MOLLER, F. DELA, *et al.* 2004. Effect of hyperglycemia and hyperinsulinemia on the response of IL-6, TNF-alpha, and FFAs to low-dose endotoxemia in humans. Am. J. Physiol. Endocrinol. Metab. **286:** E766–E772.
85. NAPPO, F., K. ESPOSITO, M. CIOFFI, *et al.* 2002. Postprandial endothelial activation in healthy subjects and in type 2 diabetic patients: role of fat and carbohydrate meals. J. Am. Coll. Cardiol. **39:** 1145–1150.
86. ESPOSITO, K., F. NAPPO, F. GIUGLIANO, *et al.* 2003. Meal modulation of circulating interleukin 18 and adiponectin concentrations in healthy subjects and in patients with type 2 diabetes mellitus. Am. J. Clin. Nutr. **78:** 1135–1140.
87. VON KANEL, R., P.J. MILLS & J.E. DIMSDALE. 2001. Short-term hyperglycemia induces lymphopenia and lymphocyte subset redistribution. Life Sci. **69:** 255–262.
88. SAMPSON, M., I. DAVIES, J. GAVRILOVIC, *et al.* 2004. Plasma matrix metalloproteinases, low density lipoprotein oxidisability and soluble adhesion molecules after a glucose load in type 2 diabetes. Cardiovasc. Diabetol. **3:** 7.
89. MANNING, P.J., W.H. SUTHERLAND, G. HENDRY, *et al.* 2004. Changes in circulating postprandial proinflammatory cytokine concentrations in diet-controlled type 2 diabetes and the effect of ingested fat. Diabetes Care **27:** 2509–2511.
90. GUDMUNDSSON, A., W.B. ERSHLER, B. GOODMAN, *et al.* 1997. Serum concentrations of interleukin-6 are increased when sampled through an indwelling venous catheter. Clin. Chem. **43:** 2199–2201.
91. ESNAULT, S. & J.S. MALTER. 1999. Primary peripheral blood eosinophils rapidly degrade transfected granulocyte-macrophage colony-stimulating factor mRNA. J. Immunol. **163:** 5228–5234.
92. MCFAUL, S.J., P.D. BOWMAN, V.M. VILLA, *et al.* 1994. Hemoglobin stimulates mononuclear leukocytes to release interleukin-8 and tumor necrosis factor alpha. Blood **84:** 3175–3181.
93. JOHNSON, K., Y. CHOI, E. DEGROOT, *et al.* 1998. Potential mechanisms for a proinflammatory vascular cytokine response to coagulation activation. J. Immunol. **160:** 5130–5135.
94. HARTEL, C., G. BEIN, M. MULLER-STEINHARDT, *et al.* 2001. *Ex vivo* induction of cytokine mRNA expression in human blood samples. J. Immunol. Methods **249:** 63–71.
95. MA, S.W., B. TOMLINSON & I.F. BENZIE. 2005. A study of the effect of oral glucose loading on plasma oxidant:antioxidant balance in normal subjects. Eur. J. Nutr. **44:** 250–254.

96. VAN OOSTROM, A.J., T.P. SIJMONSMA, C. VERSEYDEN, *et al.* 2003. Postprandial recruitment of neutrophils may contribute to endothelial dysfunction. J. Lipid Res. **44:** 576–583.
97. DRENICK, E.J. & L.C. ALVAREZ. 1971. Neutropenia in prolonged fasting. Am. J. Clin. Nutr. **24:** 859–863.
98. BABIC, A.M., H.W. WANG, M.J. LAI, *et al.* 2004. ICAM-1 and beta-2 integrin deficiency impairs fat oxidation and insulin metabolism during fasting. Mol. Med. **10:** 72–79.
99. WALRAND, S., K. MOREAU, F. CALDEFIE, *et al.* 2001. Specific and nonspecific immune responses to fasting and refeeding differ in healthy young adult and elderly persons. Am. J. Clin. Nutr. **74:** 670–678.

Functional Capacity of Macrophages Determines the Induction of Type 1 Diabetes

EPK MENSAH-BROWN,[a] A. SHAHIN,[b] KHATIJA PAREKH,[a] A. AL HAKIM,[b] M. AL SHAMISI,[b] D.K. HSU,[c] AND M.L. LUKIC[b]

[a]*Department of Anatomy, Faculty of Medicine and Health Sciences, UAE University, Al Ain, UAE*

[b]*Department of Microbiology and Immunology, Faculty of Medicine and Health Sciences, UAE University, Al Ain, UAE*

[c]*Department of Dermatology, University of California-Davis, School of Medicine Sacramento, California 95817, USA*

ABSTRACT: Macrophages are potent immune regulators and are critical in the development and pathogenesis of autoimmune diabetes. They are said to be the first cell type to infiltrate the pancreatic islet, serve as antigen-presenting cells, and are important as effector cells during diabetogenesis. The article examines the role of macrophages in autoimmune diabetes with particular emphasis on the role of galectin-3, a β-galactoside-binding lectin, and T1/ST2, an IL-1 receptor-like protein, both of which play significant roles in the immunomodulatory functions of macrophages. Multiple low-dose streptozotocin (MLD-STZ) induces infiltration of mononuclear cells in the islets of susceptible strains leading to insulitis. Deletion of the galectin-3 gene from C57BL/6 mice significantly attenuates this effect as evaluated by quantitative histology of mononuclear cells and loss of insulin-producing β cells. In contrast, deletion of the ST2 gene enhanced insulitis after MLD-STZ treatment when compared with relatively resistant wild-type BALB/c mice. Thus, it appears that functional capacity of macrophages influences their participation in T helper (Th) 1-mediated autoimmunity and the development of autoimmune diabetogenesis.

KEYWORDS: autoimmunity; galectin-3; ST2; multiple low-dose streptozotocin

Address for correspondence: Prof. M.L. Lukic, Department of Microbiology and Immunology, Faculty of Medicine and Health Sciences, UAE University, PO Box 17666, Al Ain, United Arab Emirates. Voice: +97137137511; fax: +97137671966.
e-mail: m.lukic@uaeu.ac.ae

Ann. N.Y. Acad. Sci. 1084: 49–57 (2006). © 2006 New York Academy of Sciences.
doi: 10.1196/annals.1372.014

INTRODUCTION

Macrophages are potent immune regulators and are critical in the development and pathogenesis of autoimmune diabetes. They are the first cells to infiltrate the islet where they act as antigen-presenting as well as effector cells.[1–3] These roles in the immune process have been the subject of several studies in recent times with regard to two molecules namely, galectin-3[4] and T1/ST2 (reviewed in Ref. 5) that have varied modulatory effects on macrophage function.

Galectin-3 is a 32-kDa β-galactosidase-binding lectin that is widely distributed in tissues and cells including inflammatory cells, especially those of the monocyte/macrophage lineage[6] and is considered as a positive regulator of macrophage-dependent inflammatory response (reviewed in Ref. 7). When added exogenously, galectin-3 induces production of interleukin-1 (IL-1)[8] and is chemoattractant for macrophages.[9] Furthermore, galectin-3 contributes to phagocytosis by macrophages through an intracellular mechanism suggesting an important role in innate and adaptive immunity by contributing to phagocytic clearance of apoptotic cell.[10] Galectin-3 has also been implicated in the innate immune response and has been considered as a possible modulator of T cell activation.[11] Enhanced expression of galectin-3 has been associated with the inflammatory processes in rheumatoid arthritis and activation of synovial fibroblasts.[12] Thus galectin-3 appears to act as a "proinflammatory cytokine."[4]

T1/ST2, an IL-1 receptor like protein, which has been shown to be expressed on Th2 cells also binds to macrophages and unlike galectin-3, suppresses synthesis and secretion of proinflammatory cytokine.[13]

Our aim in this article is to analyze chronic inflammatory process in C57Bl/6 mice deficient in galectin-3 and in BALB/c mice deficient in the T1/ST2 genes due to targeted disruption of the genes encoding these molecules. To this end, the model of disease used was the multiple low-dose streptozotocin (MLD-STZ)-induced diabetes.[2] The control groups comprised "wild-type" C57BL/6, which are susceptible and BALB/c mice, which are relatively resistant to induction of diabetes. Using immunohistological techniques, we have assessed the effect of deletion of these molecules on the level of mononuclear cellular infiltration and the percentage of insulin immunopositive β cells.

MATERIALS AND METHODS

Generation of Galectin-3 Null Mice

A vector used for homologous recombination was constructed from the cloned galectin-3 genomic DNA.[14] A segment from exon 4 to exon 5 within the mouse galectin-3 gene was inserted into pIMC1Neo (Stratagene, La Jolla, CA) upstream of the thymidine kinase promotor-Neo cassette. Another segment from exon 5 to exon 6 followed downstream from the Neo cassette. Thus exon 6 followed downstream from the Neo cassette and exon 5 was interrupted by the Neo gene in this vector construct. Murine stem cells, DC, were electroporated with this vector, using procedures previously described.[15] GA 18-resistant cells were screened for homologous recombination by polymerase chain reaction (PCR) and Southern blotting using procedures described below. Screening of 894 clones resulted in two successful homologous recombinations.

One clone was propagated and injected into 3.5-day-old blastocytes from C57BL/6. Mice and the injected blastocytes were implanted into pseudopregnant CD1 mothers. Male chimeric mice were bred to C57BL/6 females to produce mice hemizygous for the galectin-3 null mutant (gal $3^{+/-}$). Interbreeding (gal $3^{+/-}$) mice resulted in mice homozygous for the galectin-3- null condition (gal $3^{-/-}$). Gal $3^{-/-}$ mice were viable and fertile. For experimentation, wild-type (gal $3^{+/+}$) mice produced by gal $3^{+/-}$ interbreeding were carried in a separate lineage as controls. Both gal $3^{+/+}$ and gal $3^{-/-}$ were maintained in FMHS animal facilities according to the transfer of technology agreement between FMHS and the University of California. In experiments, 6- to 8-week-old female mice were used.

Generation of T1/ST2 Null Mice

As previously described by Townsend *et al.*, targeted disruption of mouse T1/ST2 gene was done performed in BALB/c embryonic stem cells and mice homozygous for disrupted gene were obtained.[15] They were provided by Professor F.Y. Liew (University of Glasgow, UK) and maintained in FMHS animal facilities.

Diabetes Induction

STZ was dissolved in citrate buffer of pH 4.5 and administered intraperitoneally at a dose of 40 mg/kg/day for 5 consecutive days in four groups of mice. The groups were:

(i) Galectin-3 “knockout” mice on C57BL/6 background.
(ii) Galectin-3 “wild-type” C57BL/6 mice.
(iii) T1/ST2 “knockout” mice on BALB/c background.
(iv) T1/ST2 “wild-type” BALB/c mice.

Each group comprised eight mice.

The levels of glycemia and weights of mice were determined weekly over a period of 18 days. Pancreata of all groups were taken 18 days post induction and placed in 10% buffered formaldehyde fixative solution overnight at room temperature.

Immunohistology

Immunohistochemistry for insulin-containing β cells

Sections of paraffin wax-embedded pancreata of thickness 5–7 μm were stained by the direct immunofluorescence technique. The sections were counterstained with propidium iodide (PI, 1 mg/mL). The percentage of insulin immunopositivity was then established by calculating the number of FITC-immunoreactive cells per total number of PI-stained nuclei in nonconsecutive sections. PI- stained infiltrating mononuclear cells were excluded in the quantification by staining the same sections with hematoxylin and eosin and the number of infiltrating cells were counted. We have previously described the methodology.[16]

Quantitative histology of infiltrating cells

After examination of the insulin immunofluorescent-stained slides, coverslips were gently removed and the slides were rehydrated and stained with hematoxylin and eosin. The number of infiltrating cells per islet was then quantified in nonconsecutive sections by light microscopy with a 40× oil immersion objective. To remove discrepancies due to variations in islet size, the mean perimetric size ± standard error of mean (SEM) of all islets in five nonconsecutive sections from the pancreata of three mice per experimental and control groups was computed with an Axiocam digital camera attached to a Zeiss Axiophot (Jena, Germany). The mean value in μm was then used as the "standard size islet" to calculate the number of cells per islet. Any islet larger or smaller than the mean ± SEM was excluded. All values were expressed as mean ± SEM.

RESULTS

Targeted Disruption of Galectin-3 Gene Is Associated with Insulitis and Low Insulin Immunopositivity

Diabetogenesis after MLD-STZ treatment is mediated by an early influx of macrophages into the pancreatic islets,[1,2] efficient presentation of released diabetogenic antigens, and recruitment of T cells. As evaluated on day 18 after diabetes induction, there was a higher level of mononuclear cellular infiltration in galectin-3 wild-type mice than in knockout mice indicating insulitis (FIG. 1 A) in the former in comparison to the single cell infiltrates of islets in the "knockout" mice (FIG. 1 B). Quantitative analysis of islets of similar size

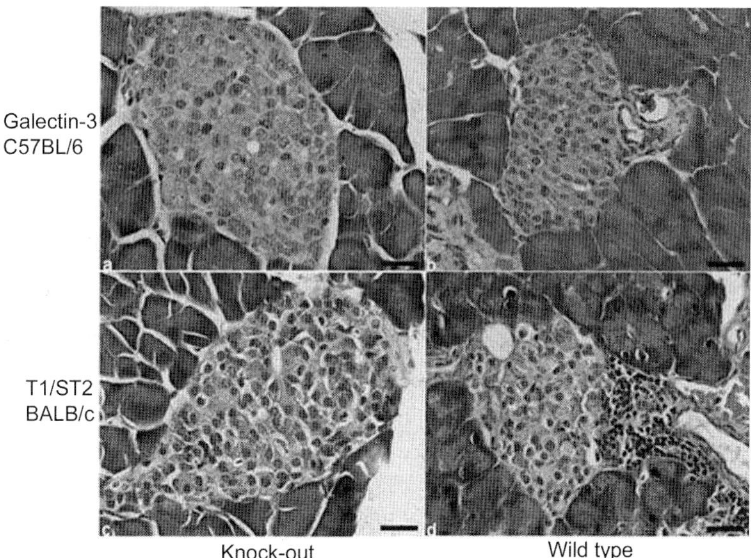

FIGURE 1. Light micrograph of pancreata of C57BL/6 galectin-3$^{-/-}$ "knockout" (A), galectin-3$^{+/+}$ "wild-type" (B) BALB/c, T1/ST2 "knockout" (C), and wild-type (D) mice showing cellular infiltration into and around islets. Note the higher level of infiltration associated with a wild-type galectin-3 and knockout T1/ST2 islets. Note also the peri-insulitis (star) around the islet of T1/ST2 wild-type (D) islets. Bar = 20 μm.

(492.24 ± 68.5 μm) confirmed the significant increase in the influx of inflammatory cells in wild-type animals versus knockouts (TABLE 1). As shown in TABLE 1 and FIGURE 1 C, insulin content was of a significantly lower concentration ($P < 0.005$) in galectin-3 wild-type (FIG. 1 B) compared to their knockout counterparts (FIG. 1 D).

TABLE 1. Quantitative analysis of mononuclear cells and insulin-positive cells in islets

Strain of mice	Infiltrating cells	Insulin immunopositivity
C57BL/6 Galectin -3$^{+/+}$	43 ± 6	38.1 ± 1.7%
C57BL/6 Galectin -3$^{-/-}$	29 ± 4**	50.7 ± 1.5**
BALB/c T1/ST2$^{+/+}$	35 ± 5	56.7 ± 4.73
BALB/c T1/ST2$^{-/-}$	46 ± 4*	46.6 ± 3.74*

Animals received subdiabetogenic (5 × 40 mg/kg b. w.) MLD-STZ treatment (see "Materials and Methods"). Data are shown as a mean ± SEM per islet of standard size 492.24 ± 68.5 μm. *$P < 0.05$; **$P < 0.005$.

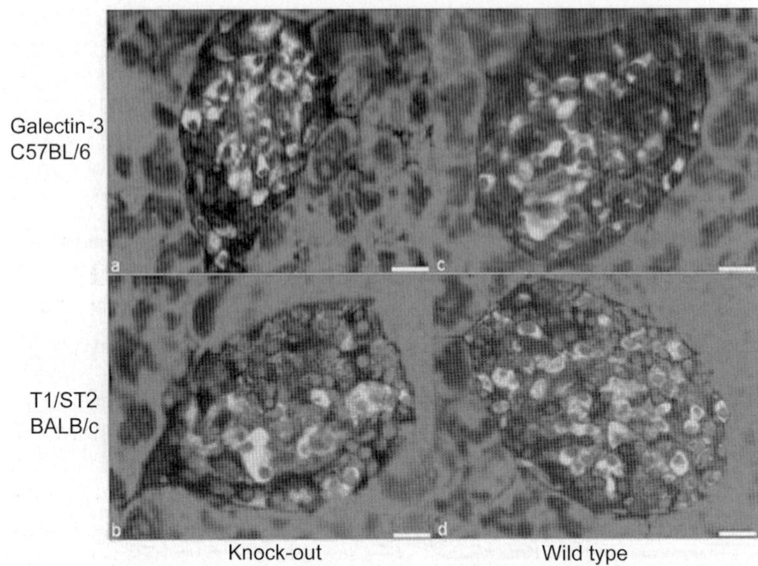

FIGURE 2. Light micrograph of pancreata of C57BL/6 galectin-3$^{-/-}$ (A), galectin-3 wild-type (B), BALB/c T1/ST2$^{-/-}$ knockout (C), and T1/ST2 "wild-type" (D) mice showing immunoreactivity to insulin-containing β cells after MLD-STZ treatment. Note the lower level of insulin immunopositivity in the galectin-3 "wild-type" and T1/ST2 "knockout" mice. Note the peri-insulitis (star) associated with islets of "wild-type" mice. Bar = 20 μm.

Targeted Disruption of T1/ST2 Gene Is Associated with Insulitis and Low Insulin Immunopositivity

In contrast to galectin-3 knockout mice, target deletion of the T1/ST2 gene led to increased infiltration of mononuclear cells in islets compared with wild-type controls (Fig. 2 A versus B). It is also noteworthy that islets of the T1/ST2 "wild-type" revealed a significant level of peri-insulitis (FIG. 1 B). Quantitative analysis also confirmed the increase in the influx of inflammatory cells in the knockout mice (TABLE 1). T1/ST2 knockout (FIG. 2 D) animals also possessed a significantly lower concentration ($P < 0.05$) of insulin immunopositive cells compared to their wild-type counterparts, respectively (FIG. 2 A).

DISCUSSION

T helper (Th) lymphocytes are the principal cells that regulate the autoimmune process through the production of cytokines. Depending on the type of cytokines secreted, the autoimmune process has been categorized as either Th1 or Th2. Th1 lymphocytes together with macrophages produce interferon-γ (IFN-γ) and tumor necrosis factor-α (TNF-α) mainly whereas Th2 cells secrete mainly IL-4 and IL-10.[17] The former cytokines together with the recently discovered IL-17[18] are critical for the development of autoimmune type 1 diabetes[16] but they may require macrophages that serve the role of antigen-presenting cells by which autoantigens are presented to naïve T cells in the draining lymph nodes and also as effector cells.[19]

While the direct effect of galectin-3 on macrophage function in the autoimmune process has not been demonstrated, it acts as a chemoattractant for monocytes and macrophages, and targeted disruption of the gene has led to the reduction of macrophage infiltration inflammatory response after thioglycollate-induced peritonitis.[20] Disruption of the galectin-3 gene in mice deleteriously influenced the phagocytic clearance capacity of peritoneal macrophages[9] as evidenced in the reduced phagocytosis of IgG opsonized erythrocytes and apoptotic thymocytes *in vivo*.[9] It might also be probable although not demonstrated that galectin-3 also contributes to the interaction between macrophages and naïve T cells as it does with the interaction between dendritic cells and naïve T lymphocytes in T cell-dependent areas of lymph nodes.[21] Even more significant is the fact that galectin-3 potentiates lipopolysaccharide (LPS)-induced production of IL-1[8] and triggers the production of superoxide anion by human peripheral blood monocytes[6] and neutrophils.[22] Macrophages elicit their diabetogenic effect by indirectly generating nitric oxide[23,24] via their production of inflammatory cytokines, such as IL-1 and TNF.[23] Indeed, it has been demonstrated that a combination of IFN-γ, TNF-α, and IL-1 and generation of nitric oxide are responsible for the β cell damage in MLD-STZ-induced diabetes in Dark Agouti rats.[2] In concordance with the above observations, we demonstrate here that MLD-STZ-induced diabetes is attenuated in mice in which galectin-3 gene is disrupted. The attenuation was associated with significant reduction of infiltrating cells in pancreatic islets compared to wild-type galectin-3 islets. We suggest that although not directly demonstrated, deleting galectin-3 gene (gal-$3^{-/-}$) attenuates MLD-STZ-induced diabetogenesis probably through its multifaceted effects but especially due to the altered macrophage-effector function.

T1/ST2 is a selective surface marker of Th2 cells that secrete IL-4, IL-5, IL-10, and IL-13.[25] In addition to several effects, Th2 cells deactivate macrophages.[13,26] However, it has been shown that the action of ST2 may not necessarily involve the effects of Th2 type cytokines and using LPS-induced inflammation, Sweet *et al.*[13] demonstrated conclusively that T1/ST2 gene immunoregulates the inflammatory process by directly inhibiting macrophages. LPS-induced inflammation involves the activation of macrophage secretion of IL-1-β and TNF-α via toll-like receptor 4, which then activate fibroblasts and other cells to secrete soluble ST2. Soluble ST2 then selectively suppresses macrophage-induced secretion of the proinflammatory cytokines TNF-α, IL-6, and IL-12.[13] Consistent with this mechanism is our observation that deletion of the T1/ST2 gene enhanced the MLD-STZ-induced inflammatory response associated with diabetogenesis as evidenced by the increased cellular infiltration in pancreatic islets and reduction in insulin immunopositivity. In the light of the observation by Leung *et al.*,[27] that soluble St2 suppresses the progression of acute-to-chronic inflammation *in vivo*, it is noteworthy that several islets of T1/ST2 " wild-type " BALB/c revealed significant peri- but not intrainsulitis implying that macrophages and disease-causing T cells are unable to infiltrate islets to initiate the disease.

In summary, while galectin-3 and T1/ST2 regulate immunoregulatory function of macrophages, and while the effect of galectin-3 leads to Th1-derived disease including autoimmune type 1 diabetes, T1/ST2 promotes Th2 reaction and prevents the enhancement of Th1 disease at the effector phase. Target disruption of the genes encoding these molecules leads either to attenuation in the former or the development of the disease in the latter. Further studies examining the molecular mechanisms by which these molecules induce or inhibit type 1 diabetes are ongoing.

ACKNOWLEDGMENT

This work is supported by Sheikh Hamdam award for the Medical Research Foundation Grant MRG-25/03-04 to MLL.

REFERENCES

1. Kolb, H., V. Burkart, B. Appels, *et al.* 1990. Essential contribution of macrophages to islet cell destruction *in vivo* and *in vitro*. J. Autoimmun. Suppl 1:117–120.
2. Lukic, M.L., S. Stosic-Grujicic & A. Shahin. 1998. Effector mechanisms in low-dose streptozotocin-induced diabetes. Dev. Immunol. **6:** 119–128.
3. Homo-Delarche, F. & H.A. Drexhage. 2004. Immune cells, pancreas development, regeneration and type 1 diabetes. Trends Immunol. **25:** 222–229.
4. Hsu, D.K., R.Y. Yang, Z. Pan, *et al.* 1994. Targeted disruption of the galectin-3 gene results in attenuated peritoneal inflammatory responses. Am. J. Pathol. **156:** 1073–1083.
5. Trajkovic, V., M. Sweet & X. Damo. 2004. T1/ST2—an IL-1 receptor-like modulator of immune responses. Cytokine Growth Factor Rev. **15:** 87–95.
6. Liu, F.T., D.K. Hsu, R.I. Zuberi, *et al.* 1995. Expression and function of galectin-3, a beta galactoside-binding lectin, in human monocytes and macrophages. Am. J. Pathol. **147:** 1016–1028.
7. Dumic, J., S. Dabelic & M. Flögel. 2006. Galectin-3: an open story. Biochim. Biophys. Acta **1760:** 616–635.
8. Jeng, K.C., L.G. Frigeri & F.T. Liu. 1994. An endogenous lectin, galectin-3(epsilon BP/Mac-2) potentiates IL-1 production by human monocytes. Immunol. Lett. **42:** 113–116.
9. Sano, H., D.K. Hsu, L. Yu, *et al.* 2000. Human galectin-3 is a novel chemoattractant for monocytes and macrophages. J. Immunol. **165:** 2156–2164.

10. SANO, H., D.K. HSU, J.R. APGAR, *et al.* 2003. Critical role of galectin-3 in phagocytosis by macrophages. J. Clin. Invest. **112:** 389–397.
11. SATO, S. & J. NIEMINEM. 2004. Seeing strangers or announcing "danger" galectin-3 in two models of innate immunity. Glycoconj. J. **19:** 583–591.
12. OSHIMA, S., S. KUCHEN & C.A. SEEMAYER, *et al.* 2003. Galectin-3 and its binding protein in rheumatoid arthritis. Arthritis Rheum. **48:** 2788–2795.
13. SWEET, M.J., B.P. LEUNG, D. KANG, *et al.* 2001. A novel pathway regulating lipopolysaccharide-induced shock by ST2/T1 via inhibition of toll-like receptor 4 expression. J. Immunol. **166:** 6633–6639.
14. GRITZMACHER, C.A., V.S. MEHL & F.T. LIU. 1992. Genomic cloning of the gene for an IgE binding lectin reveals unusual utilization of 5′ untranslated regions. Biochemistry **31:** 9533–9538.
15. TOWNSEND, M.J., P.G. FALLON, D.J. MATTHEWS, *et al.* 2000. T1/ST2 -deficient mice demonstrate the importance of T1/ST2 in developing primary T helper cell 2 responses. J. Exp. Med. **191:** 9069–9076.
16. MENSAH-BROWN, E.P.K., A. SHAHIN, M. AL SHAMSI, *et al.* 2006. IL-23 leads to diabetes induction after subdiabetogenic treatment with multiple doses of streptozotocin. Eur. J. Immunol. **26:** 216–223.
17. MUELLER, R., M. LEE. S.P. SAWYER, *et al.* 1996. Transgenic expression of interleukin 10 in the pancreas renders resistant mice susceptible to low dose streptozotocin-induced diabetes. J. Autoimmunity **9:** 151–158.
18. BETTELLI, E. & V.K. KUCHROO. 2005. IL-12 and IL-23-induced T helper cell subsets: birds of the same feather flock together. J. Exp. Med. **201:** 169–171.
19. JANSEN, A., F. HOMO-DELARCHE, H. HOOIJKAAS, *et al.* 1994. Immunohistochemical characterization of monocytes-macrophages and dendritic cells involved in the initiation of the insulitis and beta cell destruction in NOD mice. Diabetes **43:** 667–675.
20. COLNOT, C., M.A. RIPOCHE, G. MILON, *et al.* 1998. Maintenance of granulocyte numbers during acute peritonitis is defective in galectin-3-null mutant mice. Immunology **94:** 290–296.
21. SWARTE, V.V., R.E. MEBIUS, D.H. JOZIASSE, *et al.* 1998. Lymphocyte triggering via L-selectin leads to enhanced galectin-3 mediated binding to dendritic cells. Eur. J. Immunol. **28:** 2846–2871.
22. YAMAKO, A., I. KUWABARA, L.G. FRIGERI, *et al.* 1995. A human lectin, galectin-3 (epsilon bp/Mac-2) stimulates superoxide production by neutrophils. J. Immunol. **154:** 3479–3487.
23. KRÖNCKE, K., V. KOLB-BACHOFEN, B. BERSCHICK, *et al.* 1991. Activated macrophages kill pancreatic syngeneic islet cells via arginine-dependent nitric oxide generation. Biochem. Biophys. Res. Commun. **175:** 752–758.
24. LUKIC, M.L., S. STOSIC-GRUJICIC, N. OSTOJIC, *et al.* 1991. Inhibition of nitric oxide generation affects the induction of diabetes by streptozotocin in mice. Biochem. Biophys. Res. Commun. **178:** 913–920.
25. MOSSMAN, T.R. & S. SAD. 1996. The expanding universe of T-cell subsets: Th1, Th2, and more. Immunol. Today **17:** 138–146.
26. TRAJKOVIC, V., M.J. SWEET & D. XU. 2004. T1/ST2 -an IL-1 receptor modulator of immune responses. Cytokines Growth Factors Rev. **15:** 87–95.
27. LEUNG, B.P., D. XU, S. CULSHAW, *et al.* 2004. A novel therapy of murine collagen-induced arthritis with soluble T1/ST2. J. Immunol. **173:** 145–150.

Effect of Insulin on Acetylcholine-Evoked Amylase Release and Calcium Mobilization in Streptozotocin-Induced Diabetic Rat Pancreatic Acinar Cells

REKHA PATEL,[a] JOSÉ A. PARIENTE,[b] MARIA A. MARTINEZ,[b] GINÉS M. SALIDO,[b] AND JAIPAUL SINGH[a]

[a]*Department of Biological Sciences, University of Central Lancashire, Preston, Lancashire, PR1 2HE UK*

[b]*Department of Physiology, University of Extremadura, Caceres, 10071 Spain*

ABSTRACT: This article investigated the effect of acetylcholine (ACh) on amylase secretion and cellular calcium homeostasis $[Ca^{2+}]_i$ in streptozotocin (STZ; 60 mg kg^{-1}, intraperitoneally)-induced diabetic rats compared to age-matched controls in an attempt to understand the cellular mechanism of exocrine pancreatic insufficiency. ACh-evoked marked dose-dependent increases in amylase release from isolated pancreatic acini and acinar cells in healthy control rats. In diabetic acini and acinar cells, the ACh-evoked amylase release was significantly ($P < 0.05$) reduced compared to healthy acini and acinar cells. Insulin (10^{-6}M) stimulated amylase release in both control and diabetic acini and acinar cells but with a much reduced effect in diabetic tissues. Combining insulin with ACh had no significant effect on amylase release compared to the effect of ACh alone. In fura-2 loaded pancreatic acinar cells of normal rats, ACh (10^{-5}M) evoked a large initial rise (peak) in $[Ca^{2+}]_i$ followed by a decline into a plateau phase. This effect of ACh was significantly ($P < 0.05$) reduced in fura-2 loaded diabetic acinar cells. In control cells, insulin had no significant effect on either basal or ACh evoked $[Ca^{2+}]_i$ compared to the effect of ACh alone. In contrast, in diabetic acinar cells, insulin significantly ($P < 0.05$) attenuated the effect of ACh. In a normally free extracellular Ca^{2+} medium $[Ca^{2+}]_o$ containing 1 mM EGTA, the ACh-evoked $[Ca^{2+}]_i$ in normal healthy fura-2 loaded acini was similar to the response obtained with ACh in fura-2 loaded diabetic acini. Together, the results indicated that exocrine pancreatic insufficiency is associated with decreased $[Ca^{2+}]_i$ due to less Ca^{2+} released from internal stores and less Ca^{2+} entering the cell from the extracellular medium.

KEYWORDS: rats; acetylcholine; insulin; amylase; calcium; diabetes

Address for corresspondence: Prof. Jaipaul Singh, Department of Biological and Forensic Sciences, University of Central Lancashire, Preston, Lancashire, PR1 2HE UK. Voice: 0044-1772-893515; fax: 0044-1772-892929.
e-mail: jsingh3@uclan.ac.uk

**Ann. N.Y. Acad. Sci. 1084: 58–70 (2006). © 2006 New York Academy of Sciences.
doi: 10.1196/annals.1372.027**

INTRODUCTION

The exocrine pancreas secretes an isotonic fluid that is rich in digestive enzymes and bicarbonate.[1,2] Pancreatic juice secretion is controlled by the gut hormones cholecystokinin and secretin and predominantly by the parasympathetic neurotransmitter acetylcholine (ACh).[1–4] Upon stimulation of the vagal nerve, ACh is released and activates muscarinic receptors on acinar cells, resulting in the metabolism of inositol bisphosphate (PIP2) leading to the production of inositol trisphosphate (IP3), inositol tetraphosphate (IP4), and diacylglycerol (DG). IP3 in turn stimulates Ca^{2+} release from intracellular stores, whereas IP4 with IP3 induce Ca^{2+} influx into pancreatic acinar cells.[5,6] Ca^{2+} in turn activates calmodulin that phosphorylates regulatory proteins on zymogen granules resulting in the influx of fluid into the granules that swell and migrate to the luminal pole of acinar cells where they release enzymes by exocytosis. Similarly, DG stimulates protein kinase C that also activates zymogen granules to release digestive enzymes.[7,8]

There is now much evidence that the endocrine hormone insulin can interact with the parasympathetic neurotransmitter ACh both *in vivo* and *in vitro* to produce voluminous and sustained digestive enzyme secretion.[9] In the *in vitro* studies we had previously employed pancreatic segments to measure amylase output.[10] However, this interaction between insulin and ACh is impaired during diabetes mellitus (DM) leading to the long-term condition that is referred to as exocrine pancreatic insufficiency.[11] This derangement in pancreatic secretion is believed to be associated with a decrease in the synthesis and production of amylase.[12] The precise mechanism for exocrine pancreatic insufficiencies is still not fully understood. Some workers have suggested that gene expression for amylase synthesis is impaired while others have shown that diabetic acinar cells are unable to take up glucose and there is also a decrease in Na/K-ATPase activity.[11] In a preliminary study employing pancreatic acinar cells, we have shown that pancreatic insufficiency is associated with a decrease in CCK-evoked Ca^{2+} homeostasis.[12] Since ACh uses the same stimulus-secretion coupling mechanism as CCK, we have decided to investigate the effect of ACh on Ca^{2+} mobilization and amylase release in single acini and acinar cells of diabetic and age-matched control rats.

METHODS

General Procedures

All experiments were performed on adult male Wistar rats weighing about 150–450 g and relevant ethical approvals were obtained from the Ethics Committees of the University of Extremadura and University of Central Lancashire for the use of animals in experimental research. Young adult rats

(150–200 g) were rendered diabetic by using a single intraperitoneal (i.p.) injection of streptozotocin (STZ) (60 mg kg^{-1} body weight) dissolved in a citrate buffer.[13] Age-matched control animals received an equivalent volume of citrate buffer i.p. Both control and DM-induced rats were tested for diabetes 4 days following STZ injection and 6–8 weeks later on the day of the experiment using a Glucometer (Accu Chek; Roche Diagnostic, East Sussex, UK). Blood glucose concentration in excess of 300 mg dL^{-1} confirmed DM.

Both age-matched control and STZ-induced diabetic animals were humanely killed by a blow on the head followed by cervical dislocation and the pancreas was quickly removed and placed in a modified Krebs–Henseleit (K–H) solution of the following composition (mM): NaCl, 103; KCl, 4.7; $CaCl_2$, 2.6; $MgCl_2$, 1.1; $NaHCO_3$, 25; NaH_2PO_4, 1.1; D-glucose, 2.8; sodium pyruvate, 4.9; sodium fumarate, 2.7; and sodium glutamate, 4.9. The solution was kept at pH 7.4 while being continuously gassed with a mixture of 95% O_2–5% CO_2 and maintained at 37°C.

Preparation of Isolated Pancreatic Acini

Pancreatic acinar cells were isolated as described previously.[14] The pancreas was incubated in the presence of collagenase for 10 min at 37°C. This enzymatic digestion of the tissue was followed by gently pipetting the cell suspension through tips of decreasing diameter for mechanical dissociation of the acinar cells. After centrifugation, cells were resuspended in HEPES-buffered saline (HBS) containing (in mM): HEPES, 10; NaCl, 140; KCl, 4.7; $CaCl_2$, 1.3; $MgCl_2$, 1.1; and glucose, 10 (pH 7.4). With this isolation procedure, single cells as well as small clusters consisting of up to five cells were obtained. Cell viability monitored with trypan blue was greater than 95%.

Measurement of Amylase Release

For the measurement of amylase secretion, aliquots (500 μL) of fresh acinar cells were incubated with ACh at 37°C for 30 min followed by centrifugation at 500 g for 2 min (4°C). Acini exposed to the incubation medium alone served as unstimulated controls (basal release). Amylase release and activities in the supernatant were determined using the Phadebas blue starch method[15] and expressed as a percentage of total amylase content at the beginning that was released into the extracellular medium during the incubation.

Cell Loading and Ca^{2+} Analysis

The cell suspension was incubated with 2 μM fura-2-AM in the presence of 0.025% pluronic acid at room temperature for 25 min using an established method.[14] Following loading, the cells were centrifuged for 3 min at 700 rpm and resuspended in fresh HBS and used within 2–3 h. For the determination of fluorescence, 200–300 μL of cell suspension was placed on a poly-D-lysine (20 μg mL^{-1}) coated thin glass cover slip attached to a Perspex perfusion chamber, which was continuously perfused with HBS containing 2.5 mM $CaCl_2$ (approx. at a rate of 1.5 mL min^{-1}) at room temperature.[14] The perfusion chamber was placed on the stage of an inverted fluorescence microscope (Nikon Diaphot 200; Yokohama, Tokyo, Japan). The cells (50 individual cells were chosen) were alternatively excited at 340 and 380 nm by computer-controlled filter wheel (Lambda-2; Sutter Instruments, Novato, CA) and the emitted images (>515 nm) were captured by a high-speed cooled digital CCD camera (C-4880-81; Hamamatsu Photonics, Hamamatsu City, Japan), and recorded using appropriate software (Argus-HiSca; Hamamatsu Photonics). In some experiments extracellular Ca^{2+} ($[Ca^{2+}]_o$) was removed from the superfusing medium but the solution contained 1 mM EGTA. Cells were superfused with different concentrations of ACh alone (10^{-8}–10^{-4} M) or in combination with insulin. All values were measured in ratio units (F340/F380) and subsequently converted into concentrations using an established method.[16]

Statistical Analysis

All data provided were expressed as means ± standard error of the mean (SEM). Data were compared by analysis of variance (ANOVA) and only values with $P < 0.05$ were accepted as significant.

RESULTS

General Characteristics of Control and Diabetic Rats

TABLE 1 shows the general characteristics of age-matched and STZ-induced diabetic rats. The results show that diabetic rats and the pancreas weighed

TABLE 1. General characteristics of age-matched control and STZ-induced diabetic rats

Experimental conditions	Age-matched control	STZ-induced DM
Weight of animals (g)	391.83 ± 37.91 (n = 10)	190.12 ± 5.41 (n = 10)*
Blood glucose level (mg dL^{-1})	92.40 ± 2.42 (n = 10)	>500 (n = 10)*
Weight of the pancreas	1.30 ± 0.07 (n = 10)	1.02 ± 0.05 (n = 10)*
Plasma insulin (ng mL^{-1})	20.63 ± 7.52 (n = 10)	4.80 ± 1.28 (n = 10)*
Basal $(Ca^{2+})_i$ (nM)	246.09 ± 7.53 (n = 98 cells)	169 ± 4.62 (n = 138 cells)*
% of Amylase release with 10^{-6}M insulin	9.01 ± 1.19 (n = 8)	3.25 ± 2.1 (n = 8)*

Data are mean ± SEM with n values shown in brackets except for $[Ca^{2+}]_i$, which indicates cells from 8–10 animals. *$P < 0.05$ comparing control with diabetic animals.

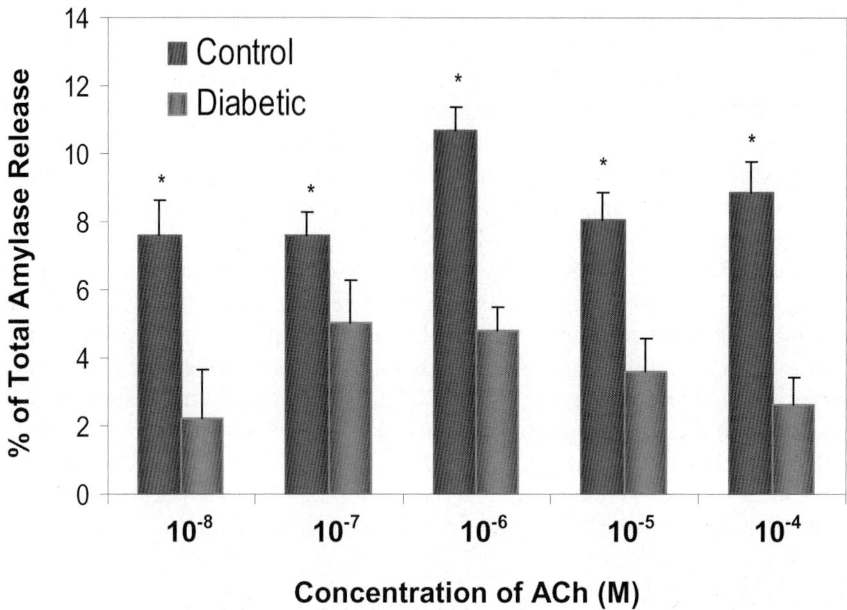

FIGURE 1. Dose–response bar charts showing the effect of 10^{-8}–10^{-4} M ACh on total amylase output from superfused healthy control and STZ-induced diabetic pancreatic acinar cells. Each point is mean ± SEM. $n = 6$–10 rats for each, $^*P < 0.05$ (independent samples Student's *t*-test). Note that stimulation with all ACh concentrations resulted in a significant difference between control and diabetic groups in the % of total amylase released.

significantly ($P < 0.05$) less compared to the age-matched control. Moreover, the diabetic animals have significantly elevated blood glucose levels ($P < 0.05$) and significantly reduced ($P < 0.05$) plasma insulin concentration compared to the age-matched control. Basal $[Ca^{2+}]_i$ in single diabetic pancreatic acinar cells decreased significantly ($P < 0.05$) compared to control. Similarly, amylase release following incubation with 10^{-6} M insulin was significantly ($P < 0.001$) less in diabetic acini compared to age-matched control acinar cells.

Measurement of Amylase Release

FIGURE 1 shows the effect of different concentrations (10^{-8}–10^{-4}M) of ACh on the percentage of amylase release from age-matched healthy control and STZ-induced diabetic pancreatic acini and acinar cells. The results show that control acinar cells released significantly ($P < 0.05$) higher levels of amylase compared to STZ-induced diabetic rats at all concentrations of ACh. Maximum total amylase release was achieved following incubation of acini with 10^{-6}M ACh.

FIGURE 2 shows the effect of different ACh concentrations (10^{-7}–10^{-4}M) on amylase release in diabetic and control pancreatic acinar cells in the absence

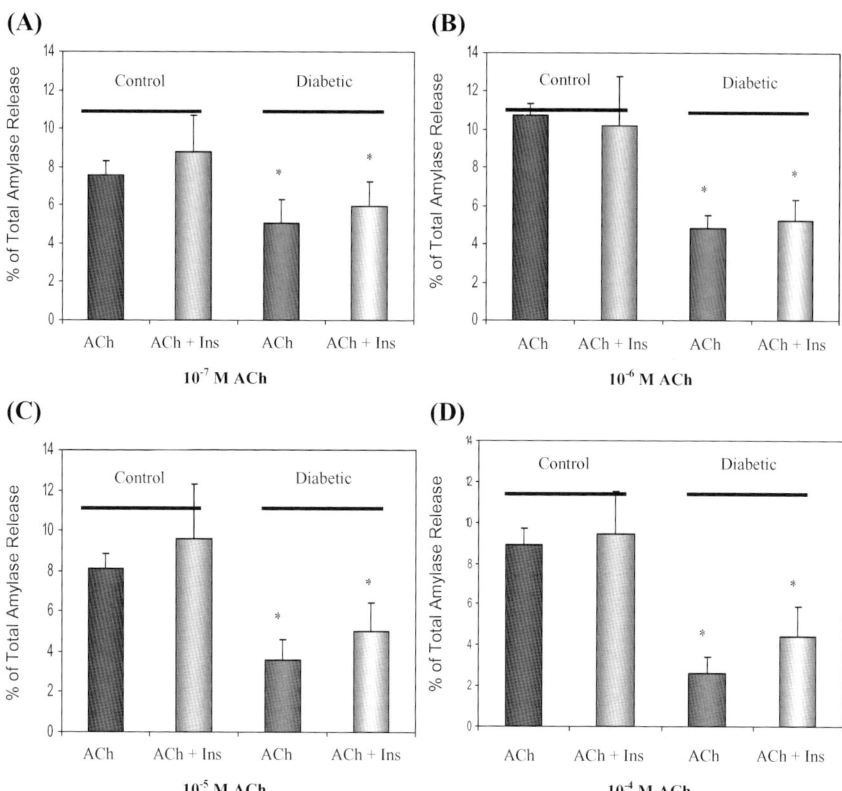

FIGURE 2. Bar charts showing the effect of combining 10^{-6} M insulin with different concentrations of ACh (10^{-7}–10^{-4} M) on total amylase output from healthy age-matched control and STZ-induced diabetic pancreatic acinar cells. Each bar is mean ± SEM. $n =$ 6–10 rats for each, $^{*}P < 0.05$ as compared to the respective control cells (independent samples Student's t-test).

and presence of 10^{-6}M insulin. The results show that ACh alone can elicit a marked increase in amylase output. Combining ACh with insulin resulted in only a slightly larger increase (but not significant) in amylase release compared to the effect of ACh alone. In diabetic acinar cells either ACh or ACh in combination with 10^{-6}M insulin evoked significantly ($P < 0.05$) less amylase release compared to the amylase release from age-matched control cells.

Measurement of $[Ca^{2+}]_i$

FIGURE 3 shows original chart recordings of time course mean changes in $[Ca^{2+}]_i$ in STZ-induced diabetic and age-matched control pancreatic acini following stimulation with either 10^{-5}M ACh alone (**A**), or ACh in combination with 10^{-6}M insulin (**B**). The results show that ACh evoked a

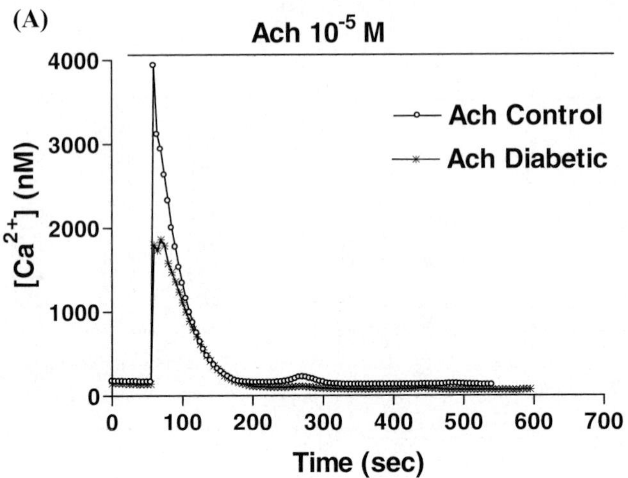

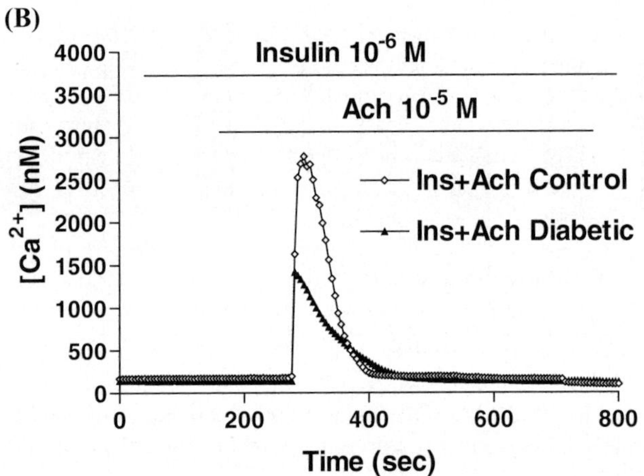

FIGURE 3. (**A**) Original chart recording of the time course of mean changes in $[Ca^{2+}]_i$ before and after ACh (10^{-5} M) application in healthy control and STZ-induced diabetic single acini in the absence (**A**) and presence (**B**) of 10^{-6} M insulin (IN). Traces are typical of 26–29 cells taken from 5–6 control and 5–6 diabetic rats.

rapid increase (initial peak) in $[Ca^{2+}]_i$ and followed a slow time course decline (plateau phase) to almost control level after 6–7 min to ACh application.

The mean ($\pm$ SEM) basal, ACh-evoked peak and plateau phases of the Ca^{2+} transient in the absence and presence of 10^{-6}M insulin are shown in FIGURE 4. The control $[Ca^{2+}]_i$ in the absence and presence of 10^{-6}M insulin is also shown in FIGURE 4 for comparison. The results show that ACh can evoke a marked and significant ($P < 0.05$) increase in the peak $[Ca^{2+}]_i$ either in the absence or

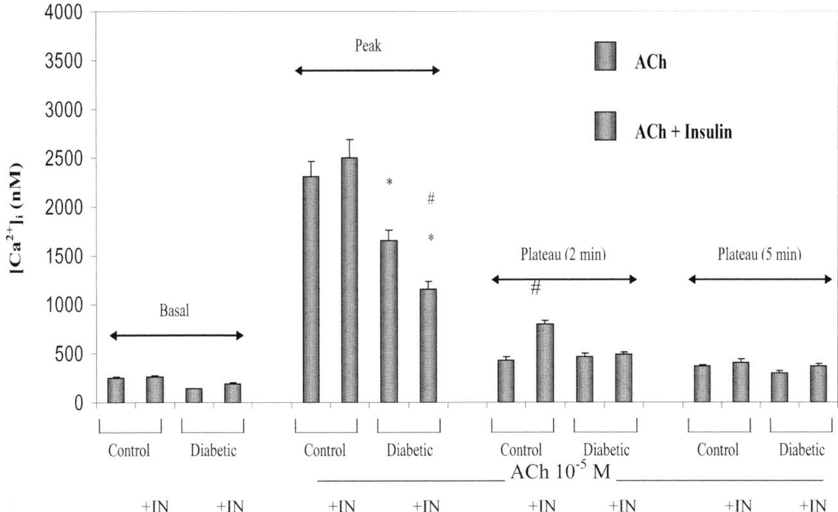

FIGURE 4. Bar charts showing mean (± SEM) basal, ACh (10^{-5} M)-evoked peak and plateau phases (2 min and 5 min after the peak response) of $[Ca^{2+}]_i$ in normal and diabetic single acini in the absence and presence of 10^{-6} M insulin (+IN). Each bar is mean ± SEM. $n = 26$–29 acinar cells taken from 5–6 rats for each. $^*P < 0.05$ as compared to the respective control and $^\# P < 0.05$ as compared to the respective effect of insulin (independent samples Student's *t*-test).

presence of 10^{-6}M insulin in control pancreatic acinar cells. In diabetic acinar cells, the ACh-induced $[Ca^{2+}]_i$ transient was significantly reduced ($P < 0.05$) either in the absence or presence of insulin compared to age-matched control pancreatic acinar cells. Insulin (10^{-6} M) was shown to significantly increase the ACh-evoked plateau response 2 min after the peak response (794.2 ± 41.8 nM, $n = 26$ in healthy control acini compared to the effect of ACh (10^{-6} M) administration alone (434.3 ± 30.3 nM, $n = 26$).

In zero $[Ca^{2+}]_o$ basal $[Ca^{2+}]_i$ was 144.20 ± 44.72 nM ($n = 29$) and 44.72 ± 9.44 nM ($n = 26$) in control and diabetic acinar cells, respectively. The ACh-evoked peak $[Ca^{2+}]_i$ was 1744.20 ± 315.17 nM ($n = 29$) in control and 747.74 ± 7.41 nM ($n = 26$) in diabetic acinar cells, respectively. The ACh-evoked plateau phase after 2 min in zero $[Ca^{2+}]_o$ was 125.56 ± 7.75 nM ($n = 29$) and 8.31 ± 1.32 nM ($n = 26$) in control and diabetic acinar cells, respectively.

FIGURE 5 shows the integral rise (area under the traces) in $[Ca^{2+}]_i$ above basal following 5 min of the ACh (10^{-5}M) stimulation of age-matched healthy and STZ-induced diabetic acinar cells in the absence and presence of 10^{-6}M insulin during normal (1.2 mM) $[Ca^{2+}]_o$ and in a nominally free $[Ca^{2+}]_o$ + 1mM EGTA. The results show that diabetic acinar cells contain significantly ($P < 0.05$) less amount of $[Ca^{2+}]_i$ compared to control in normal $[Ca^{2+}]_o$. However, when $[Ca^{2+}]_o$ was removed and 1 mM EGTA was added to the

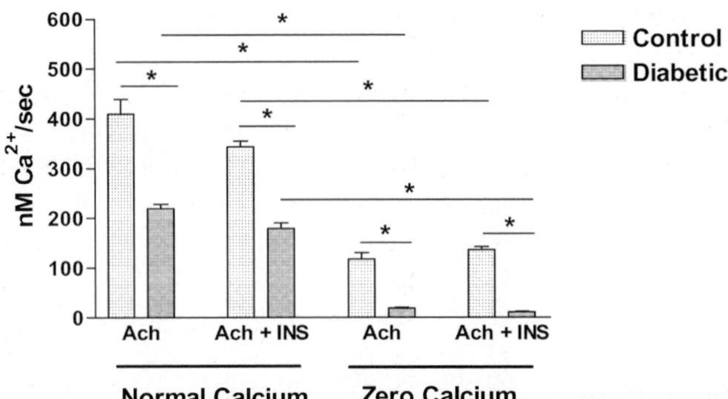

FIGURE 5. Bar charts showing the integral of rise above basal in $[Ca^{2+}]_i$ following 5 min of 10^{-5} M ACh stimulation of age-matched healthy control and STZ-induced diabetic acinar cells in the absence and presence of 10^{-6} M insulin (INS) during normal $[Ca^{2+}]_0$ and nominally free $[Ca^{2+}]_0 + 1$ mM EGTA. Data are mean $\pm$ SEM. $n = 26$–29 in each bar chart taken from 5–6 control and 5–6 diabetic rats.

superfusing medium, $[Ca^{2+}]_i$ was also significantly ($P < 0.05$) reduced in age-matched control acinar cells similar to that seen in diabetic acinar cells in normal $[Ca^{2+}]_o$. The results suggest that diabetes is associated with an decrease in cytosolic Ca^{2+} in pancreatic acinar cells and this may be due to both its release from intercellular stores and its influx into pancreatic cells.

DISCUSSION

The results of this study have shown marked differences in the characteristics of age-matched healthy control and STZ-induced diabetic rats and the functions of the pancreas. Like other investigations,[12,17] the present results show that diabetic rats and the pancreas weigh significantly less and the animals have elevated blood glucose (hyperglycemia) and reduced plasma insulin levels compared to the healthy control. It is well known that diabetic rats eat less and moreover, they produce less digestive enzymes, especially amylase, for the digestion of food stuffs.[11,12,17–20] This in turn will naturally lead to weight loss and atrophy as well as other long-term complications resulting from the hyperglycemia.[21]

The results have shown that ACh can elicit marked dose-dependent increases in amylase release from control healthy pancreatic acinar cells. In contrast, in diabetic acinar cells, the effect of ACh was significantly reduced at all concentrations of ACh employed in this study. These data support previous findings by other workers who have shown that STZ-rendered DM is associated with reduced amylase secretion.[9,11,12,22–24] The reduction in ACh-evoked amylase output in the diabetic pancreatic acinar cells is not due to a direct effect of STZ since it has no effect on amylase secretion when it is applied either alone or in combination with secretagogues.[25]

In contrast to previous studies employing either isolated pancreatic segments,[9,26] intact isolated pancreas[27–29] or the anaesthetized rat,[17] the present results have shown that insulin at 10^{-6} M can stimulate amylase release from single pancreatic acinar cells. When insulin was combined with ACh, amylase release increased only slightly compared to the effect of ACh alone. This is in contrast to previous studies employing isolated pancreatic segments and the isolated intact pancreas in which insulin potentiated the effects of secretagogues.[1,9,26,27,29] One possible explanation for this discrepancy is that pancreatic acinar cells respond differently to insulin compared to segments or the intact pancreas. This may be due to the fact that insulin has more access to cell surface receptors.

This study also measured $[Ca^{2+}]_i$ in single fura-2 loaded pancreatic acinar cells in order to determine the precise role of Ca^{2+} in the stimulus-secretion coupling process in normal and diabetic conditions. The results have shown that basal $[Ca^{2+}]_i$ was markedly reduced in diabetic acinar cells compared to control. ACh alone evoked a rapid and large increase in $[Ca^{2+}]_i$ in control and diabetic acinar cells reaching a peak within 15–20 s followed by a rapid decline to a plateau phase that remained above basal level throughout the time course response. In diabetic acinar cells, the ACh-evoked peak and plateau phases of the responses were significantly reduced compared to control. Insulin alone had no significant effect on $[Ca^{2+}]_i$ in either the control or diabetic acinar cells compared to the respective controls in the absence of insulin. Combining insulin with ACh resulted in only a small increase in $[Ca^{2+}]_i$ compared to the effect of ACh alone in normal healthy acinar cells. In contrast, insulin significantly attenuated the ACh-evoked peak and plateau phases of the Ca^{2+} transient in diabetic acinar cells compared with the effect of ACh and insulin in control cells. These results are in complete agreement employing suspensions of pancreatic acinar cells.[9,12,19]

This study has also shown that in the absence of extracellular Ca^{2+} $[Ca^{2+}]_o$, ACh evoked significantly less $[Ca^{2+}]_i$ compared to the response obtained with ACh in normal $[Ca^{2+}]_o$. These results are similar to those obtained with ACh in diabetic acinar cells. It is now well known that $[Ca^{2+}]_o$ plays a major role in filling up the intracellular stores and in elevating $[Ca^{2+}]_i$ during stimulation to enhance sustained enzyme secretion. It is also well known that in the absence of $[Ca^{2+}]_o$ ACh produces significantly less amylase output.[20] These interesting findings reveal a close relationship between amylase release and the levels of $[Ca^{2+}]_i$ available in the cytoplasm to mediate enzyme secretion.

The question that now arises is: what is responsible for the reduced $[Ca^{2+}]_i$ and amylase secretion during the diabetic state? In a previous study we have shown that both $[Ca^{2+}]_i$ and $[Mg^{2+}]_i$ are reduced in diabetic acinar cells following secretagogue stimulation compared to control.[12] It is possible that cellular Ca^{2+} homeostasis is directly linked to changes in $[Mg^{2+}]_i$.[30] Moreover, Mg^{2+}

plays a major role in cellular regulation by controlling ion transport and Ca^{2+}-dependent enzyme systems.[30] Another possible explanation is that amylase mRNA is reduced during DM leading to less synthesis and less release.[31,32] Moreover, in diabetic conditions pancreatic acinar cells are unable to take up either glucose or amino acids that are associated with reduced $Na^{+}K^{+}$ATPase activity.[33] It is conceivable that reduced $[Ca^{2+}]_i$ may be linked to all these processes since it is the mediator and promotor in cellular regulation.[34]

In conclusion, the results have demonstrated that both ACh and insulin can stimulate amylase release from age-matched control and diabetic acinar cells with much reduced effect in diabetic acinar cells. Similarly, ACh can also elevate $[Ca^{2+}]_i$ in fura-2 loaded control and diabetic acinar cells with less effect in diabetic cells. The responses in diabetic acinar cells resemble those obtained with ACh in a nominally free $[Ca^{2+}]_i$ in combination with 1 mM EGTA. The results indicate that cellular Ca^{2+} homeostasis is decreased in DM and this in turn may result in reduced amylase secretion and exocrine pancreatic insufficiency.

REFERENCES

1. Williams, J.A. & I.D. Goldfine. 1993. The insulin acinar relationship. *In* The Exocrine Pancreas: Biology, Pathobiology, and Disease, 2nd ed. V.L.M. Go, E.P. DiMagno, J.D. Gardner, *et al.*, Eds.: 789–802. Raven Press. N.Y.
2. Vander, A., J. Sherman & D. Luciano. The digestion and absorption of food. 1998. *In* Human Physiology, The Mechanisms of Body Function, 7th ed. A. Vander, J. Sherman & D. Luciano, Eds.: 551–556, 576–577. WCB McGraw-Hill. Boston.
3. Richins, C.A. 1945. The innervation of the pancreas. J. Comp. Neurol. **82:** 223–236.
4. Brown, J.H. & P.M. McDonough. 1989. Muscarinic cholinergic receptors of inositol phospholipids metabolism and calcium mobilization. *In* The Muscarinic Receptors. J.H. Brown, Ed.: 259–307. Humana Press. NJ.
5. Berridge, M.J. 1993. Inositol trisphosphate and calcium signalling. Nature **361:** 315–325.
6. Putney, J.W., Jr. 1988. The role of phosphoinositide metabolism in signal transduction in secretory cells. J. Exp. Biol. **139:** 135–150.
7. Jensen, R.T. & J.D. Gardner. 1981. Identification and characterization of receptors for secretagogues on pancreatic acinar cells. Fed. Proc. **40:** 2486–2496.
8. Nishizuka, Y. 1988. Studies and prospectives of protein kinase C in signal transduction. Nippon Ketsueki Gakkai Zasshi **51:** 1321–1326.
9. Singh, J. & E. Adeghate. 1998. Effects of islet hormones on nerve-mediated and acetylcholine-evoked secretory responses in the isolated pancreas of normal and diabetic rats. Int. J. Mol. Med. **1:** 627–634.
10. Juma, L.M., J. Singh, D.J. Pallot, *et al.* 1997. Interactions of islet hormones with acetylcholine in the isolated rat pancreas. Peptides **18:** 1415–1422.
11. Singh, J., E. Adeghate, S. Aparico, *et al.* 2004. Exocrine pancreatic insufficiency in diabetes mellitus. Int. J. Diabetes Metab. **12:** 35–43.

12. PATEL, R., M.D. YAGO, M. MANAS, *et al.* 2004a. Mechanism of exocrine pancreatic insufficiency in streptozotocin-induced diabetes mellitus in rat: effect of cholecystokinin-octapeptide. Mol. Cell. Biochem. **261:** 83–89.
13. SHARMA, A.K., I.G. DUGUID, D.S. BLANCHARD, *et al.* 1985. The effect of insulin treatment on myelinated nerve fibre maturation and integrity and on body growth in streptozotocin-diabetic rats. J. Neurol. Sci. **67:** 285–297.
14. PARIENTE, J.A., P.C. REDONDO, M.P. GRANADOS, *et al.* 2003. Calcium signalling in non-excitable cells. E. C. Qua. L. **1:** 29–43.
15. GARDNER, J.D. & M.J. JACKSON. 1977. Regulation of amylase release from dispersed pancreatic acinar cells. J. Physiol. **270:** 439–454.
16. GRYNKIEWICZ, G., M. POENIE & R.Y. TSIEN. 1985. A new generation of Ca^{2+} indicators with greatly improved fluorescence properties. J. Biol. Chem. **260:** 3440–3450.
17. PATEL, R., J. SINGH, M.D. YAGO, *et al.* 2004b. Effect of insulin on exocrine pancreatic secretion in healthy and diabetic anaesthetised rats. Mol. Cell. Biochem. **261:** 105–110.
18. AHMED, I., E. ADEGHATE, A.K. SHARMA, *et al.* 1998. Effects of Momordica charantia fruit juice on islet morphology in the pancreas of the streptozotocin-diabetic rat. Diabetes Res. Clin. Pract. **40:** 145–151.
19. SINGH, J., L.M.O. JUMA, E. ADEGHATE, *et al.* 1999. Interactive adaptation of endocrine and exocrine pancreas: effects of islet hormones and secretagogues. *In* Adaptation Biology and Medicine. K.B. Pandolf, N. Takeda & P.K. Singal, Eds.: 223–235. Narosa Publishing House. New Delhi, India.
20. SINGH, J., M.D. YAGO & E. ADEGHATE. 2001. Involvement of cellular calcium in exocrine pancreatic insufficiency during streptozotocin-induced diabetes mellitus. Arch. Physiol. Biochem. **109:** 252–259.
21. KUMAR, P.J. & M.L. CLARK. 2002. Diabetes mellitus and other disorders of metabolism. *In* Clinical Medicine. P.J. Kumar & M.L. Clark, Eds.: 1069–1122. WB Saunders. London.
22. SOFRANKOVA, A. & G.J. DOCKRAY. 1983. Cholecystokinin- and secretin-induced pancreatic secretion in normal and diabetic rats. Am. J. Physiol. **244:** G370–G374.
23. OTSUKI, M., T. AKIYAMA, H. SHIROHARA, *et al.* 1995. Loss of sensitivity to cholecystokinin stimulation of isolated pancreatic acini from genetically diabetic rats. Am. J. Physiol. **268:** E531–E536.
24. YAGO, M.D., E. ADEGHATE & J. SINGH. 1999. Interactions between the endocrine and exocrine pancreas. Effects of islet hormones, secretagogues, and nerve stimulation. *In* Neural Regulation in the Vertebrate Endocrine System: Neuroendocrine Regulation. R.A. Prasada Rao, R. Peters Eds.: 197–217. Kluwer Academic/Plenum. N.Y.
25. MAHAY, S., E. ADEGHATE, M.Z. LINDLEY, *et al.* 2004. Streptozotocin-induced type 1 diabetes mellitus alters the morphology, secretory function and acyl lipid contents in the isolated rat parotid salivary gland. Mol. Cell. Biochem. **261:** 175–181.
26. SINGH, J. & G.T. PEARSON. 1984. Effects of nerve stimulation on enzyme secretion from the *in vitro* rat pancreas and 3H-release after preincubation with catecholamines. Naunyn Schmiedebergs Arch Pharmacol. **327:** 228–233.
27. KANNO, T. & A. SAITO. 1976. The potentiating influences of insulin on pancreozymin-induced hyperpolarization and amylase release in the pancreatic acinar cell. J. Physiol. **261:** 505–521.

28. SAITO, A., J.A. WILLIAMS & T. KANNO. 1980a. Potentiation of cholecystokinin-induced exocrine secretion by both exogenous and endogenous insulin in isolated and perfused rat pancreata. J. Clin. Invest. **65:** 777–782.
29. SAITO, A., J.A. WILLIAMS & T. KANNO. 1980b. Potentiation by insulin of acetylcholine-induced secretory response of the perfused rat pancreas. Biomed. Res. **1:** 101–103.
30. YAGO, M.D., M. MANAS & J. SINGH. 2000. Intracellular magnesium: transport and regulation in epithelial secretory cells. Front. Biosci. **5:** D602–D618.
31. DUAN, R.D. & C. ERLANSON-ALBERTSSON. 1990. Altered synthesis of some secretory proteins in pancreatic lobules isolated from streptozotocin-induced diabetic rats. Pancreas **5:** 136–143.
32. DUAN, R.D. & C. ERLANSON-ALBERTSSON. 1992. The effect of pretranslational regulation on synthesis of pancreatic colipase in streptozotocin-induced diabetes in rats. Pancreas **7:** 465–471.
33. YANG, Y.K. & W.Y. ZHU. 1995. Effect of insulin on the function of pancreatic exocrine. Sheng. Li. Xue. Bao. **47:** 238–244.
34. BERRIDGE, M.J. 1995. Inositol trisphosphate and calcium signalling. Ann. N. Y. Acad. Sci. **766:** 31–43.

Mechanism of Exocrine Pancreatic Insufficiency in Streptozotocin-Induced Type 1 Diabetes Mellitus

REKHA PATEL,[a] AMIL SHERVINGTON,[a] JOSE A. PARIENTE,[b] MARIA A. MARTINEZ-BURGOS,[b] GINES M. SALIDO,[b] ERNEST ADEGHATE,[c] AND JAIPAUL SINGH[a]

[a]*Department of Biological Sciences, University of Central Lancashire, Preston PR1 2HE, UK*

[b]*Department of Physiology, University of Extremadura, 10071 Caceres, Spain*

[c]*Department of Anatomy, Faculty of Medicine and Health Sciences, UAE University, Al-Ain, United Arab Emirates*

ABSTRACT: Diabetes mellitus (DM) is a major health problem at present affecting about 180 million people worldwide. DM is associated with many metabolic abnormalities in the body including the indigestion of carbohydrates leading to malnutrition and weight loss. In this article we investigate the cellular and molecular mechanisms of exocrine pancreatic insufficiency in streptozotocin (STZ, 60 mg kg^{-1}, i.p.)-induced DM in male rats compared to healthy age-matched controls. Either electrical field stimulation (EFS) or cholecystokinin octapeptide (CCK-8, 10^{-8} M) can elicit large and significant ($P < 0.05$) increases in amylase output from pancreatic segments compared to basal secretion. Insulin (10^{-6} M) alone has no significant effect on amylase output compared to basal but it enhanced the secretory responses to either EFS or CCK-8. When rats were rendered diabetic with STZ, either EFS or CCK-8-evoked amylase output was significantly ($P < 0.01$) decreased compared to the responses obtained with either EFS or CCK-8 alone in healthy age-matched control pancreas. In addition, CCK-8 can elicit large dose-dependent release of amylase in age-matched control and diabetic acinar cells with significantly ($P < 0.05$) reduced responses in diabetic acinar cells. CCK-8 evoked a large rapid increase in peak cytosolic free calcium concentration ($[Ca^{2+}]_c$) followed by a decrease to a plateau phase in age-matched control fura-2-loaded pancreatic acinar cells. These responses were significantly ($P < 0.05$) decreased in STZ-induced diabetic acinar cells. In the presence of 10^{-6} M insulin, CCK-8 evoked a much larger increase in the Ca^{2+} transient compared to the response obtained with CCK-8 alone. These effects were significantly ($P < 0.01$) inhibited in STZ-induced

Address for correspondence: Ernest Adeghate, M.D., M.F.M., Ph.D., Department of Anatomy, Faculty of Medicine and Health Sciences, UAE University, P.O. Box 17666, Al Ain, United Arab Emirates. Voice: +971-3-7137496; fax: +971-3-7672033.
e-mail: eadeghate@uaeu.ac.ae

Ann. N.Y. Acad. Sci. 1084: 71–88 (2006).
doi: 10.1196/annals.1372.038

diabetic acinar cells. Similarly, in zero extracellular Ca^{2+} $[Ca^{2+}]\hat{c}$, the CCK-8-evoked $[Ca^{2+}]_c$ was significantly ($P < 0.05$) reduced in both diabetic and age-matched control acinar cells, but with more pronounced reduction in diabetic acinar cells. CCK_A receptor mRNA levels remained unchanged in diabetic rat acinar cells compared to age-matched healthy control. In contrast, amylase mRNA was significantly ($P < 0.05$) reduced in diabetic acinar cells compared to control. The results indicate that reduced amylase secretion in response to either EFS or CCK-8 in the diabetic pancreas may be due to reduced $[Ca^{2+}]_c$ and gene expression for amylase and not to the gene expression of CCK_A receptor in pancreatic acinar cells.

KEYWORDS: cholecystokinin; amylase; insulin; calcium; gene expression; diabetes

INTRODUCTION

The pancreas is often described as two separate organs comprising smaller endocrine and larger exocrine portions.[1–4] Cholecystokinin octapeptide (CCK), secretin, and the autonomic nerves, which release ACh and noradrenaline as well as other peptide neurotransmitters, predominantly control amylase secretion from the exocrine pancreas.[3–13] Both morphological and functional evidences indicate marked interactions between the exocrine and endocrine parts of the pancreas in order to produce an adequate amount of pancreatic juice secretion for the efficient digestion of food.[3,4,14] In diabetes mellitus (DM), the exocrine pancreas is unable to secrete sufficient amylase for the digestion of carbohydrates leading to exocrine pancreatic insufficiency, malnutrition, and weight loss.[15] Moreover, the interaction between the exocrine and endocrine pancreas is also impaired during DM.[2,4,16]

The cellular and molecular mechanisms underlying the impairment of pancreatic acinar cells to secrete an adequate amount of amylase in diabetic conditions are still not fully understood. Several mechanisms have been proposed for diabetic-induced exocrine pancreatic insufficiency including insensitivity of pancreatic acinar cell receptors to CCK,[4,17,18] magnesium deficiency,[12] and a decrease in cytosolic free Ca^{2+} concentration ($[Ca^{2+}]\hat{c}$).[4,9,12,16] These previous studies have undertaken receptor binding studies for CCK_A and suspension of pancreatic acinar cells to measure either $[Ca^{2+}]_c$ and $[Mg^{2+}]_c$. Since amylase accounts for 20% of total protein secreted by the pancreas[10,14] and its production is mediated by CCK through the CCK_A receptor, it was hypothesized that alterations in these messages may be, at least in part, responsible for pancreatic insufficiency. Therefore, the aim of this article was to measure $[Ca^{2+}]_c$ and mRNA gene expressions for CCK_A receptor and amylase in single pancreatic acinar cells of healthy age-matched control and diabetic rats in order to identify if reduced transcription of these proteins are responsible for pancreatic insufficiency in streptozotocin (STZ)-induced type 1 DM. Amylase secretion was also measured for comparison in control and diabetic pancreas. A preliminary account of some aspect of this work was presented to the Physiological Society.[19]

METHODS

General Procedures

All experiments were performed on adult male Wistar rats weighing about 150–450 g and relevant ethical approvals were obtained from the Ethics Committees of the University of Extremadura and the University of Central Lancashire for the use of animals in experimental research. Young adult rats (150–200 g) were rendered diabetic by using a single intraperitoneal (i.p.) injection of STZ (60 mg kg^{-1} body weight) dissolved in a citrate buffer.[20] Age-matched control animals received an equivalent volume of citrate buffer i.p. Both control and DM-induced rats were tested for diabetes 4–5 days following STZ injection and 6–8 weeks later on the day of the experiment using a One Touch II Glucometer (Johnson & Johnson, Skipton, UK). Blood glucose concentration in excess of 300 mg dL^{-1} confirmed DM.

Both age-matched control and STZ-induced diabetic animals were humanely killed by a blow to the head followed by cervical dislocation and the pancreas was quickly removed and placed in a modified Krebs–Henseleit (K–H) solution of the following composition (mM): NaCl, 103; KCl, 4.7; $CaCl_2$, 2.6; $MgCl_2$, 1.1; $NaHCO_3$, 25; NaH_2PO_4, 1.1; D-glucose, 2.8; sodium pyruvate, 4.9; sodium fumarate, 2.7; and sodium glutamate, 4.9. The solution was kept at a pH 7.4 while being continuously gassed with a mixture of 95% O_2–5% CO_2 and maintained at 37°C.

Measurement of Amylase Output in Pancreatic Segments

The pancreas was cut into small segments (5–10 mg) and a total weight of 50–100 mg was placed in a Perspex flow chamber (vol = 1 mL) and superfused with K–H solution at a rate of 1 mL min^{-1}. The amylase concentration in the effluent from the chamber was measured using an online fluorimetric assay by a previously described method.[21] Throughout an experiment, the generation of fluorescence that is a linear function of amylase concentration was continuously monitored on a pen recorder. The electrical field stimulation (EFS) and secretagogue-evoked amylase release were routinely expressed in terms of the output at the peak of the response in units (U) mL^{-1} $(100 \text{ mg tissues})^{-1}$. One unit of amylase is defined as the amount of amylase that will liberate 1.0 mg of maltose from starch in 3 min at pH 6.9 and 20°C. In this study, α-amylase (Sigma type II a; Sigma, Poole, UK) was used as a standard for calibration.

Either CCK-8 (10^{-8} M) or insulin (10^{-6} M; natural, from bovine pancreas) was added directly to the superfusing solution. EFS was achieved via silver wire electrodes embedded in the Perspex flow chamber (EFS parameters were 10 Hz, 50 V, and 1 ms pulse width). The tissue was stimulated with either CCK-8 or EFS for 6 min in either the absence or presence of insulin. The tissue was pretreated with insulin for 5 min prior to secretagogue application.

Preparation of Isolated Pancreatic Acini

Pancreatic acinar cells were isolated as described previously.[22,23] Briefly, the pancreas was incubated in the presence of collagenase for 10 min at 37°C. This enzymatic digestion of the tissue was followed by gently pipetting the cell suspension through tips of decreasing diameter for mechanical dissociation of the acinar cells. After centrifugation, cells were resuspended in HEPES-buffered saline (HBSS) containing (in mM): HEPES, 10; NaCl, 140; KCl, 4.7; $CaCl_2$, 1.3; $MgCl_2$, 1.1; glucose, 10 (pH 7.4). With this isolation procedure, single cells as well as small clusters consisting of up to five cells were obtained. Cell viability monitored with trypan blue [24] was greater than 95%.

Measurement of Amylase Release

For the measurement of amylase release, aliquots (500 μL) of fresh acini and acinar cells were incubated with different concentrations (10^{-11}–10^{-8}) of CCK-8 at 37°C for 30 min followed by centrifugation at 500 *g* for 2 min (4°C). Acini and cells exposed to the incubation medium alone served as unstimulated controls (basal release). Amylase release and activities in the supernatant were determined using the Phadebas blue starch method[25] and expressed as a percentage of total amylase content at the beginning that was released into the extracellular medium during the incubation.

Cell Loading and Ca^{2+} Analysis

The cell suspension was incubated with 2 μM fura-2-AM in the presence of 0.025% pluronic acid at room temperature for 25 min using an established method.[23] Following loading, the cells were centrifuged for 3 min at 700 rpm and resuspended in fresh HBSS and used within 2–3 h. For determination of fluorescence, 200–300 μL of cell suspension was placed on a poly-D-lysine (20 μg mL^{-1}) coated thin glass cover slip attached to a Perspex perfusion chamber, which was continuously perfused with HBSS containing 1.3 mM $CaCl_2$ (approximately at a rate of 1.5 mL min^{-1}) at room temperature.[22,23] The perfusion chamber was placed on the stage of an inverted fluorescence microscope

(Nikon Diaphot 200; Nikon, Surrey, UK). The cells were alternatively excited at 340 and 380 nm by computer-controlled filter wheel (Lambda-2; Sutter Instruments Novato, CA) and the emitted images (>515 nm) were captured by a high-speed cooled digital CCD camera (C-4880-81; Hamamatsu Photonics Hertfordshire, UK), and recorded using appropriate software (Argus-HiSca; Hamamatsu Photonics). In some experiments extracellular Ca^{2+} ($[Ca^{2+}]_c$) was removed from the superfusing medium but the solution contained 1 mM EGTA. Cells were superfused with either 10^{-8} M CCK-8 alone or 10^{-6} M insulin alone or insulin in combination with CCK-8. All values were measured in ratio units (F340/F380) and subsequently converted into concentrations using an established method.[26]

Measurements of mRNA Gene Expressions for CCK_A Receptor and α-Amylase

Age-matched control and STZ-induced diabetic rat pancreas were rapidly excised and frozen immediately in liquid nitrogen aseptically and stored at –80°C. Total RNA was isolated from pancreatic tissue using Tri-Reagent (Sigma), based on the acid guanidinium thiocyanate-phenol-chloroform RNA extraction method.[27] The integrity of the isolated RNA from both control and STZ-induced diabetic pancreatic tissue was analyzed using spectroscopy and agarose gel electrophoresis.

For cDNA synthesis, 1 μg of RNA was incubated using Oligo-p$[dT]_{15}$ as a hexamer primer in a reaction mixture with AMV reverse transcriptase (RT) using a First Strand cDNA Synthesis Kit (Roche Diagnostics, Sussex, UK). First strand cDNA synthesis was carried out at 25°C for 10 min followed by 42°C for 60 min (primer annealing) and then 99°C for 5 min (denaturing), and then cooling to 4°C for 5 min. The resulting single-stranded cDNA was amplified using a real time PCR together with CCK_A receptor and α-amylase-specific primers. SYBR green (LightCycler FastStart DNA Master^{PLUS} SYBR Green 1 Kit, Roche Diagnostics) was used for the amplifications. Reaction mixtures contained 2 μL of the first-strand cDNA, 0.5 μM gene-specific primers (TIB Molbiol), dNTP, Taq DNA polymerase, 1.5 mM $MgCl_2$, reaction buffer, and SYBR Green 1 dye provided in the reaction mix kit. The primers for the amplification of α-amylase cDNA were designed on the basis of the mRNA sequence of rat pancreas amylase.[28] The designed primers were: 5′TGGCCTTCTGGATCTTGCACTC and 5′AGGCTGACCGTTGACTACATTCCT (antisense), corresponding to nucleotides 540–561 and 1243–1266 of the amylase cDNA sequence. Thermal cycling conditions were denaturation at 95°C for 10 min, amplification (54°C/10s; 72°C/9 s; 64°C/40s), and a final elongation at 40°C for 30s for 40 cycles. Commercially available kit DNA was used to evaluate total DNA input.

For amplification of the coding region of the CCK_A receptor, RT-PCR was carried out using designed primers, which were 5′GGCATT GCTGTCCAGGTATT and 5′ATGACCCCACCTTAGGTTCC (antisense), corresponding to nucleotides 1484–1503 and 1685–1704, respectively, of the CCK_A receptor cDNA sequence. Thermal cycling conditions were denaturation at 95°C for 10 s, amplification (95°C/10s; 54°C/10s; 72°C/9s), and a final elongation at 40°C for 30 s for 45 cycles. At the end of each cycle, the fluorescence was measured in a single step in channel F1 (gain 1). After the 45th cycle, the specimens were heated to 95°C and rapidly cooled down to 65°C for 15s. All heating and cooling steps were performed with a slope of 20°C/s. The temperature was then raised to 95°C in slope of 0.1°C/s and fluorescence was measured continuously (channel F1, gain 1) to obtain data for the melting curve analysis. Again the control kit DNA was used as a positive control for RT-PCR reactions.

To confirm that the correct amylase and CCK_A receptor mRNA had been amplified, gel electrophoresis analysis of the RT-PCR amplicons was carried out. The PCR products were separated electrophoretically. A single band corresponding to the correct amplicon size was observed for α-amylase and CCK_A receptor of 220 and 221 bp, respectively.

Statistical Analysis

All data provided were expressed as mean ± standard error of the mean (SEM). Data were compared by analysis of variance (ANOVA) and only values with $P < 0.05$ were accepted as significant.

RESULTS

Diabetic rats and the pancreas weigh significantly ($P < 0.05$) less [195.12 ± 4.40 g ($n = 20$) and 1.02 ± 0.05 g ($n = 20$), respectively] compared to age-matched controls [395.63 ± 25.91 ($n = 20$) and 1.30 ± 0.07 g ($n = 20$), respectively] after 6–8 weeks of STZ treatment. Blood glucose level was in excess of 500 mg dL^{-1} ($n = 27$) in diabetics rats compared to age-matched control (92.40 ± 2.42 mg dL^{-1}, $n = 44$). In contrast, plasma insulin level decreased significantly ($P < 0.05$) in diabetic rats (4.80 ± 1.28 ng mL^{-1}, $n = 20$) compared to control (20.63 ± 7.52 ng mL^{-1}, $n = 20$).

Amylase Secretion

FIGURE 1 shows the effect of 10 Hz EFS and 10^{-8} M CCK-8 on amylase output from superfused pancreatic segments of age-matched control and STZ-induced diabetic rats in the absence and presence of 10^{-6} M insulin. The

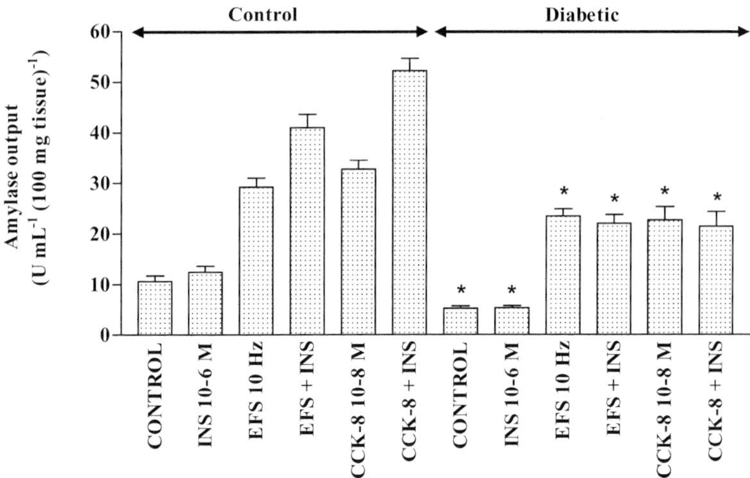

FIGURE 1. Effects of EFS and CCK-8 on pancreatic amylase secretion. Bar charts showing mean (± SEM) amylase output (U mL^{-1} (100 mg $tissue)^{-1}$) from superfused pancreatic segments of age-matched control and STZ-induced diabetic rats in response to either EFS (10 Hz, 50 V, 1 ms pulse width) or 10^{-8} M CCK-8 in the absence and presence of 10^{-6} M insulin (INS). The control response and the effect of INS alone are also shown for comparison. Either EFS or CCK-8 was applied for 6 min. Tissues were pretreated with INS for 6 min followed by either EFS or CCK-8 in the continuous presence of INS (n = 10 animals in each groups). $^{*}P < 0.05$ for diabetic compared to control. Note that insulin failed to potentiate the effect of either EFS or CCK-8 in diabetic rats.

control responses in the absence and presence of insulin are also shown for comparison. The results show that either EFS or CCK-8 can evoke a significant ($P < 0.05$) increase in amylase output from healthy control superfused pancreatic segments. Insulin alone had little or no effect on amylase output compared to basal, but it enhanced the secretory effects of either EFS or CCK-8 compared to the response obtained with either EFS or CCK-8 alone. In STZ-induced diabetic pancreatic segments both the basal and EFS and CCK-8-evoked pancreatic secretion was significantly ($P < 0.05$) decreased compared to amylase output from age-matched control animals. Furthermore, insulin failed to enhance the secretory effects of either EFS or CCK-8 in the diabetic pancreas.

In another series of experiments, amylase release was measured using the Phadebas test following stimulation of isolated age-matched control and diabetic acinar cells with 10^{-11}–10^{-8} M CCK-8 (FIG. 2). The results show that CCK-8 can evoke large increases in total amylase release from pancreatic acinar cells at all doses tested. However, the responses were significantly ($P < 0.05$) decreased in diabetic acinar cells compared to age-matched control acinar cells.

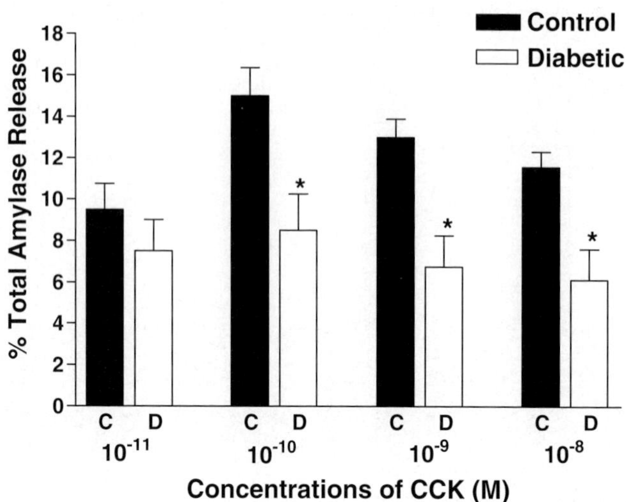

FIGURE 2. Effect of CCK-8 on amylase release. Bar charts showing the effects of different concentrations (10^{-11}–10^{-8} M) of CCK-8 on amylase release from isolated pancreatic acini and acinar cells in age-matched control and diabetic rats. Data are mean ± SEM ($n = 6$–8 rats). $^{*}P < 0.05$ for diabetic compared to control. Note that diabetic pancreas secreted significantly less amylase in response to CCK-8 compared to control.

$[Ca^{2+}]_c$ in Normal and Diabetic Pancreatic Acinar Cells

FIGURE 3A shows original chart recordings of the mean time course of CCK-8 (10^{-8} M)-evoked $[Ca^{2+}]_c$ in fura-2-loaded pancreatic acinar cells of age-matched control and diabetic rats. The results show that CCK-8 can evoke a rapid initial peak response followed by a decline to a plateau phase of $[Ca^{2+}]_c$. The mean (± SEM; $n = 40$ cells from 6 control and 6 diabetic rats) basal, peak, and plateau phases of $[Ca^{2+}]_c$ are shown in FIGURE 3 B. The results show a small decrease in basal $[Ca^{2+}]_c$ in diabetic pancreatic acinar cells (169.5 ± 4.6 nM; $n = 138$) compared to control (246.9 ± 7.5 nM; $n = 98$). The initial peak response in the presence of CCK-8 in control pancreatic acinar cells was significantly ($P < 0.05$) higher (3297.8 ± 349.5 nM; $n = 40$ cells) compared to diabetic cells (2052.9 ± 146.6 nM; $n = 40$ cells). Similarly, the plateau values for control and diabetic acinar cells 5 min following CCK-8 application was 360.7 ± 22.3 nM ($n = 40$ cells) and 271.5 ± 14.8 nM ($n = 40$ cells), respectively.

FIGURE 4 A shows mean original chart recording of CCK-8 (10^{-8} M)-evoked $[Ca^{2+}]_c$ in the continuous presence of 10^{-6} M insulin in age-matched control and diabetic pancreatic acinar cells. The mean (± SEM) basal, peak, and plateau phases of $[Ca^{2+}]_c$ are shown in FIGURE 4 B. The results show that insulin alone had no significant effect on $[Ca^{2+}]_c$ in either control or diabetic

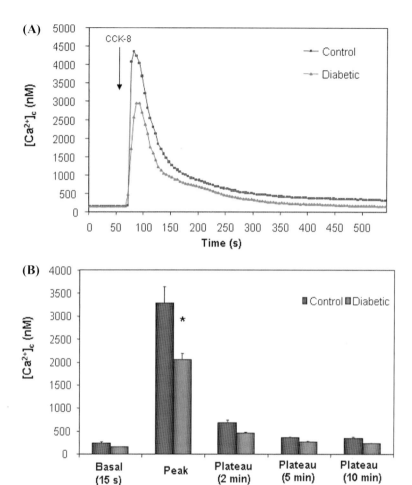

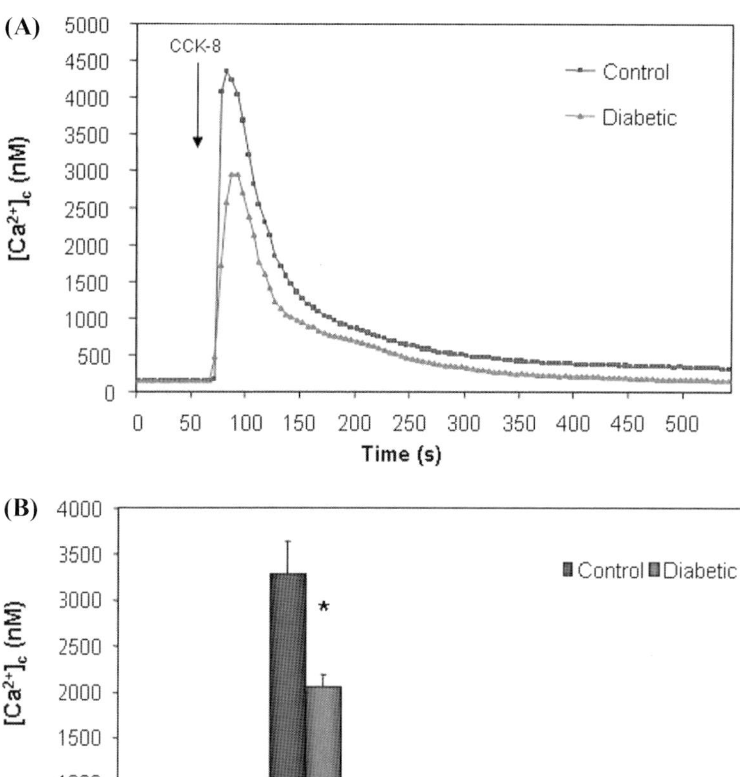

FIGURE 3. Effect of CCK-8 on $[Ca^{2+}]_c$. (**A**) Mean time course of CCK-8 (10^{-8} M)-evoked $[Ca^{2+}]_c$ in fura-2-loaded pancreatic acinar cells in age-matched control and STZ-induced diabetic rats. Traces are average of 40 different cells each from 6 control and 6 diabetic rats, respectively. (**B**) Bar charts showing the CCK-8-evoked (mean ± SEM) peak and plateau phases of $[Ca^{2+}]_c$ in age-matched control and diabetic rats (n = 6–8). $^*P < 0.05$.

acinar cells. However, in healthy age-matched control acinar cells, insulin significantly ($P < 0.05$) enhanced the effect of CCK-8 (4087.8 ± 524.4 nM; $n = 25$ cells) compared to CCK-8 application alone (3297.8 ± 349.5 nM; $n =$ 40 cells). In diabetic pancreatic acinar cells the CCK-8-evoked peak response was significantly ($P < 0.05$) less (1856.0 ± 250.1 nM, $n = 25$ cells) in the presence of insulin compared to healthy control. Insulin had little or no effect on the CCK-8-evoked plateau phase of the Ca^{2+} transient.

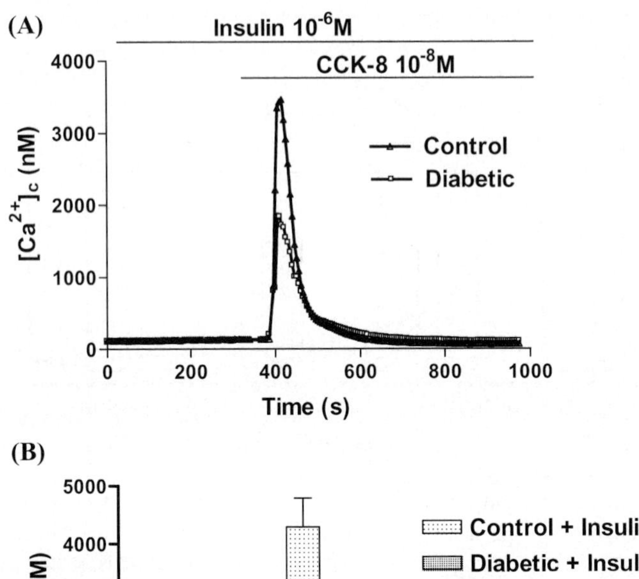

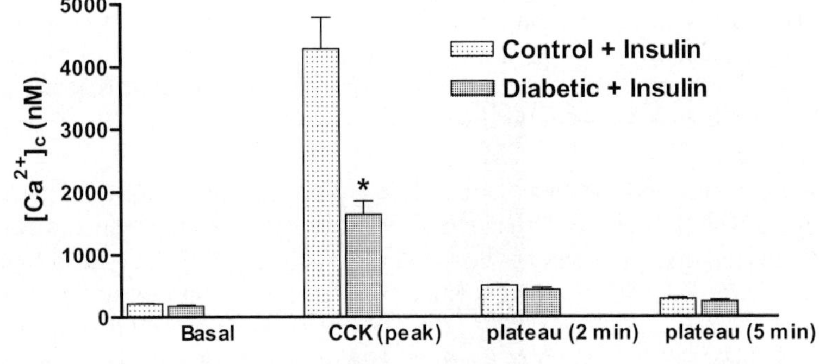

FIGURE 4. Effect of insulin and CCK-8-evoked $[Ca^{2+}]_c$ in normal and diabetic pancreatic acinar cells. (**A**) Mean time course of CCK-8 (10^{-8} M)-evoked $[Ca^{2+}]_c$ in fura-2-loaded pancreatic acinar cells in age-matched control and STZ-induced diabetic rats in the presence of 10^{-6} M insulin. Traces are average of 25 cells each from 6–8 control and 6–8 diabetic rats, respectively. (**B**) Bar charts showing the CCK-8-evoked (mean $\pm$ SEM) peak and plateau phases of $[Ca^{2+}]_c$ in normal and diabetic rats in the presence of 10^{-6} M insulin. ($n = 6$–8). $^*P < 0.05$.

In another series of experiments, extracellular Ca^{2+} concentration ($[Ca^{2+}]_o$) was nominally reduced and 1 mM EGTA was added to the superfusing medium. Basal $[Ca^{2+}]_c$ in zero $[Ca^{2+}]_c$ was 226.10 $\pm$ 14.40 nM , $n = 40$ and 161.90 $\pm$ 16.91 nM, $n = 40$ in control and diabetic acinar cells, respectively. The mean ($\pm$ SEM) CCK-8- evoked peak $[Ca^{2+}]_c$ was 2456.5 $\pm$ 228.2 nM ($n = 40$ cells) and 988.4 $\pm$ 120.5 nM ($n = 40$ cells) in control and diabetic pancreatic acinar cells, respectively. The plateau phases of $[Ca^{2+}]_c$ in control and diabetic state returned rapidly to control level and remained more or less the same as the prestimulated basal value.

The areas under the original traces were calculated to determine the total amount of $[Ca^{2+}]_c$ elevated above basal level following 5 min of CCK-8

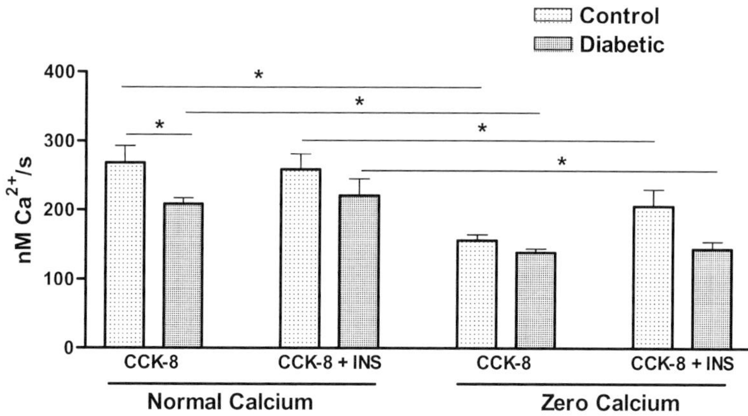

FIGURE 5. Integral of rise above basal in $[Ca^{2+}]_c$ during 5 min of CCK-8 stimulation. Bar charts showing the integral of rise above basal in $[Ca^{2+}]_c$ following 5 min of CCK-8 stimulation of age-matched healthy control and STZ-induced diabetic acinar cells in the absence and presence of 10^{-6} M insulin (INS) during normal $[Ca^{2+}]_o$ and nominally free $[Ca^{2+}]_o$ + 1 mM EGTA. Data are mean ± SEM, $n = 25$–40 cells in each bar chart taken from 6 control and 6–8 diabetic rats. $^*P < 0.05$.

stimulation under the different experimental conditions. FIGURE 5 shows the mean (± SEM) total $[Ca^{2+}]_c$ during stimulation of age-matched control and STZ-induced diabetic acinar cells with either 10^{-8} M CCK-8 alone or in combination with 10^{-6} M insulin in normal $[Ca^{2+}]_o$ and in a nominally free $[Ca^{2+}]_o$ medium containing 1 mM EGTA. The results show that diabetic acinar cells contain significantly ($P < 0.05$) less amount of $[Ca^{2+}]_c$ compared to control in normal $[Ca^{2+}]_o$. However, when $[Ca^{2+}]_o$ was removed and 1 mM EGTA was added to the superfusing medium, $[Ca^{2+}]_c$ was significantly ($P < 0.05$) reduced in age-matched control acinar cells similar to that seen in diabetic acinar cells in normal $[Ca^{2+}]_o$. These results clearly show that diabetes is associated with not only a significant ($P < 0.05$) decrease in CCK-8-evoked Ca^{2+} release from intracellular stores, but also a reduction in its influx into pancreatic acinar cells.

Gene Expression for CCK$_A$ Receptor and α-Amylase

FIGURE 6 A shows blots of CCK_A receptor cDNA in control and diabetic rat pancreas. The RT-PCR amplification product of CCK_A receptor is shown in FIGURE 6 B. There are no differences between the diabetic and the control animal in the intensity of bands of the amplified CCK_A receptor from the electrophoresis results, nor in the crossing over values obtained from the real time PCR of 20.92 ± 0.04 ($n = 8$) and 21.52 ± 0.18 ($n = 7$) for control and diabetic rats, respectively. These results show that STZ-induced diabetes is not

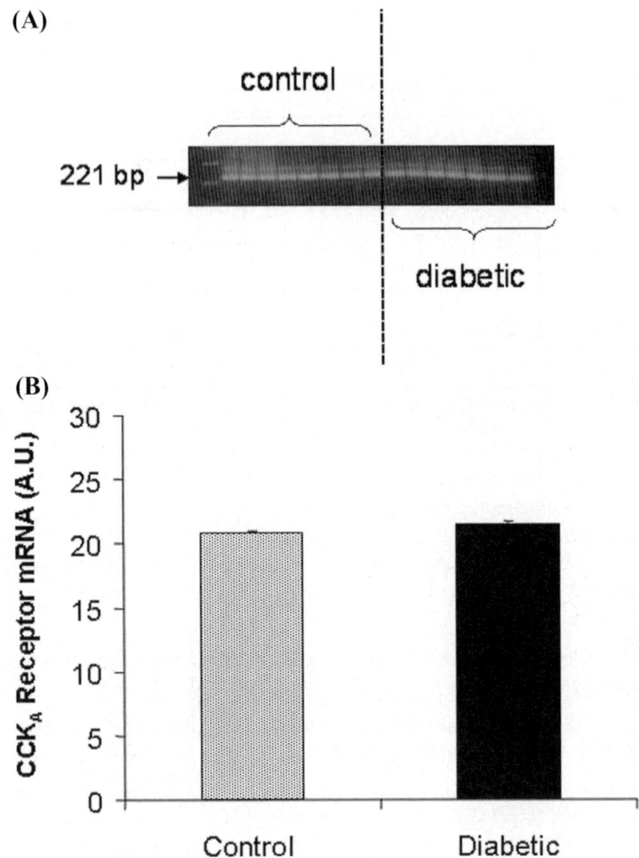

FIGURE 6. Gene expression for CCK_A receptor mRNA in control and diabetic pancreas. (**A**) Electrophoresis of PCR products stained with ethidium bromide showing unchanged CCK_A receptor cDNA between diabetic and control pancreas ($n = 8$). (**B**) Quantitative lightcycler output showing pancreatic CCK_A receptor mRNA is unchanged following 6–8 weeks of STZ-induced diabetes compared to age-matched control ($n = 7$).

associated with a decrease in CCK_A receptor mRNA levels since the values were the same in both control and diabetic conditions. Since diabetes has no effect on the gene expression of the CCK_A receptor in pancreatic acinar cells, the next logical step was to measure gene expression for α-amylase since its output is decreased during diabetes. FIGURE 7 shows the blots for α-amylase cDNA (panel A) and the quantitative light cycler output of α-amylase mRNA (panel B) in healthy control and STZ-induced diabetic acinar cells. The results show that diabetes is associated with a significant ($P < 0.05$) decrease in gene expression (transcription) of α-amylase. Healthy control pancreas had significantly ($P < 0.05$) more crossover value (17.96 ± 0.27, $n = 8$) compared to the diabetic pancreas (8.54 ± 0.13, $n = 7$)

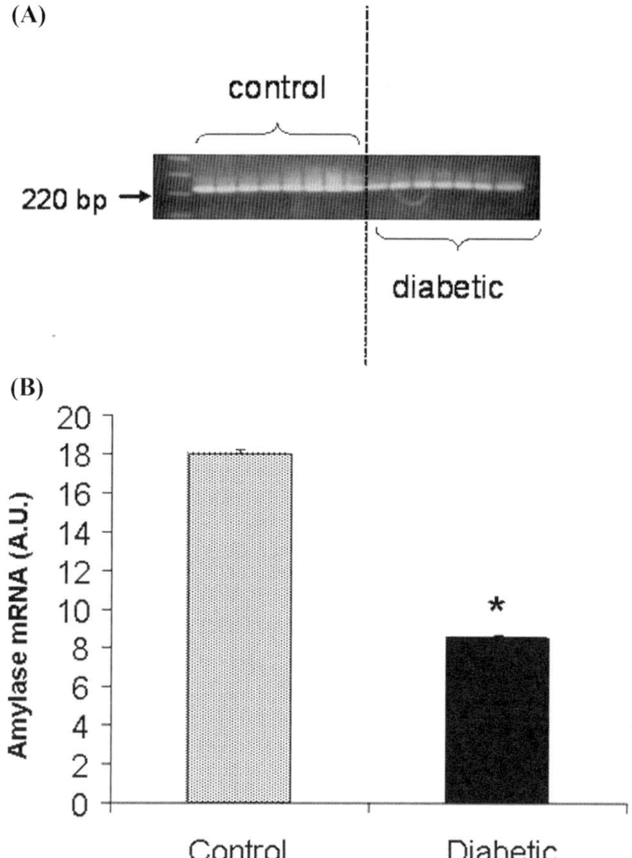

FIGURE 7. Gene expression for amylase mRNA in control and diabetic pancreas. (**A**) Electrophoresis of PCR products stained with DNA binding ethidium bromide showing less amylase cDNA in diabetic samples compared to control ($n = 8$). (**B**) Quantitative lightcycler output showing that amylase mRNA is reduced greater than twofold after 6–8 weeks of STZ-induced diabetes compared to control ($n = 7$). $^{*}P < 0.05$.

DISCUSSION

The results of this investigation have shown marked differences in the characteristics of the diabetic rats compared to healthy age-matched control. STZ is a diabetogenic agent that elevated blood glucose (hyperglycemia) within 4–5 days following its injection.[20] This is due to partial destruction of β cells of the endocrine pancreas.[29] Blood glucose remained elevated throughout the time course of the diabetes and this was associated with reduced plasma insulin levels.[12] Diabetic rats and the pancreas gained significantly less weight compared to control. Diabetic animals eat less and this in turn may lead to reduced body and pancreatic weights.[29] The results have also demonstrated marked functional changes in the pancreas during the induction of diabetes mellitus compared to healthy controls.

Amylase is produced mainly by the exocrine pancreas (40%) and the salivary parotid (55%) glands.[3,4,12,30–33] Amylase is responsible for the digestion of carbohydrates. Failure of the exocrine pancreas to secrete an adequate amount of amylase will result in exocrine pancreatic insufficiency leading to maldigestion, malnutrition, and subsequently weight loss.[15] The results of this study have shown that both EFS and CCK-8 can evoke marked increases in amylase output from the pancreas. Combining insulin with either EFS or CCK-8 resulted in an enhancement of amylase output. These responses were significantly reduced when the animals were rendered diabetic with STZ. It is particularly noteworthy that the diabetogenic agent when applied either alone or in combination with secretagogue has no effect on amylase secretion suggesting that reduced amylase output in not due to STZ but rather to the diabetes itself.[31] Taken together, the results clearly indicate that STZ-induced diabetes is associated with either an impairment of the amylase-releasing mechanism (exocytosis) and/or its synthesis and that endogenous insulin is the mainstay in the processes since short-term insulin treatment *in vivo* can reverse the pancreatic insufficiency in diabetic animals.[34,35]

The cellular and molecular mechanisms for reduced amylase output or exocrine pancreatic insufficiency are still not fully understood. Previous studies have suggested a number of mechanisms including the impairment of cellular Ca^{2+} and Mg^{2+} homeostasis,[4,9,12] insensitivity of CCK-8 receptors on pancreatic acinar cells,[17,18] decreases in amylase mRNA content,[36–39] and a reduction in ^{3}H-glucose uptake and incorporation of ^{3}H-leucine and the activity of Na^+:K^+ ATPase in pancreatic acinar cells.[40]

This study employed single acinar cells to study CCK-8-evoked Ca^{2+} homeostasis in control and diabetic pancreas. The results have clearly demonstrated that both the basal and CCK-8-evoked $[Ca^{2+}]_c$ either in the absence or presence of exogenous insulin are markedly increased in healthy control pancreatic acinar cells. In contrast, in STZ-induced diabetic pancreatic acinar cells, both the basal and CCK-8- induced $[Ca^{2+}]_c$ were significantly attenuated compared to acinar cells from healthy age-matched control pancreas. These results obtained in diabetic acinar cells are more or less similar to those obtained in control acinar cells in a nominally free $[Ca^{2+}]_o$ during the presence of 1 mM EGTA. These data suggest that diabetes interferes with cellular Ca^{2+} homeostasis, both its release from intracellular stores and its entry into pancreatic acinar cells. These results are in agreement with our previous studies employing suspension of acinar cells and in which, genistein, an inhibitor of tyrosine kinase inhibited the ACh and CCK-8-evoked Ca^{2+} transient.[4,16,41]

Since Ca^{2+} is the trigger and the initiator of the stimulus-secretion coupling process in pancreatic acinar cells,[42,43] it is tempting to suggest that diabetes interferes with the exocytosis mechanisms. Ca^{2+} in combination with Mg^{2+} and insulin may also be involved with not only the release mechanism of amylase but also with its synthesis. In a previous study, we have shown that $[Mg^{2+}]_c$ was significantly reduced during STZ-induced diabetes mellitus.[12] Moreover, both insulin and CCK are growth factors during cellular regulation.[44–46] It is conceivable that either insensitivity and/or expression of the CCK-8 receptors on acinar cells or insulin deficiency can lead to reduced amylase synthesis and subsequent release.

The results of the present study have demonstrated that diabetes has no significant effect on the gene expression of CCK_A receptors in pancreatic acinar cells. These findings indicate that the diabetic pancreas can synthesize CCK_A receptors similar to healthy control animals. However, although the receptors are present in normal amount, they may still be insensitive to CCK as demonstrated by other workers.[17,18] Finally, the results of this study have shown that diabetes is associated with a significant reduction in amylase mRNA compared to control suggesting that the gene expression for amylase is decreased during diabetes. These data are in agreement with other studies in which levels of pancreatic amylase mRNA progressively decreased in rats rendered diabetic with STZ and that the administration of insulin could reverse this effect.[35–37,47] The mechanism whereby insulin exerts its effect on amylase transcription is still unknown. It is possible that both Ca^{2+} and Mg^{2+} are involved in the process since both of them are decreased during diabetes. Mg^{2+} is involved in several biochemical and physiological processes including the synthesis and replication of DNA and RNA and it is also a cofactor for over 300 enzymes.[48–50] In addition to reduced amylase transcription, it is possible that reduced translation of amylase mRNA and CCK_A receptor mRNA may also occur in diabetes. CCK-8 has been shown to activate the PI3 kinase pathway, which mediates translation initiation. If the level of CCK is reduced in diabetes then this in turn will have adverse effect on amylase synthesis and possible release.

In conclusion, the results of this study have shown that STZ-induced diabetes mellitus is associated with significant decreases in amylase secretion, cytosolic free Ca^{2+} concentrations, and gene expression for amylase mRNA but not for CCK_A receptor. It is postulated that the decrease in cellular Ca^{2+} may lead to a derangement in amylase gene expression and synthesis and subsequently its release from pancreatic acinar cells.

ACKNOWLEDGMENTS

This work was supported by MEC (Grant BFU2004-00165) and Junta de Extremadura-FEDER (Grant 2PR04A009).

REFERENCES

1. WILLIAMS, J.A. & I.D. GOLDFINE. 1993. The insulin-acinar relationship. *In* The Exocrine Pancreas: Biology, Pathology and Disease. V.L.W. Go, E.P. DiMango, J.D. Gardner, E. Lebenthal & G.A. Scheele, Eds.: 789–792. Raven Press. New York.

2. YAGO, M.D., E. ADEGHATE & J. SINGH. 1998. Interactions between the endocrine and exocrine pancreas. Effects of islet hormones, secretagogues and nerve stimulation. *In* Neural Regulation in the Vertebrate Endocrine System: neuroendocrine Regulation. R.A. Prasada Rao & R. Peters, Eds.: 197–217. Kluwer Academic Publishers/Plenum Press. New York.
3. PATEL, R., M. D. YAGO, M. MANAS, *et al.* 2004. Interactions of islet peptides with cholecystoknin-octapeptide in normal and diabetic pancreas. Curr. Top. Rep. Prot. Res. **6:** 47–56.
4. SINGH, J., E. ADEGHATE, S. APARICIO & R. HOPKIN. 2004. Exocrine pancreatic insufficiency in diabetes mellitus. Int. J. Diabetes Metab. **12:** 35–43.
5. RICHENS, C.A. 1945. The innervation of the pancreas. J. Comp. Neurol. **82:** 223–236.
6. LENNINGER, S. 1974. The autonomic innervation of the endocrine pancreas. Med. Clin. North Am. **58:** 1311–1318.
7. PEARSON, G.T., J. SINGH & O.H. PETERSEN. 1984. Adrenergic control of cyclic AMP-mediated amylase secretion in rat pancreas. Am. J. Physiol. **246:** 6563–6573.
8. SINGH, J., R. LENNARD, G.M. SALIDO, *et al.* 1992. Interaction between secretin and cholecystokinin-octapeptide in the exocrine pancreas *in vivo* and *in vitro*. Exp. Physiol. **77:** 191–204.
9. SINGH, J., M.D. YAGO & E. ADEGHATE. 2001. Involvement of cellular calcium in exocrine pancreatic insufficiency during streptozotocin-induced diabetes mellitus. Arch. Physiol. Biochem. **109:** 252–259.
10. CHEY, W.Y. 1993. Hormonal control of exocrine pancreatic secretion. *In* The Exocrine Pancreas: Biology, Pathology and Disease, V.L.W. Go, E.P. DiMango, J.D. Gardener, E. Lebenthal & G. Scheele, Eds.: 301–314. Raven Press. New York.
11. HOLST, J.D. 1993. Neural regulation of the exocrine pancreas. *In* The Exocrine Pancreas: Biology, Pathology and Disease. V.L.W. Go, E.P. DiMango, J.D. Gardener, E. Lebenthal and G.A. Scheele, Eds.: 381–402. Raven Press. New York.
12. PATEL, R., M.D. YAGO, M. MANAS, *et al.* 2004. Mechanism of pancreatic insufficiency in streptozotocin-induced diabetes mellitus in rat: effect of cholecystokinin octapeptide. Mol. Cell. Biochem. **261:** 83–89.
13. PATEL, R., J. SINGH, M.D. YAGO, *et al.* 2004. Effect of insulin on pancreatic juice secretion in healthy and diabetic anaesthetized rat. Mol. Cell. Biochem. **261:** 105–110.
14. OWYANG, C. 1993. Endocrine changes in pancreatic insufficiency. *In* The Exocrine Pancreas: Biology, Pathology and Disease. V.L.W. Go, E.P. DiMango, J.D. Gardener, E. Lebenthal & G.A. Scheele, Eds.: 803–813. Raven Press. New York.
15. KUMAR, P.J. & M. CLARK. 2002. Diabetes mellitus and other disorders of metabolism. *In* Clinical Medicine. P.J. Kumar & M. Clark, Eds.: 1069–1121. Saunders. London.
16. SINGH, J., E. ADEGHATE, G.M. SALIDO, *et al.* 1999. Interactions of islet hormones with cholecystokinin-octapeptide in the isolated pancreas of normal and diabetic rats. Exp. Physiol. **84:** 299–318.
17. OTSUKI, M., T. AKIYAMA, H. SHIROHARA, *et al.* 1995. Loss of sensitivity to cholecystokinin stimulation of isolated pancreatic acini from genetically diabetic rats. Am. J. Physiol. **268:** E531–E536.
18. OKABAYASHI, Y., M. OTSUKI, T. NAKAMURA, *et al.* 1990. Regulatory effect of cholecystokinin on subsequent insulin binding to pancreatic acini. Am. J. Physiol. **288:** E562–E568.

19. PATEL, R., J.A. PARIENTE, A.L. LAJAS, *et al.* 2005. CCK-8-evoked calcium transport and gene expression for α-amylase and CCK_A receptor mRNA in pancreatic acinar cells of control and diabetic rats. J. Physiol. 565P, PC111.
20. SHARMA, A.K., I.G.M. DUGUID, D.S. BLANCHARD & P.K. THOMAS. 1985. The effects of insulin treatment on myelinated nerve fibre maturation and integrity and on body growth in streptozotocin-diabetic rats. J. Neurol. Sci. **67:** 285–297.
21. RINDERKNECHT, H. & E.P. MARBACH. 1972. A new automated method for the determination of serum alpha-amylase. Clin. Chim. Acta **29:** 107–110.
22. GONZALEZ, A., P.J. CAMELLO, J.A. PARIENTE & G.M. SALIDO. 1997. Free cytosolic calcium levels modify intracellular pH in rat acini. Biochem. Biophys. Res. Commun. **230:** 652–656.
23. PARIENTE, J.A., C. CAMELLO, P.J. CAMELLO & G.M. SALIDO. 2001. Release of calcium from mitochondrial and non-mitochondrial intracellular stores in mouse pancreatic acinar cells by hydrogen peroxide. J. Membr. Biol. **179:** 27–35.
24. HERZOG, V., H. SIES & F. MILLER. 1976. Exocytosis in secretory cells of rat lacrimal gland. J. Cell Biol. **70:** 692–706.
25. CESKA, M., K. BIRATH & B. BROWN. 1969. A new and rapid method for the clinical determination of alpha-amylase activities in human serum and urine. Optimal conditions. Clin. Chim. Acta **26:** 437–444.
26. GRYNKIEWICZ, G., M. POENIE & R.Y. TSIEN. 1985. A new generation of Ca^{2+} indicators with greatly improved fluorescence properties. J. Biol. Chem. **260:** 3440–3450.
27. MACDONALD, R.J., M.M. CRERAR, W.F. SWAIN, *et al.* 1980. Structure of a family of rat amylase genes. Nature **11:** 117–122.
28. CHOMCZYNSKI, P. & N. SACCHI. 1987. Single-step method of RNA isolation by acid guanidinium thiocyanate-phenol-chloroform extraction. Anal. Biochem. **162:** 156–159.
29. AHMED, I., E. ADEGHATE, A.K. SHARMA, *et al.* 1998. Effect of *Momordica charantia* fruit juice in islet morphology in the pancreas of streptozotocin-induced diabetic rat. Diab. Res. Clin. Pract. **40:** 145–151.
30. VANDER, A., J. SHERMAN & D. LUCIANIO. 2001. The digestion and absorption of food. *In*: Human Physiology: The Mechanism of Body Function. 553–592. McGraw Hill. London.
31. MAHAY, S., E. ADEGHATE, M.Z. LINDLEY, *et al.* 2004a. Streptozotocin-induced type 1 diabetes mellitus on the morphology, secretory function and acyl lipid contents in the isolated rat parotid salivary gland. Mol. Cell. Biochem. **261:** 175–181.
32. MAHAY, S., J.A. PARIENTE, A.I. LAJAS, *et al.* 2004b. Effects of ageing on morphology, amylase release, cytosolic Ca^{2+} signals and acyl lipids in isolated rat parotid gland tissues. Mol. Cell. Biochem. **266:** 199–208.
33. MATA, A.D., D. MARQUES, S. ROCHA, *et al.* 2004. Effects of diabetes mellitus in salivary secretion and its composition in humans. Mol. Cell. Biochem. **261:** 137–142.
34. VERCH, R.L., S. WALLACH, R. TAYLOR & R. AGRAWAL. 1984. Pancreatic exocrine function and cyclic nucleotides in the diabetic rat. J. Am. Coll. Nutr. **3:** 61–67.
35. SANKARAN, H., Y. IWAMOTO, M. KORC, *et al.* 1981. Insulin action in pancreatic acini from streptozotocin-induced diabetic rats: Binding of ^{125}Insulin to receptors. Am. J. Physiol. **240:** G63–G68.
36. DUAN, R.D. & C. ERLANSON-ALBERTSSON. 1990. Altered synthesis of some secretory proteins in pancreatic lobules isolated from streptozotocin-induced diabetic rats. Pancreas **5:** 136–143.

37. DUAN, R.D. & C. ERLANSON-ALBERTSSON. 1992. The effect of pretranslational regulation on synthesis of pancreatic colipase in streptozotocin-induced diabetes in rat. Pancreas **7:** 465–471.
38. KIM, S.K., L.M. CUZZORT & E.D. ALLEN. 1991. Effects of age on diabetes- and insulin-induced changes in pancreatic levels of alpha-amylase and its mRNA. Mech. Ageing Dev. **58:** 151–161.
39. DUAN, R.D., Y. CHENG & C. ERLANSON-ALBERTSSON. 1992. Effect of emertamine on exocrine and endocrine pancreatic function in normal and diabetic rats. Scand. J. Clin. Lab. Invest. **52:** 579–584.
40. YANG, Y.K. & W.Y. ZHU. 1995. Effect of insulin on the function of the exocrine pancreas. Sheng. Li. Xue. Bao. **47:** 238–244.
41. Juma, L.M., J. SINGH, D.J. PALLOT, *et al.* 1997. Interactions of islet hormones with acetylcholine in the isolated rat pancreas. Peptides **18:** 1415–1422.
42. PETERSEN, O.H. 1992. Stimulus-secretion coupling: cytoplasmic calcium signals and control of channels in exocrine acinar cells. J. Physiol. **448:** 1–51.
43. PARIENTE, J.A., P.C. REDONDO, M.P. GRANADOS, *et al.* 2003. Calcium signalling in non-excitable cells. J. E. C. Qua. L. **1:** 29–43.
44. FUNAKOSHI, A. 1996. Cholecystokinin and cholecystokinin receptor. Nippon. Rinsho. **4:** 1097–1103.
45. FUNAKOSHI, A., K. MIYASAKA, A. JIMI, *et al.* 1994. Little or no expression of the cholecystokinin-A receptor gene in the pancreas of diabetic rats (Otsuka Long-Evans Tokushima Fatty = OLETF rats). Biochem. Biophys. Res. Comm. **199:** 482–488.
46. SESTI, G., M. FEDERECI, M.L. HRIBAL, *et al.* 2001. Defects of insulin receptors substrate (IRS) system in human metabolic disorders. FASEB J. **15:** 2099–2111.
47. TSAI, A., M.R. COWAN, D.G. JOHNSON & P.M. BRANNON. 1994. Regulation of pancreatic amylase and lipase gene expression by diet and insulin in diabetic rats. Am. J. Physiol. **267:** G575–G583.
48. FLATMAN, P.W. 1984. Magnesium transport across cell membranes. J. Membr. Biol. **80:** 1–14.
49. BIRCH, N.J. 1993. Magnesium and the Cell. Academic Press. London.
50. YAGO, M.D., M. MANAS & J. SINGH. 2000. Intracellular magnesium Transport and regulation in epithelial secretory cells. Front. Biosci. **5:** 602–618.

Inflammatory Process in Type 2 Diabetes

The Role of Cytokines

KRYSTALLENIA ALEXANDRAKI,[a] CHRISTINA PIPERI,[a] CHRISTOS KALOFOUTIS,[a] JAIPAUL SINGH,[b] ANTONIS ALAVERAS,[a] AND ANASTASIOS KALOFOUTIS[a]

[a]*Laboratory of Biological Chemistry, University of Athens Medical School, Goudi 11527, Athens, Greece*

[b]*Department of Biological Sciences, University of Central Lancashire, Preston PR1 2HE, UK*

ABSTRACT: Population-based studies have shown strong relationship between inflammatory markers and metabolic disturbances, obesity, and atherosclerosis, whereas inflammation has been considered as a "common soil" between these clinical entities and type 2 diabetes (T2D). The accumulation of macrophages in adipose tissue (AT), the common origin of macrophages and adipocytes, the prevalent presence of peripheral mononuclear cells, and apoptotic β cells by themselves seem to be the sources of inflammation present in T2D, since they generate the mediators of the inflammatory processes, namely cytokines. The main cytokines involved in the pathogenesis of T2D are interleukin-1β (IL-1β), with an action similar to the one present in type 1 diabetes, tumor necrosis factor-α (TNF-α), and IL-6, considered as the main regulators of inflammation, leptin, more recently introduced, and several others, such as monocyte chemoattractant protein-1, resistin, adiponectin, with either deleterious or beneficial effects in diabetic pathogenesis. The characterization of these molecules targeted diabetes treatment beyond the classical interventions with lifestyle changes and pharmaceutical agents, and toward the determination of specific molecular pathways that lead to low grade chronic inflammatory state mainly due to an immune system's unbalance.

KEYWORDS: type 2 diabetes mellitus; inflammation; cytokines

INTRODUCTION

In the last decade it has been suggested that mechanisms involved in the acute-phase inflammatory response and the activation of the innate immune

Address for correspondence: Christina Piperi, Laboratory of Biological Chemistry, University of Athens Medical School, M. Asias 75, Goudi 11527, Athens, Greece. Voice: 30-210-7462610; fax: 30-210-8037372.
e-mail: cpiperi@med.uoa.gr

**Ann. N.Y. Acad. Sci. 1084: 89–117 (2006). © 2006 New York Academy of Sciences.
doi: 10.1196/annals.1372.039**

system may underlie the pathological processes of type 2 diabetes (T2D) as well as the clinical entities associated with T2D, such as insulin resistance, dyslipidemia, hypertension, atherosclerosis, and central obesity.[1] Acute-phase response consists of a series of physiological reactions initiated in response to tissue damage and infection and it is carried out by acute-phase proteins secreted primarily from hepatocytes, mainly represented by the C-reactive protein (CRP).[2] CRP is considered an independent predictor of cardiovascular complications with a potential role in the pathogenesis of atherosclerotic lesions,[3–8] and has been extensively evaluated for its association with risk factors for development of T2D.[9] These original observations have led to further studies of inflammation presence and contribution in T2D pathology.

Inflammation in T2D

In the last decade, besides the known involvement of inflammatory process in the pathogenesis of type 1 diabetes, increasing evidence suggests that individuals who progress to T2D display features of inflammation years before the disease onset and low-grade inflammation has been proposed to be involved in the pathogenetic processes causing T2D.[10–17] Population-based studies have shown strong relationship between inflammatory markers and carbohydrate and lipid metabolism abnormalities, obesity, and atherosclerosis.[18–23] Obesity and sedentary lifestyle are considered the main environmental causes for the development of insulin resistance and T2D.[24,25] Considering that T2D is a polygenic disease, defects in many molecular pathways have been demonstrated or implicated. Recent evidence suggests common molecular mechanisms between inflammatory and insulin signaling pathways,[26–28] both of which cause insulin resistance and endothelial dysfunction that synergize to predispose for cardiovascular disorders,[29] establishing the idea that diabetes and atherosclerotic diseases both come from a "common soil."[30] The presence of chronic low-grade inflammation in obese states,[31–34] in insulin resistance/T2D,[1,22,33–37] and in the early stages of atherogenesis[22,34] enhances the notion that inflammation may be the putative link that connects adipose tissue (AT) dysfunction with the metabolic and vascular pathologies.[38,39]

T2D is characterized by progressive β-cell failure and increased apoptosis, which have been considered as the main causes of reduced β-cell mass in T2D.[40] There is evidence that inflammatory mediators may not only represent markers of metabolic aberrations in T2D[5,41] but may also contribute energetically to β-cell death due to impaired function and progressive decline in β-cell function and mass.[40,42] Additionally, apoptotic cells by themselves can provoke the activation of the innate immune system[43,44] and hyperglycemia can induce β-cell expression of several molecules involved in immunological processes.[45,46] Notably, AT, which comprises several cell types (adipocytes, preadipocytes, tissue matrix, nerve tissue, stromal–vascular cells, macrophages, endothelial cells, fibroblasts[47]), was for long considered a passive tissue but, recently, its endocrine activity has been revealed. AT expresses proinflammatory mediators with auto-/paracrine or endocrine properties,[48–51] which have been found increased in human obesity and have been causally linked to insulin resistance, possibly representing mediators of the ongoing process of β-cell destruction occurring in T2D.

Regarding the investigation of the origin of the inflammatory process in T2D, recent reports have been conducted demonstrating the accumulation of macrophages in the AT of obese subjects as well as their participation in the inflammatory pathways activated in adipocytes.[52,53] Macrophages reside in human AT and their number has been found positively related with body mass index (BMI), suggesting their contribution to the dysregulation of AT as well as to the impairment of adipocytes function. These macrophages besides being source of proinflammatory factors, may also modulate the activity of adipocytes in their products secretion, a hypothesis that has been supported by both animal and human studies.[52,53] In the AT of obese mice, macrophages from multinucleated giant cells are reminiscent of those present in granulomas, suggesting an activated phenotype.[52,53] On the other hand, another source of the circulating inflammatory proteins of tissue macrophages could be mononuclear cells since the latter are derived from the former. The peripheral blood mononuclear cells of obese subjects, have been shown to be in an inflammatory state, expressing increased amounts of proinflammatory cytokines and related factors with an increase in the transcription of proinflammatory genes regulated by the nuclear factor-κB (NF-κB),[54] the central proinflammatory transcription factor as well as an increase in the intranuclear expression of p65 (Rel A), the major protein component of NF-κB. These cells also express diminished amounts of the inhibitor κB (IκB) β, which is the inhibitor of NF-κB activation.[55] Another interesting finding consists in the similarities noticed between macrophages and adipocytes.[56] In fact, preadipocytes, the progenitors of mature adipocytes, could be transdifferentiated into macrophages under experimental conditions.[57] This hypothesis fits well with the observation that monocyte chemoattractant protein-1 (MCP-1), a proinflammatory chemokine mainly produced by macrophages and endothelial cells, can be secreted from isolated adipocytes.[58,59] However, adipose macrophages were shown to be predominantly derived from bone marrow and developed from circulating monocytes infiltrating AT.[52] Consequently, the enlarged adipocytes can become inflammatory and increase their secretion of cytokines which, in turn, can lead to the recruitment of macrophages to the AT.[60] More than 90% of all macrophages in white AT of obese mice and humans have been reported to form multinucleate giant cells, a hallmark of chronic inflammation.[61] Consequently, adipose inflammation in obesity appears to have features of a typical macrophage-mediated chronic inflammatory response[62] and the macrophage-mediated inflammation in obesity appears to take place prevalently in AT.[53] Therefore, cytokines and chemokines secreted from AT are the larger source of inflammatory factors leading to the systemic inflammation.[9] These findings, altogether, underline the AT dysregulation in the pathogenesis of insulin resistance and the resulting low-grade chronic systemic inflammation in insulin-resistance states, such as T2D.

Cytokines Involvement in T2D

From all the above hypotheses, T2D has been suggested to compose the final result of an acute-phase reaction during which cytokines are released in large amounts from AT,[1] as well as from macrophages recruited into AT, sustaining inflammation and impaired adipocyte function.[53] In turn, cytokines also inhibit the differentiation of the preadipocytes and induce an inflammatory phenotype in these cells, which, can attract and recruit inflammatory cells to AT.[60]

Cytokines are a group of pharmacologically active low molecular weight proteins that possess autocrine and paracrine effects[63] and are known products and effectors of the inflammatory and immune system.[64] When they are produced locally in the inflamed plaques, as frequently seen in patients with not well-controlled diabetes they exert prothrombotic effects on endothelial cells, may increase directly capillary permeability and cause oxidative stress and endothelial dysfunction, further aggravating the atherosclerotic process.[11]

On the other hand, AT represents an endocrine organ that secretes large numbers of cytokines, called adipokines (including tumor necrosis factor-α [TNF-α], interleukin-6 [IL-6], IL-8, MCP-1, CRP, plasminogen activator inhibitor type 1 [PAI-1], adiponectin, haptoglobin, complement proteins like complement 3, adipsin[60]), which communicate with brain and peripheral tissues to regulate energy homeostasis and metabolism.[1,65] These cytokines induce the liver to produce acute-phase proteins and at the same time may act on the pancreatic islets and impair β-cell secretory function.[11]

Obesity-mediated cytokines release is probably pivotal in increasing the circulating levels of CRP and IL-6 and in turn, both IL-6 and TNF-α increase hepatic synthesis of CRP.[11] In obesity, the proinflammatory effects of cytokines through intracellular signaling pathways involve the NF-κB and Janus kinase (JNK) systems. In diabetes, after adjustment for obesity, cytokines levels have been found consistently high,[11] implying an additive but not exclusive role of obesity on inflammatory state of diabetes.

Finally, cytokines involvement seem to have a central role in another source of inflammatory state, the apoptotic cells that can provoke an immune response when present in high enough numbers or when apoptosis is the consequence of exposure to cytokines.[43,44,66] An intense activation of the acute-phase response has been associated with islet cell autoantibodies production in patients with T2D.[67] In some T2D, when apoptosis is induced by glucose or FFA, a mobilization of T cells reactive to β-cells antigens may be shown, which depends from their age and from genetic and/or environmental factors, resulting in autoimmune destruction of β-cells similar to type 1 diabetics.[68] In this way, a vicious cycle can be created since proinflammatory cytokines, and in particular IL-1β, are thought to be important pathogenic effectors responsible for the induction of β-cell apoptosis in both types of diabetes. IL-1β, TNF-α, and interferon-γ (IFN-γ) most likely act synergically during the immune infiltration of the pancreas to induce β-cell damage and apoptosis. IL-1β secreted by activated macrophages, has been found to be also secreted by β-cells under certain circumstances.[45,69] TNF-α is solely produced and secreted by macrophages, whereas IFN-γ is secreted by T-helper cells. *In vitro*, IL-1β appears the most β-cell cytotoxic cytokine sufficient to cause inhibition of β-cell function and often sufficient to promote an apoptotic response.[68] However, massive induction of apoptosis in β-cells usually requires a combination of IL-1β plus IFN-γ and/or TNF-α.[45,46,69–72]

MAIN CYTOKINES INVOLVED IN T2D

*IL-1*β

IL-1 is the prototypical inflammatory cytokine and a critical early mediator of inflammation.[73] IL-1 has not been implicated in β-cell apoptosis in human islets as in animal experiments.[74,75] It is not clear whether this relates to the culture conditions or to the secretion of cytokines (TNF-α or IFN-γ) in these particular islet preparations. IL-1 receptor antagonist also has been suggested as physiological regulator of β-cell viability and small interfering RNAs directed against the IL-1 receptor antagonist have increased the apoptotic rate.[76] Additionally, a common signaling pathway has been suggested between glucose- and IL-1-induced β-cell apoptosis, since reduced levels of Fas-associated death domain protein-like IL-1b have been detected when apoptosis is induced by glucose in pancreases of T2D. This protein further converts the enzyme-inhibitory protein (FLIP)[77] which determines whether Fas signaling results in apoptosis or cell proliferation.[78] IL-1 also has been implicated as enhancer in the documented toxicity of NEFA.[79]

From the clinical point of view, in a prospective study it was shown that elevated concentrations of both IL-6 and IL-1β were associated with a threefold increased risk of developing diabetes compared to the control group, but when only IL-6 levels were increased and IL-1β levels undetectable, no increased risk was documented.[28,80]

TNF-α

TNF-α as well as IL-6 are considered the major adipocyte cytokines.[55] Both can impair insulin action[81] by interfering with insulin signaling[10,15,82–84] after their binding to their cognate receptor on muscle cells or on hepatocytes.

AT is the major source of TNF-α, a proinflammatory cytokine, which influences the synthesis, secretion, and activity of others cytokines[85] and has been shown to be abundantly expressed by AT as well as by endothelial, smooth muscle cells, and macrophages. It is hyperexpressed in obesity, can impair insulin sensitivity, and may stimulate lipolysis in animal models of obesity[49,86,87] as well as in obese subjects. Finally, there is evidence that in combination with other cytokines, accelerates dysfunction and destruction of the β-cells.[75,88]

An improvement of insulin sensitivity has been observed after the neutralization of TNF-α with the soluble TNF-α receptors in obese rats.[49] Mice lacking TNF-α or TNF receptors loci were protected from obesity-induced insulin resistance[28,89,90] while, TNF-α infusion caused insulin resistance *in vivo*.[91] However, the infusion of soluble TNF-α receptors in the human did not reproduce the results observed in mice.[49,92–94] This fact may be due to the administration of not sufficiently high concentrations of TNF-α antagonist or to the participation of immune mediators other than TNF-α with major role in the induction of insulin resistance in humans. It has been speculated that TNF-α is associated with the downregulation of GLUT 4 mRNA and with reduction in insulin receptor substrate-1 (IRS-1).[95,96] TNF-α has been also implicated in endothelial dysfunction pathogenesis since it has been shown to increase leukocyte adhesion to endothelium,[97] activate NFκB-dependent inflammatory pathways,[98] induce endothelial cell expression of vascular cell adhesion molecule-1 (VCAM-1) and endothelin-1 (ET-1),[99,100] induce smooth muscle expression of matrix metalloproteinases contributing in plaque destabilization[101] and suppress the expression of nitric oxide synthase (NOS).[102]

From the clinical point of view, even if it is not clear whether AT releases sufficient amounts of TNF-α into the circulation,[81] in humans, TNF-α levels are negatively related with insulin sensitivity assessed by euglycemic–hyperinsulinemic clamp.[103]

IL-6

IL-6 belongs to the IL-6 family of cytokines, which are characterized by the common use of the IL-6Rβ receptor. IL-6 receptors, IL-6Rβ, and IL-6Rα, belong to the type I cytokine receptor family.[104] Several cell types are reported to produce IL-6 including cells of the immune system, endothelial cells, skeletal and smooth muscle cells, adipocytes, islet β-cells, hepatocytes, microglial cells, astrocytes, and other cell types.[104] In the adaptive and innate immune systems, IL-6 is involved in both the amplification of and protection against inflammation.[104,105] Inappropriate regulation of IL-6 may play protective as well as deleterious role in antigen-specific immune-mediated diseases characterized by low-grade inflammation state.[5,41,104,105]

IL-6 exerts multiple stimulatory effects on cell growth and inflammation,[106] being involved in the initiation and the maintenance of the acute-phase inflammatory response, in the immunoregulation and in nonimmune events in cell types and tissues outside the immune system.[104] IL-6 affects also glucose homeostasis and metabolism directly and indirectly by action on skeletal muscle cells, adipocytes, hepatocytes, pancreatic β-cells, and neuroendocrine cells.[107] It is considered the principal procoagulant cytokine since it increases plasma concentrations of fibrinogen, PAI-1, and CRP.[108] IL-6 seems to induce hypertriglyceridemia by increasing lipolysis and hepatic triglyceride secretion *in vivo*[109] and studies have shown that IL-6 inhibits glucose-stimulated insulin secretion from rodent islets,[110–114] but the role of IL-6 in insulin resistance remains controversial.[115] IL-6 is expressed in and released from both the subcutaneous and visceral AT but with a two- to threefold higher *in vitro* release of IL-6 from visceral compared to subcutaneous adipocytes *in vitro*.[48,116] In rodents, obesity has been associated with macrophage accumulation in AT, but IL-6 has been found expressed in adipocytes more than in macrophages.[52] Its expression is thought to be stimulated in a paracrine fashion by proinflammatory mediators released. *In vitro* studies on adipocyte cell lines,[26,117–119] strongly support a role of IL-6 as causing insulin resistance in adipocyte cell lines. The suppressor's of cytokine signaling (SOCS)-3 expression has been also found increased in adipocyte cell lines exposed to IL-6 *in vitro*[83,120,121] as well as in AT of obese insulin-resistant nondiabetic individuals and it has been strongly correlated with IL-6 expression *in vivo*.[122] *In vivo* and *in vitro* studies in rodents and *in vitro* studies in human cell line provide evidence for the ability of IL-6 to reduce insulin sensitivity in hepatocytes by hampering insulin signaling.[83,123–126] Angiotensin II also has been found to increase hepatic IL-6 production in parallel with increased insulin resistance.[11] During exercise, IL-6 is released from muscle tissue beds,[127,128] and has been proposed to participate in glucose homeostasis.[122,123,128] It could be speculated that the impact of IL-6 on insulin sensitivity in skeletal muscle cells may be dependent of dose and time of exposure on IL-6.[122,124] Generally, it has been suggested that elevated levels of IL-6 may reduce insulin sensitivity by inhibiting GLUT4.[129]

A dual effect of IL-6 is also present regarding its role in apoptosis. It has been observed an *in vitro* antiapoptotic effect of IL-6 on islets and β-cell line exposed to inflammatory cytokines since IL-6 increased transcriptional activities of genes encoding mainly proapoptotic but also some antiapoptotic molecules.[113] When in combination with other cytokines, it was observed to possess cytotoxic effects on β-cells[130] and synergizes with IL-1,[112] however, increased apoptosis was not observed in transgenic mice expressing IL-6 in islets.[131,132] Additionally, IL-6$^{-/-}$ mice had identical fasting insulin levels when compared with pair-fed IL-6$^{+/+}$ littermates,[133] arguing against an independent *in vivo* effect of IL-6 on β-cell function. In healthy males challenged with IL-6,[134,135] there was no effect on serum insulin levels compared to controls and consequently an acute increase in IL-6 does not alone seem to affect β-cell function in humans.

From the clinical point of view, the positive correlation between serum levels of IL-6 and obesity[136] can be in part explained by the fact that the *in vivo* release of IL-6 from fat contributes as much as 30–35% to the basal circulating levels in humans,[116,137] and circulating levels of IL-6 are elevated years before onset of T2D, without being clarified whether this is involved in precipitating T2D. AT IL-6 mRNA has been shown to be elevated in insulin-resistant humans,[115,138] and its levels correlated with reduced rates of insulin-stimulated glucose disposal.[139] Elevated levels of IL-6 predict future risk of T2D development[20,140,141] but CRP remains a stronger predictor. Therefore, the dual effects of IL-6, result in the suggestion that the association between IL-6 and progression to T2D development may reflect an attempt to counter-regulate low-grade inflammation induced by other inflammatory mediators.

IL-6 has also effects on cerebral centers involved in regulation of energy expenditure and the hypothalamic-pituitary-adrenal axis,[142,143] and obesity in IL-6$^{-/-}$ mice was partly reversed by IL-6 replacement,[144] when administrated intracerebroventricularly, but not intraperitoneally.[143] Interestingly, in obese humans IL-6 levels in cerebrospinal fluid correlate negatively with total body fat and the cerebrospinal fluid levels are of the same magnitude or even higher than in serum,[143] suggesting that cerebrospinal fluid IL-6 is at least in part regulated independently of serum IL-6, possibly by local production in the brain.

IL-6 and TNF-α have recently been shown to induce SOCS-3.[83,120] SOCS proteins are a family of potent inhibitors of cytokine signaling involved in negative feedback loops. SOCS-1 and SOCS-6 were shown to inhibit insulin receptor signaling in adipocytes.[145] SOCS-3 expression was found increased in AT of obese mice, and it was suggested to be induced by insulin stimulation in adipocytes.[120] In liver, activation of SOCS-1 and SOCS-3 by TNF-α led to upregulation of transcription factor SREBP-1c, which in turn increased fatty acid synthesis and resulted in the development of fatty liver.[146] SOCS-3 was also found to be induced by IL-6 in hepatocytes.[107]

Leptin

Leptin, is a 16-kDa nonglycosylated peptide cytokine-like hormone, member of the IL-6 cytokine family,[147] encoded by the obese (ob) gene and mainly produced by adipocytes.[51,148] Leptin receptor (LR) is a member of the class I cytokine receptor superfamily.[149,150] Leptin possesses pleiotropic actions, being a major hormone regulating energy homeostasis[51] and is considered an anorexic peptide, having additional roles as a regulator of sexual function and of immune system, since it is has been demonstrated to be proinflammatory and to promote aggregation of platelets.[151–153] Circulating leptin levels have been correlated to AT mass and act at hypothalamic central level decreasing food intake and increasing energy consumption.[154,155] Exogenous leptin administration leads to neuroendocrine normalization and decrease in food intake both in rodents and in leptin-deficient human obese patients. However, in human clinical trials with obese subjects, the effect of exogenous leptin administration was modest.[156]

The coexistence of insulin resistance and obesity in humans has suggested an intercorrelation between leptin and insulin signaling.[157–159] In rodent islets, leptin induces β-cell proliferation and protects from FFA-induced β-cell apoptosis[160–163] but chronic exposure of human islets to leptin leads to β-cell apoptosis by reducing levels of IL-1 receptor antagonist and by increasing IL-1β synthesis and secretion.[164] In rats, overfeeding leads to insulin and leptin resistance, which both seem to be causally related.[165] Insulin seems to influence leptin mRNA expression and to increase leptin secretion by adipocytes.[166,167] Leptin can also inhibit insulin's effects on lipid oxidation and synthesis[168–170] and enhance insulin sensitivity and insulin's inhibition of hepatic glucose production in rats.[171,172] Leptin has been shown to have antidiabetic effects in diabetic rodent models.[173–175] The lipolytic effect of leptin in peripheral tissues may protect pancreatic β-cells against overaccumulation of intracellular lipids, resulting in reducing development of T2D.[176] Ob/ob leptin-deficient mice are hyperglycemic and insulin resistant, but it has not been clarified if this is a direct result of leptin deficiency or a result of increased fat mass, since peripheral administration of leptin reverses hyperglycemia and hyperinsulinemia before weight loss.[177] Ob/ob mice are resistant against diet-induced atherosclerosis[178] but atherosclerotic lesions can be induced after leptin administration.[179] Leptin also has direct effects on blood pressure[180] but its effects differ since chronic intravenous injection of leptin results in increased, and acute intravenous injection in decreased arterial pressure in rat models.[181,182] However, intracerebroventricular leptin administration in rats or in rabbits increases blood pressure through increased sympathetic nerve activity.[183,184] A positive correlation has been noticed between mean blood pressure and leptin serum levels in lean subjects with essential hypertension.[185] LR is found on the endothelium,[186] macrophages and foam cells,[187] on platelets[188] and on vascular smooth muscle cells[189] and leptin seems to affect the function of each of these cell types, carrying a proatherogenic role in almost every step of atheroma formation.[150]

Resistance to leptin action has been attributed to its reduced transport into the brain across the blood–brain barrier due to a deficit in LR isoforms.[190] An additional mechanism could be the overexpression of different leptin target genes, such as SOCS-3, which limit leptin actions both *in vitro* and *in vivo*.[191,192]

From the clinical point of view, high circulating leptin levels were shown to be an independent predictor of cardiovascular morbidity and mortality,[193–195] and hyperleptinemia has been suggested to play a central role in metabolic syndrome.[196] In population-based studies, serum leptin concentrations are positively correlated with BMI, and fasting insulin concentrations.[197] Additionally, human plasma leptin concentrations are independently associated with structural and functional vascular abnormalities.[198,199] The reduced response to leptin in obese people could be suggested by the fact that high leptin levels have no effect in appetite suppression.[149]

Leptin expression is mainly regulated by food intake and hormones. Glycolytic substrates are necessary to maintain basal leptin secretion but are not sufficient to stimulate leptin secretion as does insulin.[200] Leptin, in turn, has direct action also on lipid metabolism regulating fatty acid oxidation by interfering with a number of enzymes in hypothalamic as well as on skeletal muscle and hepatic level.[156,201] Leptin levels present positive correlation with insulin[202] and negative with glucocorticoid levels.[203] Leptin and LRs are expressed in the pituitary, particularly in corticotropic cells.[204] *In vitro* leptin reduces corticotropin-releasing hormone release induced by hypoglycemia without altering the adrenocorticotropin (ACTH) secretion[205] and in the adrenal reduces cortisol synthesis by downregulating the steroid-producing enzyme cascade in the cortical cell.[206] In turn, *in vitro* studies showed a stimulatory effect of glucocorticoids on leptin synthesis and secretion by isolated adipocytes[207] and their peripheral infusion to rats induced ob gene expression in AT.[208] In patients with leptin deficiency, plasma ACTH and cortisol levels are slightly elevated with abolition of their circadian rhythm.[209] Leptin secretion also exhibits a circadian rhythm, increasing during night, inversely related to that of cortisol and ACTH[210] and a central effect on leptin gene expression has been suggested.[201]

Additionally, leptin is regulated by immune processes[211] and infections as well as inflammatory mediators increase leptin synthesis.[210,212] Circulating leptin levels increase promptly in experimental models of acute inflammation.[211] However, a chronic stimulation with proinflammatory cytokines causes its suppression.[213,214] Inflammatory mediators like lipopolysaccharide, regulate leptin mRNA expression and its circulating levels[215]and leptin can be produced by inflammatory regulatory cells.[216] Leptin from AT is stimulated by proinflammatory cytokines, such as TNF-α and IL-1β, suggesting a short-term release of stored leptin. On the other hand, long-term treatments with proinflammatory cytokines may lower plasma leptin concentrations.[213] On the other hand, leptin is considered as an immune modulator, since LR-deficient (db/db) mice suffer from thymus atrophy.[211,217–219] Regarding innate immunity, leptin promotes phagocytic function and induces synthesis of eicosanoid, nitric oxide, and several proinflammatory cytokine production in macrophages and monocytes[220,221] while stimulates growth hormone production by peripheral blood mononuclear cells.[222] Leptin increases also IFN-γ-induced expression of NOS in murine macrophages,[223] induces chemotaxis and reactive oxygen species (ROS) release in neutrophils,[224,225] and regulates natural killer cells proliferation, differentiation, activation, and cytotoxicity.[226] Regarding adaptive immunity[219] leptin can prevent glucocorticoid-induced thymocytes apoptosis and increase thymic cellularity.[227] Leptin may also induce T cell activation and modify T cell cytokines production pattern by favoring a Th1 T cell differentiation.[228,229] Leptin administration reverts immune suppression in ob/ob mice, in acute starvation and in reduced caloric intake.[229] Consequently, leptin acts also itself as a proinflammatory cytokine regulating several cytokines secretion and macrophage activation.[230] Finally, increased serum leptin levels have been reported preceding the onset of the diabetes in nonobese diabetic (NOD) female mice[231] and leptin administration seems to increase both inflammatory infiltrates and IFN-γ production in peripheral T cells, accelerating pancreatic β-cells impairment.[232] These data also suggest that acute cytokines may provoke a rise in leptin, which in turn supports the inflammatory process through para- or autocrine actions.

MCP-1

Chemoattractant factors, such as MCP-1 and macrophage stimulatory factor, attract monocytes into vessel walls, promotes synthesis and release of proinflammatory cytokines that enhance attachment of monocytes and macrophages to vessel walls and their genes transcription is activated by NF-κB.[233] MCP-1 is one of the key chemokines responsible for monocyte recruitment into AT.[9] As other chemoattractant molecules, it activates the resident macrophages to secrete cytokines and chemokines to recruit additional monocytes and macrophages into fat resulting in a vicious cycle amplifying the inflammatory status. In mice, the expression of MCP-1 has been found increased after a high-fat diet and this rise preceded the development of hyperglycemia and hyperinsulinemia.[53,234] It has been documented that proinflammatory states that enhance innate immune signaling result in activation of NF-κB which, in turn, activates transcription of genes encoding chemoattractant factors, such as MCP, resulting in monocytes recruitment into vessel walls.[235] Angiotensin II also induces MCP-1 expression in cell culture.[236]

Others Inflammatory Mediators

Adiponectin is an adipose-specific plasma protein,[237] considered as anti-inflammatory and potentially antiatherogenic.[238] Circulating adiponectin levels are decreased in subjects with obesity-related insulin resistance, T2D, and coronary heart disease and has been found downregulated in obese/diabetic states.[238–240] Adiponectin inhibits liver neoglucogenesis, promotes fatty acid oxidation in skeletal muscle, and improves insulin sensitivity.[241] At the same time it stimulates production of nitric oxide,[242] reduces expression of adhesion molecules in endothelial cells, and decreases cytokine production from macrophages by inhibiting NF-κB signaling. It further counteracts proinflammatory effects of TNF-α on the arterial wall and suppresses the transformation of macrophages in foam cells.[230,243,244] IL-6 inhibits adiponectin expression and secretion in adipocytes.[245]

Resistin is another major adipocyte-derived hormone, expressed predominantly in white AT but also detectable in serum.[246] Studies about insulin sensitivity imply its role to insulin resistance.[245,246] Interestingly, resistin administration has been demonstrated to markedly increase SOCS-3 expression in adipocytes.[247]

The proinflammatory mediator CD40 ligand (CD40L) is expressed on CD4$^+$ T cells and activated platelets and has an important role in a cascade of inflammatory and proatherothrombotic functions.[248]

POSSIBLE THERAPEUTIC APPROACHES TO REDUCE INFLAMMATORY PROCESSES IN T2D

The documented central role of inflammation in pathogenesis of T2D resulted in extended studies and interventions to reduce the low-grade chronic inflammation. A first approach involved evaluation of pharmaceutical and nonpharmaceutical interventions already used in diabetes treatment. Another approach was to target new approaches based on newly documented molecules implicated in pathogenesis of T2D.

Body weight reduction through diet, exercise, or surgery has been proven beneficial in lowering inflammation and improving insulin sensitivity.[9] Lifestyle modifications including weight loss, exercise, or Mediterranean-style diet reduced serum concentrations of cytokines, such as TNF-α, IL-6, IL-7, IL-18, and increased adiponectin levels in diabetic or obese subjects.[249–251]

Insulin sensitizers of the thiazolidinedione class[252–254] have been shown to exert an anti-inflammatory effect in addition to their glucose-lowering effect in patients with diabetes, reducing inflammatory markers, such as TNF-α plasma levels.[255] Rosiglitazone reduces plasma MCP-1 and CRP in obese patients and diabetics.[254,256] Rosiglitazone or pioglitazone therapy significantly increases adiponectin levels in diabetic subjects[257,258] and experimental models.[259] On the other hand, it was observed that, rosiglitazone does not reduce IL-6 levels in patients with T2D compared with placebo.[256] Interestingly, rosiglitazone and troglitazone significantly potentiate TNF-α–induced production of IL-6 and/or IL-8 in epithelial cells. Although there is evidence that thiazolidinediones exert a direct anti-inflammatory effect on macrophages *in vitro*, it is possible that *in vivo*, their effect could be mediated through insulin sensitization.[55] Metformin also causes a reduction in the plasma concentrations of MIF in obese subjects.[260]

The anti-inflammatory effect of antilipidemic agents has been recently studied extensively in an effort to explain the high rates of survivals after treatment particularly with statins. TNF-α plasma levels decreased after simvastatin treatment in hyperlipidemia.[261] Simvastatin has been found to significantly lower serum IL-6 levels.[262] Exercise, either alone or in combination with pravastatin, reduces IL-8 and MCP-1 levels after 12 weeks in subjects with metabolic syndrome.[263] Fibrates, also, reduce CRP-induced expression of MCP-1 in human umbilical vein endothelial cells[264] and clinically, in patients with dyslipidemia, fenofibrate therapy decreases circulating levels of IL-6[265] and significantly increases plasma adiponectin levels and insulin sensitivity.[266]

In hypertensive patients, candesartan therapy significantly reduces plasma levels of MCP-1 compared to placebo.[267] Treatment with temocapril and candesartan significantly increases adiponectin levels as well as insulin sensitivity without affecting the degree of adiposity.[268] Losartan attenuates the effect of CRP on upregulating AT1 receptors in vascular smooth muscle cells.[269] The combination of simvastatin with ramipril or losartan significantly reduces CRP and MCP-1 levels more than monotherapy in hypercholesterolemic diabetic or in hypercholesterolemic hypertensive patients,[270–272] while the same combination increased plasma adiponectin levels.[271]

Insulin also could be anti-inflammatory and consequently antiatherogenic, since it has been shown to suppress several proinflammatory transcription factors, such as NF-κB, Egr-1, and activating protein-1 (AP-1) and their corresponding genes, to increase IκB expression in mononuclear cells as well as to suppress plasma concentrations of intercellular adhesion molecule-1 (ICAM-1) and MCP-1.[273,274] Impaired insulin action and following insulin resistance are considered to induce atherogenesis resulting in the activation of proinflammatory transcription factors. Hyperinsulinemia could be seen as a compensatory attempt to suppress the inflammation and overcome the insulin resistance.[275] In humans, infusion of low doses of insulin in obese individuals promptly reduced the production of ROS in leukocytes, increased anti-inflammatory nitric oxide bioavailability, and reduced the CRP and other inflammatory markers in serum.[11,275] Additionally, treatment of T2D with insulin for 2 weeks caused a reduction in CRP and MCP-1[276] and the treatment of severe hyperglycemia with insulin resulted in a rapid marked decrease in the concentration of inflammatory mediators.[277] Insulin seems to exhibit also an antiapoptotic effect.[278,279]

Regarding the newly introduced pharmaceutical agents targeting inflammatory molecules the studies conducted have not concluded to an acceptable treatment. Treatment with TNF-α antibody, has not yet been proved beneficial.[280–282] IL-1 synthesis and secretion and high-glucose-induced β-cell apoptosis have been shown to be prevented by an IL-1 receptor antagonist[75]; a clinical trial testing the efficacy of IL-1 receptor antagonist (IL-1a) in T2D was conducted but without final results.[41] Inhibitors of JNK1 and IKKβ are under active investigation.[28,283] Targeting macrophage infiltration by an inhibitor of CCR2, the MCP-1 receptor, has been suggested and other key molecules mediating inflammation are under investigation.[284] Finally, taking into consideration the detrimental effect of the increased circulating leptin on inflammation, it could be suggested that a specific soluble receptor could reverse undesired leptin actions. The blockade of LR, by using monoclonal humanized antibodies or leptin mutants able to bind LR without its activation,[285] could be another potential way to antagonize leptin actions. Antileptin treatment is currently under investigation. However, caution should be addressed for serious undesirable adverse effects since the role of each molecule has not been extensively clarified and inflammatory genes or pathways implicated are also participating in the normal regulation of inflammation and energy omeostasis, such as insulin signaling.

CONCLUSIONS

T2D is a disease with accelerated prevalence and its recognition as a low-grade inflammation disease can be proved an important pass to a better follow-up, as well as prediction and even more treatment of patients particularly in early stages. Immune mediators have been shown to affect insulin sensitivity by direct or indirect mechanisms in clinical as well as in experimental studies. Therefore, it can be concluded that the metabolic and the immunological unbalance are correlated and the presence of one of these parameters may lead to the other resulting in a vicious cycle, which if not interrupted can provoke the known deleterious long-term complications of diabetes.

ACKNOWLEDGMENT

Dr. K. Alexandraki has been awarded with a scholarship from Alexander S. Onassis, public benefit foundation.

REFERENCES

1. Pickup, J.C. & M.A. Crook. 1998. Is type II diabetes mellitus a disease of the innate immune system? Diabetologia **41:** 1241–1248.
2. Gabay, C. & I. Kushner. 1999. Acute-phase proteins and other systemic responses to inflammation. N. Engl. J. Med. **340:** 448–454.
3. Blake, G.J. & P.M. Ridker. 2002. Inflammatory bio-markers and cardiovascular risk prediction. J. Intern. Med. **252:** 283–294.
4. Torres, J.L. & P.M. Ridker. 2003. Clinical use of high sensitivity C-reactive protein for the prediction of adverse cardiovascular events. Curr. Opin. Cardiol. **18:** 471–478.
5. Pickup, J.C. 2004. Inflammation and activated innate immunity in the pathogenesis of type 2 diabetes. Diabetes Care **27:** 813–823.
6. Tracy, R.P. Diabetes and atherothrombotic disease: linked through inflammation? Semin. Vasc. Med. **2:** 67–73.
7. Ferroni, P. *et al.* 2004. Inflammation, insulin resistance, and obesity. Curr. Atheroscler. Rep. **6:** 424–431.
8. Pearson, T.A. *et al.* 2003. Markers of inflammation and cardiovascular disease: application to clinical and public health practice: a statement for healthcare

professionals from the Centers for Disease Control and Prevention and the American Heart Association. Circulation **107:** 499–511.

9. CHEN, H. 2006. Cellular inflammatory responses: novel insights for obesity and insulin resistance. Pharmacol. Res. **53:** 469–477.
10. DANDONA, P., A. ALJADA & A. BANDYOPADHYAY. 2004. Inflammation: the link between insulin resistance, obesity and diabetes. Trends Immunol. **25:** 4–7.
11. DANDONA, P. *et al.* 2003. The potential influence of inflammation and insulin resistance on the pathogenesis and treatment of atherosclerosis-related complications in type 2 diabetes. J. Clin. Endocrinol. Metab. **88:** 2422–2429.
12. BIONDI-ZOCCAI, G.G. *et al.* 2003. Atherothrombosis, inflammation, and diabetes. J. Am. Coll. Cardiol. **41:** 1071–1077.
13. BLOOMGARDEN, Z.T. 2003. Inflammation and insulin resistance. Diabetes Care **26:** 1922–1926.
14. PITTAS, A.G., N.A. JOSEPH & A.S. GREENBERG. 2004. Adipocytokines and insulin resistance. J. Clin. Endocrinol. Metab. **89:** 447–452.
15. FERNANDEZ-REAL, J.M. & W. RICART. 2003. Insulin resistance and chronic cardiovascular inflammatory syndrome. Endocr. Rev. **24:** 278–301.
16. PRADHAN, A.D. & P.M. RIDKER. 2002. Do atherosclerosis and type 2 diabetes share a common inflammatory basis? Eur. Heart J. **23:** 831–834.
17. HAN, T.S. *et al.* 2002. Prospective study of C-reactive protein in relation to the development of diabetes and metabolic syndrome in the Mexico City Diabetes Study. Diabetes Care **25:** 2016–2021.
18. DUNCAN, B.B. *et al.* Low-grade systemic inflammation and the development of type 2 diabetes: the atherosclerosis risk in communities study. Diabetes **52:** 1799–1805.
19. PRADHAN, A.D. *et al.* 2003. C-reactive protein is independently associated with fasting insulin in nondiabetic women. Arterioscler. Thromb. Vasc. Biol. **23:** 650–655.
20. PRADHAN, A.D. *et al.* 2001. C-reactive protein, interleukin 6, and risk of developing type 2 diabetes mellitus. JAMA **286:** 327–334.
21. FREEMAN, D.J. *et al.* 2002. C-reactive protein is an independent predictor of risk for the development of diabetes in the West of Scotland Coronary Prevention Study. Diabetes **51:** 1596–1600.
22. FESTA, A. *et al.* 2000. Chronic subclinical inflammation as part of the insulin resistance syndrome: the Insulin Resistance Atherosclerosis Study (IRAS). Circulation **102:** 42–47.
23. FESTA, A. *et al.* 2002. Elevated levels of acute-phase proteins and plasminogen activator inhibitor-1 predict the development of type 2 diabetes: the insulin resistance atherosclerosis study. Diabetes **51:** 1131–1137.
24. ENGELGAU, M.M. *et al.* 2004. Prevention of type 2 diabetes: issues and strategies for identifying persons for interventions. Diabetes Technol.Ther. **6:** 874–882.
25. LEAHY, J.L. 2005. Pathogenesis of type 2 diabetes mellitus. Arch. Med. Res. **36:** 197–209.
26. ROTTER, V., I. NAGAEV & U. SMITH. 2003. Interleukin-6 (IL-6) induces insulin resistance in 3T3-L1 adipocytes and is, like IL-8 and tumor necrosis factor-alpha, overexpressed in human fat cells from insulin-resistant subjects. J. Biol. Chem. **278:** 45777–45784.
27. HIROSUMI, J. *et al.* 2002. A central role for JNK in obesity and insulin resistance. Nature **420:** 333–336.

28. YUAN, M. *et al.* 2001. Reversal of obesity- and diet-induced insulin resistance with salicylates or targeted disruption of Ikkbeta. Science **293:** 1673–1677.
29. KIM, J.A., K.K. KOH & M.J. QUON. 2005. The union of vascular and metabolic actions of insulin in sickness and in health. Arterioscler. Thromb. Vasc. Biol. **25:** 889–891.
30. STERN, M.P. 1995. Diabetes and cardiovascular disease. The "common soil" hypothesis. Diabetes **44:** 369–374.
31. BAYS, H., L. MANDARINO & R.A. DEFRONZO. 2004. Role of the adipocyte, free fatty acids, and ectopic fat in pathogenesis of type 2 diabetes mellitus: peroxisomal proliferator-activated receptor agonists provide a rational therapeutic approach. J. Clin. Endocrinol. Metab. **89:** 463–478.
32. YUDKIN, J.S. *et al.* 2000. Inflammation, obesity, stress and coronary heart disease: is interleukin-6 the link? Atherosclerosis **148:** 209–214.
33. YUDKIN, J.S. *et al.* 1999. C-reactive protein in healthy subjects: associations with obesity, insulin resistance, and endothelial dysfunction: a potential role for cytokines originating from adipose tissue? Arterioscler. Thromb. Vasc. Biol. **19:** 972–978.
34. HAK, A.E. *et al.* 1999. Associations of C-reactive protein with measures of obesity, insulin resistance, and subclinical atherosclerosis in healthy, middle-aged women. Arterioscler. Thromb. Vasc. Biol. **19:** 1986–1991.
35. HANSSON, G.K. *et al.* 1989. Immune mechanisms in atherosclerosis. Arteriosclerosis **9:** 567–578.
36. PICKUP, J.C. *et al.* 1997. NIDDM as a disease of the innate immune system: association of acute-phase reactants and interleukin-6 with metabolic syndrome X. Diabetologia **40:** 1286–1292.
37. HOEKSTRA, T. *et al.* 2005. Relationship of C-reactive protein with components of the metabolic syndrome in normal-weight and overweight elderly. Nutr. Metab. Cardiovasc. Dis. **15:** 270–278.
38. DUNCAN, B.B. & M.I. SCHMIDT. Chronic activation of the innate immune system may underlie the metabolic syndrome. Sao Paulo Med. J. **119:** 122–127.
39. SCHMIDT, M.I. & B.B. DUNCAN. 2003. Diabesity: an inflammatory metabolic condition. Clin. Chem. Lab. Med. **41:** 1120–1130.
40. BUTLER, A.E. *et al.* 2003. Beta-cell deficit and increased beta-cell apoptosis in humans with type 2 diabetes. Diabetes **52:** 102–110.
41. KOLB, H. & T. MANDRUP-POULSEN. 2005. An immune origin of type 2 diabetes? Diabetologia **48:** 1038–1050.
42. DONATH, M.Y. *et al.* 1999. Hyperglycemia-induced beta-cell apoptosis in pancreatic islets of Psammomys obesus during development of diabetes. Diabetes **48:** 738–744.
43. BELLONE, M. *et al.* 1997. Processing of engulfed apoptotic bodies yields T cell epitopes. J. Immunol. **159:** 5391–5399.
44. TRUDEAU, J.D. *et al.* 2000. Neonatal beta-cell apoptosis: a trigger for autoimmune diabetes? Diabetes **49:** 1–7.
45. MAEDLER, K. *et al.* 2002. Glucose-induced beta cell production of IL-1beta contributes to glucotoxicity in human pancreatic islets. J. Clin. Invest. **110:** 851–860.
46. MAEDLER, K. *et al.* 2001. Glucose induces beta-cell apoptosis via upregulation of the Fas receptor in human islets. Diabetes **50:** 1683–1690.

47. FRAYN, K.N. *et al.* 2003. Integrative physiology of human adipose tissue. Int. J. Obes. Relat. Metab. Disord. **27:** 875–888.
48. FRIED, S.K., D.A. BUNKIN & A.S. GREENBERG. 1998. Omental and subcutaneous adipose tissues of obese subjects release interleukin-6: depot difference and regulation by glucocorticoid. J. Clin. Endocrinol. Metab. **83:** 847–850.
49. HOTAMISLIGIL, G.S., N.S. SHARGILL & B.M. SPIEGELMAN. 1993. Adipose expression of tumor necrosis factor-alpha: direct role in obesity-linked insulin resistance. Science **259:** 87–91.
50. MEIER, C.A. *et al.* 2002. IL-1 receptor antagonist serum levels are increased in human obesity: a possible link to the resistance to leptin? J. Clin. Endocrinol. Metab. **87**: 1184–1188.
51. ZHANG, Y. *et al.* 1994. Positional cloning of the mouse obese gene and its human homologue. Nature **372:** 425–432.
52. WEISBERG, S.P. *et al.* 2003. Obesity is associated with macrophage accumulation in adipose tissue. J. Clin. Invest. **112:** 1796–1808.
53. XU, H. *et al.* 2003. Chronic inflammation in fat plays a crucial role in the development of obesity-related insulin resistance. J. Clin. Invest. **112:** 1821–1830.
54. GHANIM, H. *et al.* 2004. Circulating mononuclear cells in the obese are in a proinflammatory state. Circulation **110:** 1564–1571.
55. DANDONA, P. *et al.* 2005. Metabolic syndrome: a comprehensive perspective based on interactions between obesity, diabetes, and inflammation. Circulation **111:** 1448–1454.
56. WELLEN, K.E. & G.S. HOTAMISLIGIL. Inflammation, stress, and diabetes. J. Clin. Invest. **115:** 1111–1119.
57. CHARRIERE, G. *et al.* 2003. Preadipocyte conversion to macrophage. Evidence of plasticity. J. Biol. Chem. **278:** 9850–9855.
58. CHRISTIANSEN, T., B. RICHELSEN & J.M. BRUUN. Monocyte chemoattractant protein-1 is produced in isolated adipocytes, associated with adiposity and reduced after weight loss in morbid obese subjects. Int. J. Obes. (Lond.) **29:** 146–150.
59. GERHARDT, C.C. *et al.* 2001. Chemokines control fat accumulation and leptin secretion by cultured human adipocytes. Mol. Cell. Endocrinol. **175:** 81–92.
60. MURDOLO, G. & U. SMITH. 2006. The dysregulated adipose tissue: a connecting link between insulin resistance, type 2 diabetes mellitus and atherosclerosis. Nutr. Metab. Cardiovasc. Dis. **16**(Suppl 1): S35–S38.
61. CINTI, S. *et al.* Adipocyte death defines macrophage localization and function in adipose tissue of obese mice and humans. J. Lipid Res. **46:** 2347–2355.
62. FUJIWARA, N. & K. KOBAYASHI. 2005. Macrophages in inflammation. Curr. Drug Targets Inflamm. Allergy **4:** 281–286.
63. COPPACK, S.W. 2001. Pro-inflammatory cytokines and adipose tissue. Proc. Nutr. Soc. **60:** 349–356.
64. ALDHAHI, W. & O. HAMDY. 2003. Adipokines, inflammation, and the endothelium in diabetes. Curr. Diab. Rep. **3:** 293–298.
65. KERSHAW, E.E. & J.S. FLIER. 2004. Adipose tissue as an endocrine organ. J. Clin. Endocrinol. Metab. **89:** 2548–2556.
66. MATHIS, D., L. VENCE & C. BENOIST. 2001. beta-Cell death during progression to diabetes. Nature **414:** 792–798.
67. PIETROPAOLO, M. *et al.* 2000. Evidence of islet cell autoimmunity in elderly patients with type 2 diabetes. Diabetes **49:** 32–38.

68. DONATH, M.Y. *et al.* Inflammatory mediators and islet beta-cell failure: a link between type 1 and type 2 diabetes. J. Mol. Med. **81:** 455–470.
69. GIANNOUKAKIS, N. *et al.* 1999. Adenoviral gene transfer of the interleukin-1 receptor antagonist protein to human islets prevents IL-1beta-induced beta-cell impairment and activation of islet cell apoptosis *in vitro*. Diabetes **48:** 1730–1736.
70. LOWETH, A.C. *et al.* 1998. Human islets of Langerhans express Fas ligand and undergo apoptosis in response to interleukin-1beta and Fas ligation. Diabetes **47:** 727–732.
71. RABINOVITCH, A. *et al.* 1990. Cytotoxic effects of cytokines on human pancreatic islet cells in monolayer culture. J. Clin. Endocrinol. Metab. **71:** 152–156.
72. STASSI, G. *et al.* 1997. Nitric oxide primes pancreatic beta cells for Fas-mediated destruction in insulin-dependent diabetes mellitus. J. Exp. Med. **186:** 1193–1200.
73. KOH, K.K., S.H. HAN & M.J. QUON. 2005. Inflammatory markers and the metabolic syndrome: insights from therapeutic interventions. J. Am. Coll. Cardiol. **46:** 1978–1985.
74. MANDRUP-POULSEN, T. 1996. The role of interleukin-1 in the pathogenesis of IDDM. Diabetologia **39:** 1005–1029.
75. EIZIRIK, D.L. & T. MANDRUP-POULSEN. 2001. A choice of death–the signal-transduction of immune-mediated beta-cell apoptosis. Diabetologia **44:** 2115–2133.
76. MAEDLER, K. *et al.* 2004. Leptin modulates beta cell expression of IL-1 receptor antagonist and release of IL-1beta in human islets. Proc. Natl. Acad. Sci. USA **101:** 8138–8143.
77. MAEDLER, K. *et al.* 2002. FLIP switches Fas-mediated glucose signaling in human pancreatic beta cells from apoptosis to cell replication. Proc. Natl. Acad. Sci. USA **99:** 8236–8241.
78. MAEDLER, K. *et al.* 2004. Glucose- and interleukin-1beta-induced beta-cell apoptosis requires $Ca2^{+}$influx and extracellular signal-regulated kinase (ERK) 1/2 activation and is prevented by a sulfonylurea receptor 1/inwardly rectifying K^{+}channel 6.2 (SUR/Kir6.2) selective potassium channel opener in human islets. Diabetes **53:** 1706–1713.
79. AARNES, M., S. SCHONBERG & V. GRILL. 2002. Fatty acids potentiate interleukin-1beta toxicity in the beta-cell line INS-1E. Biochem. Biophys. Res. Commun. **296:** 189–193.
80. KIM, J.K. *et al.* 2001. Prevention of fat-induced insulin resistance by salicylate. J. Clin. Invest. **108:** 437–446.
81. HOTAMISLIGIL, G.S. *et al.* 1995. Increased adipose tissue expression of tumor necrosis factor-alpha in human obesity and insulin resistance. J. Clin. Invest. **95:** 2409–2415.
82. RUAN, H. & H.F. LODISH. 2003. Insulin resistance in adipose tissue: direct and indirect effects of tumor necrosis factor-alpha. Cytokine Growth Factor Rev. **14:** 447–455.
83. SENN, J.J. *et al.* 2003. Suppressor of cytokine signaling-3 (SOCS-3), a potential mediator of interleukin-6-dependent insulin resistance in hepatocytes. J. Biol. Chem. **278:** 13740–13746.
84. PERALDI, P. & B.B. SPIEGELMAN. 1998. TNF-alpha and insulin resistance: summary and future prospects. Mol. Cell. Biochem. **182:** 169–175.

85. MOHAMED-ALI, V. *et al.* 1999. Production of soluble tumor necrosis factor receptors by human subcutaneous adipose tissue *in vivo*. Am. J. Physiol. **277:** E971–E975.
86. ARNER, P. 2001. Regional differences in protein production by human adipose tissue. Biochem. Soc. Trans. **29:** 72–75.
87. ZHANG, H.H. *et al.* 2002. Tumor necrosis factor-alpha stimulates lipolysis in differentiated human adipocytes through activation of extracellular signal-related kinase and elevation of intracellular cAMP. Diabetes **51:** 2929–2935.
88. MANDRUP-POULSEN, T. 2001. Beta-cell apoptosis: stimuli and signaling. Diabetes **50**(Suppl 1): S58–S63.
89. UYSAL, K.T. 1997. Protection from obesity-induced insulin resistance in mice lacking TNF-alpha function. Nature **389:** 610–614.
90. UYSAL, K.T., S.M. WIESBROCK & G.S. HOTAMISLIGIL. 1998. Functional analysis of tumor necrosis factor (TNF) receptors in TNF-alpha-mediated insulin resistance in genetic obesity. Endocrinology **139:** 4832–4838.
91. RASK-MADSEN, C. *et al.* 2003. Tumor necrosis factor-alpha inhibits insulin's stimulating effect on glucose uptake and endothelium-dependent vasodilation in humans. Circulation **108:** 1815–1821.
92. OFEI, F. *et al.* 1996. Effects of an engineered human anti-TNF-alpha antibody (CDP571) on insulin sensitivity and glycemic control in patients with NIDDM. Diabetes **45:** 881–885.
93. PAQUOT, N. *et al.* 2000. No increased insulin sensitivity after a single intravenous administration of a recombinant human tumor necrosis factor receptor: Fc fusion protein in obese insulin-resistant patients. J. Clin. Endocrinol. Metab. **85:** 1316–1319.
94. DI ROCCO, P. *et al.* 2004. Lowered tumor necrosis factor receptors, but not increased insulin sensitivity, with infliximab. Obes. Res. **12:** 734–739.
95. STEPHENS, J.M. & P.H. PEKALA. 1991. Transcriptional repression of the GLUT4 and C/EBP genes in 3T3-L1 adipocytes by tumor necrosis factor-alpha. J. Biol. Chem. **266:** 21839–21845.
96. HOTAMISLIGIL, G.S. *et al.* 1996. IRS-1-mediated inhibition of insulin receptor tyrosine kinase activity in TNF-alpha- and obesity-induced insulin resistance. Science **271:** 665–668.
97. ZENG, M. *et al.* 2002. Tumor necrosis factor-alpha-induced leukocyte adhesion and microvessel permeability. Am. J. Physiol. Heart Circ. Physiol. **283:** H2420–H2430.
98. ASHTON, A.W. *et al.* 2003. Inhibition of tumor necrosis factor alpha-mediated NFkappaB activation and leukocyte adhesion, with enhanced endothelial apoptosis, by G protein-linked receptor (TP) ligands. J. Biol. Chem. **278:** 11858–11866.
99. PATEL, J.N. *et al.* 2002. Effects of tumour necrosis factor-alpha in the human forearm: blood flow and endothelin-1 release. Clin. Sci. (Lond.) **103:** 409–415.
100. WEBER, C. *et al.* 1995. Inhibitors of protein tyrosine kinase suppress TNF-stimulated induction of endothelial cell adhesion molecules. J. Immunol. **155:** 445–451.
101. UZUI, H. *et al.* Increased expression of membrane type 3-matrix metalloproteinase in human atherosclerotic plaque: role of activated macrophages and inflammatory cytokines. Circulation **106:** 3024–3030.
102. FARD, A. *et al.* 2000. Acute elevations of plasma asymmetric dimethylarginine and impaired endothelial function in response to a high-fat meal in patients with type 2 diabetes. Arterioscler. Thromb. Vasc. Biol. **20:** 2039–2044.

103. KATSUKI, A. *et al.* 1998. Serum levels of tumor necrosis factor-alpha are increased in obese patients with noninsulin-dependent diabetes mellitus. J. Clin. Endocrinol. Metab. **83:** 859–862.
104. KAMIMURA, D., K. ISHIHARA & T. HIRANO. 2003. IL-6 signal transduction and its physiological roles: the signal orchestration model. Rev. Physiol. Biochem. Pharmacol. **149:** 1–38.
105. JONES, S.A. *et al.* 2001. The soluble interleukin 6 receptor: mechanisms of production and implications in disease. FASEB J. **15:** 43–58.
106. SCHELLER, J. *et al.* 2006. Interleukin-6 trans-signalling in chronic inflammation and cancer. Scand. J. Immunol. **63:** 321–329.
107. KRISTIANSEN, O.P. & T. MANDRUP-POULSEN. 2005. Interleukin-6 and diabetes, or the indifferent? Diabetes **54**(Suppl 2): S114–S124.
108. WILLERSON, J.T. & P.M. RIDKER. 2004. Inflammation as a cardiovascular risk factor. Circulation **109**(Suppl 2): II2–II10.
109. NONOGAKI, K. *et al.* 1995. Interleukin-6 stimulates hepatic triglyceride secretion in rats. Endocrinology **136:** 2143–2149.
110. SOUTHERN, C., D. SCHULSTER & I.C. GREEN. 1990. Inhibition of insulin secretion from rat islets of Langerhans by interleukin-6. An effect distinct from that of interleukin-1. Biochem. J. **272:** 243–245.
111. SANDLER, S. *et al.* 1990. Interleukin-6 affects insulin secretion and glucose metabolism of rat pancreatic islets *in vitro*. Endocrinology **126:** 1288–1294.
112. WADT, K.A. *et al.* 1998. Ciliary neurotrophic factor potentiates the beta-cell inhibitory effect of IL-1beta in rat pancreatic islets associated with increased nitric oxide synthesis and increased expression of inducible nitric oxide synthase. Diabetes **47:** 1602–1608.
113. CHOI, S.E. *et al.* 2004. IL-6 protects pancreatic islet beta cells from pro-inflammatory cytokines-induced cell death and functional impairment *in vitro* and *in vivo*. Transpl. Immunol. **13:** 43–53.
114. CAMPBELL, I.L. *et al.* 1989. Evidence for IL-6 production by and effects on the pancreatic beta-cell. J. Immunol. **143:** 1188–1191.
115. CAREY, A.L. & M.A. FEBBRAIO. 2004. Interleukin-6 and insulin sensitivity: friend or foe? Diabetologia **47:** 1135–1142.
116. MOHAMED-ALI, V. *et al.* 1997. Subcutaneous adipose tissue releases interleukin-6, but not tumor necrosis factor-alpha, *in vivo*. J. Clin. Endocrinol. Metab. **82:** 4196–4200.
117. STOUTHARD, J.M., R.P. OUDE ELFERINK & H.P. SAUERWEIN. Interleukin-6 enhances glucose transport in 3T3-L1 adipocytes. Biochem. Biophys. Res. Commun. **220:** 241–245.
118. LAGATHU, C. *et al.* 2003. Chronic interleukin-6 (IL-6) treatment increased IL-6 secretion and induced insulin resistance in adipocyte: prevention by rosiglitazone. Biochem. Biophys. Res. Commun. **311:** 372–379.
119. FASSHAUER, M. *et al.* 2003. Adiponectin gene expression and secretion is inhibited by interleukin-6 in 3T3-L1 adipocytes. Biochem. Biophys. Res. Commun. **301:** 1045–1050.
120. EMANUELLI, B. *et al.* 2001. SOCS-3 inhibits insulin signaling and is up-regulated in response to tumor necrosis factor-alpha in the adipose tissue of obese mice. J. Biol. Chem. **276:** 47944–47949.
121. SHI, H. *et al.* 2004. Suppressor of cytokine signaling 3 is a physiological regulator of adipocyte insulin signaling. J. Biol. Chem. **279:** 34733–34740.

122. Rieusset, J. *et al.* 2004. Suppressor of cytokine signaling 3 expression and insulin resistance in skeletal muscle of obese and type 2 diabetic patients. Diabetes **53:** 2232–2241.

123. Kim, H.J. *et al.* 2004. Differential effects of interleukin-6 and -10 on skeletal muscle and liver insulin action *in vivo*. Diabetes **53:** 1060–1067.

124. Klover, P.J. *et al.* Chronic exposure to interleukin-6 causes hepatic insulin resistance in mice. Diabetes **52:** 2784–2789.

125. Kanemaki, T. *et al.* 1998. Interleukin 1beta and interleukin 6, but not tumor necrosis factor alpha, inhibit insulin-stimulated glycogen synthesis in rat hepatocytes. Hepatology **27:** 1296–1303.

126. Senn, J.J. *et al.* 2002. Interleukin-6 induces cellular insulin resistance in hepatocytes. Diabetes **51:** 3391–3399.

127. Febbraio, M.A. *et al.* 2004. Interleukin-6 is a novel factor mediating glucose homeostasis during skeletal muscle contraction. Diabetes **53:** 1643–1648.

128. Pedersen, B.K. *et al.* 2004. The metabolic role of IL-6 produced during exercise: is IL-6 an exercise factor? Proc. Nutr. Soc. **63:** 263–267.

129. Strassmann, G. *et al.* 1993. The role of interleukin-6 in lipopolysaccharide-induced weight loss, hypoglycemia and fibrinogen production, *in vivo*. Cytokine **5:** 285–290.

130. Eizirik, D.L. *et al.* 1994. Cytokines suppress human islet function irrespective of their effects on nitric oxide generation. J. Clin. Invest. **93:** 1968–1974.

131. DiCosmo, B.F., D. Picarella & R.A. Flavell. 1994. Local production of human IL-6 promotes insulitis but retards the onset of insulin-dependent diabetes mellitus in non-obese diabetic mice. Int. Immunol. **6:** 1829–1837.

132. Campbell, I.L. *et al.* 1994. Islet inflammation and hyperplasia induced by the pancreatic islet-specific overexpression of interleukin-6 in transgenic mice. Am. J. Pathol. **145:** 157–166.

133. Di Gregorio, G.B. *et al.* Lipid and carbohydrate metabolism in mice with a targeted mutation in the IL-6 gene: absence of development of age-related obesity. Am. J. Physiol. Endocrinol. Metab. **287:** E182–E187.

134. Tsigos, C. *et al.* 1997. Dose-dependent effects of recombinant human interleukin-6 on glucose regulation. J. Clin. Endocrinol. Metab. **82:** 4167–4170.

135. van Hall, G. *et al.* 2003. Interleukin-6 stimulates lipolysis and fat oxidation in humans. J. Clin. Endocrinol. Metab. **88:** 3005–3010.

136. Pedersen, M. *et al.* 2003. Circulating levels of TNF-alpha and IL-6-relation to truncal fat mass and muscle mass in healthy elderly individuals and in patients with type-2 diabetes. Mech. Ageing Dev. **124:** 495–502.

137. Mohamed-Ali, V. *et al.* 2001. beta-Adrenergic regulation of IL-6 release from adipose tissue: *in vivo* and *in vitro* studies. J Clin Endocrinol Metab. **86:** 5864–5869.

138. Carey, A.L. *et al.* 2004. Interleukin-6 and tumor necrosis factor-alpha are not increased in patients with Type 2 diabetes: evidence that plasma interleukin-6 is related to fat mass and not insulin responsiveness. Diabetologia **47:** 1029–1037.

139. Bastard, J.P. *et al.* 2002. Adipose tissue IL-6 content correlates with resistance to insulin activation of glucose uptake both *in vivo* and *in vitro*. J. Clin. Endocrinol. Metab. **87:** 2084–2089.

140. Spranger, J. *et al.* 2003. Inflammatory cytokines and the risk to develop type 2 diabetes: results of the prospective population-based European Prospective

Investigation into Cancer and Nutrition (EPIC)-Potsdam Study. Diabetes **52:** 812–817.
141. Hu, F.B. *et al.* 2004. Inflammatory markers and risk of developing type 2 diabetes in women. Diabetes **53:** 693–700.
142. Kamimura, D., K. Ishihara & T. Hirano. 2003. IL-6 signal transduction and its physiological roles: the signal orchestration model. Rev. Physiol. Biochem. Pharmacol. **149:** 1–38.
143. Wallenius, K., J.O. Jansson & V. Wallenius. 2003. The therapeutic potential of interleukin-6 in treating obesity. Expert Opin. Biol. Ther. **3:** 1061–1070.
144. Wallenius, V. *et al.* 2002. Interleukin-6-deficient mice develop mature-onset obesity. Nat. Med. **8:** 75–79.
145. Mooney, R.A. *et al.* 2001. Suppressors of cytokine signaling-1 and -6 associate with and inhibit the insulin receptor. A potential mechanism for cytokine-mediated insulin resistance. J. Biol. Chem. **276:** 25889–25893.
146. Ueki, K., T. Kadowaki & C.R. Kahn. 2005. Role of suppressors of cytokine signaling SOCS-1 and SOCS-3 in hepatic steatosis and the metabolic syndrome. Hepatol. Res. **33:** 185–192.
147. Maedler, K. *et al.* Leptin modulates beta cell expression of IL-1 receptor antagonist and release of IL-1beta in human islets. Proc. Natl. Acad. Sci. USA **101:** 8138–8143.
148. Ahima, R.S. & J.S. Flier. 2000. Leptin. Annu. Rev. Physiol. **62:** 413–437.
149. Otero, M. *et al.* 2006. Towards a pro-inflammatory and immunomodulatory emerging role of leptin. Rheumatology. (Oxford) **45:** 944–950.
150. Peelman, F. *et al.* 2004. Leptin: linking adipocyte metabolism with cardiovascular and autoimmune diseases. Prog. Lipid. Res. **43:** 283–301.
151. La Cava, A., C. Alviggi & G. Matarese. 2004. Unraveling the multiple roles of leptin in inflammation and autoimmunity. J. Mol. Med. **821:** 4–11.
152. Huang, L. & C. Li. Leptin: a multifunctional hormone. Cell. Res. **10:** 81–92.
153. Nakata, M. *et al.* 1999. Leptin promotes aggregation of human platelets via the long form of its receptor. Diabetes **48:** 426–429.
154. Ahima, R.S. *et al.* 1996. Role of leptin in the neuroendocrine response to fasting. Nature **382:** 250–252.
155. Chan, J.L. *et al.* 2003. The role of falling leptin levels in the neuroendocrine and metabolic adaptation to short-term starvation in healthy men. J. Clin. Invest. **111:** 1409–1421.
156. Zhang, F. *et al.* 2005. Leptin: structure, function and biology. Vitam. Horm. **71:** 345–372.
157. Cohen, B. *et al.* 1996. Modulation of insulin activities by leptin. Science **274:** 1185–1188.
158. Szanto, I. & C.R. Kahn. 2000. Selective interaction between leptin and insulin signaling pathways in a hepatic cell line. Proc. Natl. Acad. Sci. USA **97:** 2355–2360.
159. Kim, Y.B. *et al.* 2000. *In vivo* administration of leptin activates signal transduction directly in insulin-sensitive tissues: overlapping but distinct pathways from insulin. Endocrinology **141:** 2328–2339.
160. Islam, M.S., A. Sjoholm & V. Emilsson. 2000. Fetal pancreatic islets express functional leptin receptors and leptin stimulates proliferation of fetal islet cells. Int. J. Obes. Relat. Metab. Disord. **24:** 1246–1253.
161. Okuya, S. *et al.* 2001. Leptin increases the viability of isolated rat pancreatic islets by suppressing apoptosis. Endocrinology **142:** 4827–4830.

162. SHIMABUKURO, M. *et al.* 1998. Protection against lipoapoptosis of beta cells through leptin-dependent maintenance of Bcl-2 expression. Proc. Natl. Acad. Sci. USA **95:** 9558–9561.
163. TANABE, K. *et al.* 1997. Leptin induces proliferation of pancreatic beta cell line MIN6 through activation of mitogen-activated protein kinase. Biochem. Biophys. Res. Commun. **241:** 765–768.
164. MAEDLER, K. & M.Y. DONATH. 2004. Beta-cells in type 2 diabetes: a loss of function and mass. Horm. Res. **3**(62 Suppl): 67–73.
165. WANG, J. *et al.* 2001. Overfeeding rapidly induces leptin and insulin resistance. Diabetes **50:** 2786–2791.
166. WABITSCH, M. *et al.* 1996. Insulin and cortisol promote leptin production in cultured human fat cells. Diabetes **45:** 1435–1438.
167. RUSSELL, C.D. *et al.* 1998. Leptin expression in adipose tissue from obese humans: depot-specific regulation by insulin and dexamethasone. Am. J. Physiol. **275**(3 Pt 1): E507–E515.
168. BAI, Y. *et al.* 1996. Obese gene expression alters the ability of 30A5 preadipocytes to respond to lipogenic hormones. J. Biol. Chem. **271:** 13939–13942.
169. MULLER, G. *et al.* 1997. Leptin impairs metabolic actions of insulin in isolated rat adipocytes. J. Biol. Chem. **272:** 10585–10593.
170. REIDY, S.P. & J. WEBER. 2000. Leptin: an essential regulator of lipid metabolism. Comp. Biochem. Physiol. A. Mol. Integr. Physiol. **125:** 285–298.
171. SIVITZ, W.I. *et al.* 1997. Effects of leptin on insulin sensitivity in normal rats. Endocrinology **138:** 3395–3401.
172. ROSSETTI, L. *et al.* 1997. Short term effects of leptin on hepatic gluconeogenesis and *in vivo* insulin action. J. Biol. Chem. **272:** 27758–27763.
173. PELLEYMOUNTER, M.A. *et al.* 1995. Effects of the obese gene product on body weight regulation in ob/ob mice. Science **269:** 540–543.
174. CHINOOKOSWONG, N., J.L. WANG & Z.Q. SHI. 1999. Leptin restores euglycemia and normalizes glucose turnover in insulin-deficient diabetes in the rat. Diabetes **48:** 1487–1492.
175. SHIMOMURA, I. *et al.* 1999. Leptin reverses insulin resistance and diabetes mellitus in mice with congenital lipodystrophy. Nature **401:** 73–76.
176. UNGER, R.H. 2002. Lipotoxic diseases. Annu. Rev. Med. **53:** 319–336.
177. KAMOHARA, S. *et al.* 1997. Acute stimulation of glucose metabolism in mice by leptin treatment. Nature **389:** 374–377.
178. YEN, T.T. *et al.* 1977. Dissociation of obesity, hypercholesterolemia and diabetes from atherosclerosis in ob/ob mice. Experientia **33:** 995–996.
179. SCHAFER, K. *et al.* 2004. Leptin promotes vascular remodeling and neointimal growth in mice. Arterioscler. Thromb. Vasc. Biol. **24:** 112–117.
180. MATSUMURA, K. *et al.* 2003. Neural regulation of blood pressure by leptin and the related peptides. Regul. Pept. **114:** 79–86.
181. SHEK, E.W., M.W. BRANDS & J.E. HALL. 1998. Chronic leptin infusion increases arterial pressure. Hypertension **31**(1 Pt 2): 409–414.
182. LEMBO, G. *et al.* 2000. Leptin induces direct vasodilation through distinct endothelial mechanisms. Diabetes **49:** 293–297.
183. DUNBAR, J.C., Y. HU & H. LU. 1997. Intracerebroventricular leptin increases lumbar and renal sympathetic nerve activity and blood pressure in normal rats. Diabetes **46:** 2040–2043.
184. MATSUMURA, K. *et al.* 2000. Central effects of leptin on cardiovascular and neurohormonal responses in conscious rabbits. Am. J. Physiol. Regul. Integr. Comp. Physiol. **278:** R1314–R1320.

185. AGATA, J. *et al.* 1997. High plasma immunoreactive leptin level in essential hypertension. Am. J. Hypertens. **10**(10 Pt 1): 1171–1174.
186. SIERRA-HONIGMANN, M.R. *et al.* 1998. Biological action of leptin as an angiogenic factor. Science **281:** 1683–1686.
187. PARK, H.Y. *et al.* Potential role of leptin in angiogenesis: leptin induces endothelial cell proliferation and expression of matrix metalloproteinases *in vivo* and *in vitro*. Exp. Mol. Med. **33:** 95–102.
188. BODARY, P.F. *et al.* 2002. Effect of leptin on arterial thrombosis following vascular injury in mice. JAMA **287:** 1706–1709.
189. ODA, A., T. TANIGUCHI & M. YOKOYAMA. 2001. Leptin stimulates rat aortic smooth muscle cell proliferation and migration. Kobe J. Med. Sci. **47:** 141–150.
190. VAN HEEK, M. *et al.* 1997. Diet-induced obese mice develop peripheral, but not central, resistance to leptin. J. Clin. Invest. **99:** 385–390.
191. BJORBAEK, C. *et al.* 1998. Identification of SOCS-3 as a potential mediator of central leptin resistance. Mol. Cell. **1:** 619–625.
192. BJORBAEK, C. *et al.* 1999. The role of SOCS-3 in leptin signaling and leptin resistance. J. Biol. Chem. **274:** 30059–30065.
193. SODERBERG, S. *et al.* 1999. Leptin is associated with increased risk of myocardial infarction. J. Intern. Med. **246:** 409–418.
194. WALLACE, A.M. *et al.* 2001. Plasma leptin and the risk of cardiovascular disease in the west of Scotland coronary prevention study (WOSCOPS). Circulation **104:** 3052–3056.
195. SODERBERG, S. *et al.* 1999. Leptin is a risk marker for first-ever hemorrhagic stroke in a population-based cohort. Stroke **30:** 328–337.
196. ZIMMET, P. *et al.* 1999. Etiology of the metabolic syndrome: potential role of insulin resistance, leptin resistance, and other players. Ann. N. Y. Acad. Sci. **892:** 25–44.
197. DE COURTEN, M. *et al.* 1997. Hyperleptinaemia: the missing link in the, metabolic syndrome? Diabet. Med. **14:** 200–208.
198. CICCONE, M. *et al.* 2001. Plasma leptin is independently associated with the intima-media thickness of the common carotid artery. Int. J. Obes. Relat. Metab. Disord. **25:** 805–810.
199. SINGHAL, A. *et al.* 2002. Influence of leptin on arterial distensibility: a novel link between obesity and cardiovascular disease? Circulation **106:** 1919–1924.
200. CAMMISOTTO, P.G. *et al.* 2005. Regulation of leptin secretion from white adipocytes by insulin, glycolytic substrates, and amino acids. Am. J. Physiol. Endocrinol. Metab. **289:** E166–E171.
201. FLIERS, E. *et al.* 2003. White adipose tissue: getting nervous. J. Neuroendocrinol. **15:** 1005–1010.
202. BODEN, G. *et al.* 1997. Effects of prolonged hyperinsulinemia on serum leptin in normal human subjects. J. Clin. Invest. **100:** 1107–1113.
203. ZAKRZEWSKA, K.E. *et al.* 1997. Glucocorticoids as counterregulatory hormones of leptin: toward an understanding of leptin resistance. Diabetes **46:** 717–719.
204. JIN, L. *et al.* 199. Leptin and leptin receptor expression in normal and neoplastic human pituitary: evidence of a regulatory role for leptin on pituitary cell proliferation. J. Clin. Endocrinol. Metab. **84:** 2903–2911.
205. HEIMAN, M.L. *et al.* 1997. Leptin inhibition of the hypothalamic-pituitary-adrenal axis in response to stress. Endocrinology **138:** 3859–3863.

206. KRUSE, M. *et al.* 1998. Leptin down-regulates the steroid producing system in the adrenal. Endocr. Res. **24:** 587–590.
207. WABITSCH, M. *et al.* 1996. Insulin and cortisol promote leptin production in cultured human fat cells. Diabetes **45:** 1435–1438.
208. DE VOS, P. *et al.* 1995. Induction of ob gene expression by corticosteroids is accompanied by body weight loss and reduced food intake. J. Biol. Chem. **270:** 15958–15961.
209. OZATA, M. I.C. OZDEMIR & J. LICINIO. 1999. Human leptin deficiency caused by a missense mutation: multiple endocrine defects, decreased sympathetic tone, and immune system dysfunction indicate new targets for leptin action, greater central than peripheral resistance to the effects of leptin, and spontaneous correction of leptin-mediated defects. J. Clin. Endocrinol. Metab. **84:** 3686–3695.
210. SARRAF, P. *et al.* 1997. Multiple cytokines and acute inflammation raise mouse leptin levels: potential role in inflammatory anorexia. J. Exp. Med. **185:** 171–175.
211. OTERO, M. *et al.* 2005. Leptin, from fat to inflammation: old questions and new insights. FEBS Lett. **579:** 295–301.
212. GUALILLO, O. *et al.* 2000. Elevated serum leptin concentrations induced by experimental acute inflammation. Life Sci. **67:** 2433–2441.
213. POPA, C. *et al.* 2005. Markers of inflammation are negatively correlated with serum leptin in rheumatoid arthritis. Ann. Rheum. Dis. **64:** 1195–1198.
214. ZHANG, H.H. *et al.* 2000. Tumour necrosis factor-alpha exerts dual effects on human adipose leptin synthesis and release. Mol. Cell. Endocrinol. **159:** 79–88.
215. FAGGIONI, R., K.R. FEINGOLD & C. GRUNFELD. 2001. Leptin regulation of the immune response and the immunodeficiency of malnutrition. FASEB J. **15:** 2565–2571.
216. SANNA, V. *et al.* 2003. Leptin surge precedes onset of autoimmune encephalomyelitis and correlates with development of pathogenic T cell responses. J. Clin. Invest. **111:** 241–250.
217. KIMURA, M. *et al.* 1998. T lymphopenia in obese diabetic (db/db) mice is nonselective and thymus independent. Life Sci. **62:** 1243–1250.
218. LA CAVA, A. & G. MATARESE. 2004. The weight of leptin in immunity. Nat. Rev. Immunol. **4:** 371–379.
219. MATARESE, G., S. MOSCHOS & C.S. MANTZOROS. 2005. Leptin in immunology. J. Immunol. **174:** 3137–3142.
220. ZARKESH-ESFAHANI, H. *et al.* 2001. High-dose leptin activates human leukocytes via receptor expression on monocytes. J. Immunol. **167:** 4593–4599.
221. MANCUSO, P. *et al.* 2004. Leptin augments alveolar macrophage leukotriene synthesis by increasing phospholipase activity and enhancing group IVC iPLA2 (cPLA2gamma) protein expression. Am. J. Physiol. Lung Cell. Mol. Physiol. **287:** 497–502.
222. DIXIT, V.D. *et al.* 2003. Leptin induces growth hormone secretion from peripheral blood mononuclear cells via a protein kinase C- and nitric oxide-dependent mechanism. Endocrinology **144:** 5595–5603.
223. RASO, G.M. *et al.* 2002. Leptin potentiates IFN-gamma-induced expression of nitric oxide synthase and cyclo-oxygenase-2 in murine macrophage J774A.1. Br. J. Pharmacol. **137:** 799–804.
224. CALDEFIE-CHEZET, F. *et al.* 2001. Leptin: a potential regulator of polymorphonuclear neutrophil bactericidal action? J. Leukoc. Biol. **69:** 414–418.

225. CALDEFIE-CHEZET, F., A. POULIN & M.P. VASSON. 2003. Leptin regulates functional capacities of polymorphonuclear neutrophils. Free Radic. Res. **37:** 809–814.
226. TIAN, Z. *et al.* 2002. Impaired natural killer (NK) cell activity in leptin receptor deficient mice: leptin as a critical regulator in NK cell development and activation. Biochem. Biophys. Res. Commun. **298:** 297–302.
227. HOWARD, J.K. *et al.* 1999. Leptin protects mice from starvation-induced lymphoid atrophy and increases thymic cellularity in ob/ob mice. J. Clin. Invest. **104:** 1051–1059.
228. FAROOQI, I.S. *et al.* 2002. Beneficial effects of leptin on obesity, T cell hyporesponsiveness, and neuroendocrine(metabolic dysfunction of human congenital leptin deficiency. J. Clin. Invest. **110:** 1093–1103.
229. LORD, G.M. *et al.* 1998. Leptin modulates the T-cell immune response and reverses starvation-induced immunosuppression. Nature **394:** 897–901.
230. BASTARD, J.P. *et al.* 2006. Recent advances in the relationship between obesity, inflammation, and insulin resistance. Eur. Cytokine Netw. **17:** 4–12.
231. MATARESE, G. *et al.* 2002. Leptin accelerates autoimmune diabetes in female NOD mice. Diabetes **51:** 1356–1361.
232. SANNA, V. *et al.* 2003. Leptin surge precedes onset of autoimmune encephalomyelitis and correlates with development of pathogenic T cell responses. J. Clin. Invest. **111:** 241–250.
233. KOH, K.K. 2002. Effects of estrogen on the vascular wall: vasomotor function and inflammation. Cardiovasc. Res. **55:** 714–726.
234. CHEN, A. *et al.* 2005. Diet induction of monocyte chemoattractant protein-1 and its impact on obesity. Obes. Res. **13:** 1311–1320.
235. KOH, K.K., S.H. HAN & M.J. QUON. 2005. Inflammatory markers and the metabolic syndrome: insights from therapeutic interventions. J. Am. Coll. Cardiol. **46:** 1978–1985.
236. FUNAKOSHI, Y. *et al.* 2001. Rho-kinase mediates angiotensin II-induced monocyte chemoattractant protein-1 expression in rat vascular smooth muscle cells. Hypertension **38:** 100–104.
237. SCHERER, P.E. *et al.* 1995. A novel serum protein similar to C1q, produced exclusively in adipocytes. J. Biol. Chem. **270:** 26746–26749.
238. KUBOTA, N. *et al.* 2002. Disruption of adiponectin causes insulin resistance and neointimal formation. J. Biol. Chem. **277:** 25863–25866.
239. UKKOLA, O. & M. SANTANIEMI. 2002. Adiponectin: a link between excess adiposity and associated comorbidities? J. Mol. Med. **80:** 696–702.
240. HOTTA, K. *et al.* 2000. Plasma concentrations of a novel, adipose-specific protein, adiponectin, in type 2 diabetic patients. Arterioscler. Thromb. Vasc. Biol. **20:** 1595–1599.
241. BERG, A.H. *et al.* 2001. The adipocyte-secreted protein Acrp30 enhances hepatic insulin action. Nat. Med. **7:** 947–953.
242. CHEN, H. *et al.* 2003. Adiponectin stimulates production of nitric oxide in vascular endothelial cells. J. Biol. Chem. **278:** 45021–45026.
243. OUCHI, N. *et al.* 1999. Novel modulator for endothelial adhesion molecules: adipocyte-derived plasma protein adiponectin. Circulation **100:** 2473–2476.
244. OUCHI, N. *et al.* 2000. Adiponectin, an adipocyte-derived plasma protein, inhibits endothelial NF-kappaB signaling through a cAMP-dependent pathway. Circulation **102:** 1296–1301.

245. FASSHAUER, M. *et al.* 2003. Adiponectin gene expression and secretion is inhibited by interleukin-6 in 3T3-L1 adipocytes. Biochem. Biophys. Res. Commun. **301:** 1045–1050.
246. STEPPAN, C.M. *et al.* 2001. The hormone resistin links obesity to diabetes. Nature **409:** 307–312.
247. STEPPAN, C.M. *et al.* 2005. Activation of SOCS-3 by resistin. Mol. Cell. Biol. **25:** 1569–1575.
248. SCHONBECK, U. & P. LIBBY. 2001. CD40 signaling and plaque instability. Circ. Res. **89:** 1092–1103.
249. ESPOSITO, K. *et al.* 2003. Effect of weight loss and lifestyle changes on vascular inflammatory markers in obese women: a randomized trial. JAMA **289:** 1799–1804.
250. ESPOSITO, K. *et al.* 2004. Effect of a mediterranean-style diet on endothelial dysfunction and markers of vascular inflammation in the metabolic syndrome: a randomized trial. JAMA **292:** 1440–1446.
251. MONZILLO, L.U. *et al.* 2003. Effect of lifestyle modification on adipokine levels in obese subjects with insulin resistance. Obes. Res. **11:** 1048–1054.
252. GHANIM, H. *et al.* 2001. Suppression of nuclear factor-kappaB and stimulation of inhibitor kappaB by troglitazone: evidence for an anti-inflammatory effect and a potential antiatherosclerotic effect in the obese. J. Clin. Endocrinol. Metab. **86:** 1306–1312.
253. ALJADA, A. *et al.* 2001. Nuclear factor-kappaB suppressive and inhibitor-kappaB stimulatory effects of troglitazone in obese patients with type 2 diabetes: evidence of an antiinflammatory action? J. Clin. Endocrinol. Metab. **86:** 3250–3256.
254. MOHANTY, P. *et al.* 2004. Evidence for a potent antiinflammatory effect of rosiglitazone. J. Clin. Endocrinol. Metab. **89:** 2728–2735.
255. KATSUKI, A. 2000. Troglitazone reduces plasma levels of tumour necrosis factor-alpha in obese patients with type 2 diabetes. Diabetes Obes. Metab. **2:** 189–191.
256. HAFFNER, S.M. *et al.* 2002. Effect of rosiglitazone treatment on nontraditional markers of cardiovascular disease in patients with type 2 diabetes mellitus. Circulation **106:** 679–684.
257. YU, J.G. *et al.* 2002. The effect of thiazolidinediones on plasma adiponectin levels in normal, obese, and type 2 diabetic subjects. Diabetes **51:** 2968–2974.
258. HIROSE, H. *et al.* 2002. Effects of pioglitazone on metabolic parameters, body fat distribution, and serum adiponectin levels in Japanese male patients with type 2 diabetes. Metabolism **51:** 314–317.
259. MAEDA, N. *et al.* 2001. PPARgamma ligands increase expression and plasma concentrations of adiponectin, an adipose-derived protein. Diabetes **50:** 2094–2099.
260. DANDONA, P. *et al.* Increased plasma concentration of macrophage migration inhibitory factor (MIF) and MIF mRNA in mononuclear cells in the obese and the suppressive action of metformin. J. Clin. Endocrinol. Metab. **89:** 5043–5047.
261. KOH, K.K. *et al.* 2002. Comparative effects of diet and simvastatin on markers of thrombogenicity in patients with coronary artery disease. Am. J. Cardiol. **91:** 1231–1234.
262. KOH, K.K. *et al.* 2002. Statin attenuates increase in C-reactive protein during estrogen replacement therapy in postmenopausal women. Circulation **105:** 1531–1533.

263. TROSEID, M. *et al.* 2004. Exercise reduces plasma levels of the chemokines MCP-1 and IL-8 in subjects with the metabolic syndrome. Eur. Heart J. **25:** 349–355.
264. PASCERI, V. *et al.* 2001. Modulation of C-reactive protein-mediated monocyte chemoattractant protein-1 induction in human endothelial cells by anti-atherosclerosis drugs. Circulation **103:** 2531–2534.
265. STAELS, B. *et al.* 1998. Activation of human aortic smooth-muscle cells is inhibited by PPARalpha but not by PPARgamma activators. Nature **393:** 790–793.
266. KOH, K.K. *et al.* 2005. Beneficial effects of fenofibrate to improve endothelial dysfunction and raise adiponectin levels in patients with primary hypertriglyceridemia. Diabetes Care **28:** 1419–1424.
267. KOH, K.K. *et al.* 2003. Pleiotropic effects of angiotensin II receptor blocker in hypertensive patients. J. Am. Coll. Cardiol. **42:** 905–910.
268. FURUHASHI, M. *et al.* 2003. Blockade of the renin-angiotensin system increases adiponectin concentrations in patients with essential hypertension. Hypertension **42:** 76–81.
269. WANG, C.H. *et al.* 2003. C-reactive protein upregulates angiotensin type 1 receptors in vascular smooth muscle. Circulation **107:** 1783–1790.
270. KOH, K.K. *et al.* 2005. Vascular and metabolic effects of combined therapy with ramipril and simvastatin in patients with type 2 diabetes. Hypertension **45:** 1088–1093.
271. KOH, K.K. *et al.* 2004. Additive beneficial effects of losartan combined with simvastatin in the treatment of hypercholesterolemic, hypertensive patients. Circulation **110:** 3687–3692.
272. KOH, K.K. *et al.* 2004. Simvastatin combined with ramipril treatment in hypercholesterolemic patients. Hypertension **44:** 180–185.
273. DANDONA, P. *et al.* 2001. Insulin inhibits intranuclear nuclear factor kappaB and stimulates IkappaB in mononuclear cells in obese subjects: evidence for an anti-inflammatory effect? J. Clin. Endocrinol. Metab. **86:** 3257–3265.
274. ALJADA, A. *et al.* 2002. Insulin inhibits the pro-inflammatory transcription factor early growth response gene-1 (Egr)-1 expression in mononuclear cells (MNC) and reduces plasma tissue factor (TF) and plasminogen activator inhibitor-1 (PAI-1) concentrations. J. Clin. Endocrinol. Metab. **87:** 1419–1422.
275. DANDONA, P. & A. ALJADA. 2002. A rational approach to pathogenesis and treatment of type 2 diabetes mellitus, insulin resistance, inflammation, and atherosclerosis. Am. J. Cardiol. **90:** 27G–33G.
276. TAKEBAYASHI, K., Y. ASO & T. INUKAI. 2004. Initiation of insulin therapy reduces serum concentrations of high-sensitivity C-reactive protein in patients with type 2 diabetes. Metabolism **53:** 693–699.
277. STENTZ, F.B. *et al.* 2004. Proinflammatory cytokines, markers of cardiovascular risks, oxidative stress, and lipid peroxidation in patients with hyperglycemic crises. Diabetes **53:** 2079–2086.
278. CHAUDHURI, A. *et al.* 2004. Anti-inflammatory and profibrinolytic effect of insulin in acute ST-segment–elevation myocardial infarction. Circulation **109:** 849–854.
279. JONASSEN, A.K. *et al.* 2001. Myocardial protection by insulin at reperfusion requires early administration and is mediated via Akt and p70s6 kinase cell-survival signaling. Circ. Res. **89:** 1191–1198.
280. Di ROCCO, P. *et al.* 2004. Lowered tumor necrosis factor receptors, but not increased insulin sensitivity, with infliximab. Obes. Res. **12:** 734–739.

281. PAQUOT, N. *et al.* 2000. No increased insulin sensitivity after a single intravenous administration of a recombinant human tumor necrosis factor receptor: Fc fusion protein in obese insulin-resistant patients. J. Clin. Endocrinol. Metab. **85:** 1316–1319.
282. OFEI, F. *et al.* 1996. Effects of an engineered human anti-TNF-alpha antibody (CDP571) on insulin sensitivity and glycemic control in patients with NIDDM. Diabetes **45:** 881–885.
283. KANETO, H. *et al.* 2004. Possible novel therapy for diabetes with cell-permeable JNK-inhibitory peptide. Nat. Med. **10:** 1128–1132.
284. KANETO, H. *et al.* 2004. Oxidative stress and the JNK pathway as a potential therapeutic target for diabetes. Drug News Perspect. **17:** 447–453.
285. PEELMAN, F. *et al.* 2004. Mapping of the leptin binding sites and design of a leptin antagonist. J. Biol. Chem. **279:** 41038–41046.

Beneficial Effect of Supplemental Lipoic Acid on Diabetes-Induced Pregnancy Loss in the Mouse

RENGASAMY PADMANABHAN,[a] SHAFIULLAH MOHAMED,[b] AND SARABJIT SINGH[c]

[a]*Department of Anatomy, Faculty of Medicine and Health Sciences, UAE University, Al Ain, United Arab Emirates*

[b]*Department of Pharmacology, Faculty of Medicine and Health Sciences, UAE University, Al Ain, United Arab Emirates*

[c]*Department of Physiology, Faculty of Medicine and Health Sciences, UAE University, Al Ain, United Arab Emirates*

ABSTRACT: Uncontrolled diabetes mellitus (DM) is an etiological factor for recurrent pregnancy loss, fetal growth disorders, and major congenital malformations in the offspring. Antioxidant therapy has been advocated to overcome the oxidant–antioxidant disequilibrium inherent in diabetes. The objective of this article was to evaluate the beneficial effects of α-lipoic acid (LA) on fetal outcome in a mouse model of streptozotocin (STZ)-induced DM. Timed pregnant mice were made diabetic by intraperitoneal (IP) injection of a single dose of STZ (200 mg/kg) on gestation day (GD) 2. Diabetic animals were supplemented daily with an IP injection of 15 mg/kg of LA starting on GD 4 and continued through GD 12. Fetuses were examined on GD 18 for malformations and growth restriction. Some diabetic mice injected with Evans blue were examined on GD 3.5 and GD 6.5 to evaluate frequency of implantations. STZ-treated mice had all cardinal signs of DM. LA treatment did not normalize blood glucose levels of DM mice. Rates of pregnancy in saline control, DM, and DM + LA groups were 90%, 28%, and 64%, respectively, indicating that LA promotes pregnancy in DM animals. However, postimplantation resorption showed a threefold increase in the DM + LA group. Rates of intrauterine growth restriction and major congenital malformations were also augmented thus indicating that the interaction between DM and LA has deleterious effects on postimplantation embryos.

KEYWORDS: pregnancy loss; diabetes; fetal anomalies; fetal growth restriction; postimplantation resorption; supplemental lipoic acid

Address for correspondence: Rengasamy Padmanabhan, M.S., Ph.D., CBiol FIBiol (Lond), D.Sc. (med), Department of Anatomy, Faculty of Medicine and Health Sciences, UAE University, P.O. Box 17666, Al Ain, United Arab Emirates. Voice: 00-971-3-7137-494; fax: 00-971-3-7672-033.
e-mail: padmanabhanr@uaeu.ac.ae

**Ann. N.Y. Acad. Sci. 1084: 118–131 (2006). © 2006 New York Academy of Sciences.
doi: 10.1196/annals.1372.015**

INTRODUCTION

The steadily increasing trend in the prevalence of diabetes mellitus (DM) is of global concern.[1] This noncommunicable disease brings with it a staggering toll in cardiovascular, renal, and retinal complications and mortality.[2] Women are reported to be more prone to type 1 DM than men.[3] About 5% of all pregnancies occur among diabetic women, and DM is often diagnosed in women during pregnancy. With increasing longevity and changes in life style, the number of women who grew poorly in early life, presenting transgenerational health problems for their offspring is also found to be increasing. There is a two- to threefold increased incidence of major congenital malformations (MCM) in the offspring of diabetic women compared to that of the general population.[4] The nature of MCM observed in type 1, type 2, and gestational diabetes (GDM) are similar. High rates of stillbirths, preterm deliveries, perinatal mortality, and MCM have also been reported among diabetic women. Because congenital malformations are known to enhance perinatal mortality in general, it can be argued that the increased rates of perinatal death in the offspring of diabetic women might be due to structural malformations.[5–7] Associated with these complications is the need for caesarean operation among diabetic women that might impose considerable economic burden on health administration. Uncontrolled diabetes has been implicated as an etiological factor for recurrent pregnancy loss, and there is an estimated incidence of 17% spontaneous abortion in DM pregnancies.[8,9] Prevention of fetal complications in maternal DM requires a thorough understanding of the underlying pathophysiology of pregnancy in diabetes.

Poor maternal metabolic control during pregnancy is attributed to be the major cause for the augmented malformation rate.[6–10] Major organ system anomalies arise in embryos of diabetic women during the period of organogenesis and affect various systems rather nonspecifically.[4] Fetal macrosomia and poor growth outcome at birth are reported frequently in diabetic pregnancies.[11,12] Experimental studies on maternal diabetes in laboratory animals on the other hand have reported a consistent intrauterine growth restriction (IUGR) and fetoplacental abnormalities.[13–15] The mechanisms of diabetic embryopathy are not clearly understood as yet. There is some strong evidence that there is oxidant–antioxidant disequilibrium in DM.[16] Antioxidant therapy (e.g., vitamin E) has been reported to partially rescue the embryos from being malformed in diabetic environment, both *in vivo* and *in vitro*.[17]

α-Lipoic acid (LA) has been described as an ideal or universal antioxidant.[18] However, the only study that used LA as an antioxidant to prevent congenital malformations[19] claimed beneficial effects of LA against neural tube defects (NTD) in the streptozotocin (STZ) rat model. However, the results of their experiments have not been confirmed by other investigators. The TO mouse model of STZ-induced diabetes developed in our laboratory has NTD, skeletal malformations, and IUGR in a substantial proportion of embryos[20] in addition to a high incidence of pregnancy failure. The objective of the present article was to determine if exogenous LA had any protective effect against maternal diabetes-related pregnancy loss, embryonic death, fetal malformations, and IUGR in the mouse. We also studied histologically the decidua of DM and DM + LA group of animals characterized by profound loss of post-implantation embryos.

MATERIALS AND METHODS

The TO strain of mice used in this study were from a colony raised from a breeding nucleus obtained from Harlan Olac, England, UK. Adult females, about 30 g in weight and about 6 weeks of age were mated overnight with males in the evening and a vaginal plug identified in the following morning was taken to be a sign of successful mating. Plug positive day was designated as gestation day (GD) 0. All animals were housed in rooms at a temperature of $21 \pm 1^{\circ}$C and a relative humidity of 65% with 12:12 h light–dark cycle. A commercial chow and tap water were made available *ad libitum* to all animals throughout the study.

Diabetes was induced on GD 2 by intraperitoneal (IP) injection of a single dose of 200 mg/kg of STZ (Sigma-Aldrich Corp., St. Louis, MO) dissolved freshly in citrate buffer (pH 4.7). The controls received a proportionate volume of buffer. A blood glucose level of 200 mg/dL or more determined photometrically 24 h later was considered to confirm presence of DM. LA (Sigma) was dissolved in saline buffered to pH 7.2. One half of the DM animals were administered daily (IP) a single dose of 15 mg/kg LA (DM + LA), while the other half received IP an equal volume of saline (DM + Saline) starting on GD 4 and continued through GD 12—the major period of organogenesis. The citrate buffer group was also divided into two subgroups and treated (IP) with LA (Buffer + LA) or a proportionate volume of saline (Buffer + Saline) during GD 4–12. Thus, there were four groups in all and all animals had an equal number of injections. Their plasma glucose levels, food and water consumption, and body weight gain with time were recorded. All animals were killed by cervical dislocation on GD 18. Fetal deaths/resorptions were recorded and live fetuses collected. They were weighed, examined for external malformations with a dissecting microscope, fixed in 95% ethanol, and subsequently evaluated for visceral and skeletal malformations according to the procedures of Sterz and Lehmann[21] and Inouye[22] slightly modified in our laboratory. Another set of similarly treated animals were injected in the tail vein with 0.5% of Evans blue in saline on GD 3.5 and 6.5, killed after 5 min, their uteri collected, and number of implantations counted.[23]

Statistics

The data were analyzed using the Statistical Packages for Social Sciences (SPSS). Student's *t*-test was used to ascertain the significances between mean values of two continuous variables and Mann-Whitney *U*-test was used for nonparametric distribution. One-way analysis of variance (ANOVA) was employed for comparison of several group means. Resorption, fetal weight, and malformations were analyzed by ANOVA. The level of significance was set at $P < 0.05$.

RESULTS

Maternal Effects

For the sake of simplicity, henceforth, the four treatment groups of this study will be referred to as: (1) Diabetes-alone group (DM + Saline), (2) LA-alone group (buffer + LA), (3) LA-supplemented diabetic group (DM + LA), and (4) Saline control group (Buffer + Saline). Only those animals that were vaginal plug positive were used in this study. Both the LA-supplemented diabetic and diabetes-alone groups of mice exhibited all cardinal signs of diabetes, such as hyperglycemia, polyuria, polyphagia, and polydipsia. The diabetic animals gained in body weight rather poorly unlike the nontreated or saline controls. The LA-supplemented diabetic animals consumed moderately greater amounts of food and water but this did not impact significantly on their body weight gain.

The maternal blood sugar levels recorded on GD 4, 12, and 18 indicated that both in LA-alone and saline control groups, the blood sugar levels were comparable and as low as that of the nontreated controls. In diabetes-alone animals, however, the sugar levels went up by three to four times the values of the nontreated control group, and LA treatment was found to have no impact at all on controlling glucose levels of diabetic animals (FIG. 1). Plasma concentration of glucose in LA-supplemented DM group was consistently high and similar to that of the nonsupplemented DM group of mice.

On laparotomy on GD 18, about 90% of saline control animals and LA group were found to be pregnant, whereas only 28% of the DM-alone animals were found to carry fetuses. About 64% of the LA-supplemented DM group animals were found to be pregnant indicating a statistically significant effect ($P < 0.05$) of LA in rescuing mice from DM-induced early pregnancy loss (TABLE 1).

Resorption

The total number of implantations per litter ranged from 10 to 12 in saline, LA, and LA-supplemented DM groups similar to that of the nontreated control. Most striking is the fact that pregnancy failure occurred more frequently in the DM group, and supplemental LA substantially rescued the mice from this failure (TABLE 1). However, postimplantation embryo toxicity was higher in

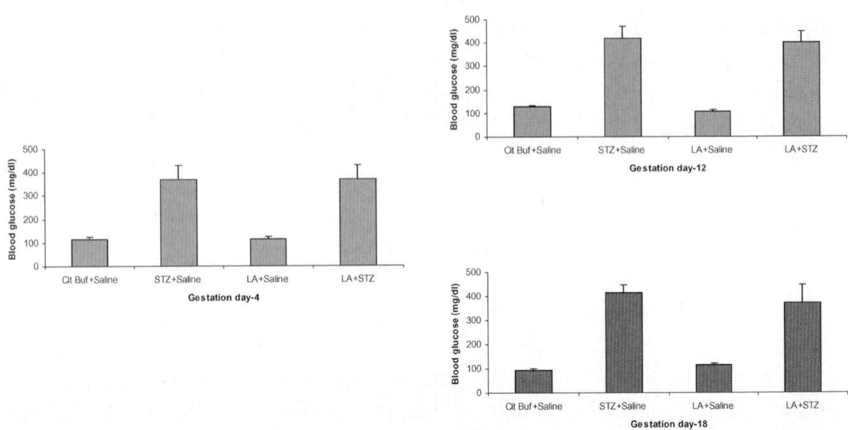

FIGURE 1. Effect of LA treatment on blood sugar levels of diabetic mice.

the LA-supplemented DM groups of mice. There was a threefold increase in the incidence of resorption when the diabetic animals were supplemented with LA. About 8% of LA-supplemented animals had their entire litters resorbed, indicating the high level of embryo toxicity of this dose of LA in diabetic pregnancy (TABLE 1). The LA-induced resorption in the nondiabetic pregnancy was as low as 2.3%. These data indicate how abnormal fuel metabolism disturbs normal implantation and how extensively postimplantation survival of mouse embryos could be affected. The data also indicate that there is some interaction between LA and diabetic condition, which is toxic to the postimplantation embryos.

Malformations

Both the nontreated and saline control animals had a low frequency of minor malformations. Maxillary, mandibular hypoplasia, low-set ears, etc., generally registered a modest increase in incidence in DM + LA group. Exencephaly was confined to LA-supplemented DM group (1.5%) and LA (1.0%) group. The difference was not significant. Holoprosencephaly (HPE) occurred in one litter of the DM group and in three litters of LA-supplemented DM group. This complex malformation sequence comprised mandibular micrognathism and agnathism, severe upper-midface hypoplasia, undivided hypoplastic cerebral vesicle without corpus callosum, agenesis of the olfactory bulbs, asymmetric growth of the forebrain vesicle, hypoplasia or agenesis of the cerebellum, low-anteriorly set microtia, edema, astomia/microstomia, anophthalmia, occasional cyclopia, and proboscis (FIGS. 2 and 3). IUGR was marked in the diabetic

TABLE 1. Effect of LA supplementation on fetal toxicity in STZ-induced diabetes in the mouse

	Saline (citrate buffer + saline)	DM (STZ + saline)	LA (citrate buffer + lipoic acid)	DM + LA (STZ + lipoic acid)
No of mice treated	12	39	16	25
No of mice pregnant (a,c,d,e,f)	11 (91.7)	11 (28.2)	14 (87.5)	16 (64.0)
Nonpregnant (a,c,d,e,f)	1 (8.3)	32 (82.1)	2 (12.5)	7 (28.0)
Average implantations	9.8	10	9.1	8.4
Resorptions (a,c,d,e,f)	14 (13.0)	18 (18.2)	3 (2.3)	68 (50.9)
Live fetuses (c,e,f)	94 (87.0)	92 (83.6)	125 (97.7)	67 (49.6)
No of litters malformed (a,c,d,f)	1 (9.1)	6 (54.6)	1 (7.1)	11 (68.8)
Fetal weight (g) (mean ± SD) (a,c,d,e,f)	1.266±0.056	0.897 ± 0.136	1.354 ± 0.104	0.864 ± 0.115
IUGR at 2 SD (c,e,f)	0	92 (100.0)	0	67 (100.0)

NOTE: IUGR = intrauterine growth restriction; STZ = streptozotocin; LA = lipoic acid; DM = diabetes mellitus parentheses contain percentage; $P < 0.05$, when comparisons are made as follows: a = DM vs Saline; b = LA vs Saline; c = DM + LA vs Saline; d = LA vs DM; e = DM + LA vs DM; f = DM + LA vs LA.

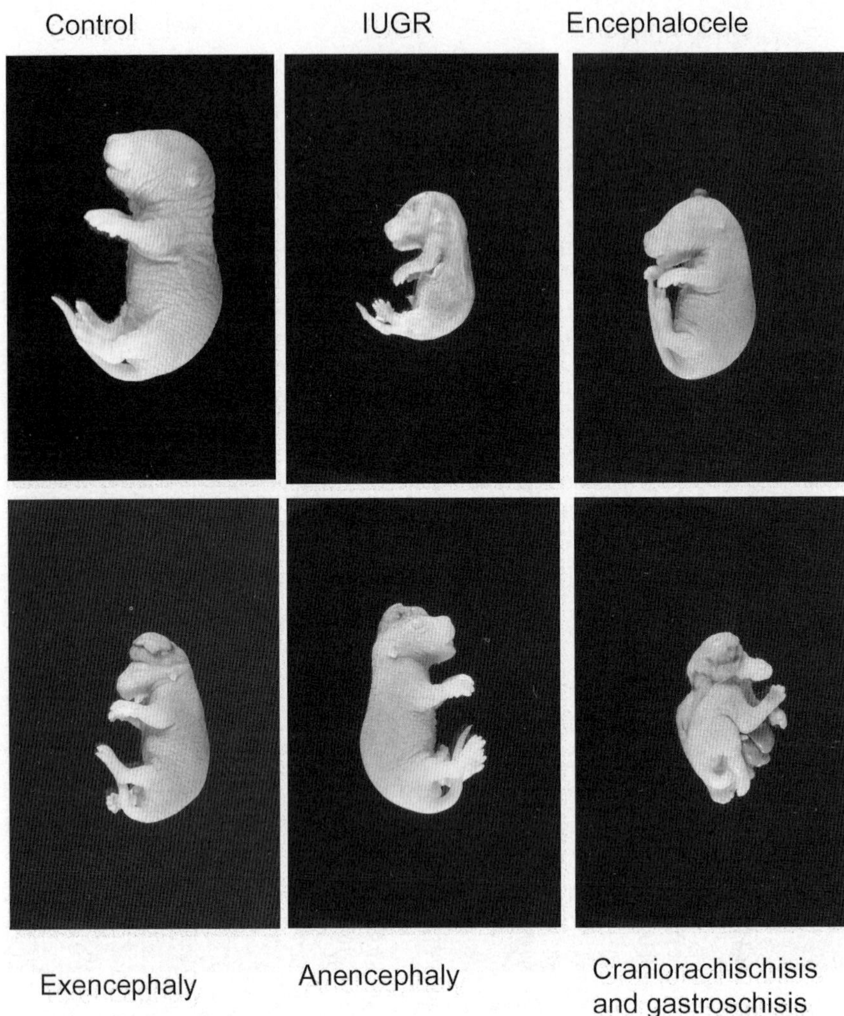

FIGURE 2. IUGR and CNS malformations in LA-supplemented diabetes group mouse embryos of gestation day 18.

group and both severity and frequency of IUGR were found to be enhanced by LA supplementation. Diabetic-group fetuses had a generalized retardation of skeletal growth, most marked as hypoplasia of the caudal vertebrae and bones of the hands and feet (data not presented here). LA supplementation did not have any preventative impact on the malformation rate. Craniofacial skeletal malformations of the fetuses of diabetic animals supplemented with LA were similar in nature and comparable in frequency to those of the diabetes-alone group.

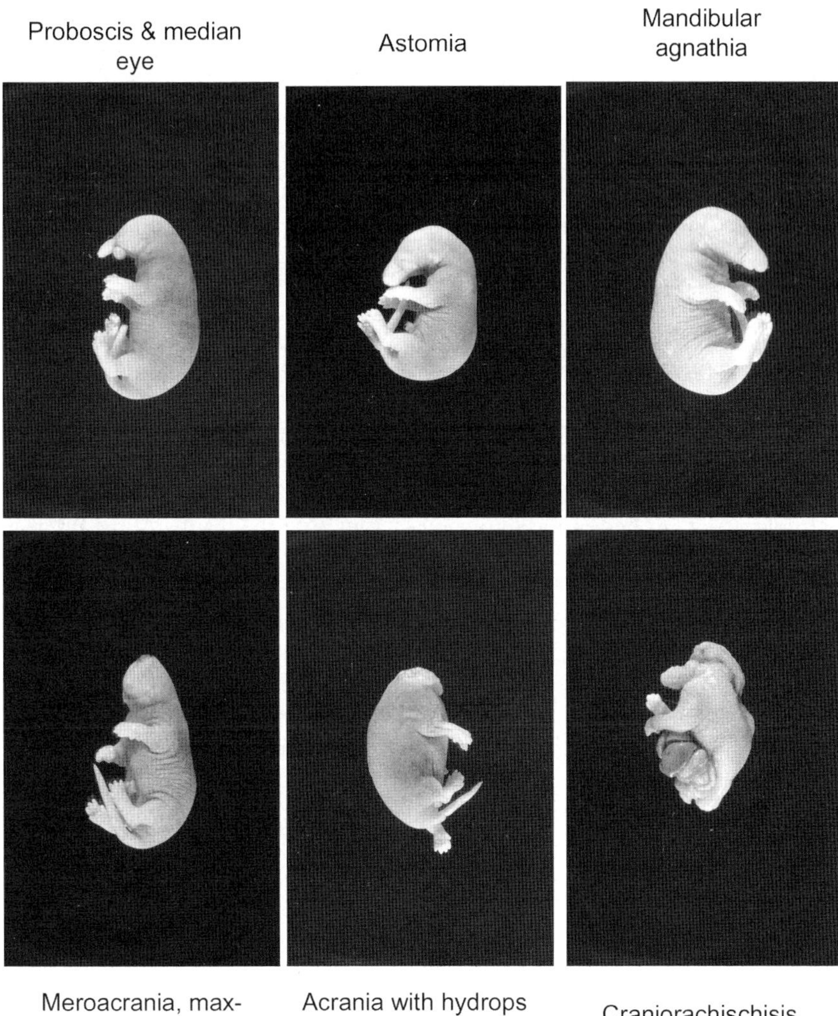

FIGURE 3. HPE sequence, acrania and gastroschisis in LA-supplemented diabetic group mouse embryos of gestation day 18.

Intrauterine Growth Restriction

Fetuses weighing 2 SD less than the mean body weight of the age-matched controls were regarded as growth restricted.[24] Fetuses of diabetic animals were much lighter in weight than those of the saline control (TABLE 2, IUGR in FIG. 2). LA-alone-treated animals had fetuses that weighed significantly more than the saline controls. When diabetic animals were supplemented with LA, the fetal body weight was found to be reduced further, more than that of the DM-alone group. The IUGR incidence was greatly pronounced in comparison to buffer or LA-alone groups indicating a possible interaction between maternal diabetic state with the antioxidant LA administered. Thus LA appears to have a synergic effect on diabetes-related IUGR. In other words, LA supplementation did not rescue the embryos from diabetes-induced IUGR but only aggravated the growth restriction.

DISCUSSION

Previous studies from our laboratory have shown that both in rats and mice, maternal diabetes during gestation can result in significant resorption of embryos, major structural malformations, and placental abnormalities.[20,25–27] The current study is an effort to determine whether these DM-related complications could be reduced by an antioxidant, namely, LA. The rationale is the observation that DM causes an oxidant–antioxidant imbalance.[16] Although NTD are not particularly common in our rat studies,[13,27] the results of the present experiments showed that there was only a low incidence of exencephaly in the DM group of mice. Although HPE did not occur at all in rats, the present study had a significant incidence of both the typical form of HPE (cyclopia, undivided forebrain with no corpus callosum, cerebellar hypoplasia, etc.) and a milder form of HPE-like phenotype (partial absence of forebrain, unilateral hypoplasia and folding of cerebral tissue, microcephaly, absence of olfactory bulbs and tracts, hypoplasia or agenesis of corpus callosum, and moderate to severe midline facial hypoplasia). A 7% incidence of HPE in DM group was found to be accentuated to about 21% incidence in LA-supplemented DM group, which strongly suggests an interaction of LA with maternal DM state. HPE is the most common of forebrain malformations. Failure of or defective induction signals from the prechordal plate and deficiency of midline mesoderm in the area around forebrain vesicle are thought to result in persistence of an embryonic condition of an undivided prosencephalon.[28] This precursor tissue deficiency might also explain the spectrum of midline facial malformations associated with HPE. Several human and mouse studies have recently established the strong roles that sonic hedgehog (SHH), SIX3, TGIF, and ZIC gene families play in the pathogenesis of this MCM spectrum.[29–34] A high incidence of HPE in our mouse model of DM during pregnancy implies that DM possibly modifies the functions of these developmental genes. HPE is reported to occur at a rate of 1:250 in the nonselected population of early human embryos and decreasing throughout gestation and is reduced to a frequency of 1:16,000/1:20,000 in live-born infants,[28,34,35] indicating the lethal nature of this anomaly to the developing embryos. The present study revealed a high incidence of resorption in the DM (18%) and DM + LM groups (51%), which suggests that at least some of these embryos were severely malformed before they died.

TABLE 2. Effect of LA supplementation on fetal malformations in STZ-induced diabetes in the mouse

	Saline (citrate buffer + saline)	DM (STZ + saline)	LA (citrate buffer + lipoic acid)	STZ + LA (STZ + lipoic acid)
Total number of embryos	94	92	125	67
Malformed embryos	1 (1.1)	15 (16.3)	1 (0.8)	23 (34.3)
Mandible hypoplasia	1 (1.1)	8 (8.7)	1 (0.8)	15 (22.4)
Maxilla hypoplasia	0	8 (8.7)	1 (0.8)	14 (20.9)
Exencephaly	0	2 (2.2)	1 (0.8)	1 (1.5)
Holoprosencephaly	0	6 (6.5)	0	14 (20.9)
Eye open	0	1 (1.1)	0	6 (9.0)
Exomphalos	0	0	0	5 (7.5)
Astomia	0	4 (4.4)	0	4 (6.0)
Microstomia	0	1 (1.1)	0	3 (4.5)
Gastroschisis	0	1 (1.1)	0	2 (3.0)
Unascended Kidney	0	1 (1.1)	0	3 (4.5)
Hydrops	0	3 (3.3)	0	1 (1.5)
Anteriorly set ears	0	3 (3.3)	0	0
Proboscis	0	3 (3.3)	0	1 (1.5)
Madian eye	0	2 (2.2)	0	0
Low set microtia	0	2 (2.2)	0	0
Acrania	0	2 (2.2)	0	0
Exophthalmia	0	1 (1.1)	0	1 (1.5)
*Other abnormalities	0	10 (10.9)	0	5 (7.5)

*__Other abnormalities:__ encephalocele, cyclopia, cleft palate, single ventricle, anophthalmia, kinky tail, anterior half face absent protruding tongue, craniorachischisis, undescended testes, open eye, single nostril.

Our study has also shown that DM produces a primary pregnancy failure in about 70% of animals in this model. Evans blue preparation showed that the embryos of diabetic dams landed in the uterus after considerable delay suggesting that the damage to embryos of DM dams occurs as the embryos traverse the Fallopian tube. Exogenous LA administered from GD 4 through GD 12 enhanced pregnancy rate in mice with DM to 64%. In addition to affirming the beneficial effects of supplemental LA in promoting pregnancy rate, these data also show that most of the pregnancy loss occurred before GD 4, the first day of LA supplementation, thus establishing the vulnerability of early embryos to altered maternal metabolic status. The exact mechanism by which LA prevents embryo loss is unknown, but it can be safely assumed that LA possibly protected preimplantation embryos against DM-related apoptosis and growth inhibition. That the average implantation rate did not differ statistically in different treatment groups of this study (TABLE 1) suggests that LA followed an "all or none" effect in terms of the number of embryos it would support survival until implantation. A noteworthy outcome of this study is a threefold increased incidence of embryo resorption in the LA-supplemented DM pregnancies over that of the DM-alone group. This enhanced postimplantation embryo loss in DM + LA group shows that although LA at this dosage regimen has a direct beneficial effect on preimplantation embryos, at early postimplantation stages maternal mediation of LA is rather deleterious to the conceptus. The trophectoderm of the ectoplacental cone and the decidua contribute to the definitive placenta, which becomes interposed between the embryonic and the maternal compartments in the postimplantation embryos. It is important to try and understand the responses of these tissues to maternal DM in the peri-implantation period and whether LA modified these responses thus leading to embryonic resorption. We are currently working on this project. The increased rates of IUGR and major structural anomalies observed in the DM + LA group in comparison to those of the nonsupplemented DM group would point to and further strengthen the view that LA and DM interact in some unknown way in producing augmented postimplantation embryo loss, malformation rate, and IUGR.

Data from our previous studies indicate that IUGR is almost a rule in our rat and mouse models of DM.[13,15,20] We have not encountered any instance of fetal macrosomia in these studies. This observation is at variance with clinical reports of fetal macrosomia for which maternal DM is a significant risk factor.[36,37] Most of the experimental studies on DM have focussed attention on congenital malformations in animal models but growth disorders have not received yet the attention they deserve. Since Hales and Barker[38] proposed the "thrifty phenotype" hypothesis in 1992, numerous clinical and laboratory studies have adduced evidence that IUGR confers increased risk on affected offspring for developing later in adult life both chronic and fatal diseases through the effects of prenatal programming.[39,40] As a result, studies into the causes, mechanisms, and manifestations of prenatal growth restriction have assumed greater importance recently than ever before. Fetal growth disturbances in diabetic pregnancies are well recognized. Besides maternal DM, other factors including maternal obesity, increased BMI, and weight gain during pregnancy are also attributed to fetal macrosomia.[41] Macrosomic fetuses are reported to attain accelerated growth during early second trimester.[41] However, some ultrasonographic studies have indicated early on that even those fetuses that are found to be normal in size at term in diabetic pregnancies are in fact growth restricted during early stages of the development.[42,43]

SUMMARY AND CONCLUSIONS

STZ-induced maternal DM results in a significant reduction in the frequency of successful pregnancies in vaginal plug positive mice. The offspring of DM mice are growth restricted and about 16% of them are severely malformed. Craniofacial, urogenital, and skeletal anomalies were the most common abnormalities. Supplementation with LA substantially enhanced pregnancy rate but augmented the rates of postimplantation resorption, malformation, and IUGR. These results indicate that the antioxidant-related rescue effects are limited to the preimplantation development and that the LA interaction with DM is rather deleterious to postimplantation embryos. Because the decidua and trophectoderm contribute to the placenta development in mice, future studies must be directed at the immunologic and morphologic changes that occur in the embryo and uterine environment during the process of implantation and during the period that immediately follows to obtain some insight into the role of these tissues in embryonic resorption after LA supplementation in DM mice.

REFERENCES

1. Steering Committee of the National Health Initiative and women's Health, Centers for disease control and prevention, Report from the CDC. The National Public Health Initiative on Diabetes and Women's Health: leading the way for women with and at risk for diabetes. J. Women's Health (Larchmt.) 2004: **13:** 962–967.
2. Steinbrook, R. 2006. Facing the diabetes epidemic—mandatory reporting of glycosylated hemoglobin values in New York City. N. Engl. J. Med. **354:** 545–548.
3. Pishdad, G.R. 2005. Low incidence of type 1 diabetes in Iran. Diabetes Care **28:** 927–928.
4. Greene, M.F. 2001. Diabetic embryopathy 2001: moving beyond the "diabetic milieu". Teratology **63:** 116–118.
5. Brydon, P., T. Smith, M. Proffitt, *et al.* 2000. Pregnancy outcome in women with type 2 diabetes mellitus needs to be addressed. Int. J. Clin. Pract. **54:** 418–419.

6. JENSEN, D.M., P. DAMM, L. MOELSTED-PEDERSEN, *et al.* 2004. Outcomes in type 1 diabetic pregnancies: a nationwide, population-based study. Diabetes Care **27:** 2819–2823.
7. NGAI, C.W., W.L. MARTIN, A. TONKS & M.P. KILBY. 2005. Are isolated facial cleft lip and palate associated with increased perinatal mortality? A cohort study from the West Midlands Region, 1995–1997. J. Matern. Fetal Neonatal Med. **17:** 203–206.
8. CASSON, I.F., C.A. CLARKE, C.V. HOWARD, *et al.* 1997. Outcomes of pregnancy in insulin dependent diabetic women: results of a five year population cohort study. Br. Med. J. **315:** 275–278.
9. ARREDONDO, F. & L.S. NOBLE. 2006. Endocrinology of recurrent pregnancy loss. Semin. Reprod. Med. **24:** 33–39.
10. SUHONEN, L., V. HIILESMAA & K. TERAMO. 2000. Glycemic control during early pregnancy and fetal malformations in women with type 1 diabetes mellitus. Diabetologia **43:** 79–82.
11. TAMURA, R.K., R.E. SABBAGHA, R. DEPP, *et al.* 1986. Diabetic macrosomia: accuracy of third trimester ultrasound. Obstet. Gynoncol. **67:** 828–832.
12. LAMPL, M. & P. JEANTY. 2004. Exposure to maternal diabetes is associated with altered fetal growth patterns: a hypothesis regarding metabolic allocation to growth under hyperglycemic-hypoxemic conditions. Am. J. Hum. Biol. **16:** 237–263.
13. PADMANABHAN, R. & A.G.H. AL-ZUHAIR. 1988. Congenital malformation and intrauterine growth retardation in streptozotocin induced diabetes during gestation in the rat. Reprod. Toxicol. **1:** 117–125.
14. KALTER, H.A. 1999. Flawed experiment, again. Am. J. Obstet. Gynecol. **181:** 1039–1040.
15. PADMANABHAN, R. & M. SHAFIULLAH. 2001. Intrauterine growth retardation in experimental diabetes: possible role of the placenta. Arch. Physiol. Biochem. **109:** 260–271.
16. MOINI, H., L. PACKER & N.E. SARIS. 2002. Antioxidant and pro-oxidant activities of alpha-lipoic acid and dihydrolipoic acid. Toxicol. Appl. Pharmacol. **182:** 84–90.
17. ZAKEN, V., R. KOHEN & A. ORNOY. 2001. Vitamin C and E improve rat embryonic antioxidant defense mechanism in diabetic culture medium. Teratology **64:** 33–34.
18. PACKER, L., K. KRAEMER & G. RIMBACH. 2001. Molecular aspects of lipoic acid in the prevention of diabetes complications. Nutrition **17:** 888–895.
19. WIZNITZER, A., N. AYALON, R. HERSHKOVITZ, *et al.* 1999. Lipoic acid prevention of neural tube defects in offspring of rats with streptozocin-induced diabetes. Am. J. Obstet. Gynecol. **80:** 188–193.
20. PADMANABHAN, R. & M. SHAFIULLAH. 2004. Effect of maternal diabetes and ethanol interactions on embryo development in the mouse. Mol. Cell. Biochem. **261:** 43–56.
21. STERZ, H. & H. LEHMANN. 1985. A critical comparison of the free hand razor blade dissection method according to Wilson with an in situ sectioning method for rat fetuses. Teratog. Carcinog. Mutagen **5:** 347–354.
22. INOUYE, M. 1976. Differential staining of cartilage and bone in fetal mouse skeleton by alcian blue and alizarin red-S. Cong. Anom. **16:** 171–173.
23. CHAVEZ, D.J. 1986. Cell surface of mouse blastocysts at the trophectoderm-uterine interface during the adhesive stage of implantation. Am. J. Anat. **176:** 153–158.
24. WILSON, J.G. 1973. Environment and Birth Defects. Academic Press. New York.

25. PADMANABHAN, R., A.G.H. AL-ZUHAIR & H. AIDA. 1988. Histopathological changes of the placenta in diabetes induced by maternal administration of streptozotocin during pregnancy in the rat. Cong. Anom. **28:** 1–15.
26. PADMANABHAN, R. & M. SHAFIULLAH. 2001. Intrauterine growth retardation in experimental diabetes. Possible role of the placenta. Arch. Physiol. Biochem. **109:** 260–271.
27. AL GHAFLI, M.H., R. PADMANABHAN, H.H. KATAYA & B. BERG. 2004. Effects of alpha-lipoic acid supplementation on maternal diabetes-induced growth retardation and congenital anomalies in rat fetuses. Mol. Cell. Biochem. **261:** 123–135.
28. YAMADA, S., C. UWABE, S. FUJII & K. SHIOTA. 2004. Phenotypic variability in human embryonic holoprosencephaly in the Kyoto Collection. Birth Defects Res. A Clin. Mol. Teratol. **70:** 495–508.
29. DUBOURG, C., L. LAZARO, L. PASQUIER, *et al.* 2004. Molecular screening of SHH, ZIC2, SIX3, and TGIF genes in patients with features of holoprosencephaly spectrum: mutation review and genotype-phenotype correlations. Hum. Mutat. **24:** 43–51.
30. BENDAVID, C., C. DUBOURG, I. GICQUEL, *et al.* 2006. Molecular evaluation of fetuses with holoprosencephaly shows high incidence of microdeletions in the HPE genes. Hum. Genet. **119:** 1–8.
31. HAYHURST, M. & S.K. MCCONNELL. 2003. Mouse models of holoprosencephaly. Curr. Opin. Neurol. **16:** 135–141.
32. GRINBERG, I. & K.J. MILLEN. 2005. The ZIC gene family in development and disease. Clin. Genet. **67:** 290–296.
33. MAITY, T., N. FUSE & P.A. BEACHY. 2005. Molecular mechanisms of Sonic hedgehog mutant effects in holoprosencephaly. Proc. Natl. Acad. Sci. USA **102:** 17026–17031.
34. BROWN, L., M. PARASO, R. ARKELL & S. BROWN. 2005. In vitro analysis of partial loss-of-function ZIC2 mutations in holoprosencephaly: alanine tract expansion modulates DNA binding and transactivation. Hum. Mol. Genet. **14:** 411–420.
35. MATSUNAGA, E. & K. SHIOTA. 1977. Holoprosencephaly in human embryos: epidemiologic studies of 150 cases. Teratology **16:** 261–272.
36. OLSEN, C.L., J.P. HUGHES, L.G. YOUNGBLOOD & M. SHARPE-STIMAC. 1997. Epidemiology of holoprosencephaly and phenotypic characteristics of affected children: New York State, 1984-1989. Am. J. Med. Genet. **73:** 217–226.
37. HEISKANEN, N., K. RAATIKAINEN & S. HEINONEN. 2006. Fetal macrosomia—a continuing obstetric challenge. Biol. Neonate **90:** 98–103.
38. HALES, C.N. & D.J. BARKER. 1992. Type 2 (non-insulin-dependent) diabetes mellitus: the thrifty phenotype hypothesis. Diabetologia **35:** 595–601.
39. HALES, C.N. & S.E. OZANNE. 2003. For debate: fetal and early postnatal growth restriction lead to diabetes, the metabolic syndrome and renal failure. Diabetologia **46:** 1013–1019.
40. MONK, D. & G.E. MOORE. 2004. Intrauterine growth restriction–genetic causes and consequences. Semin. Fetal Neonatal Med. **9:** 371–378.
41. WONG, S.F., F.Y. CHAN, J.J. OATS & D.H. MCINTYRE. 2002. Fetal growth spurt and pregestational diabetic pregnancy. Diabetes Care **25:** 1681–1684.
42. PEDERSEN, J.F. & L. MOLSTED-PEDERSEN. 1979. Early growth retardation in diabetic pregnancy. Br. Med. J. **1:** 18–19.
43. PEDERSEN, J.F. & L. MOLSTED-PEDERSEN. 1981. Early fetal growth delay detected by ultrasound marks increased risk of congenital malformation in diabetic pregnancy. Br. Med. J. **283:** 269–271.

Audit of Pregnancies Complicated by Diabetes from One Center Five Years Apart with Selective versus Universal Screening

M. EZIMOKHAI,[a] ANNIE JOSEPH,[b] AND P. BRADLEY-WATSON[b]

[a]*Department of Obstetrics and Gynaecology, Faculty of Medicine and Health Sciences, UAE University, Al Ain, United Arab Emirates*

[b]*General Authority for Health Services, Al Ain Hospital, Al Ain, United Arab Emirates*

ABSTRACT: The article compares the effect of selective and universal screening on detection rate and outcomes of pregnancies complicated by diabetes mellitus (DM) in a multiethnic population. The method used was to review the pregnancy and delivery of two 18-month periods, 5 years apart. In the year 1996–1997 when selective screening was used 315 (5.7%) of 5506 delivered women had diabetes during pregnancy. The rates of diabetes in the different ethnic groups were: UAE (4.4%), Peninsula Arabs (4.0%), Chami Arabs (4.5%), North African Arabs (6.7%), Indian subcontinent (7.5%), and Somalis and Sudanese (9.7%). The rate of diabetes among the different ethnic groups for the year 2001–2002 when screening was universal but diagnosis made by the same criteria were 590 (9.7%) of 6232 delivered women, UAE (9.2%), Peninsula Arabs (8.4%), Chami Arabs (8.2%), North African Arabs (9.6%), Indian Subcontinent (11.0%), Somalis and Sudanese (11.3%). The outcome indicators and their rates in the years 1996–1997 and 2001–2002 were respectively: gestational diabetes, 86.3%, 89.0%; requirement of insulin treatment, 74.3% 82.5%; vaginal delivery, 68.2%, 75.3%; cesarean section, 30.3%, 19.8%; macrosomia, 22.2%, 6.7%; intrauterine fetal death, 2.9%, 1.1%; and preterm delivery, 22.5%, 17.5%. This article confirms the influence of ethnic background on the prevalence of gestational diabetes in a multiethnic and multicultural society. Over a period of 5 years, there was a 66.7% increase in the incidence of gestational diabetes, which was probably due to a combination of increased detection by change in screening policy and an increase in the incidence of gestational diabetes. The indicators of disease severity and control, such as insulin requirement, rates of abdominal delivery, macrosomia, and structural congenital malformations, were significantly better in a

Address for correspondence: Prof. M. Ezimokhai, Department of Obstetrics and Gynaecology, Faculty of Medicine and Health Sciences, UAE University, P.O. Box 17666, Al Ain, United Arab Emirates. Voice: +971-3-7137567; fax: +971-3-7672067.

e-mail: mezimokhai@uaeu.ac.ae

Ann. N.Y. Acad. Sci. 1084: 132–140 (2006). © 2006 New York Academy of Sciences.
doi: 10.1196/annals.1372.009

cohort identified by universal screening compared with that identified by selective screening. Universal screening seems to be a more appropriate strategy for screening in this environment.

KEYWORDS: **gestational diabetes; screening; ethnicity; pregnancy outcomes**

INTRODUCTION

Pregnancies complicated by diabetes carry high risk for both the mother and fetus.[1,2] Prenatal control of blood sugar has been shown to improve the outcomes.[3] A majority of pregnant mothers with diabetes are unaware of the disease and develop it during pregnancy.[4] To identify the affected mothers, screening programs have been suggested and widely practiced. Nonetheless, the very existence of the disease,[5] need for screening,[6] diagnostic criteria, and ideal methods for screening are all disputed.[7,8] The recent publication by the Australian Carbohydrate Intolerance Study (ACHOIS),[9] which showed improved obstetric outcomes for treated women with relatively mild disease (impaired glucose tolerance), compared with untreated women, clearly validates both screening and treatment of gestational diabetes.

Some of the many factors, which affect the decision on screening policy include prevalence, availability of resources, and perceived cost effectiveness. The prevalence of the disease is influenced by the patients' ethnic origin.[10,11]

The United Arab Emirates, as a rapidly developing economy, provides job opportunities for people from different parts of the world and consequently the healthcare system has to cater for a heterogeneous multiethnic and multinational population. Our obstetric database has 24 nationalities on record. There are no valid data to direct decision making in providing care to mothers with gestational diabetes in this environment and previous studies[12] on the population have not addressed these.

Between the years 1994 and 2000, at the Department of Obstetrics and Gynaecology, Al Ain Hospital, Al Ain, United Arab Emirates, the policy regarding gestational diabetes required administration of the 1 h 50 g glucose challenge test to pregnant women selectively on the basis of risk factors (diabetes in first-degree relative, previous history of gestational diabetes, unexplained stillbirth at term, previous macrosomic infant, weight over 100 kg, etc.) followed by a diagnostic 3 h 100 g oral glucose tolerance test[13] for those in whom the screening value was $\geq$7.8 mmol/L. This policy was modified in the year 2000 and a 1 h 50 g glucose challenge test was administered for all pregnant women followed by a diagnostic test if cutoff values were obtained. This two-step approach was again modified in the year 2004 to the one-step 75 g oral glucose tolerance test for all women. These decisions were made on the basis of resource availability rather than an audit of effectiveness and outcomes.

This article is aimed at defining the prevalence of diabetes among different ethnic groups, the effect of screening method on diagnosis and outcomes, and the temporal trend in the incidence of the disease based on our experience at the Department of Obstetrics and Gynaecology, Al Ain Hospital, United Arab Emirates. This is one of the hospitals used for teaching by the Faculty of Medicine and Health Sciences, UAE University, Al Ain, United Arab Emirates. The delivery rate at the hospital is about 4000 per annum and perinatal mortality rate is about 10 per 1000. Ninety-eight percent of all deliveries take place in the hospital.

MATERIALS AND METHODS

The demographic and obstetric records of all patients were entered in a database. After obtaining ethical approval from the Al Ain Hospital Research and Ethics Committee, demographic data, number of diagnosed gestational diabetes, insulin requirement during pregnancy, duration of pregnancy and mode of delivery, birth weight of newborns, presence of structural congenital malformation for all subjects were extracted for two 18-month periods (June 1996 to December 1997 and June 2001 to December 2002), 5 years apart.

The protocols for obstetric and medical management of gestational diabetes were unaltered during this period and the same team of endocrinologist physicians was consulted for the whole period. The incidence of diabetes among the different ethnic groups, the incidence of diabetes in the population, and the rates of the selected outcome indicators for the years 1996–1997 and 2001–2002 were compared. The outcome indicators were the route of delivery, rates of neonatal macrosomia, preterm delivery, unexplained intrauterine fetal death, structural congenital malformations, and early (first 7 days of life) neonatal deaths.

For ease of analysis, ethnic groups from close geographical areas were grouped together as follows: Peninsula Arabs (Omanis, Emiratis, Saudis, Kuwaitis, Yemenis), Chami Arabs (Lebanese, Jordanians, Palestinians, Syrians), North African Arabs (Egyptians, Moroccans, Libyans, Tunisians, Mauritanians, Algerians), East African Arabs (Somalis and Sudanese), and Indian subcontinent (Iranians, Indians, Pakistanis, Afghanis, Sri Lankans, Bangladeshis) (FIG. 1). Differences in proportions were compared using the Fischer's exact test and are considered significant if $P < 0.05$.

RESULTS

TABLE 1 shows that the distribution of the ethnic groups among the obstetric population remained relatively the same in the years 1996–1997 and 2001–2002, suggesting a stable population structure, with regards to ethnic distribution. The proportion of pregnancies complicated by diabetes has significantly increased over the 5-year period in all the obstetric patients

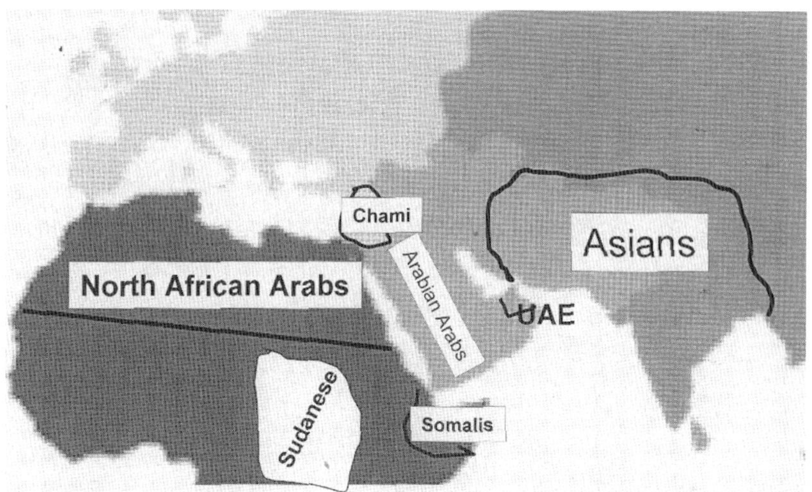

FIGURE 1. Approximate geographical location of the ethnic groups.

($P = 0.0001$) as well as among the different ethnic groups (range 16.7–110%, $P < 0.0001$).

The highest and lowest incidences were recorded for the same ethnic groupings over the 5-year period although the screening policies were different. However, the difference between the highest (9.7%) and lowest (4.0%) incidence in the year 1996–1997 had narrowed significantly and the difference between the highest (11.3%) and lowest (8.2%) rates was not statistically significant in the year 2001–2002. Consequently, the ethnic groupings with the highest incidence in the year 1996–1997 demonstrated the lowest increase by the year 2001–2002, whereas the ethnic grouping with the lowest incidence in the year 1996–1997 demonstrated the highest increase by the year 2001–2002.

The type of diabetes and the need for insulin to control blood glucose are shown in TABLE 2. A significantly higher proportion (25.7%, $P = 0.007$) of the patients diagnosed with gestational diabetes in the 1996–1997 cohort required insulin to control the blood sugar compared with the 2001–2002 cohort (17.4%). Further, the proportion of patients with gestational diabetes was more (89.8%) in the year 2001–2002 compared with 1996–1997 (86.3%) but the difference was not statistically significant.

Compared to the 1996–1997 cohort, a smaller proportion of the patients in the 2001–2002 cohort were delivered by cesarean section ($P = 0.002$), had macrosomic infants ($P = 0.000003$), or structural congenital anomalies ($P = 0.003$). There were no significant differences in the rate of preterm delivery (<37 completed weeks gestation) (TABLE 3). There were no significant differences in the incidences of these events among the nondiabetic groups in the two time periods.

TABLE 1. Incidence of gestational diabetics among the different ethnic groupings (1996–1997 and 2001–2002)

Group	1996–1997				2001–2002				% increase in DM
	Number		Diabetic		Total number		Total Diabetic		
	N_1	% of T	N	% of N_1	N_2	% of T_2	N	% of N_2	
UAE national	1,352	24.6	60	4.4	1,313	21.1	121	9.2	109.1
Peninsula Arabs	608	11.0	24	4.0	818	13.1	69	8.4	110.0
Chami Arabs	1,110	20.2	50	4.5	1,331	21.4	109	8.2	82.2
North African Arabs	565	10.3	38	6.7	676	10.9	65	9.6	43.3
Indian Subcont	1,325	24.1	99	7.5	1,550	24.9	171	11.0	46.7
Somalis and Sudanese	392	7.1	38	9.7	424	6.8	48	11.3	16.7
Others	154	2.8	6	3.9	120	1.9	7	5.8	48.7
Total	(T_1) 5,506	100	315	5.7*	(T_2) 6,232	100	590	9.5*	66.7

$^*P = 0.0000$.

TABLE 2. Types of diabetes and insulin requirements (1996–1997 and 2001–2002)

	1996–1997 (N = 5,506) Diabetics (N = 315)		2001–2002 (N = 6,232) Diabetics (N = 590)	
	Gestational diabetics	Pregestational diabetics	Gestational diabetics	Pregestational diabetics
Diet treatment	202 (74.3%)	40 (93.0%)	438 (82.6%)	56 (93.3%)
Insulin treatment	70 (25.7%)*	3 (7.0%)	92 (17.4%)*	4 (6.7%)
Total	272 (86.3%)	43 (13.7%)	530 (89.8%)	60 (10.2%)

*$P = 0.007$.

DISCUSSION

Depending on the population and diagnostic criteria, the prevalence of gestational diabetes ranges from 1% to 14%.[14] The value of 9.7% (range 9.2–11.3%) obtained in this study indicates a relatively high prevalent rate of gestational diabetes in the population in the year 2001–2002. It is probably higher now. This could be a reflection of genetic makeup and or the lifestyle of the inhabitants. Various previous reports have indicated that prevalence rates of gestational diabetes are higher among non-Caucasian populations, such as ours, when compared with Caucasians.[15] Our results show that the ethnic background significantly influences the incidence of diabetes mellitus (DM) in pregnancy as has been described in other studies.[10,11] The lowest rates in the year 1996–1997 (4.0% among the Peninsula Arabs and 4.5% among the Chami Arabs) were higher than the 1.5–2.7% recorded among Caucasian populations.[15] The highest rates were among the subjects from the Indian subcontinent (7.5%), the Sudanese and the Somalis (9.7%). A similar pattern was obtained in the year 2001–2002 but the gap between the lowest rates (8.2% and 8.4% among the Chami and Peninsula Arabs, respectively and the highest rates (11.0% and 11.3%, among the subjects from Indian subcontinent, Sudanese and Somalis, respectively) has narrowed considerably.

TABLE 3. Outcomes of pregnancy (1996–1997 and 2001–2002)

	1996–1997				2001–2002			
	Diabetic		Nondiabetic		Diabetic		Nondiabetic	
	N	%	N	%	N	%	N	%
Vaginal delivery	215	68.2	4561	88.0	444	75.3	4724	83.7
Cesarean section	94	30.3*	524	10.0	117	19.8*	587	10.4
Macrosomia	71	22.2**	402	8.0	63	10.6**	376	6.7
Intrauterine fetal death	9	2.9	53	1.0	8	1.4	62	1.1
Preterm delivery	71	22.5	298	5.8	103	17.5	381	7.0
Congenital malformation	21	6.6***	72	1.4	14	2.2***	93	1.7

*$P = 0.002$; **$P = 0.000003$; ***$P = 0.003$.

It is uncertain if similar incidences will be observed among the non-UAE national subjects in the study if they were in their own environments and in their home countries. It is possible that, in addition to genetic factors, dietary habits and lifestyle changes adopted after emigration have contributed to the high rates of gestational diabetes among these groups. It may also be a self-selection effect because the more educated segment of the population at increased risk of diabetes (because of adopted dietary habits and lifestyle) has the level of education and skills to secure external jobs. Nonetheless, the results of this study identify these ethnic groups as targets for screening if the policy is not universal screening.

It is uncertain if the increased prevalent rates obtained at the two periods, were due to the different screening policies or a true increase in the incidence of the disease in the population. In the study by Griffin *et al.*,[15] universal screening detected significantly more (2.7%) cases than the 1.45% detected in the risk factor screened group. On the other hand, in a study similar in design to ours,[16] which compared the effects of changing screening policy from selective to universal, universal screening tested more subjects, but the number diagnosed with the disease remained the same. This differs from our results where 66.7% more cases were diagnosed. It is expected that universal screening would additionally, detect patients with gestational diabetes who had no known risk factors, particularly in an environment of high prevalence rate. It is noteworthy that the proportion of preexisting diabetes was lower (though not significantly) in the year 2001–2002, suggesting that the higher rate of diagnosis in the year 2001–2002 was not a result of accumulation of cases but perhaps due to increased detection of gestational diabetes.

However, if the increased rate in the year 2001–2002 was solely due to increased detection, the interethnic differences would be maintained. Rather, the differences have narrowed such that there was no statistical significant difference between the highest and the lowest rates, suggesting increase in the incidence of the disease.

It is interesting to note that the ethnic groups with the lowest rates in the year 1996–1997 (UAE nationals and other Peninsula Arabs) had recorded the highest increase (109–110%) whereas the ethnic groups with the highest rates (Indian subcontinent, Somalis and Sudanese) had the lowest increase in the year 2001–2002. The reasons for this are obscure. It may be speculated that, the increase in incidence among the UAE national population reflects recent changes from traditional lifestyle to one, which is already prevalent among the more sophisticated expatriate population. On the other hand, it is possible that there is a prevalent rate for a population with the economic and lifestyle characteristics of the UAE, which residents of that culture will eventually achieve.

The study also shows that the severity of the disease (assessed by proportion requiring insulin) was less and perinatal outcomes were better in the 2001–2002 cohort. This is similar to the report of Griffin *et al.*[15] but contrasts with the results from a similar previous study[16] on the effect of change of policy from selective to universal screening where the perinatal outcomes were unchanged. It is not likely that changes in obstetric practice could account for our own result because there was no significant difference in the corresponding data for the nondiabetic patients over the two periods. It is possible that patients without known risk factors but who develop gestational diabetes have less severe disease and hence reduced insulin requirement and better perinatal outcomes.

It remains controversial whether screening for gestational diabetes should be universal or reserved for women who have risk factors. Most women with gestational diabetes have no symptoms and many have none of the classic risk factors associated with gestational diabetes.[17] Several published works suggest that selective screening fails to detect a significant, up to one-third of cases of gestational diabetes.[15,18–20] Others [21] suggest that selective screening is as effective as universal screening if implemented appropriately. Some expert committees, including the UK National Institute for Clinical Excellence (NICE) also advise against routine screening because of unproven cost-effectiveness.[8] The key points seem to be in the implementation and the prevalence of the disease in the concerned community. The results of this study support the recommendation of universal screening as a superior strategy to risk factor-based screening in a population with high prevalence of gestational diabetes.

CONCLUSION

This study confirms the influence of ethnic background on the prevalence of gestational diabetes in a multiethnic and multicultural society.

Over a period of 5 years, there was a 66.7% increase in the incidence of gestational diabetes, which was probably due to a combination of increased detection by change in screening policy and an increase in the incidence of gestational diabetes. The indicators of disease severity and control, such as insulin requirement, rates of abdominal delivery, macrosomia, and structural congenital malformations were all better in a cohort identified by universal screening compared with that identified by selective screening. Universal screening seems to be a more appropriate policy for screening in this environment.

REFERENCES

1. Dunne, F., P. Brydon, K. Smith, *et al.* 2003. Pregnancy in women with type 2 diabetes: 12 years outcome data 1990–2002. Diabet. Med. **20:** 734–738.
2. Watson, D., J. Rowan, L. Neale, *et al.* 2003. Admission to neonatal intensive care unit following pregnancies complicated by gestational or type 2 diabetes. Aust. N.Z. J. Obstet. Gynecol. **43:** 429–432.

3. GABBE, S.G. & C.R GRAVES. 2003. Management of diabetes mellitus complicating pregnancy. Obstet. Gynecol. **102:** 857–868.
4. GALERNEAU, F. & S.E INZUCCHI. 2004. Diabetes mellitus in pregnancy. Obstet. Gynecol. Clin. North Am. **31:** 907–933.
5. BERGER, H., J. CRANE & D. FARINE D. 2002. Screening for gestational diabetes mellitus. J. Obstet. Gynaecol. Can. **24:** 894–903.
6. SCOTT, D.A., E. LOVEMAN, L. MCINTYRE, *et al.* 2002. Screening for gestational diabetes: a systematic review and economic evaluation. Health Technol. Assess. **6(11):** 1–161.
7. HOFFMAN, L., C. NOLAN, J.D. WILSON, *et al.* 1998. Gestational diabetes mellitus—management guidelines. The Australasian Diabetes in Pregnancy Society. Med. J. Aust. **169:** 93–97.
8. NATIONAL COLLABORATING CENTRE FOR WOMEN'S AND CHILDREN'S HEALTH. 2003. Antenatal Care: routine care for the healthy pregnant woman. RCOG Press. London, United Kingdom.
9. CROWTHER, C.A., J.E. HILLIER, J.R. MOSS, *et al.* 2005. Effect of treatment of gestational diabetes mellitus on pregnancy outcomes. N. Engl. J. Med. **352:** 2477–2486.
10. NAHUM, G.G. & B.J HUFFAKER. 1993. Racial differences in oral glucose screening test results: establishing race specific criteria for abnormality in pregnancy. Obstet. Gynecol. **81:** 517–522.
11. DOOLEY, S.L., B.E. METZGER, N. CHO N, *et al.* 1991. The influence of demographic and phenotypic heterogeneity on the prevalence of gestational diabetes mellitus. Int. J. Gynecol. Obstet. **35:** 13–18.
12. AGARWAL, M.M., P.F. HUGHES, J. PUNNOSE, *et al.* 2001. Gestational diabetes screening of a multiethnic, high risk population using glycated proteins. Diab. Res. Clin. Prac. **51:** 67–73.
13. AMERICAN COLLEGE OF OBSTETRICIANS AND GYNECOLOGISTS. 1994. Management of diabetes mellitus in pregnancy. ACOG Technical Bulletin 100. Lippincott William and Williams. Parkway, MD.
14. ENGELGAN, M.M., W.H. HERMAN, P.J. SMITH, *et al.* 1995. The epidemiology of diabetes and pregnancy in the US. Diabetes Care **18:** 1029–1033.
15. GRIFFIN, M.E., M. COFFEY, H. JOHNSON, *et al.* 2000. Universal vs risk factor-based screening for gestational diabetes mellitus: detection rates, gestation at diagnosis and outcome. Diab. Med. **17:** 26–32.
16. CASEY, B.M., M.J. LUCAS, D.D. MCINTIRE, *et al.* 1999. Population impact of universal screening for gestational diabetes. Am. J. Obstet. Gynecol. **180:** 536–539.
17. MOSES, R.G., J. MOSES & W.S DAVIS. 1998. Gestational diabetes; do lean young Caucasian women need to be tested? Diabetes Care **21:** 1803–1806.
18. LAVIN, J.P. 1985. Screening of high-risk and general populations for gestational diabetes. Diabetes **34:** 24–27.
19. COUSTAN, D.R., C. NELSON, M.W. CARPENTER, *et al.* 1989. Maternal age and screening for gestational diabetes: a population based study. Obstet. Gynecol. **73:** 557–560.
20. WEEKS, J.W., C.A. MAJOR, M. DEVECIANA, *et al.* 1994. Gestational diabetes: does the presence of risk factor influence perinatal outcome? Am. J. Obstet. Gynecol. **171:** 1003–1007.
21. NAYLOR, C.D., M. SERMER, E. CHEN, *et al.* 1997. Farine D for the Toronto TriHospital Gestational Diabetes Project Investigators. Selective screening for gestational diabetes mellitus. N. Engl. J. Med. **337:** 1591–1596.

Blockade of the Renin–Angiotensin System Attenuates Sarcolemma and Sarcoplasmic Reticulum Remodeling in Chronic Diabetes

XUELIANG LIU,[a] HIDEAKI SUZUKI,[b] RAJAT SETHI,[c] PARAMJIT S. TAPPIA,[a] NOBUAKIRA TAKEDA,[b] AND NARANJAN S. DHALLA[a]

[a]*Institute of Cardiovascular Sciences, St. Boniface General Hospital Research Centre, Faculty of Medicine and Faculty of Human Ecology, University of Manitoba, Winnipeg, Canada R2H 2A6*

[b]*Aoto Hospital, Jikei University, Tokyo 125-8506, Japan*

[c]*Irma Lerma Rangel College of Pharmacy, Kingsville, Texas 78363-8202, USA*

ABSTRACT: Although the defects in the sarcolemma (SL) and sarcoplasmic reticulum (SR) membranes are known to be associated with cardiac dysfunction in chronic diabetes, very little information regarding the mechanisms of these membrane abnormalities is available in the literature. For this reason, rats were treated daily for 8 weeks with and without enalapril, an angiotensin-converting enzyme inhibitor, or losartan, an angiotensin receptor antagonist, 3 days after inducing diabetes with an injection of streptozocin. Treatment of diabetic animals with both enalapril and losartan attenuated alterations in cardiac function and the left ventricular redox potential without any changes in the increased plasma glucose or reduced plasma insulin levels. The SL Na^+–K^+ ATPase, Ca^{2+} pump, Na^+-dependent Ca^{2+}-uptake, Ca^{2+}-channel density, and low-affinity Ca^{2+}-binding activities were depressed whereas Ca^{2+} ecto-ATPase activity was increased in the diabetic heart. Furthermore, the SR Ca^{2+}-release and Ca^{2+}-pump activities in the diabetic hearts were decreased without any changes in the Mg^{2+}-ATPase activity. These alterations in SL and SR membranes in diabetic animals were partly prevented by treatments with enalapril and losartan. The results suggest that the activation of the renin–angiotensin system plays an important role in diabetes-induced changes in SL and SR membranes as well as cardiac function.

KEYWORDS: diabetic heart; sarcolemma membrane; sarcoplasmic reticulum; renin–angiotensin system; cardiac dysfunction

Address for correspondence: Dr. Naranjan S. Dhalla, Institute of Cardiovascular Sciences, St. Boniface General Hospital Research Centre, 351 Tache Avenue, Winnipeg, Manitoba, Canada R2H 2A6. Voice: 204-235-3417; fax: 204-233-6723.
e-mail: nsdhalla@sbrc.ca

Ann. N.Y. Acad. Sci. 1084: 141–154 (2006). © 2006 New York Academy of Sciences.
doi: 10.1196/annals.1372.003

INTRODUCTION

Both clinical and experimental studies have revealed the existence of cardiomyopathy and cardiac dysfunction in chronic diabetes.[1–4] Several investigators have now demonstrated the association of heart dysfunction with alterations in subcellular organelles, such as myofibrils, sarcoplasmic reticulum (SR), and sarcolemma (SL) in diabetic animals.[5–14] Whereas abnormalities in myofibrillar ATPase and SR Ca^{2+}-release and Ca^{2+}-uptake activities are considered to explain the impaired contraction and relaxation processes, changes in the SL Na^{+}–K^{+} ATPase, Ca^{2+}-pump, Na^{+}–Ca^{2+} exchange, L-type Ca^{2+} channels, and Ca^{2+} ecto-ATPase activities have been suggested to account for a defect in the excitation–contraction coupling as well as changes in cation homeostasis in the diabetic heart.[14,15] Although the occurrence of oxidative stress in diabetic myocardium has been indicated as being responsible for the development of subcellular defects in the diabetic heart,[15] the exact mechanisms of the changes in myofibrils, SR, and SL remain to be elucidated.

Since the renin–angiotensin system (RAS) has been reported to be activated in diabetes[15,16] and the blockade of RAS has been shown to improve cardiac function in diabetes,[17–19] it can be argued that subcellular abnormalities in the diabetic heart are elicited by the activation of RAS. This view is supported by our recent observations that myofibrillar remodeling (changes in the molecular structure, biochemical composition, and activities) is attenuated by the treatment of diabetic animals with enalapril, an angiotensin-converting enzyme (ACE) inhibitor as well as losartan, an angiotensin receptor antagonist.[20] Because of the lack of information regarding the role of RAS in SL and SR defects in the diabetic heart, the present article was undertaken to investigate if changes in SL and SR activities in diabetic animals are prevented by treatment with enalapril or losartan.

METHODS

Diabetes in male Sprague–Dawley rats (weighing about 200 g each) was induced by an intravenous injection of streptozotocin (65 mg/kg body weight) in a 0.1 M citrate buffer. After 3 days, these animals were divided into three groups; untreated diabetic (tap water), enalapril-treated diabetic (enalapril, 10 mg/kg), and losartan-treated diabetic (losartan, 20 mg/kg). The drugs and tap water were given daily for 8 weeks via a gastric tube. Control animals received an injection of 0.1 M citrate buffer. The methods for inducing diabetes, as well as the experimental design and doses of drugs, are the same as employed previously.[5,8,11,20] All these animals were anesthetized and assessed hemodynamically by procedures described earlier.[21–24] The hemodynamic data for the left ventricular developed pressure (LVDP), left ventricular end-diastolic pressure (LVEDP), rate of pressure development (+dP/dt), and rate of pressure decay (–dP/dt) were analyzed. Left ventricles from four animals were pooled together for isolating purified SL or SR membrane preparations.[21,22] The methods for the measurement of SL Na^+–K^+ ATPase, Mg^{2+}-ATPase, Ca^{2+}-pump ATPase, ATP-dependent Ca^{2+}-uptake, Na^+-dependent Ca^{2+}-uptake, and Ca^{2+} channel density, as well as SR Ca^{2+}-uptake, Ca^{2+}-release, Ca^{2+}-pump ATPase, and Mg^{2+}-ATPase activities were the same as described elsewhere.[10–12,14,21,22] For the measurement of low-affinity Ca^{2+}-binding and low-affinity Ca^{2+}-ATPase activities, heavy SL fraction was employed as described elsewhere.[13] Plasma glucose, plasma insulin, plasma ACE, plasma angiotensin II, left ventricular (LV) ACE, and LV-reduced glutathione/oxidized glutathione ratio (GSH/GSSG ratio) as well as malondialdehyde (MDA) content were measured according to the methods used earlier.[8,21] It should be mentioned that plasma ACE represents the activity of peripheral RAS whereas cardiac ACE represents the activity of tissue RAS. Furthermore, GSH/GSSG ratio and MDA content are indices for the degree of oxidative stress.

RESULTS

Experimental Model and Drug Treatments

The data in TABLE 1 indicate that both body weight and ventricular weight as well as plasma insulin levels were decreased, whereas plasma glucose was increased in the 8-week-old diabetic rats. Treatment of diabetic animals with either enalapril or losartan partially attenuated the changes in the body weight and ventricular weight without affecting the changes in plasma glucose or insulin levels. Hemodynamic assessment revealed depressions in the LVDP, +dP/dt, and –dP/dt without any change in the LVEDP in diabetic animals; these alterations were partly prevented by treatment with enalapril or losartan

TABLE 1. General characteristics and cardiac contractile function of control and diabetic rats with or without drug treatment

			Diabetic-treated with	
	Control	Diabetic	Enalapril	Losartan
Body wt (g)	526 ± 18.4	321 ± 16.2*	396 ± 16.9#	381 ± 14.3#
Ventricular wt (mg)	1074 ± 56.2	795 ± 31.8*	947 ± 20#	933 ± 16.6#
Plasma glucose (mg/dL)	163 ± 7.5	476 ± 15.2*	481 ± 16.3	467 ± 12.5
Plasma insulin (U/mL)	27.4 ± 2.4	10.2 ± 1.4*	12.5 ± 1.3	12.5 ± 1.2
LVDP (mm Hg)	140 ± 12.1	85 ±8.4*	119 ±7.6#	116 ± 6.9#
LVEDP (mm Hg)	3.4 ± 0.2	3.9 ± 0.3	3.9 ± 0.2	4.1 ± 0.3
+dP/dt (mm Hg/s)	8856 ± 815	5380 ± 621*	7176 ± 702#	7044 ± 516#
–dP/dt (mm Hg/s)	9072 ± 966	5148 ± 603*	6982 ± 684#	6826 ± 532#

NOTE: Values are mean ± SE of six animals in each group. *Significantly different ($P < 0.05$) from control.

#Significantly different ($P < 0.05$) from untreated diabetic.

TABLE 2. Status of RAS and oxidative stress in control and diabetic rats with or without drug treatment

	Control	Diabetic	Diabetic-treated with	
			Enalapril	Losartan
Plasma ANG II (fmol/mL)	7.2 ± 0.8	7.4 ± 0.5	6.4 ± 0.6	$10.9 \pm 0.4^{\#}$
Plasma ACE activity (nmol/min/mL)	48 ± 2.5	52 ± 3.1	49 ± 3.5	57 ± 2.6
LV ACE activity (nmol/min/mg)	0.57 ± 0.03	$0.89 \pm 0.04^{*}$	$0.56 \pm 0.3^{\#}$	0.79 ± 0.03
LV GSH/GSSG ratio	6.8 ± 0.4	$2.5 \pm 0.2^{*}$	$4.3 \pm 0.5^{\#}$	$4.8 \pm 0.2^{\#}$
MDA content (nmol/mg tissue lipids)	3.8 ± 0.13	$7.1 \pm 0.49^{\#}$	$4.9 \pm 0.46^{\#}$	5.4 ± 0.58

NOTE: Values are mean ± SE of six animals in each group. *Significantly different ($P < 0.05$) from control.

#Significantly different ($P < 0.05$) from untreated diabetic.

(TABLE 1). The level of plasma angiotensin II level or plasma ACE activity was unaltered whereas LV ACE activity was increased in diabetic animals. Treatment of diabetic animals with enalapril, unlike losartan, reduced the LV ACE activity whereas plasma angiotensin II levels were increased by losartan, unlike enalapril (TABLE 2). The depression in LV GSH/GSSG ratio and the increase in MDA content in diabetic animals were attenuated by both enalapril and losartan treatments (TABLE 2).

Alterations in SL Activities

The activities of SL Na^{+}–K^{+} ATPase, Ca^{2+}-pump ATPase, and ATP-dependent Ca^{2+} uptake were decreased whereas the activity of Mg^{2+}-ATPase was unaltered in the diabetic heart (FIGS. 1 and 2). Furthermore, the activities of SL Na^{+}-dependent Ca^{2+}-uptake, Ca^{2+}-channel density, and low-affinity Ca^{2+} binding were depressed whereas the activity of low-affinity Ca^{2+}-ATPase (Ca^{2+} ecto-ATPase) was increased in the diabetic heart (FIGS. 3 and 4). All these changes in the SL membrane were attenuated by the treatment of diabetic animals with enalapril or losartan (FIGS. 1–4).

Alterations in SR Activities

The data in FIGURES 5 and 6 indicate that the activities of both SR Ca^{2+}-uptake and Ca^{2+}-release as well as Ca^{2+}-pump ATPase were depressed, whereas the activity of Mg^{2+}-ATPase was unaltered in the diabetic heart. These alterations in SR activities were attenuated by the treatment of diabetic animals with either enalapril or losartan (FIGS. 5 and 6).

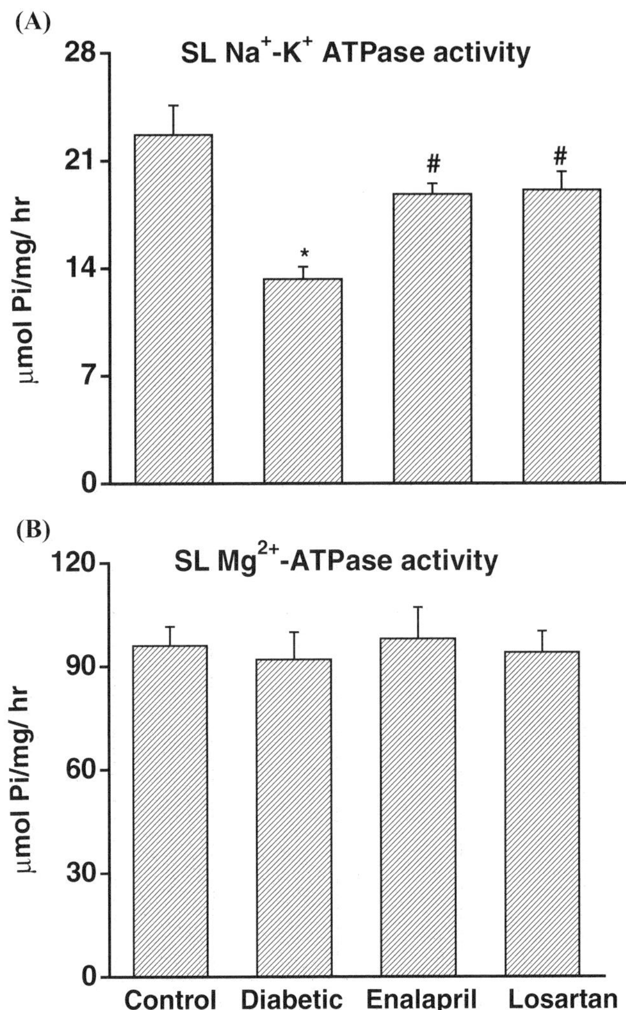

FIGURE 1. SL Na^+–K^+ ATPase and Mg^{2+}-ATPase activities in hearts from 8-week-old diabetic rats treated with and without enalapril or losartan. Each value is a mean ± SE of six preparations in each group. *Significantly ($P < 0.05$) different from control; #significantly ($P < 0.05$) different from untreated diabetic animals.

DISCUSSION

In this study we have shown that SL Na^+–K^+ ATPase, Ca^{2+}-stimulated ATPase, ATP-dependent Ca^{2+}-uptake, and Na^+-dependent Ca^{2+}-uptake activities as well as SL Ca^{2+}-channel density and low-affinity Ca^{2+}-binding were depressed in the diabetic heart. Furthermore, SR Ca^{2+}-release, Ca^{2+}-uptake,

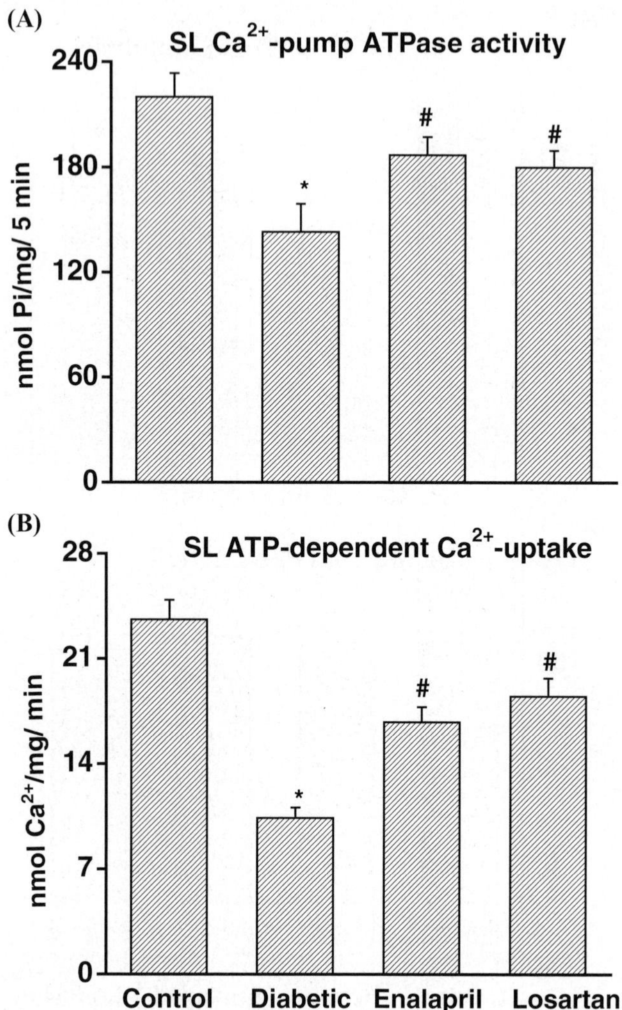

FIGURE 2. SL Ca^{2+}-pump ATPase and ATP-dependent Ca^{2+}-uptake activities in hearts from 8-week-old diabetic rats treated with and without enalapril or losartan. Each value is a mean ± SE of six preparations in each group. *Significantly ($P < 0.05$) different from control; #significantly ($P < 0.05$) different from untreated diabetic animals.

and Ca^{2+}-stimulated ATPase activities decreased in the diabetic heart. These alterations in the SL and SR membranes were not due to any artifact, because Mg^{2+}-ATPase activities in both SL and SR preparations from the diabetic heart were not altered whereas the low-affinity Ca^{2+}-ATPase activity in the SL membrane increased. These results are in agreement with previous studies from our laboratory.[8,10–14] Whereas depressed SR Ca^{2+}-release and Ca^{2+}-pump

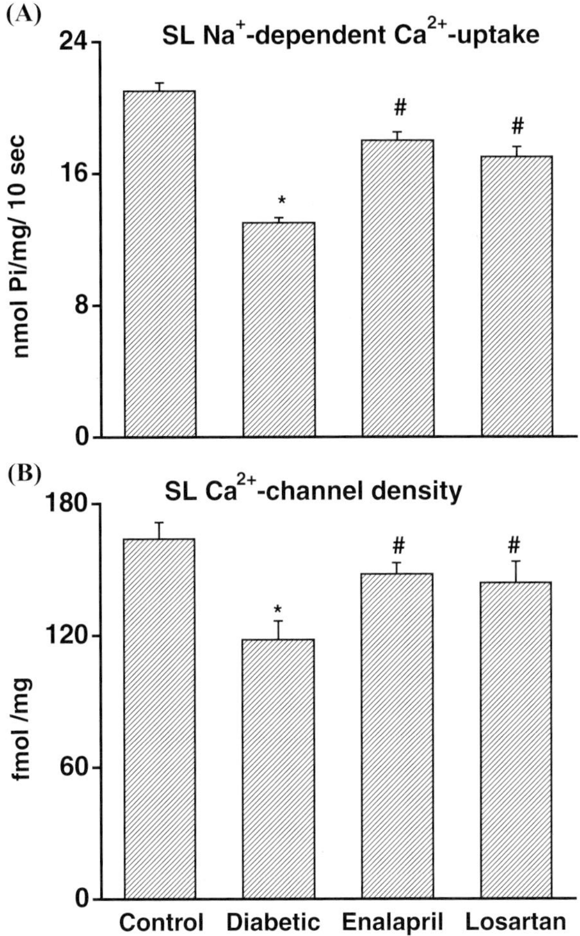

FIGURE 3. SL Na^{+}-dependent Ca^{2+}-uptake activity and Ca^{2+} channel density in the hearts from 8-week-old diabetic rats treated with and without enalapril or losartan. Each value is a mean ± SE of six preparations in each group. *Significantly ($P < 0.05$) different from control; #significantly ($P < 0.05$) different from untreated diabetic animals.

(ATP-dependent Ca^{2+}-uptake and Ca^{2+}-stimulated ATPase) activities can be seen to explain defects in the contraction and relaxation process in the diabetic heart,[8,15] decreased SL Ca^{2+}-channel density and low-affinity Ca^{2+}-binding can be seen to be associated with reduced Ca^{2+}-influx and thus, impaired cardiac contraction.[13,14] On the other hand, depressions in SL Na^{+}–K^{+} ATPase, Ca^{2+}-pump (ATP-dependent Ca^{2+}-uptake and Ca^{2+}-stimulated ATPase) as well as reduced SL Na^{+}-dependent Ca^{2+}-uptake (Na^{+}–Ca^{2+} exchange) activity may result in the occurrence of intracellular Ca^{2+}-overload in the diabetic

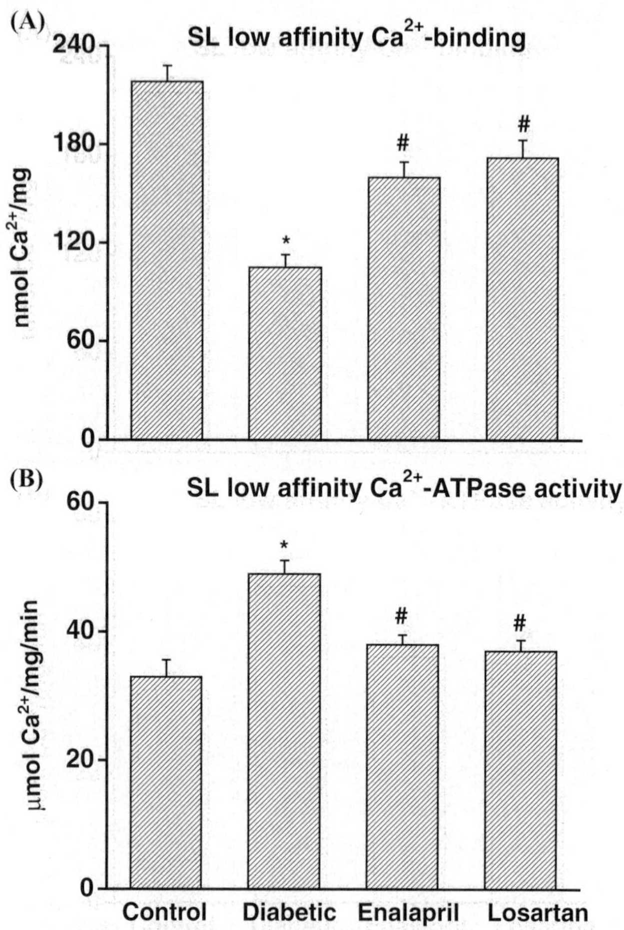

FIGURE 4. SL low-affinity Ca^{2+}-binding and low-affinity Ca^{2+}-ATPase (Ca^{2+} ecto-ATPase) in hearts from 8-week-old diabetic rats treated with and without enalapril or losartan. Each value is a mean ± SE of four preparations in each group. *Significantly ($P < 0.05$) different from control; #significantly ($P < 0.05$) different from untreated diabetic animals.

myocardium and thus produce heart dysfunction.[14,15] The role of intracellular Ca^{2+} overload in the development of cardiac dysfunction and cardiomyopathy in chronic diabetes has been emphasized previously.[25] It should be noted that alterations in both SL and SR membranes, reflecting Ca^{2+} handling abnormalities in cardiomyocytes,[15] may be complimentary to myofibrillar changes[5] in explaining cardiac dysfunction in chronic diabetes.

It was demonstrated that improvement of the cardiac function in diabetic animals was associated with the attenuation of both SL and SR abnormalities upon

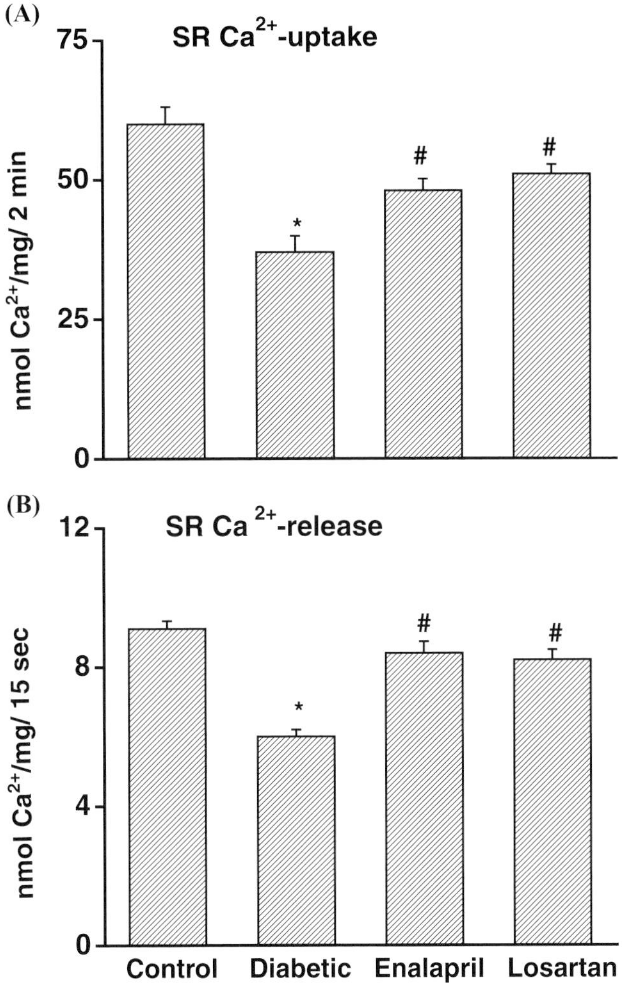

FIGURE 5. SR Ca^{2+}-release and Ca^{2+}-uptake activities in hearts from 8-week-old diabetic rats treated with and without enalapril or losartan. Each value is a mean ± SE of six preparations in each group. *Significantly ($P < 0.05$) different from control; #significantly ($P < 0.05$) different from untreated diabetic animals.

treatment with an ACE inhibitor, enalapril. Because the effects of enalapril on cardiac function as well as membrane defects in diabetic animals were simulated by treatment with an angiotensin II receptor antagonist, losartan, it appears that the beneficial effects of these drugs are elicited by the blockade of RAS. It should be noted that cardiac ACE activity, unlike plasma ACE activity and plasma angiotensin II levels, was elevated in diabetic animals and

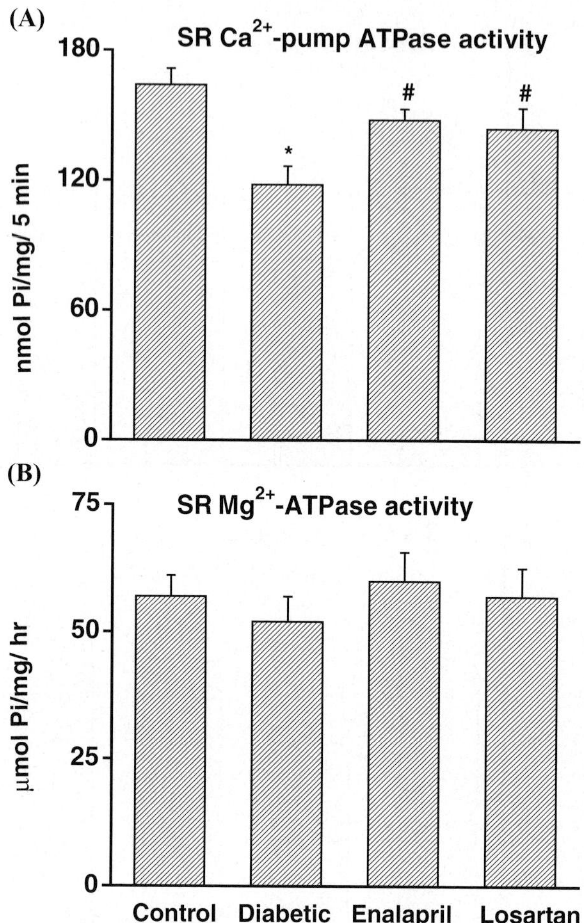

FIGURE 6. SR Ca^{2+}-pump ATPase and Mg^{2+}-ATPase activities in hearts from 8-week-old diabetic rats treated with and without enalapril or losartan. Each value is a mean ± SE of six preparations in each group. *Significantly ($P < 0.05$) different from control; #significantly ($P < 0.05$) different from untreated diabetic animals.

this change was prevented by treatment with enalapril. It is thus likely that the tissue RAS, but not the peripheral RAS, is activated in diabetes. This view as well as the observed increase in plasma angiotensin II level upon treatment of diabetic animals with losartan are consistent with earlier reports.[16,20,21] Since treatment of diabetic animals with enalapril or losartan has been observed to prevent cardiac dysfunction and myofibrillar remodeling (changes in ATPase activity, myosin isozyme content, and myosin isozyme gene expression),[20] it is possible that both enalapril and losartan produce beneficial effects of SL and

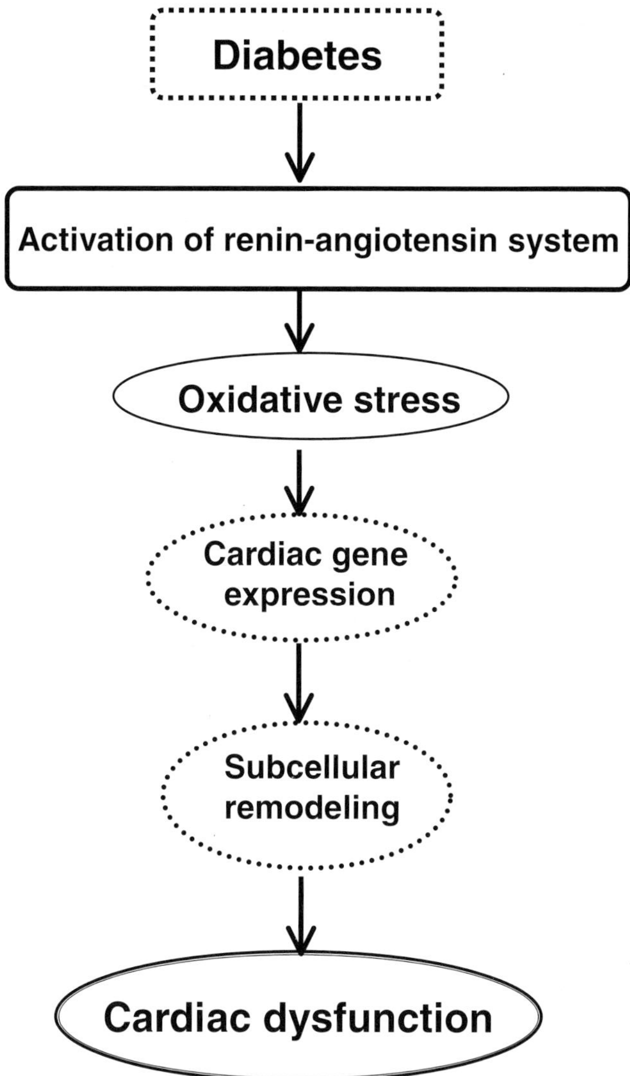

FIGURE 7. Proposed mechanisms involved in the activation of RAS, oxidative stress, and subcellular remodeling in diabetes-induced cardiac dysfunction (Modified from Ref. 20).

SR membranes by preventing their remodeling in the diabetic heart. In fact, the blockade of RAS has been shown to prevent remodeling of SL, SR, and myofibrils in congestive heart failure due to myocardial infarction.[21–24] Since the activation of RAS is known to generate oxyradicals through the release of norepinephrine and changes in mitochondrial function,[15] it is evident that the activation of RAS in the diabetic heart may produce oxidative stress. This point is supported by our observations that the LV GSH/GSSG ratio, an index of redox potential, was reduced and MDA content, a well-known index of oxidative stress, was elevated in the diabetic heart and these alterations were prevented by enalapril and losartan treatments. The role of oxidative stress in producing cardiac dysfunction and subcellular remodeling is also evident from our previous finding that these changes in the diabetic heart were partially prevented by treatment with vitamin E.[15] Accordingly, it is proposed that the activation of RAS in diabetic animals may promote the occurrence of oxidative stress that may produce remodeling of subcellular organelles such as SL, SR, and myofibrils and thus result in cardiac dysfunction (FIG. 7). Remodeling of myofibrils, SL, and SR has been shown to occur because of alterations in gene expression, protein content, and activities of these subcellular organelles in the diabetic heart.[20,26,27] Since the treatment of diabetic animals with enalapril and losartan prevented cardiac dysfunction and most of the SL and SR changes partially, it is likely that mechanisms other than the activation of RAS are also involved in the pathogenesis of subcellular remodeling and cardiac dysfunction.

ACKNOWLEDGMENTS

The research reported here was supported by a grant from the Canadian Institutes of Health Research. Both enalapril and losartan were gifts from Merck Frosst of Canada.

REFERENCES

1. FEIN, F.S. & E.H. SONNEBLICK. 1985. Diabetic cardiomyopathy. Prog. Cardiovasc. Dis. **25:** 255–270.
2. DHALLA, N.S., G.N. PIERCE, I.R. INNES & R.E. BEAMISH. 1985. Pathogenesis of cardiac dysfunction in diabetes mellitus. Can. J. Cardiol. **1:** 263–281.
3. SCHAFFER, S.W. 1991 Cardiomyopathy associated with non-insulin-dependent diabetes. Mol. Cell. Biochem. **107:** 1–20.
4. VADLAMUDI, R.V., R.L. RODGERS & J.H. MCNEILL. 1982. The effect of chronic alloxan-and streptozotocin-induced diabetes on isolated rat heart performance. Can. J. Physiol. Pharmacol. **6:** 902–911.
5. PIERCE, G.N. & N.S. DHALLA. 1985. Mechanisms of the defect in myofibrillar function during diabetes. Am. J. Physiol. Endocrin. Met. Physiol. **248:** E170–E175.
6. MALHOTRA, A., S. PENPARGKUL, F.S. FEIN, *et al.* 1981. The effect of streptozocin-induced diabetes in rats on cardiac contractile proteins. Cir. Res. **49:** 1243–1250.

7. Penpargkul, S., F.S. Fein, E.H. Sonnenblick & J. Scheuer. 1981. Depressed cardiac sarcoplasmic reticular function from diabetic rats. J. Mol. Cell. Cardiol. **13:** 303–309.
8. Ganguly, P.K., G.N. Pierce, K.S. Dhalla & N.S. Dhalla. 1983. Defective sarcoplasmic reticular calcium transport in diabetic cardiomyopathy. Am. J. Physiol. Endocrin. Met. Physiol. 244: E528–E535.
9. Lopaschuk, G.D., A.G. Tahiliani, R.V. Vadlamudi, *et al.* 1983. Cardiac sarcoplasmic reticulum function in insulin- or carnitine-treated diabetic rats. Am. J. Physiol. Heart Circ. Physiol. **245:** H969–H976.
10. Pierce, G.N. & N.S. Dhalla. 1983. Sarcolemmal Na^+-K^+ATPase activity in diabetic rat heart. Am. J. Physiol. Cell Physiol. **245:** C241–C247.
11. Makino, N., K.S. Dhalla, V. Elimban & N.S. Dhalla. 1987. Sarcolemmal Ca^{2+}-transport in streptozotocin-induced diabetic cardiomyopathy in rats. Am. J. Physiol. Endocrin. Met. Physiol. **253:** E202–E207.
12. Lee, S.L., I. Ostadalova, F. Kolar & N.S. Dhalla. 1992. Alterations in Ca^{2+}-channels during the development of diabetic cardiomyopathy. Mol. Cell. Biochem. **109:** 173–179.
13. Pierce, G.N., M.J.B. Kutryk & N.S. Dhalla. 1983. Alterations in Ca^{2+}-binding by and composition of the cardiac sarcolemmal membrane in chronic diabetes. Proc. Natl. Acad. Sci. USA **80:** 5412–5416.
14. Takeda, N., I.M.C. Dixon, T. Hata, *et al.* 1996. Sequence of alterations in subcellular organelles during the development of heart dysfunction in diabetes. Diabetes Res. Clin. Prac. **30:** S113–S122.
15. Dhalla, N.S., X. Liu, V. Panagia & N. Takeda. 1998. Subcellular remodeling and heart dysfunction in chronic diabetes. Cardiovasc. Res. **40:** 239–247.
16. Khatter, J.C., P. Sadri, M. Zhang & R.J. Hoeschen. 1996. Myocardial angiotensin II (Ang II) receptors in diabetic rats. Ann. N. Y. Acad. Sci. **793:** 466–472.
17. Rosen, P., A.F. Rump & R. Rosen. 1996. Influence of angiotensin-converting enzyme inhibition by fosinopril on myocardial perfusion in streptozotocin-diabetic rats. J. Cardiovasc. Pharmacol. **27:** 64–70.
18. Rosen, R., A.F. Rump & P. Rosen. 1995. The ACE-inhibitor captopril improves myocardial perfusion in spontaneously diabetic (BB) rats. Diabetologia **38:** 509–517.
19. Heart Outcome Prevention Evaluation (HOPE) Study Investigators. 2000. Effects of ramipril on cardiovascular and microvascular outcomes in people with diabetes mellitus: results of the HOPE study and MICRO-HOPE substudy. Lancet **355:** 253–259.
20. Machackova, J., X. Liu, A. Lukas & N.S. Dhalla. 2004. Renin-angiotensin blockade attenuates cardiac myofibrillar remodeling in chronic diabetes. Mol. Cell. Biochem. **261:** 271–278.
21. Shao, Q., B. Ren, H.K. Saini, *et al.* 2005. Sarcoplasmic reticulum Ca^{2+}-transport and gene expression in congestive heart failure are modified by imidapril. Am. J. Physiol. Heart Circ. Physiol. **288:** H1674–H1682.
22. Shao, Q., B. Ren, V. Elimban, *et al.* 2005. Modification of sarcolemmal Na^+-K^+ATPase and Na^+-Ca^{2+} exchanger expression in heart failure by blockade of renin-angiotensin system. Am. J. Physiol. Heart Circ. Physiol. **288:** H2637–H2646.

23. WANG, J., X. LIU, B. REN, *et al.* 2002. Modification of myosin expression by imidapril in failing heart due to myocardial infarction. J. Mol. Cell. Cardiol. **34:** 847–857.
24. WANG, J., X. GUO & N.S. DHALLA. 2004. Modification of myosin protein and gene expression in failing hearts due to myocardial infarction by enalapril or losartan. Biochim. Biophys. Acta **1690:** 177–184.
25. AFZAL, N., G.N. PIERCE, V. ELIMBAN, *et al.* 1989. Influence of verapamil on some subcellular defects in diabetic cardiomyopathy. Am. J. Physiol. Endocrin. Met. Physiol. **256:** E453–458.
26. KATO, K., A. LUKAS, D.C. CHAPMAN, *et al.* 2002. Differential effects of etomoxir treatment on cardiac Na^+-K^+ATPase subunits in diabetic rats. Mol. Cell. Biochem. **232:** 57–62.
27. XU, Y.-J., V. ELIMBAN, N. TAKEDA, *et al.* 1996. Cardiac sarcoplasmic reticulum function and gene expression in chronic diabetes. Cardiovasc. Pathobiol. **1:** 89–96.

Effects of Brain Natriuretic Peptide on Contraction and Intracellular Ca^{2+} in Ventricular Myocytes from the Streptozotocin-Induced Diabetic Rat

FRANK C. HOWARTH, NOURA AL SHAMSI, MARYAM AL QAYDI, MARIAM AL MAZROUEI, ANWAR QURESHI, S.I. CHANDRANATH, ELSADIG KAZZAM, AND ABDU ADEM

Faculty of Medicine and Health Sciences, United Arab Emirates University, Al Ain, UAE

ABSTRACT: **The streptozotocin (STZ)-treated rat is a widely studied experimental model of diabetes mellitus (DM). Its pathophysiology includes hypoinsulinemia, hyperglycemia, cardiac hypertrophy, and a cardiomyopathy that is characterized by the presence of diastolic and/or systolic contractile dysfunction. As part of their endocrine function cardiomyocytes in the heart produce and secrete a family of related peptide hormones called the natriuretic peptides that include A-type natriuretic peptide (ANP) and B-type natriuretic peptide (BNP). ANP and BNP levels are variously augmented in patients with hypertension, cardiac overload, in the ventricles of failing or hypertrophied heart, in cardiac heart failure, in acute myocardial infarction (MI), and in some circumstances in DM. In this article, the effects of BNP on ventricular myocyte contraction and Ca^{2+} transport in STZ-induced diabetic rats have been investigated. BNP concentration was significantly increased in blood plasma and in atrial muscle in STZ-induced diabetic rats compared to age-matched controls. BNP was 11.9 $\pm$ 0.9 ng/mL in plasma from diabetic rats compared to 6.7 $\pm$ 1.6 ng/mL in controls and 15.8 $\pm$ 2.0 ng/mg protein in diabetic atrial muscle compared to 8.5 $\pm$ 1.0 ng/mg protein in controls. The heart weight to body weight ratio, an indicator of hypertrophy, was significantly increased in diabetic rat heart (4.3 $\pm$ 0.1 mg/g) compared to controls (3.7 $\pm$ 0.04 mg/g). The amplitude of shortening was not significantly altered in diabetic myocytes (10.3 $\pm$ 0.4%) compared to controls (10.9 $\pm$ 0.4%). BNP reduced the amplitude of shortening to a greater extent in diabetic myocytes (8.1 $\pm$ 0.6%) compared to controls (10.1 $\pm$ 0.4%). The time to peak (TPK) shortening was significantly prolonged in diabetic myocytes (254 $\pm$ 8 ms) compared to controls (212 $\pm$ 5 ms) and was not additionally altered by BNP. The time to half relaxation of shortening was**

Address for correspondence: Dr. Frank C. Howarth, Department of Physiology, Faculty of Medicine and Health Sciences, United Arab Emirates University, P.O. Box 17666, Al Ain, UAE. Voice: 00-9713-7137536; fax: 00-9713-7671966.
e-mail: chris.howarth@uaeu.ac.ae

Ann. N.Y. Acad. Sci. 1084: 155–165 (2006).
doi: 10.1196/annals.1372.007

also significantly prolonged in diabetic myocytes (131 $\pm$ 8 ms) compared to controls (111 $\pm$ 5 ms). BNP (10^{-8} to 10^{-6} M) normalized the time to half relaxation of shortening in diabetic myocytes to that of controls. Time to peak (TPK) shortening of Ca^{2+} was not different between diabetic and control rats. However, BNP (10^{-7} M) increases TPK of Ca^{2+} significantly. The amplitude of the Ca^{2+} transient was significantly increased in diabetic myocytes (0.42 $\pm$ 0.02 Ratio units [RU]) compared to controls (0.36 $\pm$ 0.02 RU) and was not additionally altered by BNP. BNP may have a protective role in STZ-induced diabetic rat heart.

KEYWORDS: diabetes mellitus; heart; BNP; ventricular myocytes; contraction; calcium

INTRODUCTION

As in many other parts of the world diabetes is a major health concern in the United Arab Emirates. Epidemiological data suggest that the prevalence of diabetes among UAE nationals has increased dramatically in recent years. Data from the Emirates National Diabetic Survey 2000 suggest that 24% of UAE citizens have diabetes. Cardiovascular complications are the most common causes of morbidity and mortality in diabetic patients.[1] Both type 1 and type 2 diabetic patients have an increased risk of ischemic heart disease (IHD) and congestive heart failure (CHF). The streptozotocin (STZ)-treated rat is a widely studied experimental model of diabetes mellitus (DM). Its pathophysiology includes hypoinsulinemia, hyperglycemia, cardiac hypertrophy, and a cardiomyopathy that is characterized by the presence of diastolic and/or systolic contractile dysfunction. Defective Ca^{2+} signaling pathways including altered L-type Ca^{2+} current, Na^+/Ca^{2+} exchange, Ca^{2+}-ATPase, sarcoplasmic reticulum Ca^{2+} uptake/release mechanisms, and altered myofilament Ca^{2+} sensitivity partly underlie contractile dysfunction in the STZ-induced diabetic rat.[2–5] The heart in addition to being a very efficient pump is also an important endocrine organ. As part of its endocrine function, cardiomyocytes in the heart produce and secrete a family of related peptide hormones called the natriuretic peptides. This family includes A-type natriuretic peptide (ANP), B-type natriuretic peptide (BNP), C-type natriuretic peptide (CNP), and urodilatin. In contrast to ANP, which originates mainly from atrial tissue, BNP is expressed in both the atria and the ventricles, but is mainly released from the ventricles.[6] Ventricular proBNP production is strongly upregulated in cardiac failure and locally in the area surrounding a myocardial infarction (MI). ANP and BNP have potent diuretic, natriuretic, and vasodilatory activities via a guanylyl cyclase (GC)-coupled natriuretic peptide receptor subtype, GC-A.[7] Pathophysiologically, ANP and BNP levels are variously augmented in patients with hypertension, cardiac overload, in the ventricles of failing or hypertrophied heart, in CHF, in acute MI, and in DM under some circumstances.[6] Natriuretic peptides have emerged as important candidates for development of diagnostic tools and therapeutic agents in cardiovascular disease. The hypothesis is that BNP serves to modulate muscle contraction and has a protective role in diabetic cardiomyopathy. In this article, the levels of BNP in blood plasma and in atrial and ventricular muscle from STZ-induced diabetic rats and age-matched controls have been measured. The effects of BNP on ventricular myocyte shortening and Ca^{2+} transport in STZ-induced diabetic rat have been investigated.

METHODS

Induction of Diabetes

Diabetes was induced by a single intraperitoneal injection of STZ (60 mg/kg; Sigma, Taufkirchen, Germany) administered to young male Wistar rats (200–250 g; bred inhouse). The STZ was dissolved in a citrate buffer solution (0.1 mol/L citric acid, 0.1 mol/L sodium citrate; pH 4.5). Age-matched controls received an equivalent volume of the citrate buffer solution alone. Both groups of animals were maintained on the same diet and water *ad libitum* until they were used 8–12 weeks later. Principles of laboratory animal care were followed throughout. Approval for this project was obtained from the Faculty of Medicine and Health Sciences Ethics Committee.

Measurement of BNP in Blood Plasma and in Atria and Ventricles

The measurement of BNP from serum or plasma and tissue homogenates was performed as described by the manufacturing company (Peninsula Laboratories, San Carlos, CA). Briefly, a curve is constructed first using various dilutions of the standard concentrate provided in the kit. Twenty-five microliters of primary antisera were dispensed into each well of the immunoplate and incubated for 1 h at room temperature. Fifty microliters of the unknown samples were dispensed into the designated wells and incubated for another 2 h at room temperature. The rehydrated biotinylated peptide (25 μL) was added to each well and gently agitated. The plate was covered with an acetate plate sealer (APS) and incubated overnight at 2–8°C. The APS was removed and the contents were discarded and washed five times with assay buffer and blot dry. One hundred microliters of the diluted streptavidin-conjugated horse radish peroxidase (SA-HRP) solution was dispensed into each well and the plate was resealed with APS. After incubating for 60 min the wells were washed five times and blot dry. One hundred microliters of the tetramethyl benzidine dihydrochloride (TMB) solution was added into each well and incubated for 0.5–1 h at room temperature until the solution turned blue. The reaction was stopped by adding 100 μL of 2N HCl into each well. When the color became blue the immunoplate was loaded onto a microtiter plate reader and the absorbance was read at 450 nm.

A standard plot of optical density versus concentration was drawn. The concentration of peptide in the unknown sample was determined by locating the sample's OD on the y axis of the standard curve.

Ventricular Myocytes Isolation

Single ventricular myocytes were isolated according to the previously described technique.[3] In brief, rats were killed humanely by cervical dislocation following stunning and their hearts were removed quickly and mounted on a Langendorff apparatus. Hearts were perfused retrogradely at a constant flow of 8 mL.g heart^{-1}.min^{-1} with a HEPES-based isolation solution containing 0.75 mM Ca^{2+}. Perfusion flow rate was adjusted to allow for differences in heart weight between STZ-treated and control animals. When the coronary circulation had cleared of blood, perfusion was continued for 4 min with a Ca^{2+}-free isolation solution containing 0.1 mM EGTA, and then for 6 min with solution containing 0.05 mM Ca^{2+}, 0.75 mg/mL collagenase (type 2; Worthington, Lakewood NJ), and 0.075 mg/mL protease (type 14; Sigma). Ventricles were then excised from the heart, minced and gently shaken in collagenase-containing isolation solution supplemented with 1% BSA. Cells were filtered from this solution at 4-min intervals and resuspended in 0.75 mM Ca^{2+}-containing isolation solution. Cell viability, defined as the percentage of rod-shaped myocytes in the cell suspension was recorded within 1 h of completing the cell isolation.

Ventricular Myocyte Experiments

Freshly isolated myocytes suspended in 0.75 mM Ca^{2+}containing isolation solution were divided into two aliquots, centrifuged at low speed and the cell pellets resuspended either in normal tyrode or normal tyrode containing BNP at various concentrations (Sigma, A-8208). Cells were incubated in BNP for 1 h before the commencement of experiments. For electrophysiological studies myocytes were allowed to settle on the glass bottom of a perspex chamber mounted on the stage of an inverted microscope (Axiovert 35, Zeiss, Germany). Myocytes were superfused (3–5 mL/min) with a HEPES-based normal tyrode solution containing 1 mM Ca^{2+} or normal tyrode containing BNP. Experiments were performed in electrically stimulated myocytes (1 Hz) at room temperature (23–25°C). Unloaded myocytes shortening was followed using a video edge detection system (VED-114, Crystal Biotech, Northborough, MA). The degree of shortening (expressed as a percentage of resting cell length [RCL]), the time to peak (TPK) shortening, and the time from peak to half (THALF) relaxation of shortening were recorded. Intracellular Ca^{2+} was measured in cells loaded with the fluorescent indicator fura-2 AM (F-1221, Molecular Probes, Eugene, OR) as described previously.[3] To measure intracellular Ca^{2+} concentration, myocytes were alternately illuminated by 340 nm and 380 nm light using a monochromator (Cairn Research, Faversham, Kent, UK) that changed the excitation light every 2 ms. The resultant fluorescent emission at 510 nm was recorded by a photomultiplier tube and the ratio of the emitted fluorescence at the two excitation wavelengths (340/380 ratio) was calculated to provide an index of intracellular Ca^{2+} concentration.

Solutions

The cell isolation solution contained (in mM) 130.0 NaCl, 5.4 KCl, 1.4 $MgCl_2$, 0.4 NaH_2PO_4, 5 HEPES, 10 glucose, 20 taurine, and 10 creatine set to pH 7.3 with NaOH. The normal tyrode solution contained (in mM) NaCl 140, KCl 5, $MgCl_2$ 1, glucose 10, HEPES 5, and $CaCl_2$ 1 set to pH 7.4 with NaOH.

Statistics

Results were expressed as the mean ± SEM of "n" observations. "n" refers either to the number of rats or number of cells. Statistical comparisons were performed using either independent samples *t*-test or analysis of variance (ANOVA) followed by Bonferroni-corrected *t*-tests for multiple comparisons, as appropriate. $P < 0.05$ was considered to indicate a significant difference. Statistical analysis was carried out using SPSS (Chicago, IL).

RESULTS

General Characteristics of STZ-Induced Diabetic Rat

The general characteristics of STZ-treated rats compared with their age-matched controls are shown in TABLE 1. Diabetes was confirmed in STZ- treated rats by a significant, fivefold, elevation of blood glucose. STZ-treated rats characteristically had significantly lower body weights and heart weights compared with controls.

TABLE 1. General characteristics of STZ-induced diabetic rat

	Control	STZ
Body weight (g)	316.0 ± 16.4 (6)	266.2 ± 9.9 (5)*
Heart weight (g)	1.17 ± 0.05 (6)	1.14 ± 0.04 (5)
Blood glucose (mg/dL)	73.0 ± 5.9 (6)	327.2 ± 23.3 (5)**
Heart weight/body weight (mg/g)	3.70 ± 0.04 (6)	4.29 ± 0.11 (5)**

Data are mean ± SE. Numbers in parenthesis are numbers of animals. Statistical comparisons were performed with independent samples *t*-test. $^{*}P < 0.05$, $^{**}P < 0.01$.

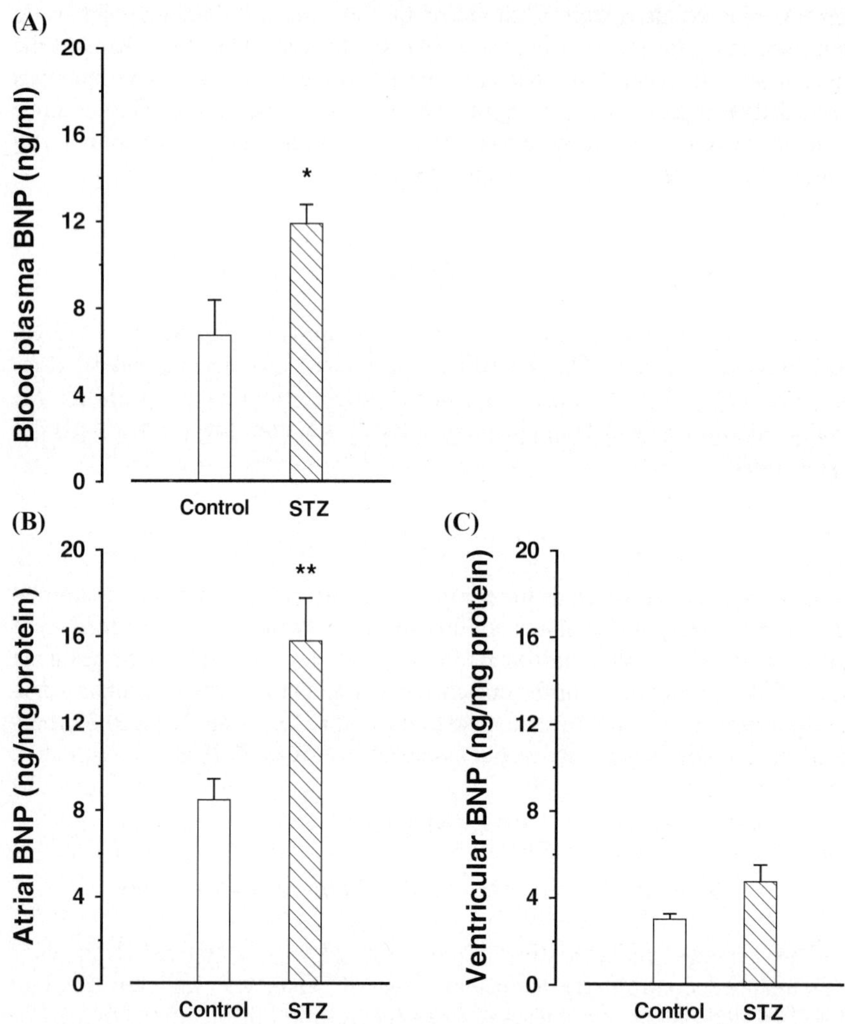

FIGURE 1. Effects of STZ-induced diabetes on BNP concentration in blood plasma (**A**), atrial muscle (**B**), and ventricular muscle (**C**). Data are mean ± SEM, $n = 4$. Statistical comparisons made with independent samples t-test ($^{*}P < 0.05$, $^{**}P < 0.01$).

Levels of BNP in Blood Plasma and in Ventricular and Atrial Muscle

The concentrations of BNP in blood plasma (panel A), and atrial (panel B), and ventricle (panel C) muscle are shown in FIGURE 1. The concentration of BNP was significantly ($P < 0.05$) increased in blood plasma and in atrial muscle and increased to a smaller extent in ventricular muscle from STZ-induced diabetic rat compared to age-matched controls. The concentration of

BNP in blood plasma from STZ-treated rats was 11.91 ± 0.89 ng/mL ($n = 4$) compared to 6.75 ± 1.64 ng/mL ($n = 4$) in controls. The level of BNP in atrial muscle from STZ-treated rats was 15.80 ± 2.00 ng/mg protein ($n = 4$ hearts) compared to 8.47 ± 0.97 ng/mg protein ($n = 4$ hearts) in controls. The level of BNP in ventricular muscle from STZ-treated rat was 4.78 ± 0.80 ng/mg protein ($n = 4$ hearts) compared to 3.03 ± 0.26 ng/mg protein ($n = 4$ hearts) in controls.

Effects of BNP on Ventricular Myocyte Shortening

A typical fast-time base recording of shortening in an electrically stimulated (1 Hz) myocyte superfused with normal tyrode containing 1 mM Ca^{2+} from a STZ-treated rat and a control rat is shown in FIGURE 2 A. The mean RCL of myocytes from STZ-treated (115.9 ± 2.9 μm, $n = 35$) was not significantly ($P > 0.05$) different from that of controls (121.9 ± 3.8 μm, $n = 33$). Exposure to 10^{-7} M BNP for at least 1 h did not significantly alter RCL. The time course of contraction was characteristically and significantly ($P < 0.05$) prolonged in diabetic myocytes compared to controls (FIG. 2 B, C). The mean TPK shortening was 254 ± 8 ms ($n = 35$) in diabetic myocytes compared to 212 ± 5 ms ($n = 33$) in controls (FIG. 2 B). Exposure of cells with 10^{-7} M BNP had no significant additional effect on TPK shortening in myocytes from either STZ-treated or control rats. The mean THALF relaxation was 131 ± 8 ms, $n = 35$ in diabetic myocytes compared to 111 ± 5 ms ($n = 33$) in controls (FIG. 2 C). Interestingly, when cells were exposed to BNP (10^{-8} to 10^{-7} M), the THALF relaxation in diabetic myocytes was normalized so that the difference in THALF relaxation between cells from diabetic myocytes and controls was no longer significant. The amplitude of shortening, expressed as a percentage of RCL, was slightly smaller in myocytes from STZ-treated (10.3 ± 0.4%, $n = 35$) rats compared to controls (10.9 ± 0.4%, $n = 33$) though the difference did not reach significance. Interestingly, exposure to BNP (10^{-7} and 10^{-6} M) produced a reduction in the amplitude of shortening (FIG. 2 D) that was significantly greater in diabetic myocytes compared to controls. At a concentration of 10^{-7} M BNP amplitudes of shortening were 8.1 ± 0.6% ($n = 22$) in diabetic myocytes compared to 10.1 ± 0.4% ($n = 38$) in controls.

Effects of BNP on Ventricular Myocyte Intracellular Ca^{2+}

Typical fast-time base recordings of Ca^{2+} transients in control and diabetic myocytes superfused with normal tyrode are shown in FIGURE 3 A. The mean resting fura-2 ratio in myocytes was not significantly altered by STZ treatment. The mean resting fura-2 ratio in diabetic myocytes was 2.43 ± 0.03 Ratio units (RU) ($n = 31$) compared to 2.34 ± 0.04 RU ($n = 28$) in controls. BNP (10^{-7} M) caused a significant reduction in mean

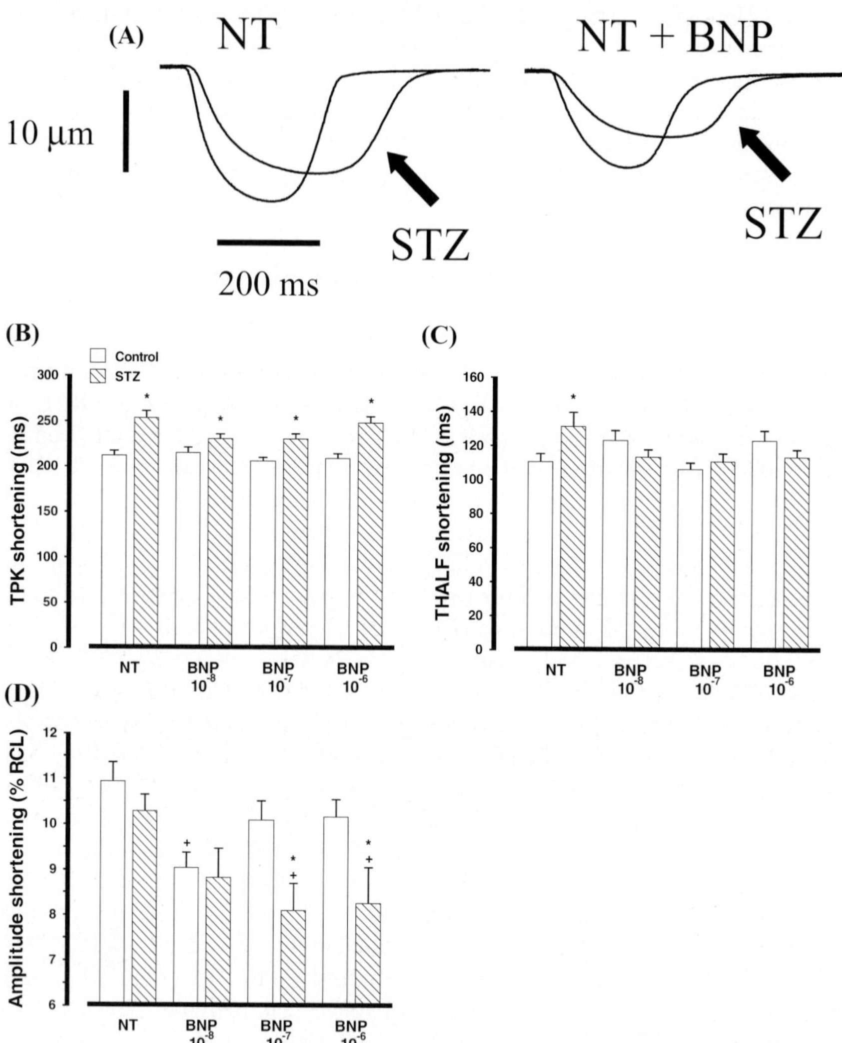

FIGURE 2. Effects of BNP on ventricular myocyte shortening. Typical records showing effects of STZ treatment and BNP on myocyte shortening (**A**). Graphs of TPK shortening (**B**), THALF relaxation of shortening (**C**), and amplitude of shortening (**D**). Data are mean ± SEM, $n = 20$–38. Means statistically compared using either independent samples t-test ($^*P < 0.05$) or ANOVA followed by Bonferroni-corrected t-tests ($^+P < 0.05$).

resting fura-2 ratio in myocytes from control rats (2.17 ± 0.03 RU, $n = 35$) though not in diabetic myocytes (2.41 ± 0.04 RU, $n = 30$). The time course of the Ca^{2+} transient was slightly prolonged in myocytes from STZ-treated rats compared to controls though the difference did not reach significance.

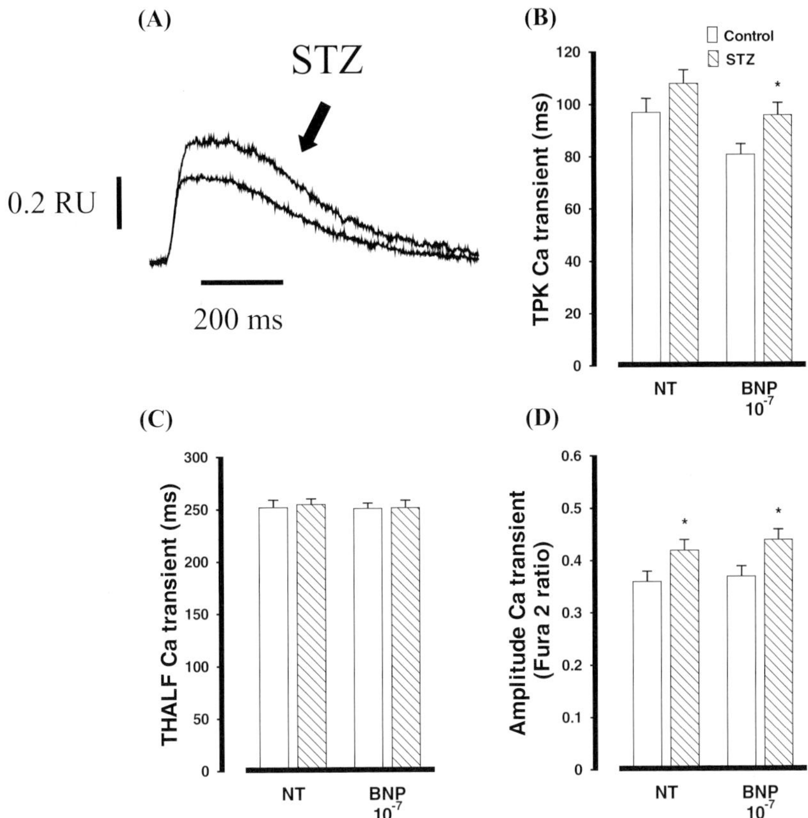

FIGURE 3. Effects of BNP on ventricular myocytes intracellular Ca^{2+}. Typical records showing effects of STZ treatment on the Ca^{2+} transient (**A**). Graphs of TPK Ca^{2+} transient (**B**), THALF relaxation of the Ca^{2+} transient (**C**), and amplitude of the Ca^{2+} transient (**D**). Data are mean ± SEM, $n = 28$–35. Mean statistically compared using Independent samples t-test ($^*P < 0.05$).

The TPK Ca^{2+} transient was 108 ± 5 ms ($n = 31$) in diabetic myocytes compared to 97 ± 5 ms ($n = 30$) in controls (FIG. 3 B). Interestingly, 10^{-7} M BNP reduced the TPK Ca^{2+} transient in both diabetic and in control myocytes. However, the reduction in TPK Ca^{2+} transient only reached significance in diabetic myocytes. The THALF relaxation of the Ca^{2+} transient was not significantly altered by either STZ treatment or by exposure to BNP. The amplitude of the Ca^{2+} transient was significantly increased (FIG. 3 D) in diabetic myocytes (0.42 ± 0.02 RU, $n = 31$) compared to controls (0.36 ± 0.02 RU, $n = 28$). Exposure to 10^{-7} M BNP had no additional effects in myocytes from either diabetic or control rats.

DISCUSSION

The study investigated the effects of STZ-induced diabetes on the distribution of BNP in plasma, and atrial and ventricular muscle. It also investigated the effects of BNP on ventricular myocyte shortening and intracellular Ca^{2+}. The major findings were that: (*a*) BNP concentrations were significantly elevated in blood plasma and atrial muscle and elevated to a smaller extent in ventricular muscle from STZ-treated rats compared to age-matched controls; (*b*) the time course, including TPK shortening and THALF relaxation of shortening was characteristically prolonged in diabetic myocytes compared to controls; (*c*) the amplitude of shortening was reduced by 10^{-7} M BNP and the effects were greater in diabetic myocytes compared to controls; and (*d*) the TPK Ca^{2+} transient was prolonged to a small extent in diabetic myocytes compared to controls and was reduced to a small extent in both diabetic and control myocytes in the presence of 10^{-7} M BNP. The reduction in TPK Ca^{2+} transient only reached significance in diabetic myocytes.

BNP concentration in plasma and atrial muscle increased significantly and to a smaller extent in ventricular muscle from diabetic rat heart compared to age-matched controls. Previous studies have demonstrated increased cardiac BNP expression in STZ-induced diabetic rat and increased expression of BNP mRNA in atrial myocardium but not in ventricular myocardium in STZ-induced diabetic pig.[8,9]

The heart weight to body weight ratio was increased in diabetic rats compared to age-matched controls. An increase in heart weight to body weight ratio is indicative of cardiac hypertrophy. Cardiac hypertrophy in STZ-induced diabetic rat has also been reported in some other studies.[10–12]

Plasma and atrial BNP were increased in diabetic rats compared to controls. This finding is consistent with previous data that have variously reported increases in ANP, ANP mRNA, and BNP expression.[10,12,13]

Contractile function is compromised in the STZ-induced diabetic rat heart. *In vivo* studies have demonstrated reduced heart rate, reduced left ventricular peak ejection rate and peak-filling rate, longer left ventricular ejection time, and isovolumic relaxation time.[2,14] Reductions in heart rate, left ventricular rate of development of systolic pressure, and rate of decline of the pressure are lower and TPK pressure and THALF relaxation from peak pressure longer in isolated perfused diabetic rat heart compared to controls.[2] Prolonged time course of contraction including prolonged TPK and THALF relaxation of contraction, seen in this study, and reduced amplitude of contraction are also frequently reported findings in ventricular myocytes from diabetic rat heart compared to controls.[2,3] Defects in Ca^{2+} transport including L-type Ca^{2+} current, sarcoplasmic reticulum Ca^{2+} release and uptake mechanisms, and Na^+/Ca^{2+} exchange partly underlie defects in contraction.[2,3] Interestingly, superfusion of myocytes with 10^{-7} M BNP reduced the amplitude of contraction in myocytes from control and from diabetic rats though the effects of BNP were greater in myocytes from diabetic rat heart.

In conclusion, the increase in BNP seen in plasma and in atrial muscle and the increased effects of BNP on amplitude of shortening and TPK Ca^{2+} transient in myocytes from diabetic heart may suggest a protective role for BNP in STZ-induced diabetic rat heart.

REFERENCES

1. AMOS, A.F., D.J. MCCARTY & P. ZIMMET. 1997. The rising global burden of diabetes and its complications: estimates and projections to the year 2010. Diabetic Med. **14:** S1–S85.
2. CHOI, K.M., Y. ZHONG, B.D. HOIT, *et al.* 2002. Defective intracellular Ca(2+) signaling contributes to cardiomyopathy in type 1 diabetic rats. Am. J. Physiol. **283:** H1398–H1408.
3. HOWARTH, F.C., M.A. QURESHI & E. WHITE. 2002. Effects of hyperosmotic shrinking on ventricular myocyte shortening and intracellular Ca(2+) in streptozotocin-induced diabetic rats. Pflugers Arch. **444:** 446–451.
4. ISHIKAWA, T., H. KAJIWARA & S. KURIHARA. 1999. Alterations in contractile properties and $Ca2^{+}$ handling in streptozotocin-induced diabetic rat myocardium. Am. J. Physiol. **277:** H2185–H2194.
5. HOWARTH, F.C., S.C. CALAGHAN, M.R. BOYETT & E. WHITE. 1999. Effect of the microtubule polymerizing agent taxol on contraction, $Ca2^{+}$ transient and L-type $Ca2^{+}$ current in rat ventricular myocytes. J. Physiol. **516:** 409–419.
6. RUSKOAHO, H. 1992. Atrial natriuretic peptide: synthesis, release, and metabolism. Pharmacol. Rev. **44:** 479–602.
7. HALL, C. 2004. Essential biochemistry and physiology of (NT-pro)BNP. Eur. J. Heart Fail. **6:** 257–260.
8. WALTHER, T., S. HERINGER-WALTHER, R. TSCHOPE, *et al.* 2000. Opposite regulation of brain and C-type natriuretic peptides in the streptozotocin-diabetic cardiopathy. J. Mol. Endocrinol. **24:** 391–395.
9. CHRISTOFFERSEN, C., J.P. GOETZE, E.D. BARTELS, *et al.* 2002. Chamber-dependent expression of brain natriuretic peptide and its mRNA in normal and diabetic pig heart. Hypertension **40:** 54–60.
10. RUZICSKA, E., G. FOLDES, Z. LAKO-FUTO, *et al.* 2004. Cardiac gene expression of natriuretic substances is altered in streptozotocin-induced diabetes during angiotensin II-induced pressure overload. J. Hypertens. **22:** 1191–1200.
11. ROSENKRANZ, A.C., S.G. HOOD & R.L. WOODS. 2003. B-type natriuretic peptide prevents acute hypertrophic responses in the diabetic rat heart: importance of cyclic GMP. Diabetes **52:** 2389–2395.
12. CANDIDO, R., J.M. FORBES, M.C. THOMAS, *et al.* 2003. A breaker of advanced glycation end products attenuates diabetes-induced myocardial structural changes. Circ. Res. **92:** 785–792.
13. HOWARTH, F.C., A. ADEM, E.A. ADEGHATE, *et al.* 2005. Distribution of atrial natriuretic peptide and its effects on contraction and intracellular calcium in ventricular myocytes from streptozotocin-induced diabetic rat. Peptides **26:** 691–700.
14. HOWARTH, F.C., M. JACOBSON, O. NASEER & E. ADEGHATE. 2005. Short-term effects of streptozotocin-induced diabetes on the electrocardiogram, physical activity and body temperature in rats. Exp. Physiol. **90:** 237–245.

Differences in Expression of Cardiovascular Risk Factors among Type 2 Diabetes Mellitus Patients of Different Age

CHRISTOS KALOFOUTIS,[a] CHRISTINA PIPERI,[a] AIKATERINI ZISAKI,[a] JAIPAUL SINGH,[b] FRED HARRIS,[c] DAVID PHOENIX,[c] ANTONIS ALAVERAS,[a] AND ANASTASIOS KALOFOUTIS[a]

[a]*Laboratory of Biological Chemistry, University of Athens Medical School, M. Asias 75, Goudi 11527, Athens, Greece*

[b]*Department of Biological Sciences, University of Central Lancashire, Preston, PR1 2HE United Kingdom*

[c]*Faculty of Science, University of Central Lancashire, Preston, PR1 2HE United Kingdom*

ABSTRACT: Atherosclerotic coronary heart disease and other forms of cardiovascular disease (CVD) are the major cause of mortality in type II diabetes (T2DM) as well as a major contributor to morbidity and lifetime costs. The purpose of this article is the identification of the biochemical parameters in plasma, which may serve as predisposition factors to CVD in T2DM patients of different ages. The variability of hyperglycemia, dyslipidemia, and inflammation with age progression was also studied for comparison. Four different diabetic groups allocated on the basis of the subjects' age (Group A: 15–25 years old; Group B: 26–40 years old; Group C: 40–60 years old; Group D: 60–80 years old) and consisting of 10 patients each, in parallel with 10 healthy controls matched for age, sex, and ethnic origin were screened for glucose, insulin, lipid profile (total cholesterol, triglycerides, LDL, and HDL), and inflammatory mediators (CRP, IL-6, and TNF-α). Significant differences were observed among the expressions of biochemical markers among different age groups. Hyperglycemia showed no variability with age whereas dyslipidemia correlated positively with age progression, as well as obesity, low physical activity, and family history of heart disease or diabetes. Marked inflammation was prominent only in Groups C and D. This article indicates that different biochemical parameters may be used for the assessment of CVD risk in T2DM patients of variable age.

Address for correspondence: Christina Piperi, Laboratory of Biological Chemistry, University of Athens Medical School, M. Asias 75, Goudi 11527, Athens, Greece. Voice: 30-210-7462610; fax: 30-210-8037372.

e-mail: cpiperi@med.uoa.gr

Ann. N.Y. Acad. Sci. 1084: 166–177 (2006).
doi: 10.1196/annals.1372.001

KEYWORDS: type 2 diabetes mellitus; cardiovascular risk factors; cytokines

INTRODUCTION

At present, about 200 million people worldwide have type 2 diabetes mellitus (T2DM), a prevalence that has been predicted to increase to 366 million by 2030.[1] Atherosclerotic coronary heart disease (CHD) and other forms of cardiovascular disease (CVD) are the major cause of mortality in T2DM as well as a major contributor to morbidity and lifetime costs.[2] A number of unfavorable conditions predisposing to CVD coexist with diabetic status, including hyperglycemia, dyslipidemia, inflammation, and coagulation, many of which may be closely associated with insulin resistance.[3,4]

Hyperglycemia is likely to contribute further to endothelial dysfunction once diabetes develops and poor glycemic control is a significant predictor of CVD mortality in diabetes.[5–7] Dyslipidemia is also likely to play a leading role in the increased CVD risk associated with diabetes since many patients show a characteristic atherogenic dyslipidemia, including hypertriglyceridemia, elevated levels of apolipoprotein B, increased prevalence of small, dense, low-density lipoprotein (LDL) cholesterol, and low levels of high-density lipoprotein (HDL) cholesterol.[8,9]

T2DM has been associated with increased oxidative stress,[10] endothelial dysfunction,[11–15] and increased proinflammatory profile. Furthermore, there is evidence that the pathophysiology of insulin resistance and atherosclerosis may share a common inflammatory basis maintaining endothelial dysfunction associated with T2DM throughout age progression.

It is recognized that the pathogenesis of insulin resistance includes low-grade inflammation[16] as characterized by elevated concentrations of various inflammatory markers in the circulation that has been reported in humans with insulin resistance, for example, interleukin- 6 (IL-6)[17]; tumor necrosis factor-α (TNF-α)[18]; soluble TNF receptors (sTNFR1, sTNFR2)[19]; and C-reactive protein (CRP).[20] In addition, adipose tissue contributes significantly to the levels of inflammatory cytokines, for example, IL-6[21] and TNF-α[22] in the circulation and accordingly, obesity is associated with elevated circulating levels of IL-6,[23] TNF-α,[18] and sTNFR2,[24] as well as CRP.[25] These cytokines may stimulate the expression of adhesion molecules on endothelial cells (e.g., vascular cell adhesion molecule-1 [VCAM-1], which participate in atherogenesis.

Although a large amount of data exists regarding hyperglycemia, dyslipidemia, and inflammation in T2DM patients, they have not been addressed systematically in relation to age progression. The effects of glycemic control on lipids, inflammatory mediators, and cytokines are inconsistent in several studies,[26,27] especially in adolescents. To our knowledge, there is no study simultaneously addressing the complicated network among hyperglycemia, dyslipidemia, and inflammation in patients with T2DM. Therefore, in order to find useful biomarkers to monitor the development of T2DM in adolescents through their age progression to elderly, this study recruited patients with T2DM of different ages to investigate the possible roles of all these parameters in the development of the disease. Therefore, the aim of the present article was to identify biochemical parameters in plasma, which may serve as predisposition factors to CVD in T2DM patients of different ages with particular emphasis on the variability of hyperglycemia, dyslipidemia, and inflammation with age progression.

METHODS

Patient Description

The 40 patients who participated in the study had T2DM and 40 healthy age-matched individuals were randomly selected. Informed consent was obtained from all subjects.

The purpose of the study, possible risks, and discomforts were explained to the subjects before obtaining written consent. The study protocol was approved by the University of Athens Medical School Ethical Committee, and was performed in accordance with the Declaration of Helsinki. The patients with T2DM were recruited using an outpatient clinic database at the Red Cross General Hospital, Athens.

Exclusion criteria included treatment with insulin, recent or ongoing infection, a history of cancer, or treatment with anti-inflammatory drugs. The nondiabetic controls were recruited among employees at the hospital.

Four different age-matched groups were eventually formed. More specifically, Group A consisted of 10 T2DM patients 15–25 years old and 10 control patients of similar age; Group B included 10 T2DM patients 26–40 years old and 10 age-matched healthy controls; Group C consisted of 10 T2DM patients 40–60 years old and 10 age-matched healthy subjects; and Group D included 10 T2DM patients 60–80 years old and 10 age-matched healthy controls.

Blood Sampling

Fasting blood was collected from each participant by standard venepuncture into evacuated tubes with and without EDTA or heparin. Blood samples were centrifuged at 1500 rpm, plasma and serum isolated, and stored at –80°C until required for analysis. The analysis was performed within 2 months from the day of storage.

Assays

Plasma glucose (mg/dL) was determined by the glucose oxidase colorimetric method (Glucose LR, GOD-PAP, Linear Chemicals, Barcelona, Spain). Insulin levels (μU/mL) were determined immunoenzymatically by using the ELISA kit from Biosource Europe SA (Nivelles, Belgium). The intra- and interassay coefficients of variation (CVs) for low and high levels, respectively, were 3.0% and 5.3%, and 4.5% and 9.5%, for insulin.

Total cholesterol (mg/dL) was measured by an enzymatic colorimetric method using cholesterol oxidase and peroxidase (Cholesterol LR, CHOD-PAP, Linear Chemicals). HDL-cholesterol (mg/dL) was assessed enzymatically using a direct method (HDL-cholesterol, DIRECT, Linear Chemicals). Triglycerides (mg/dL) were measured using an enzymatic colorimetric method based on hydrolysis of plasma triglyceride to glycerol and free fatty acids (FFA) by lipoprotein lipase (Triglycerides MR, Linear Chemicals). hsCRP (mg/L) levels were determined by ELISA (high-sensitivity CRP enzyme immunoassay test kit, LI7500; Linear Chemicals). The intra- and interassay CVs for low and high levels were, respectively 7.5 and 4.1%, and 2.3 and 2.5%, for hsCRP.

Serum IL-6 (pg/mL) and TNF-α (pg/mL) were determined using commercially available ELISA kits (IL-6: HS600B, R&D Systems, Minneapolis, MO; TNF-α: HSTA00C, R&D Systems). The sensitivities of detection levels for IL-6 and TNF-α were 2.2 and 2.0, respectively. All measurements were performed at the Chemwell Analyzer (Awareness, FL).

Statistical Methods

The results were statistically processed and values were expressed as mean ± SD. The Pearson χ^2 test was used to compare categorical variables. All data were tested at a statistical level of significance of $P < 0.05$.

RESULTS

The characteristics as well as the biochemical results of each age group for T2DM patients and controls are shown in TABLES 1–4.

TABLE 1 shows the data of Group A (15–25 years old) diabetic and age-matched control subjects. There was no significant difference in age between the two groups. There were 8 female and 2 male patients in the diabetic group whereas the control group was composed of 3 female and 7 male patients. Biochemical analysis of T2DM patients showed elevated concentrations of all the parameters measured compared to the control group but only glucose, total cholesterol, and triglyceride levels reached statistical significance ($P = 0.01$, $P = 0.001$, and $P = 0.01$, respectively).

TABLE 2 presents the main characteristics and the biochemical profile of Group B subjects (26–40 years old). Once again, there was no significant difference in age between the two groups. There were 4 female and 6 male patients in the diabetic group whereas the control group was composed of 3 female and 7 male patients. Biochemical analysis of T2DM patients showed

TABLE 1. General characteristics and biochemical analysis of Group A (15–25 years old)

	DM patients ($n = 10$)	Healthy ($n = 10$)
Gender		
Female	8	3
Male	2	7
Age	18.37 ± 2	19.12 ± 1.8
BMI	25.42 ± 1.36	23.24 ± 2.03
Insulin	8.3 ± 1.2	7.91 ± 1.3
Glucose	187.25 ± 3.26	95.49 ± 1.32*
TG	160.41 ± 3.65	88.67 ± 1.59*
Total Cholesterol	209.05 ± 3.48	120.87 ± 3.21*
HDL	43.25 ± 2.17	58.35 ± 4.16
LDL	160.26 ± 2.15	156.15 ± 2.19
CRP	3.61 ± 1.72	1.68 ± 0.57
Homocysteine	8.03 ± 2.94	6.68 ± 3.2
TNF-α	1.4	1.1
IL-6	2.1	1.23

Data are mean ± SD; $^*P < 0.05$.

elevated concentrations of statistical significance for glucose, total cholesterol, triglycerides, and CRP levels compared to the control group ($P = 0.01$, $P = 0.001$, $P = 0.01$, and $P = 0.05$, respectively).

The general characteristics and biochemical profile of Group C subjects (40–60 years old) are presented in TABLE 3. Age and body mass index (BMI) did not differ between the two groups that were composed of 5 female and

TABLE 2. General characteristics and biochemical analysis of Group B (26–40 years old)

	DM patients ($n = 10$)	Healthy ($n = 10$)
Gender		
Female	4	3
Male	6	7
Age	29.9 ± 4.1	30.5 ± 3.8
BMI	27.52 ± 2.36	24.66 ± 1.03
Insulin	9.1 ± 1.5	5.1 ± 1.1
Glucose	186.52 ± 2.42	90.88 ± 4.32*
TG	169.03 ± 2.15	94.02 ± 3.59*
Total cholesterol	230.59 ± 2.48	153.03 ± 3.11*
HDL	41.39 ± 1.47	56.69 ± 2.16
LDL	168.52 ± 3.15	160.16 ± 3.16
CRP	4.05 ± 1.37	1.78 ± 0.57*
Homocysteine	8.03 ± 1.94	6.58 ± 2.2
TNF-α	1.8	1.5
IL-6	2.5	2.1

Data are mean ± SD; $^*P < 0.05$.

TABLE 3. General characteristics and biochemical analysis of Group C (40–60 years old)

	DM patients ($n = 10$)	Healthy ($n = 10$)
Gender		
Female	5	4
Male	5	6
Age	49.18 ± 5.67	50.62 ± 4.8
BMI	27.06 ± 2.36	24.81 ± 2.13
Insulin	11.87 ± 2.1	5.7 ± 1.51
Glucose	195.15 ± 2.26	$90.89 \pm 1.32^*$
TG	187.13 ± 2.35	$95.89 \pm 5.59^*$
Total cholesterol	259.57 ± 2.23	$202.18 \pm 2.25^*$
HDL	39.42 ± 1.17	55.42 ± 3.82
LDL	172.04 ± 2.15	165.19 ± 3.29
CRP	7.02 ± 1.68	$1.69 \pm 2.37^*$
Homocysteine	9.50 ± 2.34	$6.42 \pm 2.7^*$
TNF-α	1.7	2.4
IL-6	2.3	1.4*

Data are mean ± SD; $^*P < 0.05$.

5 male patients for the diabetic group and 4 female and 6 male patients for the control group. Biochemical analysis of T2DM patients showed elevated concentrations of glucose, total cholesterol, triglycerides, and CRP levels as well as for homocysteine, and IL-6 levels compared to the control group ($P = 0.01$, $P = 0.001$, $P = 0.01$, $P = 0.05$, $P = 0.05$, and $P = 0.05$, respectively).

TABLE 4 summarizes the results of Group D subjects (60–80 years old). Age and BMI did not differ between the two groups. The T2DM group consisted of 5 female and 5 male patients and the control group consisted of 4 female and 6 male patients. Biochemical analysis showed a significant elevation in glucose, triglycerides, and total cholesterol levels compared to controls ($P = 0.01$, $P = 0.001$, $P = 0.01$, respectively). Furthermore, CRP, homocysteine, TNF-α, and IL-6 levels were also significantly increased in T2DM patients compared to controls ($P = 0.01$, $P = 0.05$, $P = 0.05$, $P = 0.05$, respectively).

DISCUSSION

Recent evidence show that people with T2DM generally carry an array of risk factors for CVD, including hyperglycemia, dyslipidemia, alterations in inflammatory mediators, and coagulation/thrombolytic parameters, as well as other "nontraditional" risk factors, many of which may be closely associated with insulin resistance. However, the effects of glycemic control on lipids, inflammatory mediators, and cytokines in relation with age progression of T2DM patients are inconsistent in several studies,[26,27] especially for adolescents. This study recruited patients with T2DM from different age groups

TABLE 4. General characteristics and biochemical analysis of Group D (60–80 years old)

	DM patients ($n = 10$)	Healthy ($n = 10$)
Gender		
Female	5	4
Male	5	6
Age	71.82 ± 4.67	70.66 ± 4.91
BMI	27.47 ± 2.61	26.16 ± 2.53
Insulin	8.21 ± 2.6	6.1 ± 1.3
Glucose	199.28 ± 3.26	94.65 ± 5.34*
TG	190.83 ± 2.59	96.28 ± 6.13*
Total cholesterol	263.37 ± 5.26	105.08 ± 6.25*
HDL	36.70 ± 3.17	52.59 ± 3.64
LDL	180.51 ± 7.14	164.92 ± 4.23
CRP	8.38 ± 1.63	1.61 ± 0.37*
Homocysteine	11.80 ± 2.74	7.41 ± 0.7*
TNF-α	2.87	1.9*
IL-6	2.9	1.7*

Data are mean ± SD; *$P < 0.05$.

in parallel with age-matched controls in order to investigate the variability of hyperglycemia, dyslipidemia, inflammation with age progression, and identify possible biochemical parameters in plasma, which may serve for monitoring the development of CVD associated with the disease.

The results of this study showed significant differences in the expression of biochemical markers among the different age groups. As expected, T2DM patients share a common hyperglycemic profile independent of age restriction compared to controls. Hyperglycemia may induce protein glycation, oxidation, glycoxidation, lipoxidation, and mediate vascular damage in DM.[28,29] Connective tissue proteins, such as collagen, may be affected by elevated glucose levels and it has been observed that in DM individuals, the gradual, age-dependent collagen glycation is impaired and accelerated two-fold or three-fold compared to non-DM.[30] Hyperglycemia also leads to the formation of advanced glycation endproducts (AGEs), such as carboxymethylysine and pentosidine, agents that are formed via the nonenzymatic, covalent modification of free proteins by reducing sugars. AGEs act through the activation of a cell surface receptor (RAGE), and have been shown to have detrimental effects in both microvascular and macrovascular endothelial cells by inducing free radical oxidation and altering the endothelial function that further contributes to CVD associated with DM.[5,30–34]

Furthermore, T2DM patients present dyslipidemia as characterized by increased total cholesterol, triglycerides, LDL, and low HDL levels independent of age. Dyslipidemia, however, seems to be a prominent feature of DM patients independent of their age and is likely to play a leading role in the increased CVD risk associated with diabetes.[5,35,36] The present data are in accordance with previous studies that have demonstrated that patients with T2DM may show a characteristic atherogenic dyslipidemia, including hypertriglyceridemia, elevated levels of apolipoprotein B, increased prevalence of small, dense, LDL cholesterol, and low levels of HDL cholesterol.[37,38] In addition to these established dyslipidemic risk factors, patients with T2DM and those who are insulin resistant are more likely to have small, dense, LDL particles. This LDL component is probably atherogenic due to high susceptibility to oxidation and its presence is an independent risk factor for CVD.[39] Several mechanisms may account for the atherogenic lipid abnormalities found in diabetic patients. Dysfunctional adipose tissue, or adiposopathy, is thought to develop via the combination of excessive fat accumulation and genetic predisposition.

Evidence suggests that this dysfunctional adipose tissue is less sensitive to insulin and has reduced hormone-sensitive lipase activity compared with normal adipose tissue.[39] As a result there is an increased breakdown of intracellular TG and increased release of FFA into the circulation, leading to fatty infiltration in the liver, muscles, and possibly pancreatic β cells. Ultimately, this contributes to, and may exacerbate, insulin resistance in the liver and muscle. After long-term exposure to FFA the function of the pancreatic β cells may also be compromised, leading to, or contributing to increased predisposition to T2DM.

Endothelial dysfunction has been proposed to be a key factor involved in the development and progression of subclinical atherosclerosis. The properties of the impaired endothelium include reduced vasoactive capability, increased ability to support thrombosis, increased permeability, and increased adhesion molecule expression.[6,31] Such changes produce increased adhesion of leukocytes and platelets, increased responsiveness to vasoconstrictor agents (e.g., angiotensin II, endothelin-1, and thrombin), and increased transmigration of leukocytes.[31,40] Endothelial dysfunction can be detected early in the prediabetic state and the progression of endothelial dysfunction to atherosclerosis parallels that of insulin resistance to T2DM.[6,31] There is a close association between inflammation and endothelial dysfunction.

In this study low-grade inflammation becomes prominent in the second group of patients between 26–40 years of age and correlated positively with age progression persisting among the groups, perhaps reflecting a widespread activation of the innate immune system, which is closely involved in the pathogenesis of T2DM dyslipidemia and atherosclerosis.[41]

Detailed evaluation of the "proinflammatory milieu" of T2DM patients as characterized by circulating inflammatory markers, showed increased CRP, IL-6, and TNF-α levels compared to healthy controls, which are capable of inducing the observed on-going acute phase response present in T2DM patients.[42] Such chronic inflammation of the endothelial cell and vascular environment impairs endothelium-dependent vasodilation, induces the expression of cell-surface adhesion molecules by endothelial cells, and increases cardiovascular risk.[43–45] In particular, CRP may play a significant role as it amplifies the inflammatory response by stimulating the production of TNF-α and IL-1 by tissue macrophages.[45] Thus, CRP has been linked with CHD mortality and the development of DM.[41,46,47] CRP also stimulates plasminogen activation inhibitor-1 (PAI-1), which inhibits fibrinolysis and also predicts CHD and DM, as well as contributes to the prothrombotic state in obesity.[42,45] The relationship between micro- or macroalbuminuria and CVD mortality may also be related to its association with endothelial dysfunction.[32]

Another protein that has been determined in T2DM patients and control groups is homocysteine, a naturally occurring amino acid in plasma. Homocysteine is produced by methionine, and it is a precursor of cystathionine. Total homocysteine levels were increased in DM patients compared to controls. The term *total plasma homocysteine* refers to the whole of the free and oxidized forms, measured after reduction of the disulfide bond to liberate the free form. When a metabolic pathway of homocysteine is inhibited, then homocysteine accumulates causing increased levels of homocysteine in plasma. Several studies have indicated that even moderately elevated plasma homocysteine is a predictor of CVD.[48] The risk of either stroke or CHD is 1.5–3 times higher, when the levels of plasma homocysteine are moderately elevated.[49] During the acute phase of myocardial infarction, an increase in homocysteine occurs, which may be connected with the increase of acute phase proteins.[50]

In summary, our results show that hyperglycemia, dyslipidemia, and low-grade inflammation are present in different age groups of T2DM patients studied and reconfirm previous observations on the role of these conditions in predisposing the development of CVD in these patients. However, among these major predisposition factors, only inflammation and associated endothelial dysfunction are age-dependent.

REFERENCES

1. FORD, E.S. *et al.* 2002. Prevalence of the metabolic syndrome among US adults: findings from the third National Health and Nutrition Examination Survey. JAMA **287:** 356–359.
2. CARO, J.J. *et al.* 2002. Lifetime costs of complications resulting from type 2 diabetes in the U.S. Diabetes Care **25:** 476–481.
3. MUNTNER, P. *et al.* 2004. Prevalence of non-traditional cardiovascular disease risk factors among persons with impaired fasting glucose, impaired glucose tolerance, diabetes, and the metabolic syndrome: analysis of the Third National Health and Nutrition Examination Survey (NHANES III). Ann. Epidemiol. **14:** 686–695.
4. PYORALA, K. *et al.* 1987. Diabetes and atherosclerosis: an epidemiologic view. Diab. Metab. Rev. **3:** 463–524.
5. NATIONAL CHOLESTEROL EDUCATION PROGRAM (NCEP) EXPERT PANEL ON DETECTION, EVALUATION AND TREATMENT OF HIGH BLOOD CHOLESTEROL IN ADULTS (ADULT TREATMENT PANEL III). 2002. Third Report of the National Cholesterol Education Program (NCEP) Expert Panel on Detection, Evaluation and Treatment of High Blood Cholesterol in Adults (Adult Treatment Panel III) final report. Circulation **106:** 3143–3421.

6. HSUEH, W.A. *et al.* 2004. Insulin resistance and the endothelium. Am. J. Med. **117:** 109–117.
7. GALL, M.A. *et al.* 1995. Albuminuria and poor glycemic control predict mortality in NIDDM. Diabetes **44:** 1303–1309.
8. BERTHEZONE, F. 2002. Diabetic dyslipidaemia. Br. J. Diab. Vasc. Dis. **2:** S12–S17.
9. BAYS, H. 2003. Atherogenic dyslipidaemia in type 2 diabetes and metabolic syndrome: current and future treatment options. Br. J. Diab. Vasc. Dis. **3:** 356–360.
10. AMMAR, R.F. *et al.* 2000. Free radicals mediate endothelial dysfunction of coronary arterioles in diabetes. Cardiovasc. Res. **47:** 595–601.
11. MCVEIGH, G.E. *et al.* 1992. Impaired endothelium-dependent and –independent vasodilation in patients with type 2 (non-insulin-dependent) diabetes mellitus. Diabetologia **35:** 771–776.
12. MAKIMATTILA, S. *et al.* 1999. Impaired endothelium dependent vasodilation in type 2 diabetes. Diabetes Care **22:** 973–981.
13. CALLES-ESCANDON, J. & M. CIPOLLA 2001. Diabetes and endothelial dysfunction: a clinical perspective. Endocr. Rev. **2:** 36–52.
14. AYDIN, A. *et al.* 2001. Oxidative stress and nitric oxide related parameters in type II diabetes mellitus: effects of glycemic control. Clin. Biochem. **34:** 65–70.
15. ABRAMS, J. 1997. Role of endothelial dysfunction in coronary artery disease. Am. J. Cardiol. **79:** 2–9.
16. RECASENS, M. *et al.* 2005. An inflammation score is better associated with basal than stimulated surrogate indexes of insulin resistance. J. Clin. Endocrinol. Metab. **90:** 112–116.
17. FERNANDEZ-REAL, J.M. *et al.* 2000. Interleukin-6 gene polymorphism and insulin sensitivity. Diabetes **49:** 517–520.
18. MISHIMA, Y. *et al.* 2001. Relationship between serum tumor necrosis factor-[alpha] and insulin resistance in obese men with Type 2 diabetes mellitus. Diab. Res. Clin. Pract. **52:** 119–123.
19. LIN, S.-Y. *et al.* 2004. Increased serum soluble tumor necrosis factor receptor levels are associated with insulin resistance in liver cirrhosis. Metabolism **53:** 922–926.
20. MCLAUGHLIN, T. *et al.* 2002. Differentiation between obesity and insulin resistance in the association with C-reactive protein. Circulation **106:** 2908–2912.
21. MOHAMED-ALI, V. *et al.* 1997. Subcutaneous adipose tissue releases interleukin-6, but not tumor necrosis factor-{alpha}, *in vivo*. J. Clin. Endocrinol. Metab. **82:** 4196–4200.
22. HOTAMISLIGIL, G.S. *et al.* 1995. Increased adipose tissue expression of tumor necrosis factor-alpha in human obesity and insulin resistance. J. Clin. Invest. **95:** 2409–2415.
23. YUDKIN, J.S. *et al.* 1999. C-reactive protein in healthy subjects: associations with obesity, insulin resistance and endothelial dysfunction: a potential role for cytokines originating from adipose tissue? Arterioscler. Thromb. Vasc. Biol. **19:** 972–978.
24. WINKLER, G. *et al.* 2003. Expression of tumor necrosis factor (TNF)-alpha protein in the subcutaneous and visceral adipose tissue in correlation with adipocyte cell volume, serum TNF-alpha, soluble serum TNF-receptor-2 concentrations and C-peptide level. Eur. J. Endocrinol. **149:** 129–135.
25. HAK, A.E. *et al.* 1999. Associations of C-reactive protein with measures of obesity, insulin resistance and subclinical atherosclerosis in healthy middle-aged women. Arterioscler. Thromb. Vasc. Biol. **19:** 1986–1991.

26. ERBAGCI, A.B. *et al.* 2002. Mediators of inflammation in children with type 2 diabetes mellitus: cytokines in type 1 diabetic children. Clin. Biochem. **34:** 645–650.
27. RAPOPORT, M.J. *et al.* 1998. Decreased secretion of Th2 cytokines precedes up-regulated and delayed secretion of Th1 cytokines in activated peripheral blood mononuclear cells from patients with insulin-dependent diabetes mellitus. J. Autoimmun. **11:** 635–642.
28. UK PROSPECTIVE DIABETES STUDY (UKPDS) GROUP. 1998. Effect of intensive blood-glucose control with metformin on complications in overweight patients with type 2 diabetes (UKPDS 34). Lancet **352:** 854–865.
29. UK PROSPECTIVE DIABETES STUDY (UKPDS) GROUP. 1998. Intensive blood-glucose control with sulphonylureas or insulin comparedwith conventional treatment and risk of complications in patients with type 2 diabetes (UKPDS 33). Lancet **352:** 837–853.
30. LYONS, T.J. *et al.* 1991. Decrease in skin collagen glycation with improved glycemic control in patients with insulin-dependent diabetes mellitus. J. Clin. Invest. **87:** 1910–1915.
31. HSUEH, W.A. *et al.* 2004. Insulin resistance and the endothelium. Am. J. Med. **117:** 109–117.
32. GALL, M.A. *et al.* 1995. Albuminuria and poor glycemic control predict mortality in NIDDM. Diabetes **44:** 1303–1309.
33. DYER, D.G. *et al.* 1993. Accumulation of Maillard reaction products in skin collagen in diabetes and aging. J. Clin. Invest. **91:** 2463–2469.
34. MCCANCE, D.R. *et al.* 1993. Maillard reaction products and their relation to complications in insulin-dependent diabetes mellitus. J. Clin. Invest. **91:** 2470–2478.
35. BERTHEZONE, F. 2002. Diabetic dyslipidaemia. Br. J. Diabetes. Vasc. Dis. **2:** S12–S17.
36. REAVEN, G.M. 2000. Insulin resistance: how important is it to treat? Exp. Clin. Endocrinol. Diabetes **108:** S274–S280.
37. BAYS, H. 2003. Atherogenic dyslipidaemia in type 2 diabetes and metabolic syndrome: current and future treatment options. Br. J. Diab. Vasc. Dis. **3:** 356–360.
38. BRUNZELL, J.D. & A.F. AYYOBI. 2003. Dyslipidemia in the metabolic syndrome and type 2 diabetes mellitus. Am. J. Med. **115:** S24–S28.
39. FONSECA, V.A. 2003. Management of diabetes mellitus and insulin resistance in patients with cardiovascular disease. Am. J. Cardiol. **92:** J50–J60.
40. MAKIMATTILA, S. & H. YKI-JDRVINEN. 2002. Endothelial dysfunction in human diabetes. Curr. Diab. Rep. **2:** 26–36.
41. PICKUP, J.C. 2004. Inflammation and activated innate immunity in the pathogenesis of type 2 diabetes. Diabetes Care **27:** 813–823.
42. HSUEH, W.A. & D. BRUEMMER. 2004. Peroxisome proliferator-activated receptor gamma: implications for cardiovascular disease. Hypertension **43:** 297–305.
43. EINHORN, D. *et al.* 2004. Glitazones and the management of insulin resistance: what they do and how might they be used. Endocrinol. Metab. Clin. North Am. **33:** 595–616.
44. HAFFNER, S.M. 2003. Pre-diabetes, insulin resistance, inflammation and CVD risk. Diab. Res. Clin. Pract. **61:** S9–S18.
45. NESTO, R. 2004. C-reactive protein, its role in inflammation, type 2 diabetes and cardiovascular disease and the effects of insulinsensitizing treatment with thiazolidinediones. Diabet. Med. **21:** 810–817.

46. KULLER, L.H. *et al.* 1996. Relation of C-reactive protein and coronary heart disease in the MRFIT nested case-control study. Multiple Risk Factor Intervention Trial. Am. J. Epidemiol. **144:** 537–547.
47. RIDKER, P.M. *et al.* 1997. Inflammation, aspirin, and the risk of cardiovascular disease in apparently healthy men. N. Engl. J. Med. **336:** 973–979.
48. TAN, S.A. & L.G. TAN 2004. Synergistic effects of simvastatin and pioglitazone on inflammatory cytokines interferon-gamma, tumor necrosis factoralpha, interleukin-6 and C-reactive protein in diabetic patients with hyperlipidemia and coronary artery disease [abstract 58]. Endocr. Pract. **10**(Suppl 1): 21.
49. CHARBONNEL, B. *et al.* 2004. The Prospective Pioglitazone Clinical Trial in Macrovascular Events (PROactive): can pioglitazone reduce cardiovascular events in diabetes? Study design and baseline characteristics of 5238 patients. Diabetes Care **27:** 1647–1653.
50. MALINOW, M. *et al.* 1999. Homocysteine, diet and cardiovascular diseases a statement for healthcare professionals from the Nutrition Committee, American Heart Association. Circulation **99:** 178–182.

Effect of Streptozotocin-Induced Type 1 Diabetes Mellitus on Contraction, Calcium Transient, and Cation Contents in the Isolated Rat Heart

JAIPAUL SINGH,[a] APURVA CHONKAR,[a] NICHOLAS BRACKEN,[a] ERNEST ADEGHATE,[b] ZAY LATT,[a] AND MUNIR HUSSAIN[c]

[a]*Department of Biological Sciences, University of Central Lancashire, Preston, Lancashire, PR1 2HE United Kingdom*

[b]*Department of Anatomy, Faculty of Medicine & Health Sciences, United Arab Emirates University, Al Ain, UAE*

[c]*Department of Medicine, University of Liverpool, Daulby Street, Liverpool, L69 7ZX United Kingdom*

ABSTRACT: Cations play major physiological and biochemical roles in the excitation–contraction coupling processes in the heart. This study investigated the effect of streptozotocin (STZ)-induced type I diabetes mellitus (DM) on contraction, calcium transient $[Ca^{2+}]_i$, and cation contents in the isolated rat heart compared to age-matched control. Diabetes rats weighed significantly ($P < 0.05$) less compared to control. They also had significantly ($P < 0.05$) elevated blood glucose compared to control. The whole heart, as well as the atria, right and left ventricles of the diabetic heart weighed significantly ($P < 0.05$) less compared to hearts from age control rats. The force of contraction and time to peak (t-pk) contraction in diabetic ventricular myocytes increased significantly ($P < 0.05$) compared to control. By contrast, these parameters did not change for the Ca^{2+} transient except for the time to half ($t\frac{1}{2}$) relaxation. The levels of sodium (Na^+), potassium (K^+), calcium (Ca^{2+}), magnesium (Mg^{2+}), iron (Fe^{2+}), copper (Cu^{2+}), and zinc (Zn^{2+}) in the hearts varied from diabetic compared to control animals. The results indicate that 6–8 weeks of STZ-induced DM is associated with marked changes in contraction and in cation contents of the heart. The delay in the $t\frac{1}{2}$ relaxation of the Ca^{2+} transient may be responsible for the elevated contraction seen in the diabetic heart. Moreover, the changes in cation contents in the heart may be responsible for abnormal cardiac rhythms and activity during DM.

Address for corresspondence: Prof. Jaipaul Singh, Department of Biological and Forensic Sciences, University of Central Lancashire, Preston, Lancashire, PR1 2HE UK. Voice: 00-44-1772-893515; fax: 00-44-1772-892929.

e-mail: jsingh3@uclan.ac.uk

Ann. N.Y. Acad. Sci. 1084: 178–190 (2006).
doi: 10.1196/annals.1372.028

KEYWORDS: **heart; diabetes mellitus; rat; cations; contraction; calcium**

INTRODUCTION

Diabetes mellitus (DM) is associated with contractile dysfunction of the heart leading subsequently to morbidity and mortality of the diabetic patient.[1–4] The precise mechanism whereby DM can lead to impairment of cardiac muscle contraction is still unknown.[5,6] The streptozotocin (STZ)-induced diabetic rat model has been used previously to study the effect of DM on cardiac dysfunction.[7,8] This model displays similar features of the human form of DM.[7] Previous studies have shown that a derangement in cellular and subcellular Ca^{2+} homeostasis may be associated with impairment of the diabetic heart.[5,6] There is much evidence that L-type Ca^{2+} channel, SERCA pump, and the Na^{+}/Ca^{2+} exchanger are all deranged as DM develops.[9–12] In addition to Ca^{2+}, other cations, such as Mg^{2+}, Na^{+}, K^{+}, Zn^{2+}, Cu^{2+}, and Fe^{2+} play major roles in the electrical activity, contraction, and physiological integrity of the heart.[1,13,14] It is possible that the levels of some of these cations change during DM and these in turn may lead to DM-induced cardiomyopathy. Therefore, the aim of this article was to measure the levels of these cations in the atria and the right and left ventricles of the heart of age-matched control and diabetic rats. In addition, force of contraction and Ca^{2+} transient were also measured in single ventricular myocytes for comparison.

METHODS

All experiments were undertaken using adult male Wistar rats weighing 150–200g. DM was induced by a single intraperitoneal injection (i.p.) of STZ (60 mg kg^{-1} body weight) dissolved in citrate acid buffer solution.[15] Age-matched control rats received an equivalent volume of the buffer alone. All the rats were caged separately and fed routinely on normal diet and water *ad libitum* until they were used 6–8 weeks later. All experiments had ethical clearance from the Ethics Committee of University of Central Lancashire. DM was confirmed 4–5 days following STZ injection and on the day prior to killing the rats humanely for the experiments using a glucose meter (One Touch II Glucometer; Lifescan, Inc. London, UK).

Rats were routinely killed by a blow on the head followed by cervical dislocation. An incision was made in the abdomen and the heart rapidly excised and placed in ice-cold buffer solution (mM): 130 NaCl; 5.2 $CaCl_2$, 1.0 $MgCl_2$, 0.4 NaH_2PO_4, 5 hepes, 10 glucose, 10 taurine, 10 creatine, and pH 7.3. In some experiments, ventricular myocytes were isolated with the buffer solution containing collagenase (0.75 mg mL^{-1}; Sigma (Dorset, UK)) as previously described.[5,8,13,14,16] Cells were used during a period of 1–8 h after isolation to measure either contraction (shortening) using a video edge system or intracellular free Ca^{2+} free concentration $[Ca^{2+}]_i$ after loading with Fura 2 (AM) using established methods.[5,8,13,14,16]

In another series of experiments, the isolated heart was weighed and then dissected into atria, and right and left ventricles. They were rinsed in Milli-Q grade deionized water, blotted, and then weighed. They were then digested overnight in either 1 mL or 2 mL of concentrated nitric acid. Appropriate dilutions were made with Milli-Q grade deionized water prior to measurement of cations. Total cardiac Ca^{2+}, Mg^{2+}, Fe^{2+}, Cu^{2+}, and Zn^{2+} concentrations were measured by atomic absorption spectrophotometery (AAS; PYE Unicam [Cambridge, UK], Model SP9) using air/acetylene and nitrous oxide/acetylene flames, respectively. Calibration standards (Ca^{2+}, Mg^{2+}, Fe^{2+}, Cu^{2+}, and Zn^{2+}) were obtained from VWR Laboratory Suppliers (Cambridge, UK). Values for cation contents were expressed as mg (100 mg of heart tissues)$^{-1}$.[14,17] Similarly, levels of Na^+ and K^+ were measured by the flame photometry method (Corning, Model 420 Flame Photometer; Sherwood Scientific, Cambridge, UK). Sample preparation was performed in exactly the same way as for AAS. Standards ranging from 5–20 mg mL^{-1} were made from a stock concentration of 20 mg mL^{-1} of either potassium or sodium. The absorbance of these standards was measured using the flame photometer and the results were plotted to give a standard curve of each of the ions. All values were expressed as mg (100 mg of heart tissue)$^{-1}$.[17,18]

Data Analysis and Statistics

All data are expressed as mean ± SEM of (n) hearts or cells. Statistical comparisons were made (SPSS software; London, UK) using independent samples Student's t-test, paired t-test, or analysis of variance (ANOVA) followed by Bonferroni *post hoc* analysis. P values of < 0.05 were considered significant, while P values of < 0.01 were considered very significant.

TABLE 1. General characteristics of rats and the hearts

Parameters	Control	Diabetic
Weight of rats (g)	507.88 ± 7.00 (9)	243.85 ± 2.85* (7)
Weight of heart (g)	0.799 ± 0.543 (9)	0.595 ± 0.030* (7)
Weight of atria (g)	0.071 ± 0.008 (6)	0.042 ± 0.002* (6)
Weight of right ventricle (g)	0.152 ± 0.117 (9)	0.105 ± 0.004* (7)
Weight of left ventricle (g)	0.568 ± 0.033 (9)	0.430 ± 0.026* (7)
Blood glucose (mM)	6.24 ± 0.08 (9)	30.71 ± 0.45* (7)

Data are mean ± SEM.

n values are shown in the table. Note that the mean (± SEM) weight of the rats on arrival in the animal house was 158.56 ± 2.68 g ($n = 16$). *($P < 0.05$).

RESULTS

TABLE 1 shows the general characteristics of the age-matched control and STZ-treated diabetic rats and their hearts. The results show that diabetic rats gained significantly ($P < 0.05$) less weight than age-matched control rats over the 8–9 weeks following purchasing. On arrival in the animal house, the rats weighed 158.56 ± 2.69 g ($n = 16$). The diabetic rats gained 34% of body weight compared to control that gained 108% of body weight over the experimental period. The results also show that the whole heart as well as the atria, and right and left ventricles of diabetic rats gained significantly ($P <$ 0.05) less weight compared to age-matched control hearts. The results also confirmed that the diabetic rats have significantly ($P < 0.05$) elevated blood glucose compared to control. Blood glucose level rises within 1 day following STZ injection and it remained elevated throughout the time course of the experiments.

TABLE 2 shows the amplitude of either contraction (% resting control length; RCL) or the peak $[Ca^{2+}]_i$ ratio units, the time to peak (t-pk) contraction or peak $[Ca^{2+}]_i$, and the time from peak to half relaxation for contraction or decay for $[Ca^{2+}]_i$ in single ventricular myocytes of age-matched control and STZ-induced diabetic rat hearts. The results show that the amplitude of shortening and time to peak contraction were significantly ($P < 0.05$) increased in diabetic ventricular myocytes compared to control. There was no significant change in the time from peak contraction to half relaxation. In contrast, there was no significant change in either the amplitude or the time to peak Ca^{2+} transient ($[Ca^{2+}]_i$ in ratio units) in control and diabetic ventricular myocytes. In contrast, the time from peak amplitude to half $[Ca^{2+}]_i$ decay was significantly ($P < 0.05$) increased in diabetic myocytes compared to age-matched control.

FIGURE 1 shows the level of (panel A) sodium and (panel B) potassium in atrial and right and left ventricles of the heart. The results show that sodium levels increased significantly ($P < 0.05$), in the atria and right ventricle of the diabetic heart compared to control. However, there was no change in sodium level in the left ventricle of the diabetic heart compared to control. In contrast, total potassium content in atria and right ventricle did not change significantly comparing control with diabetic animals. There was a small increase in potassium level in the left ventricle of the diabetic heart compared to control.

FIGURE 2 shows the total (panel A) calcium and (panel B) magnesium contents in atria and right and left ventricles of the heart. The results clearly show that all three parts of the diabetic heart contain significantly ($P < 0.05$) less calcium compared to age-matched control hearts. In contrast, magnesium level did not change significantly in either the atria, right or left ventricle comparing control with diabetes.

FIGURE 3 shows the level of (panel A) iron and (panel B) copper in atria and right and left ventricles of the heart. The results show that iron level increases

TABLE 2. Effect of 1 mM Ca^{2+} on the amplitude t-pk and time from peak to half ($t_{\frac{1}{2}}$) relaxation of contraction and calcium transient in electrically stimulated (1 Hz, 50 V 1 ms pulse width) and superfused (35–37°C) ventricular myocytes of age-matched control and diabetic rat hearts

	Contraction		Calcium transient	
Parameters	Control	Diabetic	Control	Diabetic
Shortening (% RCL) or peak $[Ca^{2+}]_i$ ratio units	5.2 ± 0.30 (15)	6.9 ± 0.40* (15)	0.061 ± 0.006 (20)	0.072 ± 0.007 (20)
t-pk contraction or peak $(Ca^{2+}]_i$ (ms)	108.2 ± 3.1 (15)	117.1 ± 2.5* (15)	91.41 ± 4.16 (20)	94.46 ± 5.54 (20)
Time for peak to half ($t_{\frac{1}{2}}$) relaxation or $[Ca^{2+}]_i$ decay (ms)	47.1 ± 3.6 (15)	43.9 ± 1.4 (15)	206.45 ± 12.90 (20)	309.60 ± 9.90* (20)

Data = mean ± SEM, n = 15–20 cells taken from 6–9 different hearts. *($P < 0.05$).

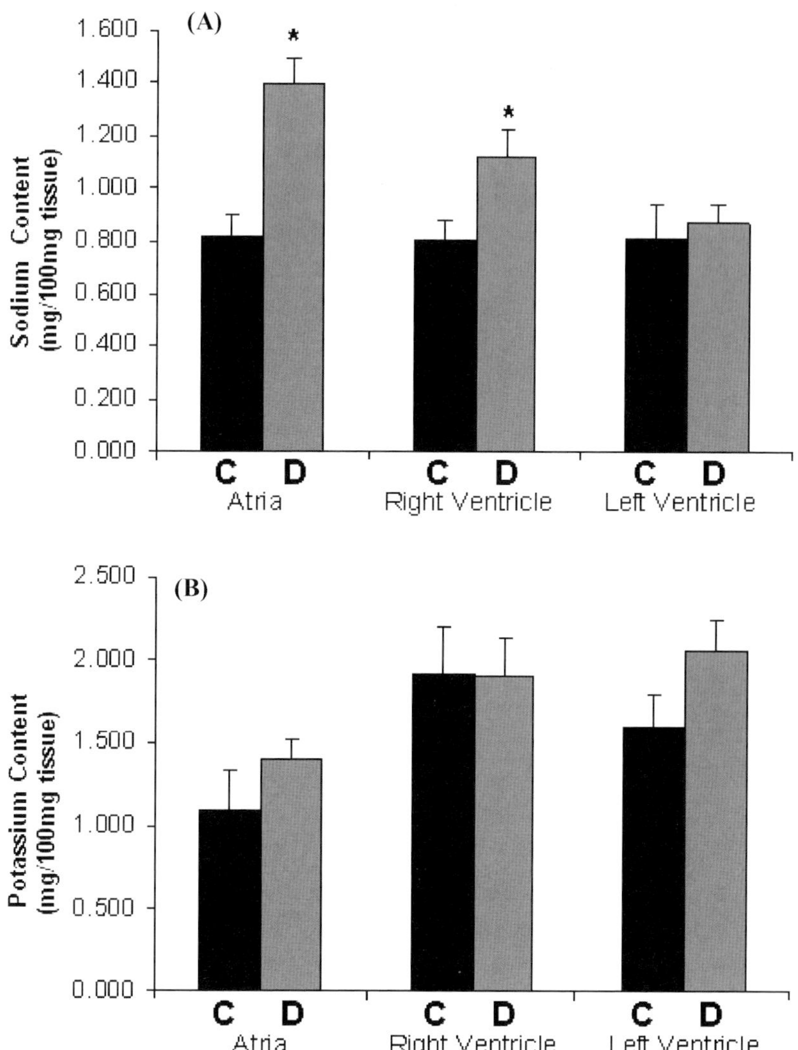

FIGURE 1. Levels of (**A**) sodium and (**B**) potassium in age-matched control (C) and STZ-treated diabetic (D) atria, and right and left ventricles of the rat heart. Data are mean ± SEM, $n = 6–9$ * $P < 0.05$.

significantly ($P < 0.05$) in the right ventricle of the diabetic heart compared to control. However, iron content remained more or less the same in the atria and left ventricle in both control and diabetic. The results also show that copper level increases significantly ($P < 0.05$) in the atria of the diabetic heart and decreases significantly ($P < 0.05$) in the left ventricle of the diabetic heart

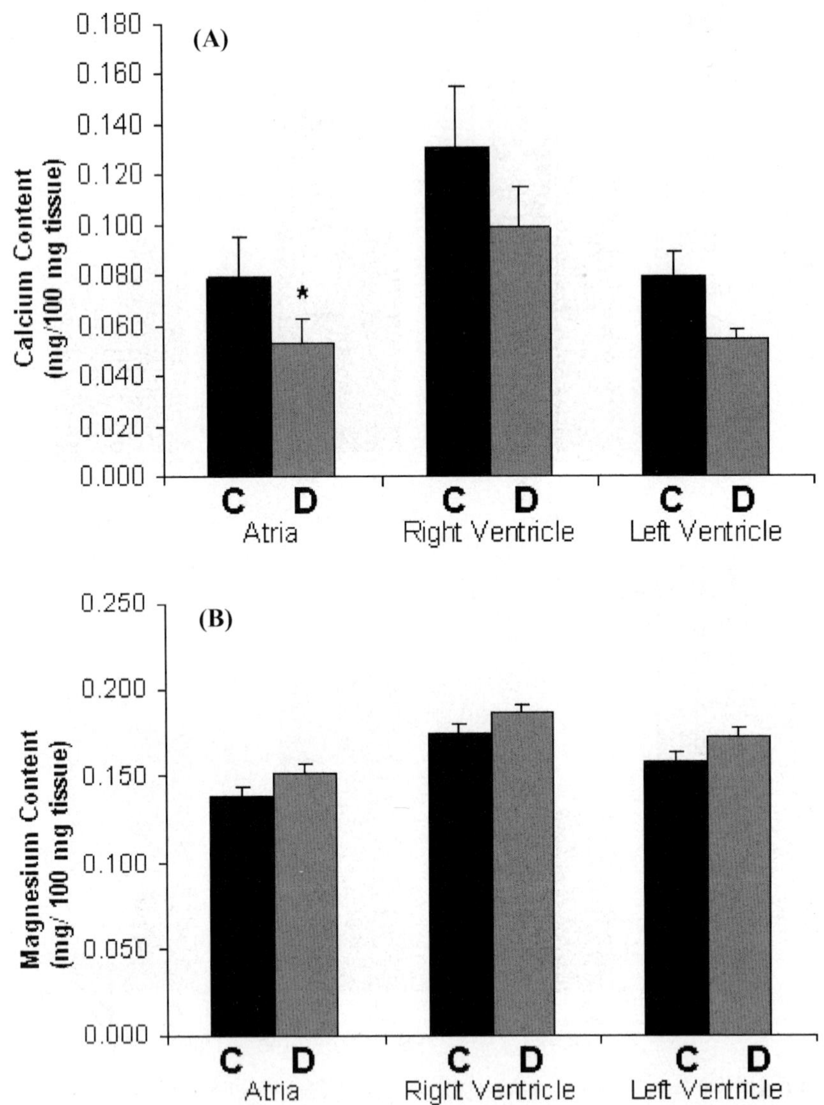

FIGURE 2. Levels of (**A**) calcium and (**B**) magnesium in age-matched control (C) and STZ-induced diabetic (D) atria, and right and left ventricles of the rat heart. Data are mean ± SEM, $n = 6$–9. $* P < 0.05$

compared to control. However, there was no change in copper content in the right ventricle in either control or diabetic heart. The level of zinc was also measured in all three parts of the heart but zinc values were undetectable.

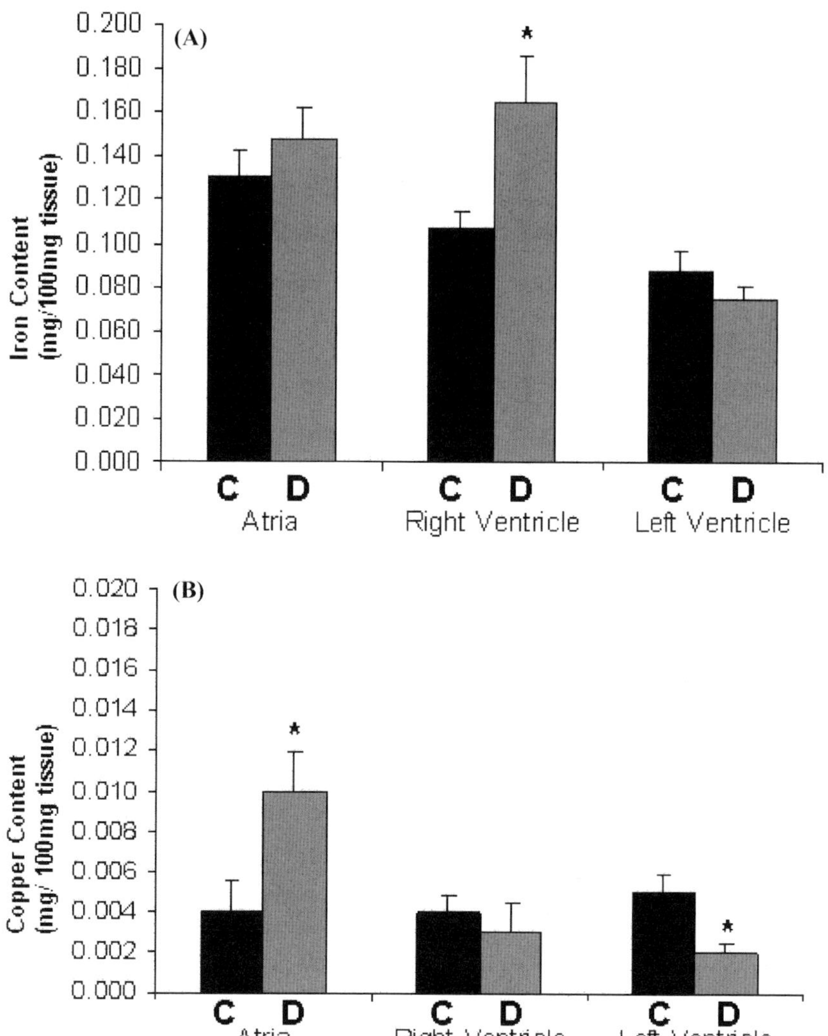

FIGURE 3. Levels of (**A**) iron and (**B**) copper in age-matched control (C) and STZ-induced diabetic (D) atria, and right and left ventricles of the rat heart. Data are mean ± SEM, $n = 6$–9 $*$ $P < 0.05$.

DISCUSSION

The results of this study have demonstrated that the diabetogenic agent STZ can elevate blood glucose sugar within 24 h following injection and the blood glucose sugar remained elevated throughout the time course of the experiments compared to control rats. When administered to young rats, STZ

(60 mg kg^{-1} body weight) destroys the insulin producing β cells of the pancreas and produces symptoms that are consistent with type 1 diabetes mellitus.[19] Moreover, the STZ-treated rats gained significantly less body weight compared to age-matched control animals. The diabetic rats only gained 34% of their body weight compared to 108% by the control rats over the experimental period. The results also show that the whole heart as well as the atria, and right and left ventricles have significantly reduced weights in the diabetic rats compared to the control animals. These results are in total agreement in previous studies employing the STZ-induced diabetic rats.[5,6,14,16] The reduction in body weight as well as the weight of the heart in diabetic animals may be due either to the diabetes itself or the animals eating less.[19]

The results of this study have also demonstrated that amplitude and time to peak contraction in STZ-treated ventricular myocytes was significantly increased compared to myocytes from age-matched control animals. In other studies, it has been reported that STZ-induced diabetes was associated with a decrease in contraction.[9,10] This contradiction regarding the results may be due either to the duration of the STZ-treatment or to the voltage at which the contraction was measured.[16] The time-dependent changes in the chronic model of diabetes may be indicative of some underlying compensatory process that is instigated within the heart to secure its integrity. The increase in contraction is due either to increased Ca^{2+} influx into the cell, increased sarcoplasmic reticulum Ca^{2+} release, increased myofilament Ca^{2+} sensitivity, or other underlying mechanisms that are associated with cellular Ca^{2+} homeostasis.[5,6] The results presented in this study show that the amplitude of the Ca^{2+} transient remained more or less the same in both control and STZ-treated ventricular myocytes. However, the time to half (t $\frac{1}{2}$)decay of the Ca^{2+} transient was significantly longer in diabetic myocytes, which may be responsible for the increase in contraction. The increase in the decay in Ca^{2+} transient may be due to a derangement in either the SERCA pump or the Na^{+}-Ca^{2+} exchange.[7–10]

The results of this study show marked elevation in sodium contents in the diabetic heart compared to control. In contrast, total potassium level remains more or less the same in diabetic hearts compared to control. Sodium plays a major role in the depolarization of the heart, especially in the atria where the beat of the heart is initiated.[20] The increase in sodium content may be responsible for abnormal heart rhythm that usually occurs during DM.[21]

The total calcium concentration following 6–8 weeks of diabetes was significantly reduced after STZ treatment. The decrease in tissue Ca^{2+} content may be due either to a decrease in Ca^{2+} influx into the heart cell during DM. It was demonstrated recently that the L-type Ca^{2+} channel is impaired during DM leading to a reduced influx of Ca^{2+} into ventricular myocytes.[14,16] These results have demonstrated an increase in contraction in the diabetic heart compared to control but there was no increase in the amplitude of the calcium transient except for a delay in the decay of $[Ca^{2+}]_i$. This dissociation between the Ca^{2+} content, the Ca^{2+} transient and contraction may be due to insensitivity of the cardiac cell myofilaments to Ca^{2+}.[14,16] In contrast to Ca^{2+}, total cardiac Mg^{2+} levels increased slightly but these values were not significantly different between control and STZ-treated rats after 6–8 weeks of treatment. The data in this study would suggest that cardiac Mg^{2+} is not affected in STZ-induced diabetes. In a previous study, it was demonstrated that experimental-induced diabetes was associated with a significant decrease in cardiac Mg^{2+} levels from STZ- and alloxan-treated animals compared to controls.[22,23] However, in another study, it has been shown that there were no significant changes in heart Mg^{2+} in STZ-induced and controls.[24] These later findings are in agreement with the results obtained in this study.

$[Mg^{2+}]_i$ and extracellular Mg^{2+} ($[Mg^{2+}]_o$) concentrations play an important role in a variety of cellular events and are also an important cofactor for ATP in many cellular enzyme systems.[25] $[Mg^{2+}]_i$ has been reported to be important in the regulation of the Na^+/Ca^{2+}-exchanger and consequently cause a reduced or increased concentration of Ca^{2+} within the cell.[25] It has also been reported that Mg^{2+} deficiency can induce the rise of $[Ca^{2+}]_i$, changes in cell membrane permeability, and transport processes in cardiac cells, whereas high Mg^{2+} has the opposite effect. It has been suggested that the reason for opposing effect of Ca^{2+} and Mg^{2+} is that there is competition for the same site of action proteins, such as troponin-C.[26] The decrease in Ca^{2+} content in the diabetic heart may be directly linked to the small elevation in Mg^{2+} content.

Total copper concentration was significantly increased in the atria of the diabetic rat heart compared to control. In contrast, it was significantly decreased in the left ventricle of diabetic heart. There was no significant change in copper contents in either diabetic or control right ventricles. It has been shown that a decrease in Cu^{2+} within the diet and subsequent Cu^{2+} deficiency leads to ischemic heart disease.[27] As a result of decreased Cu^{2+} intake, hearts would also appear to have lesser amounts of Cu^{2+}. The results of this study show both an increase in Cu^{2+} in the atria and a decrease in the diabetic left ventricle compared to control. Moreover, it has been shown[28] that elevated levels of serum Cu^{2+} concentrations may be associated with higher incidence of cardiovascular disease. There is little data available to directly link experimental diabetes with elevated levels of cardiac Cu^{2+}; however, it has been shown that Cu^{2+} is elevated in the liver of diabetic animals.[29,30] From the literature and results presented in this study, it seems unclear if there is a direct link with alterations in Cu^{2+} and an increase in diabetic-induced cardiomyopathy. The results show that total iron increased significantly in the right ventricle but its level decreased in the left ventricle. A previous study has shown that both copper and iron play an important physiological role in preventing myocardial ischemia.[29,30] Previous reports suggest that an alteration in Fe^{2+} levels is not implicated in the pathophysiology of diabetes.[31] Zinc concentration was also measured in all three tissues in this study. It was impossible to detect any trace of zinc using the AAS to measure its content in both control and diabetic hearts.

In conclusion, the results of this study have demonstrated marked characteristic changes in diabetic rats and their hearts compared to age-matched control. Moreover, diabetic hearts produce more force compared to control and this may be associated with the prolongation in the decay of the Ca^{2+} transient. The results also reveal marked variation in cation contents in either the atria, right or left ventricles of diabetic hearts compared to control. It is possible that any changes in cation imbalance during DM may lead to a disturbance in both cardiac rhythm and function.

ACKNOWLEDGMENTS

The work was supported by a grant to MH and JS from the British Heart Foundation.

REFERENCES

1. KUMAR, P. & M. CLARK. 2002. Diabetes mellitus and other disorders of metabolism. *In* Clinical Medicine. P. Kumar & M. Clark, Eds.: 1069–1121. WB Saunders. London.
2. KANNEL, W.B. & D.L. MCGEE. 1979. Diabetes and cardiovascular disease. The Framingham Study. JAMA **241:** 2035–2039.
3. MIETTENEN, H.S., S. LEHTO, V. SALOMAA, *et al.* 1998. Impact of diabetes on mortality after the first myocardial infarction. The Finmonica Myocardial Infarction Register Study Group. Diabetes Care **21:** 69–75.
4. FALLOW, G.D. & J. SINGH. 2004. The prevalence, type and severity of cardiovascular disease in diabetic and non-diabetic patients: a matched-paired retrospective analysis using coronary angiography and the diagnostic tool. Mol. Cell. Biochem. **261:** 263–269
5. BRACKEN, N.K., J. SINGH, W. WINLOW, *et al.* 2003. Mechanism underlying contractile dysfunction in streptozotocin-induced type 1 and type 2 diabetic cardiomyopathy. *In* Athersclerosis, Hypertension and Diabetes, G.N. Pierce, M Nagano, P. Zahradka & N.S. Dhalla, Eds.: 387–408. Kluwer Academic Publishers. Boston.
6. HOWARTH, F.C. & J. SINGH. 1999. Altered handling of calcium during the process of excitation-contraction coupling in the streptozotocin-induced diabetic heart: a short review. Int. J. Diabetes **7:** 52–64.
7. PANDIT, S.V., W.R. GILES & S.S. DEMIR. 2003. A mathematic model of the electrophysiological alterations in rat ventricular myocyte in type 1 diabetes mellitus. Biophys. J. **84:** 832–841.
8. QURESHI, M.A., N.K. BRACKEN, W. WINLOW, *et al.* 2001. Time dependant effects of streptozotocin-induced diabetes on contraction in rat ventricular myocytes. Emirates J. **19:** 25–41.
9. HATTORI, Y., N. MATSUDA, J. KIMURA, *et al.* 2000. Diminished function and expression of the cardiac Na^+-Ca^{2+} exchanger in diabetic rats: implication of Ca^{2+} overload. J. Physiol. **527:** 85–94.

10. CHOI, K.M., Y. ZHONG, B.D. HOIT, *et al.* 2002. Defective intracellular Ca^{2+} signalling contributes to cardiomyopathy in type 1 in diabetic rats. Am. J. Physiol. **283:** H1398–H1408.
11. GANGULY, P.K., G.N. PIERCE, K.S. DHALLA, *et al.* 1983. Defective sarcoplasmic reticular calcium transport in diabetic cardiomyopathy. Am. J. Physiol. **244:** E528–E535.
12. NETTICADAN, T., R.M. TEMSAH, A. KENT, *et al.* 2001. Depressed levels of Ca^{2+}-cycling proteins may underlie sarcoplasmic reticulum dysfunction in the diabetic heart. Diabetes **50:** 2133–2138.
13. LAGADIC-GROSSMAN, D. & D. FEUVRAY. 1991. Intracellular sodium activity in papillary muscle from diabetic rats. Exp. Physiol. **76:** 147–149.
14. BRACKEN, N.K.. 2003. Cellular mechanism of contractile dysfunction in the diabetes heart. PhD thesis, University of Central Lancashire.
15. SHARMA, A.K., I.G.M. DUGUID, D.S. BLANCHARD, *et al.* 1985. The effects of insulin treatment on myelinated nerve fibre maturation and integrity and on body growth in streptozotocin-diabetic rats. J. Neurol. Sci. **67:** 285–297.
16. BRACKEN, N.K., A.J. WOODALL, F.C. HOWARTH, *et al.* 2004. Voltage dependence of contraction in streptozotocin-diabetic myocytes. Mol. Cell. Biochem. **261:** 235–243.
17. BRACKEN, N.K., M.A. QURESHI, F.C. HOWARTH, *et al.* 2002. Effects of diabetes on cation content and on contraction in the isolated rat heart. Adap. Biol. Med. **3:** 112–121.
18. ROY, K., F. HARRIS, S.R. DENNISON, *et al.* 2005. Effects of streptozotocin-induced type I diabetes mellitus on protein and ion concentrations in ocular tissues of rat. Int. J. Diabetes Met. **13:** 154–158.
19. AHMED, I., E. ADEGHATE, A.K. SHARMA, *et al.* 1998. Effect of Momordica charantia fruit juice in islet morphology in the pancreas of streptozotocin-induced diabetic rat. Diabetes Res. Clin. Pract. **40:** 145–151.
20. GRUPP, I., I.M. WOOK-BIN, O. CHIN, *et al.* 1985. Relation of sodium pump inhibition to positive inotropy at low concentrations of ouabain in rat heart muscle. J. Physiol. **360:** 149–160.
21. HOWARTH, F.C., M.A. QURESHI, *et al.* 2002. Effects of hyperosmotic shrinking on ventricular myocyte shortening and intracellular Ca^{2+} in streptozotocin-induced diabetic rats. Pflugers Arch. **444:** 451–461.
22. BHIMJI, S., D.V. GODIN, *et al.* 1986. Insulin reversal of biochemical changes in hearts from diabetic rats. Am. J. Physiol. **251:** H670–H675.
23. BHIMJI, S. & J.H. MCNEIL. 1989. Isoproterenol-induced ultrastructural alterations in hearts of alloxan-diabetic rabbits. Gen. Pharmacol. **20:** 479–485.
24. EWIS, S.A. & M.S. ABDELRAHMAN. 1995. Effect of metformin on glutathione and magnesium in normal and streptozotocin-induced diabetic rats. J. Appl. Toxicol. **15:** 387–390.
25. HOWARTH, F.C. & A.J. LEVI. 1998. Internal free magnesium modulates the voltage dependence of contraction and Ca transient in rabbit ventricular myocytes. Pflügers Arch. **435:** 687–698.
26. CHAKRABORTI, S., T. CHAKRABORTI, *et al.* 2002. Protective role of magnesium in cardiovascular diseases: a review. Mol. Cell. Biochem. **238:** 163–179.
27. KLEVAY, L.M.. 2000. Cardiovascular disease from copper deficiency—a history. J Nutr. **130:** 489S–492S.

28. Hallmans, G. & F. Lithner. 1980. Early changes in zinc and copper metabolism in rats with alloxan diabetes of short duration after traumatization with heat. Ups. J. Med. Sci. **85:** 59–66.
29. Ford, E.S.. 2000. Serum copper concentration and coronary heart disease among U.S. adults. Am. J. Epidemiol. **151:** 1182–1188.
30. Chevion, M., Y. Jian, *et al*. Copper and iron are mobilized following myocardial ischaemia. Possible predictive criteria after tissue injury. Proc. Natl. Head Sci. **90:** 1102–1106.
31. Tuvemo, T. & M. Gebre-Medhin. 1983. The role of trace elements in juvenile diabetes mellitus. Paediatrician **12:** 213–219.

Predicting the Development of Macrovascular Disease in People with Type 1 Diabetes

A 9-Year Follow-up Study

LATIKA SIBAL,[a,b] HUONG NAI LAW,[a] JANICE GEBBIE,[a] UMESH K. DASHORA,[a,b] SHARAD C. AGARWAL,[b] AND PHILIP HOME[a,b]

[a]*Newcastle Diabetes Centre, Newcastle upon Tyne, NE4 6BE, United Kingdom*

[b]*Newcastle University, Newcastle upon Tyne, NE2 4HH United Kingdom*

ABSTRACT: The aim of the article was to use prospectively collected data on people with type 1 diabetes to assess which routinely collected clinical measures predict the development of macrovascular disease in people with type 1 diabetes. Data have been collected in a structured format at an annual review since 1985. For this study, all people with type 1 diabetes in the database in both 1992 and 2001 were ascertained. Data were extracted for a diagnosis of coronary artery disease, stroke, and peripheral vascular disease (macrovascular complications). Presence of other microvascular complications was also ascertained. Forty-one of 404 (10.1%) people had macrovascular disease at the index visit in 1992 and 61 others developed macrovascular complications during follow-up. People who developed macrovascular complications were older (48 ± 12 versus 36 ± 11 [SD] years; $P = 0.000$), had longer duration of diabetes (28 ± 12 versus 18 ± 11 years; $P = 0.000$), higher BMI (26.7 ± 4.6 versus 25.4 ± 3.6 kg/m^2; $P = 0.041$), higher base line serum cholesterol (5.9 ± 1.7 versus 5.2 ± 1.1 mmol/L, $P = 0.007$), higher median base line triglyceride levels (1.5 [IQ range 0.9–2.6] versus 1.1 [0.8–1.7] mmol/L; $P = 0.002$), higher systolic BP (145 ± 21 versus 129 ± 20 mmHg; $P = 0.000$), and higher serum creatinine (102 ± 57 versus 86 ± 17 μmol/L; $P = 0.038$) than those who did not. We found no significant difference in the base line glycated hemoglobin in the two groups. The multivariate model showed that age, duration of diabetes, systolic BP, and serum cholesterol and creatinine levels predicted the development of macrovascular complications, which were also associated with the later development of microalbuminuria. Macrovascular complications developed in 16.8% of people with type 1 diabetes over a 9-year follow-up, and were predicted by potentially modifiable factors including higher BP, BMI, and serum triglyceride and cholesterol levels.

Address for correspondence: Latika Sibal, SCMS-Diabetes, The Medical School, Framlington Place, Newcastle upon Tyne, NE2 4HH, UK. Voice: 44-191-256-3365; fax: 44-191-256-3212.
e-mail: latika.sibal@ncl.ac.uk

**Ann. N.Y. Acad. Sci. 1084: 191–207 (2006). © 2006 New York Academy of Sciences.
doi: 10.1196/annals.1372.037**

KEYWORDS: type 1 diabetes; cardiovascular risk factors; macrovascular complications

INTRODUCTION

Diabetes mellitus leads to long-term microvascular and macrovascular complications, the latter including coronary artery disease (CAD), stroke, and peripheral vascular disease. The concomitant increase in the healthcare costs associated with these complications relate not only to the index presentation, but also the subsequent increased requirement of healthcare services by the affected individuals.[1]

Type 1 diabetes confers a two- to tenfold increased risk of death and cardiovascular disease (CVD) compared with nondiabetic people.[2–8] A recent primary care database study of people with type 1 diabetes in the United Kingdom reported a hazard ratio of 4.5 (95% CI 3.8–5.4) for major CVD in people with type 1 diabetes compared with nondiabetic people. In addition, type 1 diabetic men aged 45–55 years were found to have an absolute CVD risk similar to nondiabetic men approximately 10–15 years older, a difference even greater for women.[9]

Cardiovascular complications and renal failure are the main cause of mortality in type 1 diabetes. Microalbuminuria is not just a predictor of diabetic nephropathy, but also a strong predictor of CAD, cardiac failure, cardiovascular death, and peripheral vascular complications.[3,10–20] Elevated blood pressure (BP) has also been found to be a strong risk factor for coronary heart disease.[3,17–20] Furthermore, diabetic neuropathy has been found to be associated with cardiovascular mortality.[21] Despite this, clinical management of people with type 1 diabetes tends to be centered around blood glucose control, as though the major ongoing preventative management was for microvascular disease.

In the present article we rather set out to ascertain the clinical predictors of macrovascular disease and mortality in people with type 1 diabetes that are collected in routine care and could be used by clinicians in identifying at-risk patients. We used a 9-year follow-up period using data collected in structured form prospectively, and compared these clinical predictors in people with and without microalbuminuria.

METHODS

Study Design and Population

The study design was a retrospective analysis of data collected prospectively in structured format over a 9-year period. Ethics approval for data review was obtained from the local research ethics committee. A total of 404 people

(54% male, mean age 40.5 ± 13.5 [SD], range 17–81, years) with type 1 diabetes attended the diabetes services in Newcastle upon Tyne for structured annual outpatient review in 1992, and had follow-up information available in 2001, or had died. Of those who did not have macrovascular disease ($n = 363$) at base line, 61 developed macrovascular disease during the 9-year follow-up (45 alive, 16 deceased during follow-up), 291 remained healthy in this respect, and 11 people died due to noncardiovascular causes. Overall 52 people died, 25 of whom had macrovascular disease at base line and 16 of whom developed macrovascular complications during follow-up.

Definition of Macrovascular Disease

Macrovascular disease was defined as ischemic heart disease (IHD), cerebrovascular disease, or peripheral vascular disease. IHD was defined as a history of myocardial infarction, angina, and revascularization including coronary angioplasty or coronary artery bypass grafting (CABG). Cerebrovascular disease was defined as stroke or transient ischemic attack (TIA). Peripheral arterial disease (PAD) was defined as absent peripheral pulses together with a history of claudication, peripheral ischemia, or a revascularization procedure in the legs.

Normotension was defined as systolic/diastolic BP less than 140/90 mmHg without antihypertensive therapy. Patients were classified as being hypertensive if they were on antihypertensive therapy or were not normotensive.

Biochemical Measures

base line glycated hemoglobin was Diabetes Control and Complications Trial (DCCT)-aligned by formal regression between the methods used in 1992–2001 (nondiabetic reference <6.1%). Microalbuminuria measured by nephelometry was defined as urine albumin:creatinine ratio ≥2.5 mg/mmol creatinine for men and ≥3.5 mg/mmol creatinine for women in people without proteinuria. We estimated glomerular filtration rate (GFR) by the modification of diet in renal disease (MDRD) equation.[22,23] The following base line predictors of cardiovascular risk were assessed: serum total cholesterol and triglycerides, smoking, body mass index (BMI), systolic and diastolic BP (standard sphygmomanometer, sitting); all were formal parts of the annual review process. Annual review data were entered into a computer database close to the time of collection.

Other Microvascular Complications

Diabetic retinopathy was defined as nonproliferative, preproliferative, or proliferative classified on the basis of retinal photographs, initially taken using

Polaroid film and later by digital cameras. Distal peripheral neuropathy was defined by presence of two of three measures performed as part of structured annual review: neuropathic symptoms, absence of pinprick sensation, and abnormal biothesiometer measurements and/or abnormal 10-g monofilament sensation.

Statistical Analysis

Statistical analyses were performed using Minitab14 (Minitab, Coventry, UK) and SPSS 11 (SPSS, Chicago, IL). Univariate analysis was performed using Student's *t*-test, Mann-Whitney *U*-test, and χ^2 where appropriate. Logistic regression and Cox proportional hazards model were used to assess the odds ratio for the development of macrovascular disease and mortality in this cohort of type 1 diabetes compared with the lowest odds ratio. The covariates were stratified into quarters for the Cox proportional hazards model and the results adjusted for age, glycated hemoglobin, and gender. The odds ratio for the lowest quarter of the risk factors was taken as 1.00 and the odds ratio for each quarter (i.e., second, third, and fourth quarter) compared to that of the lowest quarter. The earliest of time to death or the development of macrovascular complications was used as the dependent variable. A P value <0.05 was taken as significant; other P values are given for information only.

RESULTS

Forty-one of 404 (10.1%) people had macrovascular disease at the index visit in 1992. The remaining 363 people free of macrovascular disease at base line had a mean age of 39 ± 13 (SD) years and a mean duration of diabetes 20 ± 11 (range 1–56) years (TABLE 1). Fifty-two people died during the follow-up of whom 25 people had macrovascular disease at base line and were thus excluded from further analysis. Forty-one of 52 (79%) deceased people had macrovascular disease prior to or at the time of death. Overall, macrovascular disease developed in 61 of 363 (16.8%) people during the follow-up of whom IHD developed first in the largest proportion (49%), followed by PAD (40%), and then cerebrovascular disease (11%).

Univariate Analysis

People who developed macrovascular disease were older (48 ± 12 versus 36 ± 11 years; $P = 0.000$) and had longer duration of diabetes (28 ± 12 versus 18 ± 11 years; $P = 0.000$) than those who remained free of it (TABLE 2). BMI, serum cholesterol, triglyceride, and creatinine, and systolic BP were higher in

TABLE 1. base line characteristics of the type 1 diabetes population ($n = 363$) who did not already have macrovascular disease

Measure	Value
Age (years)	39 ± 13 (17–76)
Duration of diabetes (years)	20 ± 11 (1–56)
BMI (kg/m^2)	25.6 ± 3.8 (15.2–51.3)
Systolic BP (mmHg)	132 ± 21 (90–215)
Diastolic BP (mmHg)	76 ± 11 (40–120)
Serum cholesterol (mmol/L)	5.3 ± 1.2 (2.8–12.0)
Serum triglyceride (mmol/L)	1.2 (0.3–6.3)
HbA_{1c} (%)	9.4 ± 2.1 (2.8–16.9)
Microalbuminuria (*n* (%))	60 (20)

Mean ± SD (range), or median (interquartile range), or number (%).

the macrovascular disease group compared with the group that remained free of it (TABLE 2). In addition, although microalbuminuria at base line was not different between the two groups, progression to microalbuminuria occurred in a significantly greater number of people who developed macrovascular disease during the follow-up (TABLE 2). We found no significant difference in gender, diastolic BP, high-density lipoprotein (HDL) cholesterol, or glycated hemoglobin at base line between the two groups. Furthermore, smoking was comparable in the two groups (TABLE 2).

Mortality was associated with age, duration of diabetes, systolic BP, and serum creatinine, cholesterol, and triglyceride at base line. In addition, people who died had a higher prevalence of macrovascular disease and lower estimated GFR at base line than patients who remained alive (TABLE 3).

Microvascular Complications

Thirty-eight of 61 people who developed macrovascular disease did not have microalbuminuria at base line, of whom 10 (26%) became microalbuminuric during the follow-up. Microalbuminuria was noted to regress in four of 19 (21%) people during the follow-up. In addition, BP, serum triglyceride and cholesterol, and glycated hemoglobin were comparable when people who developed macrovascular disease were stratified based on base line microalbuminuria status (TABLE 4).

Of the 45 people who developed macrovascular disease and were alive at follow-up, distal peripheral neuropathy was present in a higher proportion compared with the group that remained free of it. Overall, there was no significant difference in the presence of nonproliferative retinopathy either at base line or during the follow-up. However, proliferative retinopathy was present in a greater proportion of people at base line who later developed macrovascular disease (20 versus 9%; $P = 0.030$) (TABLE 5).

TABLE 2. base line markers of development of macrovascular disease in people with type 1 diabetes

	Macrovascular disease	No macrovascular disease	*P*
N	61	291	
Age (years)	48 ± 12	36 ± 11	0.000
Sex (% male)	59	57	NS
Duration of diabetes (years)	28 ± 12	18 ± 11	0.000
BMI (kg/m^2)	26.7 ± 4.6	25.4 ± 3.6	0.041
Systolic BP (mmHg)	145 ± 21	129 ± 20	0.000
Diastolic BP (mmHg)	79 ± 12	76 ± 11	NS
Hypertension (*n* (%))	42 (69)	104 (36)	0.000
ACE inhibitors (*n* (%))	9 (14.8)	30 (10.3)	0.315
Serum cholesterol (mmol/L)	5.9 ± 1.7	5.2 ± 1.1	0.007
Serum triglyceride (mmol/L)	1.5 (0.9–2.6)	1.1 (0.8–1.7)	0.002
Serum HDL (mmol/L)	1.4 ± 0.7	1.5 ± 0.4	NS
Serum LDL (mmol/L)	3.4 ± 1.7	3.1 ± 0.8	0.398
Statins (*n* (%))	11 (18)	25 (8.6)	0.027
HbA_{1c} (%) in 1992	9.6 ± 2.2	9.4 ± 2.1	NS
HbA_{1c} (%) in 2001	8.6 ± 2.0	8.6 ± 1.3	0.944
Average updated HbA_{1c} (%)	9.2 ± 2.1	9.0 ± 1.6	0.567
Serum creatinine (μmol/L)	102 ± 57	86 ± 17	0.038
Microalbuminuria 1992 (*n* (%))	19/57 (33)	71/244 (29)	NS
Microalbuminuria 2001 (*n* (%)	20/43 (47)	43/256 (17)	0.000
eGFR (mL/min/1.73 m^2)	73.4 ± 22.4	81.9 ± 20.0	0.023
Smoking (*n* (%))	14 (23)	45 (15)	NS

Number (%), or mean ± SD, or median (interquartile range).
HDL data in 1992 available in 149 (41%).

Regression Analysis

The multivariate model adjusted for duration of diabetes showed that age, duration of diabetes, and presence of hypertension, systolic BP, serum cholesterol,

TABLE 3. base line markers of death in people with type 1 diabetes

	Deceased	No macrovascular disease	*P*
N	52	291	
Age (years)	54.7 ± 12.7	36.5 ± 11.7	0.000
Duration of diabetes (years)	28.6 ± 12.8	18.1 ± 10.6	0.000
Systolic BP (mmHg)	147 ± 25	128 ± 20	0.000
Serum creatinine (μmol/L)	96 (83–120)	84 (75–95)	0.000
Serum cholesterol (mmol/L)	5.9 ± 1.3	5.2 ± 1.1	0.010
Serum triglyceride (mmol/L)	1.6 (1.2–2.3)	1.1 (0.8–1.7)	0.001
eGFR (mL/min/1.73 m^2)	64.5 ± 26.4	81.9 ± 20.0	0.000
Macrovascular disease (*n* (%))	41 (79 %)	0	0.000

Mean ± SD, or median (interquartile range).
No significant difference was found for sex, BMI, diastolic BP, HbA_{1c}, HDL, or LDL cholesterol.

TABLE 4. Predictive characteristics of development of macrovascular disease by presence or absence of microalbuminuria

	No microalbuminuria	Microalbuminuria	*P*
N	38	19	
Age (years)	48 ± 11	48 ± 12	NS
Duration of diabetes (years)	27 ± 11	29 ± 13	NS
Systolic BP (mmHg)	142 ± 19	150 ± 22	NS
Diastolic BP (mmHg)	79 ± 12	80 ± 14	NS
HbA_{1c} (%)	9.8 ± 2.1	9.8 ± 1.8	NS
Serum cholesterol (mmol/L)	5.9 ± 1.2	6.0 ± 2.0	NS
Serum triglyceride (mmol/L)	1.6 (0.9–2.7)	1.6 (0.9–2.8)	NS

Mean ± SD, or median (interquartile range).

and serum creatinine predicted the development of macrovascular disease (TABLE 6). Predictors of CVD mortality included age, systolic BP, serum creatinine, and eGFR (TABLE 6). In the Cox proportional hazards regression analysis, systolic BP greater than the 50th percentile ($\geq$131 mmHg) predicted macrovascular disease after adjusting for age. After adjusting for glycated hemoglobin, systolic BP $\geq$119 mmHg, diastolic BP $\geq$ 85 mmHg, and serum cholesterol $\geq$ 6.1 predicted the development of macrovascular disease. Estimated GFR less than the 25th percentile was associated with a significantly increased risk of developing macrovascular disease (TABLE 7). In addition, development of microalbuminuria during the follow-up was associated with an odds ratio of 4.11 (95% CI 2.24–7.54) for the development of macrovascular disease.

Furthermore, systolic BP >75th percentile was strongly associated with mortality after adjusting for glycated hemoglobin and gender (TABLE 8).

DISCUSSION

The present analysis was undertaken to ascertain those factors, routinely measured in clinical practice, which could help clinicians identify higher risk of CVD in people with type 1 diabetes. Because type 1 diabetes is a hormone

TABLE 5. Retinopathy and neuropathy in relation to incident macrovascular disease

Retinopathy	Macrovascular disease (*n* (%))	No macrovascular disease (*n* (%))	*P*
All	45	291	
Background	11 (24)	81 (28)	NS
Preproliferative	0 (0)	7 (2)	–
Proliferative	9 (20)	27 (9)	0.030
Maculopathy	2 (4)	6 (3)	–
Neuropathy	10 (22)	22 (8)	0.002

Statistical calculations not performed where numbers with event very low.

TABLE 6. Logistic regression for new macrovascular disease and mortality in people with type 1 diabetes adjusted for duration of diabetes

	Regression coefficient	SE	*P*	OR
Macrovascular disease (incident)				
Age	0.054	0.019	0.005	1.06
Duration of diabetes	0.061	0.014	0.000	1.06
Hypertension	1.031	0.333	0.002	2.80
Systolic BP	0.024	0.008	0.002	1.03
Serum cholesterol	0.311	0.128	0.015	1.37
Serum creatinine	0.014	0.006	0.014	1.02
Microalbuminuria at follow-up	1.554	0.348	0.000	4.73
Death				
Age	0.074	0.029	0.011	1.08
Systolic BP	0.028	0.011	0.009	1.03
Serum creatinine	0.026	0.009	0.004	1.03
eGFR	−0.036	0.013	0.007	0.96

deficiency disease, unlike type 2 diabetes which also has a large pathogenetic metabolic component, clinical management tends to concentrate on the optimal delivery of insulin therapy to achieve blood glucose control, and indeed in the earlier decades it is prevention of microvascular disease, specific to people with hyperglycemia, that is the major focus of concern. Nevertheless these people suffer two major risks of premature mortality in middle age, namely renal failure and IHD,[2–4] the former now largely manageable by dialysis and renal transplantation. Accordingly concern over health risk reduction in type 1 diabetes has in recent years turned to prevention of CVD, with debate between treating all individuals over a certain age as high risk (requiring statins for example) and treating only those at identifiable high risk. Presently the first of these is unattractive for reasons of cost and drug toxicity, and the latter problematic because of uncertainty as to how to identify high risk, with the exception of those people with microalbuminuria.[24]

Guideline groups have suggested two means of approaching this question based on identification of conventional risk factors, and risk factors associated with the metabolic syndrome, although because identification of hyperglycemia is not an issue here, and because some factors (such as high BP) fall into both categories, the distinction can be unhelpful. Nevertheless, it is striking that systolic BP, a core component of the metabolic syndrome and one that is often not a strong independent predictor in people with type 2 diabetes, is in this analysis one of the strongest predictors identified, is confirmed by formal identification of hypertension (which includes treatment), and statistically survives adjustment for duration of diabetes. Review of quarters of BP control (TABLE 7) suggests that a cutoff of $\geq$119 mmHg carries increased risk in itself, though if age is separately considered as a risk then a cutoff of 130 mmHg might be more relevant.

Also noteworthy is serum triglyceride concentration, 36% higher in those going on to macrovascular disease compared with those who did not (TABLE 2). It is noteworthy here that serum low-density lipoprotein (LDL) cholesterol was not predictive even on univariate analysis, implying that the difference in serum total cholesterol found was secondary to the increased triglyceride levels (i.e., raised very low-density lipoprotein [VLDL] cholesterol level), rather than the conventional risk factor. Serum HDL cholesterol was, however, not predictive, but this may reflect a weakness of the study, namely that in 1992 HDL cholesterol was not measured in everyone having annual review, and that the assay used at the time was less precise. A recent study of 27,358 young people with diabetes (age up to 26 years) showed that while dyslipidemia, systolic hypertension, and diastolic hypertension were present in 28.6, 8.1, and 2.5% of the study group respectively, the percentage of people on lipid-lowering and antihypertensive agents was only 0.4 and 2.1%.[25] While triglyceride may be more useful in identifying people at risk, it may be that the proven clinical properties of statins imply that these are a better choice for reducing that risk.

A further weakness of the present analysis also derives from its 1992 index date, an inevitability in any study which derives its strength from a longer period of follow-up. At that time it was not usual to measure waist circumference or waist/hip ratio, two other factors normally regarded as core elements of the metabolic syndrome.[26] Nevertheless, body weight was predictive of CVD, and that the association of what is a fairly precise measurement is weaker than for systolic BP or serum triglycerides does suggest it might be predictive because of its association with another factor, of which abdominal adiposity might be expected to be closest.

Another association expected with body weight might be glycated hemoglobin. But in people with type 1 diabetes, inevitably treated with insulin, the association of body weight with blood glucose control is complex, if only because insulin insensitivity, as in people with type 2 diabetes, confers a degree of resistance to hypoglycemia, thereby allowing use of compensatory higher insulin dosage.

In the present study neither base line nor endpoint HbA_{1c} was predictive of macrovascular disease, consistent with the disparate finding in the literature. Thus, some authors have demonstrated an association between hyperglycemia and mortality[27,28] as well as CAD[28,29] in people with type 1 diabetes, while others are consistent with our findings that glycated hemoglobin is neither predictive of mortality nor macrovascular disease.[17,18,30–32] Furthermore, in the Pittsburgh Epidemiology of Diabetes Complications study, insulin resistance (measured by estimated glucose disposal rate) was found to be associated with CAD diagnosed by angiographic stenosis in the coronary arteries of $\geq$50%.[32] This should in no way diminish the importance of glycemic control in the management of type 1 diabetes following the publication of the results of the EDIC follow-up to the DCCT,[33] as it not only reduces microvascular complications but also lipid abnormalities linked to poor glycemic control. However,

TABLE 7. Cox proportional hazard for macrovascular disease in people with type 1 diabetes by quarters of the measured variables

	Unadjusted			Adjusted for age			Adjusted for HbA_{1c}			Adjusted for gender		
	Coefficient	*P*	OR	Coefficient	*P*	OR	Coefficient	*P*	OR	Coefficient	*P*	OR
Systolic BP (mmHg)												
≤118			1.00			1.00			1.00			1.00
119–130	1.306	0.040	3.69	1.095	0.087	2.99	1.333	0.037	3.80	1.230	0.055	3.42
131–142	1.781	0.005	5.94	1.333	0.042	3.79	1.726	0.008	5.62	1.702	0.009	5.48
≥143	2.439	0.000	11.46	1.651	0.010	5.21	2.432	0.000	11.38	2.405	0.000	11.08
Serum cholesterol (mmol/L)												
≤4.6			1.00			1.00			1.00			1.00
4.7–5.2	0.157	NS	1.17	−0.151	NS	0.86	0.152	NS	1.16	0.153	NS	1.17
5.3–6.0	0.125	NS	1.13	−0.423	NS	0.66	0.051	NS	1.05	0.056	NS	1.06
≥6.1	0.867	0.017	2.38	0.056	NS	1.06	0.899	0.013	2.46	0.875	0.017	2.40
Serum triglyceride (mmol/L)												
≤0.8			1.00			1.00			1.00			1.00
0.9–1.1	−0.395	NS	0.67	−0.305	NS	0.74	−0.406	NS	0.67	−0.402	NS	0.67
1.2–1.8	0.222	NS	1.25	0.048	NS	1.05	0.228	NS	1.26	0.210	NS	1.23
≥1.9	0.644	0.065	1.90	0.525	NS	1.69	0.650	0.063	1.92	0.585	NS	1.80

(*Continued*)

TABLE 7. Continued

	Unadjusted			Adjusted for age			Adjusted for HbA_{1c}			Adjusted for gender		
	Coefficient	*P*	OR	Coefficient	*P*	OR	Coefficient	*P*	OR	Coefficient	*P*	OR
Diastolic BP (mmHg)												
≤70			1.00			1.00			1.00			1.00
71–78	−0.116	NS	0.89	−0.155	NS	0.86	−0.031	NS	0.97	−0.036	NS	0.96
79–84	0.121	NS	1.13	−0.100	NS	0.90	0.124	NS	1.13	0.139	NS	1.15
≥85	0.742	0.021	2.10	0.592	0.070	1.81	0.781	0.017	2.18	0.823	0.013	2.28
Serum creatinine (μmol/L)												
≤76			1.00			1.00			1.00			1.00
77–85	−0.013	NS	0.98	−0.353	NS	0.70	0.199	NS	1.22	0.062	NS	1.06
86–97	0.295	NS	1.34	0.112	NS	1.12	0.504	NS	1.66	0.342	NS	1.41
≥98	0.607	NS	1.84	0.137	NS	1.15	0.828	0.050	2.29	0.614	NS	1.85
eGFR (mL/min/1.73 m^2)												
≥95.3			1.00			1.00			1.00			1.00
82.4–95.2	0.242	NS	1.27	−0.180	NS	0.84	0.218	NS	1.24	0.256	NS	1.29
71.2–82.3	0.706	NS	2.03	−0.019	NS	0.98	0.797	0.086	2.22	0.759	0.098	2.14
≤71.1	0.968	0.029	2.63	−0.106	NS	0.90	1.012	0.023	2.75	1.109	0.014	3.03

The *P* value is the comparison of the other quarters with the first index quarter.

TABLE 8. Cox proportional hazard for mortality in people with type 1 diabetes by quarters of the measured variables

	Unadjusted			Adjusted for age			Adjusted for HbA_{1c}			Adjusted for gender		
	Coefficient	*P*	OR	Coefficient	*P*	OR	Coefficient	*P*	OR	Coefficient	*P*	OR
Systolic BP (mmHg)												
≤118			1.00			1.00			1.00			1.00
119–130	0.284	NS	1.33	−0.171	NS	0.84	0.025	NS	1.03	−0.182	NS	0.83
131–142	0.790	NS	2.20	0.317	NS	1.37	0.809	NS	2.25	0.616	NS	1.85
≥143	1.469	0.023	4.34	0.600	NS	1.82	1.441	0.026	4.22	1.490	0.021	4.40
Serum cholesterol (mmol/L)												
≤4.6			1.00			1.00			1.00			1.00
4.7–5.2	0.618	NS	1.86	0.068	NS	1.07	0.527	NS	1.69	0.250	NS	1.28
5.3–6.0	0.514	NS	1.67	0.085	NS	1.09	0.624	NS	1.87	0.527	NS	1.69
≥6.1	0.996	NS	2.71	0.001	NS	1.00	1.052	NS	2.86	0.902	NS	2.46
Serum triglyceride (mmol/L)												
≤0.8			1.00			1.00			1.00			1.00
0.9–1.1	−12.361	NS	0.00	−12.396	NS	0.00	−12.414	NS	0.00	−12.359	NS	0.00
1.2–1.8	−0.286	NS	0.75	−0.361	NS	0.70	−0.176	NS	0.84	−0.235	NS	0.79
≥1.9	0.596	NS	1.82	0.482	NS	1.62	0.615	NS	1.85	0.530	NS	1.70

(Continued)

TABLE 8. Continued

	Unadjusted			Adjusted for age			Adjusted for HbA_{1c}			Adjusted for gender		
	Coefficient	*P*	OR	Coefficient	*P*	OR	Coefficient	*P*	OR	Coefficient	*P*	OR
Diastolic BP (mmHg)												
≤70			1.00			1.00			1.00			1.00
71–78	0.430	NS	1.54	−0.013	NS	0.99	0.235	NS	1.26	0.321	NS	1.38
79–84	0.058	NS	1.06	−0.074	NS	0.93	0.104	NS	1.11	0.025	NS	1.03
≥85	0.790	NS	2.20	0.515	NS	1.67	0.815	NS	2.25	0.937	NS	2.55
Serum creatinine (μmol/L)												
≤76			1.00			1.00			1.00			1.00
77–85	0.278	NS	1.32	0.343	NS	1.41	0.626	NS	1.87	0.708	NS	2.03
86–97	0.269	NS	1.31	0.442	NS	1.56	0.591	NS	1.81	0.877	NS	2.40
≥98	1.419	0.029	4.13	1.288	NS	3.63	1.719	0.027	5.60	1.820	0.026	6.17
eGFR (mL/min/1.73 m^2)												
≥95.3			1.00			1.00			1.00			1.00
82.4–95.2	1.111	NS	3.04	0.865	NS	2.37	1.097	NS	3.00	1.115	NS	3.05
71.2–82.3	1.823	0.091	6.19	1.398	NS	4.05	1.782	NS	5.94	1.856	0.086	6.40
≤71.1	2.222	0.035	9.23	1.500	NS	4.48	2.210	0.036	9.12	2.316	0.029	10.13

The *P* value is for comparison of the other quarters with the first index quarter.

it should direct us away from an essentially glucose-centered approach to one in which cardiovascular risk factors are addressed through lifestyle measures, optimized metabolic control, and pharmacotherapy if indicated in addition to the usual measures for glycemic control.[34]

During the 9-year follow-up of people with type 1 diabetes, 17% developed macrovascular complications, and development of albuminuria during the follow-up was an important predictor of macrovascular disease in the present study. Previous reports have shown the cumulative incidence of coronary heart disease to be six- to eightfold higher in people with type 1 diabetes who had nephropathy compared with people without nephropathy.[35,36] Jensen and colleagues[35] found that systolic and diastolic BP tended to be higher in people who developed nephropathy even prior to the onset of albuminuria, while as observed above, systolic BP was a good predictor in the current study from base line, suggesting that the latter variable is an earlier and initially more useful marker in people with type 1 diabetes. Interestingly, we found no suggestion of a difference in the presence of microalbuminuria at base line in people with and without macrovascular disease, and when people who developed macrovascular disease were stratified according to the base line microalbuminuria status, there was no difference in age, duration of diabetes, systolic BP, diastolic BP, glycated hemoglobin, serum cholesterol, and triglyceride. Two-thirds of the people who developed macrovascular disease did not have microalbuminuria at the base line visit.

Another factor that found to be predictive of macrovascular disease on univariate analysis was serum creatinine (TABLE 2), but its derivative, eGFR, performed even more strongly in both the univariate analysis, in predicting mortality (TABLE 3), and in the Cox model (TABLE 8), though not after adjustment for age. Nevertheless, it appears that the trend to raised risk of macrovascular disease begins at an eGFR reduction to as high as 70–80 mL/min/1.73 m^2, with more than a doubling of risk in the lower quarter ($\leq$71 mL/min/1.73 m^2) (TABLE 7). The explanation may be that this is identifying early renal arterial disease rather than diabetic nephropathy, but in any case this is an easily ascertained and monitored measure in clinical practice.

During the follow-up, 12% people died. On logistic regression, systolic BP, serum creatinine levels, and eGFR were risk factors for mortality, as well as the expected age. In the Cox proportional hazards model (TABLE 8), a systolic BP $\geq$ 143 mmHg was associated with a fourfold risk of mortality after adjusting for glycated hemoglobin and gender. Serum creatinine $\geq$98 μmol/L was associated with a three- to sixfold increased risk of mortality, and the derived eGFR in the lowest quarter was associated with a nine- to tenfold increased risk of mortality.

In contrast to previous reports that smoking is a strong predictor of CVD[32] and mortality,[30] smoking was not a risk factor in the present study. This might be due to the lower prevalence of smoking in our cohort (16%) compared with the other studies reporting a much higher prevalence of 55% and 32%, respectively, in people with and without CAD.[32] Indeed this finding highlights that our overall rate of development of macrovascular disease, and the risk of death, were low compared with previous figures, perhaps emphasizing the changes in care and health that had occurred by the time of collection of base line data in 1992.

In conclusion, identification of raised systolic BP and serum triglycerides, in the context of increasing age, developing nephropathy, and early worsening of renal function can be used to detect a risk of development of macrovascular disease over 9 years in people with type 1 diabetes.

ACKNOWLEDGMENTS

The authors wish to thank Dr. Tim J. Butler for advice. We also thank staff of the Newcastle Diabetes Centre for administrative assistance.

REFERENCES

1. CLARKE, P., A. GRAY, R. LEGOOD, *et al.* 2003. The impact of diabetes-related complications on healthcare costs: results from the United Kingdom prospective diabetes study (UKPDS Study No. 65). Diabet. Med. **20:** 442–450.
2. DORMAN, J.S., R.E. LAPORTE, L.H. KULLER, *et al.* 1984. The Pittsburgh insulin-dependent diabetes mellitus (IDDM) morbidity and mortality study. Mortality results. Diabetes **33:** 271–276.
3. KROLEWSKI, A.S., E.J. KOSINSKI, J.H. WARRAM, *et al.* 1987. Magnitude and determinants of coronary artery disease in juvenile-onset, insulin-dependent diabetes mellitus. Am. J. Cardiol. **59:** 750–755.
4. LAING, S.P., A.J. SWERDLOW, S.D. SLATER, *et al.* 1999. The British Diabetic Association cohort study 2: cause-specific mortality in patients with insulin-treated diabetes mellitus. Diabet. Med. **16:** 466–471.
5. LAING, S.P., A.J. SWERDLOW, S.D. SLATER, *et al.* 2003. Mortality from heart disease in a cohort of 23,000 patients with insulin-treated diabetes. Diabetologia **46:** 760–765.
6. PYORALA, K., M. LAAKSO & M. UUSITOPA. 1987. Diabetes and atherosclerosis: an epidemiologic view. Diabetes Metab. Rev. **3:** 463–524.
7. ROPER, N.A., R.W. BILOUS, W.F. KELLY, *et al.* 2001. Excess mortality in a population with diabetes and the impact of material deprivation: longitudinal, population based study. BMJ **322:** 1389–1393.
8. SWERDLOW, A.J. & M.E. JONES. 1996. Mortality during 25 years of follow-up of a cohort with diabetes. Int. J. Epidemiol. **25:** 1250–1261.
9. SOEDAMAH-MUTHU, S.S., J.H. FULLER, H.E. MULNIER, *et al.* 2006. High risk of cardiovascular disease in patients with type 1 diabetes in the U.K.: a cohort study using the general practice research database. Diabetes Care **29:** 798–804.
10. MATTOCK, M.B., N.J. MORRISH, G. VIBERTI, *et al.* 1992. Prospective study of microalbuminuria as predictor of mortality in NIDDM. Diabetes **41:** 736–741.
11. DAMSGAARD, E.M., A. FROLAND, O.D. JORGENSEN, *et al.* 1992. Eight to nine year mortality in known non-insulin dependent diabetics and controls. Kidney Int. **41:** 731–735.

12. Neil, A., M. Hawkins, M. Potok, *et al.* 1993. A prospective population-based study of microalbuminuria as a predictor of mortality in NIDDM. Diabetes Care **16:** 996–1003.
13. MacLeod, J.M., J. Lutale & S.M. Marshall. 1995. Albumin excretion and vascular deaths in NIDDM. Diabetologia **38:** 610–616.
14. Gall, M.A., K. Borch-Johnsen, P. Hougaard, *et al.* 1995. Albuminuria and poor glycemic control predict mortality in NIDDM. Diabetes **44:** 1303–1309.
15. Niskanen, L.K., I. Penttila, M. Parviainen, *et al.* 1996. Evolution, risk factors, and prognostic implications of albuminuria in NIDDM. Diabetes Care **19:** 486–493.
16. Borch-Johnsen, K., P.K. Andersen & T. Deckert. 1985. The effect of proteinuria on relative mortality in type 1 (insulin-dependent) diabetes mellitus. Diabetologia **28:** 590–596.
17. Deckert, T., H. Yokoyama, E. Mathiesen, *et al.* 1996. Cohort study of predictive value of urinary albumin excretion for atherosclerotic vascular disease in patients with insulin dependent diabetes. BMJ **312:** 871–874.
18. Rossing, P., P. Hougaard, K. Borch-Johnsen, *et al.* 1996. Predictors of mortality in insulin dependent diabetes: 10 year observational follow up study. BMJ **313:** 779–784.
19. Forrest, K.Y., D.J. Becker, L.H. Kuller, *et al.* 2000. Are predictors of coronary heart disease and lower-extremity arterial disease in type 1 diabetes the same? A prospective study. Atherosclerosis **148:** 159–169.
20. Fuller, J.H., L.K. Stevens & S.L. Wang. 2001. Risk factors for cardiovascular mortality and morbidity: the WHO mutinational study of vascular disease in diabetes. Diabetologia **44**(Suppl 2): S54–S64.
21. Forsblom, C.M., T. Sane, P.H. Groop, *et al.* 1998. Risk factors for mortality in type II (non-insulin-dependent) diabetes: evidence of a role for neuropathy and a protective effect of HLA-DR4. Diabetologia **41:** 1253–1262.
22. Levey, A., T. Greene, J. Kusek, *et al.* 2000. A simplified equation to predict glomerular filtration rate from serum creatinine [abstract]. J. Am. Soc. Nephrol. **11:** 155A.
23. Levey, A.S., J.P. Bosch, J.B. Lewis, *et al.* 1999. A more accurate method to estimate glomerular filtration rate from serum creatinine: a new prediction equation. Modification of diet in renal disease study group. Ann. Intern. Med. **130:** 461–470.
24. The National Collaborating Centre for Chronic Conditions. 2004. Type 1 diabetes in adults. London: Royal College of Physicians, 2004. Available at www.nice.nhs.uk (accessed July 2006).
25. Schwab, K.O., J. Doerfer, W. Hecker, *et al.* 2006. Spectrum and prevalence of atherogenic risk factors in 27,358 children, adolescents, and young adults with type 1 diabetes: cross-sectional data from the German diabetes documentation and quality management system (DPV). Diabetes Care **29:** 218–225.
26. The IDF Consensus Group. 2005. The IDF consensus worldwide definition of the metabolic syndrome. Brussels, International Diabetes Federation. Available at http://www.idf.org/webdata/docs/MetSyndrome_FINAL.pdf (accessed July 2006).
27. Moss, S.E., R. Klein, B.E. Klein, *et al.* 1994. The association of glycemia and cause-specific mortality in a diabetic population. Arch. Intern. Med. **154:** 2473–2479.

28. KLEIN, R. 1995. Hyperglycemia and microvascular and macrovascular disease in diabetes. Diabetes Care **18:** 258–268.
29. LEHTO, S., T. RONNEMAA, K. PYORALA, *et al.* 1999. Poor glycemic control predicts coronary heart disease events in patients with type 1 diabetes without nephropathy. Arterioscler. Thromb. Vasc. Biol. **19:** 1014–1019.
30. MUHLHAUSER, I., H. OVERMANN, R. BENDER, *et al.* 2000. Predictors of mortality and end-stage diabetic complications in patients with type 1 diabetes mellitus on intensified insulin therapy. Diabet Med. **17:** 727–734.
31. LLOYD, C.E., L.H. KULLER, D. ELLIS, *et al.* 1996. Coronary artery disease in IDDM. Gender differences in risk factors but not risk. Arterioscler. Thromb. Vasc. Biol. **16:** 720–726.
32. ORCHARD, T.J., J.C. OLSON, J.R. ERBEY, *et al.* 2003. Insulin resistance-related factors, but not glycemia, predict coronary artery disease in type 1 diabetes: 10-year follow-up data from the Pittsburgh epidemiology of diabetes complications study. Diabetes Care **26:** 1374–1379.
33. NATHAN, D.M., P.A. CLEARY, J.Y. BACKLUND, *et al.* 2005. Intensive diabetes treatment and cardiovascular disease in patients with type 1 diabetes. N. Engl. J. Med. **353:** 2643–2653.
34. SILVERSTEIN, J., G. KLINGENSMITH, K. COPELAND, *et al.* 2005. Care of children and adolescents with type 1 diabetes: a statement of the American Diabetes Association. Diabetes Care **28:** 186–212.
35. JENSEN, T., K. BORCH-JOHNSEN, A. KOFOED-ENEVOLDSEN, *et al.* 1987. Coronary heart disease in young type 1 (insulin-dependent) diabetic patients with and without diabetic nephropathy: incidence and risk factors. Diabetologia **30:** 144–148.
36. TUOMILEHTO, J., K. BORCH-JOHNSEN, A. MOLARIUS, *et al.* 1998. Incidence of cardiovascular disease in type 1 (insulin-dependent) diabetic subjects with and without diabetic nephropathy in Finland. Diabetologia **41:** 784–790.

Effects of Streptozotocin-Induced Diabetes on Contraction and Calcium Transport in Rat Ventricular Cardiomyocytes

NICHOLAS BRACKEN,[a] FRANK C. HOWARTH,[b] AND JAIPAUL SINGH[a]

[a]*Department of Biological Sciences, University of Central Lancashire, Preston, Lancashire, PR1 2HE UK*

[b]*Department of Physiology, F.M.H.S., United Arab Emirates University, Al-Ain, UAE*

ABSTRACT: Cardiovascular diseases are the major cause of morbidity and mortality in diabetic patients. Contractile function of the heart is frequently compromised in the clinical setting and in experimental models of diabetes mellitus (DM). This article investigated the effect of streptozotocin (STZ)-induced type 1 DM on contraction, L-type calcium (Ca^{2+}) current ($I_{Ca^{2+}L}$), and on cytosolic calcium concentrations $[Ca^{2+}]_i$ in ventricular myocytes of the rat heart. After 4–10 weeks of STZ treatment, blood glucose levels in diabetic animals were significantly ($P < 0.05$) higher compared to age-matched controls. Diabetic rats have significantly ($P < 0.05$) reduced body, reduced heart weight, and reduced viability of ventricular myocytes compared to controls. The amplitude of $I_{Ca^{2+}L}$ and amplitude of contraction were significantly reduced ($P < 0.05$) at test potentials in the range –10 mV to +20 mV and –30 mV to +40 mV, respectively, in myocytes from diabetic animals compared to age-matched controls. Moreover, there was a significant ($P < 0.05$) delay in electrically stimulated and caffeine-evoked time to half relaxation of the Ca^{2+} transient in myocytes from diabetic animals compared to controls. A similar effect was obtained in myocytes treated with a combination of caffeine and nickel chloride ($NiCl_2$). It is concluded that the diabetes-induced voltage-dependent decrease in contraction is associated with reduced Ca^{2+} channel activities and prolonged diastolic cytosolic Ca^{2+} compared to age-matched control. Taken together, the results suggest that Ca^{2+} homeostasis is deranged during DM and this may be expressed at the level of the Na^+/Ca^{2+} exchanger.

KEYWORDS: diabetes; streptozotocin; rat; heart; ventricular myocytes; calcium; contraction

Address for corresspondence: Prof. Jaipaul Singh, Department of Biological and Forensic Sciences, University of Central Lancashire, Preston, Lancashire, PR1 2HE UK. Voice: 0044-1772-893515; fax: 0044-1772-892929.
e-mail: jsingh3@uclan.ac.uk

Ann. N.Y. Acad. Sci. 1084: 208–222 (2006). © 2006 New York Academy of Sciences.
doi: 10.1196/annals.1372.018

INTRODUCTION

Contractile dysfunction is frequently reported in human patients and in experimental animals with diabetes mellitus (DM).[1–5] This metabolic disorder is now accepted as a major risk factor for cardiovascular disease rivaling cigarette smoking, stress, obesity, sedentary lifestyles, cholesterol disorders, and hypertension.[6] In the UK alone, over 33,000 people die annually from DM-induced cardiomyopathy, and it costs the National Health Service around £5–6 billion per year to treat and to care for diabetic patients.[7] With over 180 million people affected globally by DM,[8] most of whom may die from cardiovascular-related diseases, it is imperative that we understand the cellular and molecular mechanisms of DM-induced cardiomyopathy.

A variety of contractility defects have been frequently demonstrated in the STZ-induced DM rat heart including heart rhythm disturbances, prolonged time course of contraction and/or relaxation, and altered amplitude of contraction and altered electrical activity.[9–12] Defects in Ca^{2+} transport including I_{CaL}[13–16] and Na^{+}/Ca^{2+} changer,[17,18] reduce sarcoplasmic reticulum (SR) Ca^{2+} ATPase activity and Ca^{2+} regulatory proteins.[19–22] This article has investigated the effects of STZ-induced DM on the voltage dependence of contraction, the mechanisms of SR Ca^{2+} release, and Ca^{2+} transport regulatory proteins in rat heart.

METHODS

Experimental Model of Diabetes

DM was induced in male Wistar rats (200–250 g body weight) by a single intraperitoneal (i.p.) injection of streptozotocin (STZ) (60 mg kg^{-1} body weight) dissolved in a citrate acid buffer solution.[23] Age-matched control rats received an equivalent volume of citrate acid buffer solution alone. Control and STZ-treated animals were caged separately but housed under similar conditions. Both groups were fed the same diet and water *ad libitum* until they were used 4–10 weeks later. All experiments had ethical clearance from the Ethics Committees at the University of Central Lancashire and Faculty of Medicine and Health Sciences, United Arab Emirates University. Glucose was measured in whole blood with a glucose meter (One Touch II Glucometer; Lifescan Inc., London, UK) prior to administration of STZ, 3–5 days following administration of STZ to confirm a diabetic state and immediately prior to experiments.

Isolation of Ventricular Myocytes

Rats were humanely killed by a blow to the head followed by cervical dislocation in accordance with the Home Office Guidelines on the operation of

Animals (Schedule 1, Animals, Scientific Procedures Act, 1986). Ventricular myocytes were isolated with an isolation solution (see "Solutions") following collagenase (0.75 mg mL^{-1}; Sigma, Dorsett, UK) digestion of the heart, as previously described.[24–26] Cells were used during a period of 1–8 h after the isolation. Rod cell viability was measured (ratio of rod-shaped versus round-shaped cells) with a Neubauer hemocytometer within 1h after completion of the cell isolation.

Simultaneous Measurement of Ventricular Myocyte Contraction and L-Type Ca^{2+} Current

Voltage dependence of contraction was measured in patch-clamped ventricular myocytes in whole cell mode. Patch pipettes (PG1-5OT-10; Harvard, CT) were pulled (Model PP-83; Narishige, Tokyo, Japan) and fire polished (MF-79 microfuge; Narishige) to between 2 and 5 MΩ. Patch pipettes were filled with a cesium-based pipette solution (see "Solutions"). Patch-clamp recordings were made in whole cell, voltage-clamp mode using an EPC-7 patch amplifier and headstage (HEKA, Plymouth, UK). The "pipette to bath" junction potential was corrected before negative pressure was applied to cells, which were then subjected to a holding membrane potential (E_m) of –40 mV to inactivate the sodium current (I_{Na}) and T-type Ca^{2+} current ($I_{Ca,T}$).[27] Test pulses (400 ms duration) were applied at potentials between –30 mV and +50 mV in 10 mV increments. Membrane capacitance (compensated for differences in cell size using c-slow/c-fast with a slow range of 100 pF), series resistance (g-series compensation) (<15 MΩ), and capacitance compensation (30–40%) were corrected before recordings were taken. A train of four conditioning pulses were applied before each test pulse to standardize SR Ca^{2+} load.[28] $I_{Ca,L}$ was measured using WINWCP (version 3.2) electrophysiological software (John Dempster, Strathclyde University, Glasgow, UK) concurrently with contraction using a video-edge detection system. (VED-114; Crystal Biotech, Boston, MA). The amplitude of the $I_{Ca,L}$ was measured as the difference between the peak inward current at the start of the test pulse and the steady-state current at the end of the test pulse.[28–31]

Measurement of Ventricular Myocyte Intracellular Ca^{2+}

Ventricular myocytes were allowed to settle on the glass bottom of an inverted microscope (Nikon Diaphot-TMD, Tokyo, Japan). Myocytes were superfused (3–5 mL min^{-1}) with a normal tyrode (NT) solution (see "Solutions") containing 1 mM Ca^{2+} maintained at 35–37°C with a temperature controller (Medical Systems Corp, NY). Myocytes were field stimulated (S88 stimulator, Grass-Telfactor, West Warwick, RI) via two platinum electrodes located on either side of the chamber. Intracellular Ca^{2+} concentration ($[Ca^{2+}]_i$) was measured in fura-2-AM (F-1221; Molecular Probes, Zeeland, Netherlands) loaded cells using a fluorescence photometry system (Optoscan Monochrometer; Cairn Research, Kent, UK) according to previously described techniques.[24–26] In some experiments, a rapid application of 10 mM caffeine or caffeine plus 10 mM $NiCl_2$ (N-5756; Sigma) was applied to myocytes to characterize Ca^{2+} efflux on the Na^+/Ca^{2+} exchange. SIGNAL (version 1.82) software (Cambridge Electronic Design, Cambridge, UK) was used to acquire and analyze data.

Solutions

Isolation solution (in mM): 130, NaCl; 5.4, KCl; 1.4 $MgCl_2$; 0.4, NaH_2PO_4; 5, HEPES; 10, glucose; 20, taurine; 10, creatine, adjusted to pH 7.3 with 4M NaOH. This was supplemented by either EGTA or Ca^{2+} at different stages throughout the isolation procedure.[24–26] NT solution (in mM): 140, NaCl; 5, KCl; 1, $MgCl_2$; 10 HEPES, adjusted to pH 7.2 with 1 M CsoH. Patch-clamp electrode solution (in mM): 120, $CsCl_2$; 8, K_2ATP; 5, glucose; 10, NaCl; 8, $MgCl_2$; 10 HEPES, adjusted to pH 7.2 with CsOH.

Data Analysis and Statistics

All data are expressed as either mean ± standard error of the mean (SEM) of n observations. Statistical comparisons were made (SPSS, vs. 9 software; Chicago, IL) using either independent samples Student's t-test, paired t-test, or analysis of variance (ANOVA) followed by Bonferroni *post hoc* analysis as appropriate. P values of < 0.05 were considered significant, while P values of < 0.01 were considered highly significant.

RESULTS

General Characteristics of STZ-Induced Diabetic Rats and Ventricular Myocytes

The results show that diabetic rats have significantly less ($P < 0.05$) body (233.8 ± 7.2 g, $n = 6$) and heart (1.0 ± 0.03 g, $n = 5$) weights compared to age-matched control body (385.4 ± 12.5 g, $n = 5$) and heart (1.1 ± 0.05 g, $n = 5$) weights, respectively. In contrast, diabetic rats have significantly ($P < 0.01$) elevated blood glucose (407.5 ± 39.9 mg/dL, $n = 6$) compared to control (92.4 ± 2.42 mg/dL, $n = 6$). Viability (% rod cells) of ventricular myocytes was reduced significantly ($P < 0.05$) in cells from diabetic rat heart (25.3 ± 1.2 %, $n = 6$) compared to age-matched control hearts (49.4 ± 2.42 %, $n = 6$).

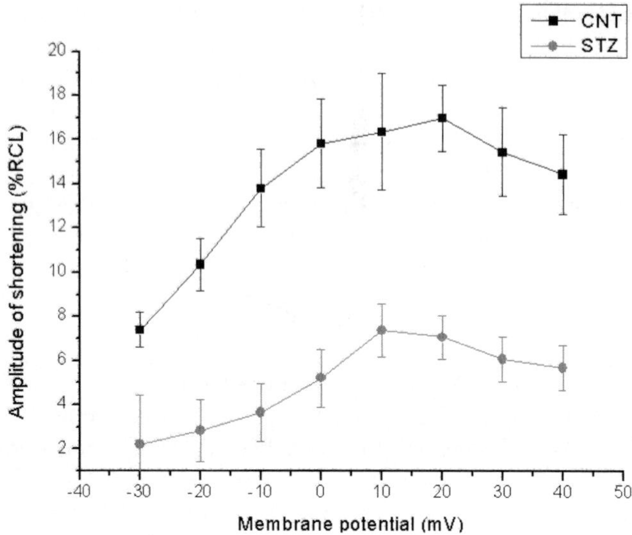

FIGURE 1. Mean voltage dependence of contraction, plotted as percentage of resting cell length for test potentials between –30 mV and +50 mV in control (CNT) and 8–12 weeks STZ-induced diabetic ventricular myocytes at room temperature. Data shown are mean ± SEM. Statistical significance was analyzed CNT ($n = 7$) versus STZ ($n = 7$) were compared using independent t-test.

Effects of STZ-Induced DM on Voltage Dependence of Contraction

The voltage dependence of contraction (amplitude of shortening expressed as a percentage of resting cell length) in ventricular myocytes from STZ-induced DM rats and controls at room temperature (22°C) is shown in FIGURE 1. The amplitude of contraction was measured at each test potential in the range –30 mV to +40 mV. The results show that contraction was significantly ($P <$ 0.05) greater in control myocytes compared to STZ-induced myocytes at all test potentials.

Effects of STZ-Induced Diabetes on L-Type Ca^{2+} Current–Voltage Relationship

FIGURE 2 A shows typical records of $I_{Ca,L}$ following a test pulse of 0 mV, from a holding potential of –40 mV in control and STZ-induced ventricular myocytes after 6–8 weeks of STZ treatment. The time to peak $I_{Ca,L}$ was 7.97 ± 0.97 ms, $n = 9$, and 9.25 ± 1.35 ms, $n = 9$ in myocytes from control and STZ-induced diabetic rat, respectively. These data are not significantly different from one another. However, the amplitude of $I_{Ca,L}$ was significantly ($P < 0.05$) reduced

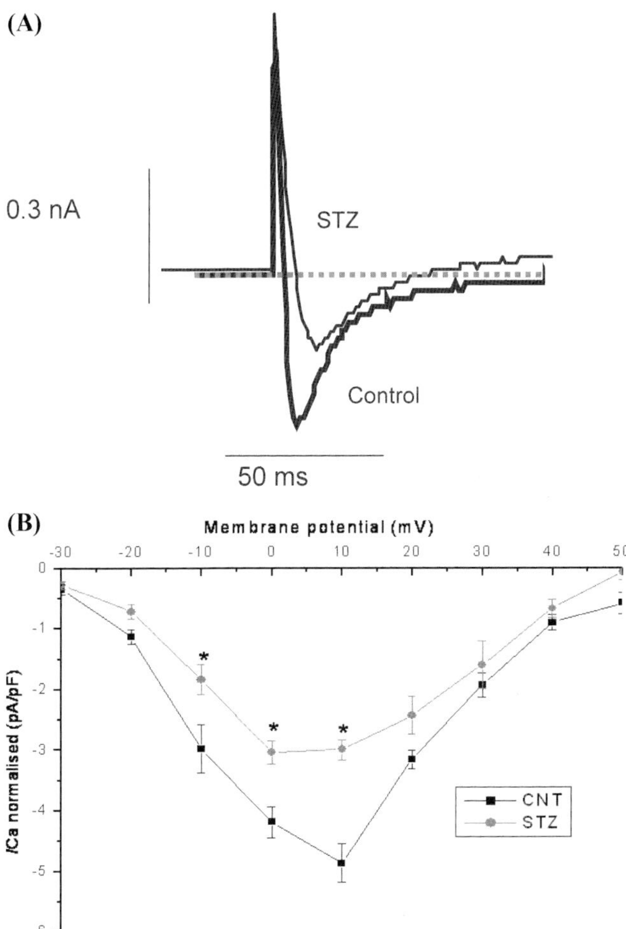

FIGURE 2. **(A)** Typical original chart traces of $I_{Ca,L}$ following test pulse of 0 mV from a holding potential of –40 mV in control and STZ-induced diabetic ventricular myocytes. Traces are typical of 8–10 different cells taken from 5–7 hearts. **(B)** Mean voltage dependence of $I_{Ca,L}$, plotted as current density (pA/pF) for test potentials between –30 mV and +50 mV between control (CNT) and STZ-induced diabetic ventricular myocytes at room temperature. Data shown are mean ± SEM. Statistical significance showing CNT ($n = 7$) versus STZ ($n = 7$) were compared using independent *t*-test. $^*P < 0.05$.

in diabetic myocytes compared to control. The current–voltage relationship in control and in ventricular myocytes from control and STZ-induced diabetic rat is shown in FIGURE 2 B, The results show that $I_{Ca,L}$ was significantly ($P <$ 0.05) reduced throughout the voltage ranges (–10 mV to +20 mV) in myocytes from STZ-induced diabetic rat compared to age-matched controls.

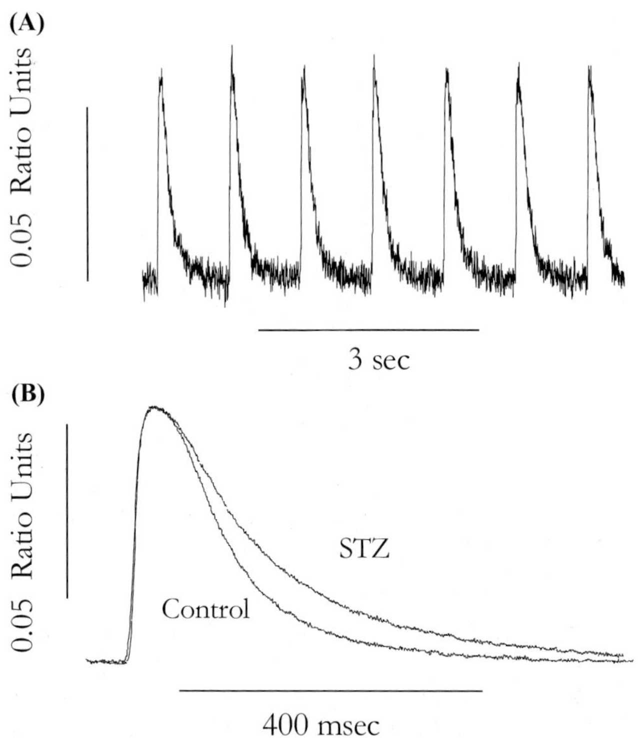

FIGURE 3. Fast-time base recordings of a train (**A**) and a single extrapolated Ca^{2+} transient (**B**) in electrically stimulated (1 Hz) ventricular myocytes isolated from age-matched control and STZ-induced diabetic rat hearts. Cells were superfused with an NT solution (1 mM Ca^{2+}) at 35–37 °C. Traces are typical of 7–10 such myocytes obtained from 3–5 hearts.

Effects of STZ-Induced DM on Intracellular Ca^{2+}

FIGURE 3 A shows typical fast-time base recordings of a train and FIGURE 3 B a typical Ca^{2+} transient after 4–8 weeks of STZ-treatment in electrically stimulated (1 Hz) ventricular myocytes. The fluorescence ratio (340/380), the indicator of intracellular Ca^{2+}, was significantly ($P < 0.01$) increased in STZ-induced diabetic myocytes following 4–6 weeks of treatment compared to control (0.738 ± 0.017 ratio units, $n = 10$ versus 0.472 ± 0.07 ratio units, $n = 10$), respectively. The amplitude and t_{pk} of Ca^{2+} transient were not significantly ($P < 0.05$) altered in myocytes from STZ-induced DM rats (98.6 ± 8.4 ms, $n = 7$) compared to controls (109.6 ± 7.5 ms, $n = 10$). However, the decay of the Ca^{2+} transient measured as the rate of ratio units/s was significantly ($P < 0.05$) longer in myocytes from STZ-induced diabetic rats (166.5 ± 12.9 ms, $n = 9$) compared to controls (91.8 ± 4.8 ms, $n = 9$).

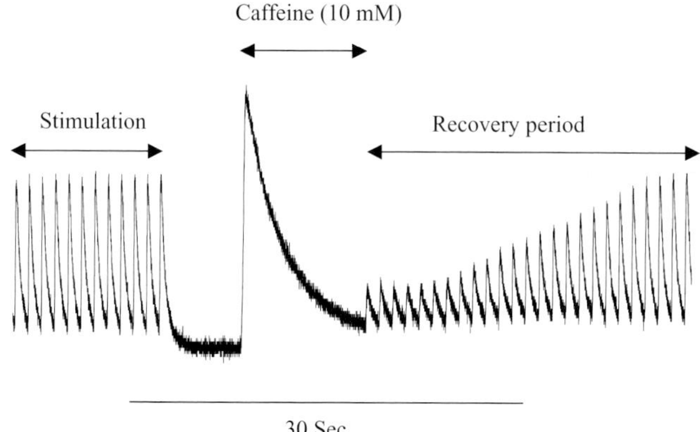

FIGURE 4. An original trace showing the time course protocol for caffeine-induced Ca^{2+} release and recovery in rat ventricular myocyte. Myocytes were stimulated and superfused with normal tyrode solution (1 mM Ca^{2+}) at 35–37°C. The trace is typical of 18 such myocytes from 6 hearts from either control or diabetic rats.

Effect of STZ-Induced Diabetes on SR Ca^{2+} Transport

FIGURE 4 shows an original chart recording of the effects of caffeine (10 mM) on SR Ca^{2+} transport. Myocytes were electrically stimulated at 1 Hz before stimulation was abbreviated and the myocytes were rapidly superfused with 10 mM caffeine. Following a 10 s application of caffeine, myocytes were restimulated and superfused with NT solution (1 mM Ca^{2+}) until Ca^{2+} transients reached precaffeine levels. The results are shown in TABLE 1. The amplitude of caffeine-induced Ca^{2+} release and fractional release were not significantly ($P > 0.05$) altered by STZ treatment. The t_{pk} of the Ca^{2+} transient was not significantly ($P > 0.05$) altered between control and STZ induced. However, the $t_{1/2}$ decay of the Ca^{2+} transient following the application of caffeine was

TABLE 1. The effects of 6–8 weeks STZ-induced diabetes on caffeine-induced Ca^{2+} release in isolated ventricular myocytes obtained from rat heart at 35–37 °C

	Age-matched control	STZ-induced (6–8 weeks)
Amplitude of Ca^{2+} release (% rise vs. basal)	25.7 1.9 (18)	25.9 2.2 (17)
Fractional Ca^{2+} release	89.7 41.8 (18)	83.5 8.8 (17)
t_{pk} of Ca^{2+} transient (ms)	250.3 50.1 (18)	330.1 48.2 (17)
Rate of Ca^{2+} decay (ratio units/s)	0.73 0.07 (18)	0.56 0.04 (17)*
t_{pk} Ca^{2+} decay (ms)	91.8 4.8 (18)	156.1 8.4 (17)*

Data are ± SEM. Number in parenthesis indicates number of cells. Controls vs. STZ were compared using Student's independent samples *t*-test. $^{*}P < 0.05$.

significantly ($P < 0.05$) longer and the rate of relaxation was significantly ($P < 0.05$) smaller in myocytes from STZ-induced DM rats compared to age-matched controls.

Effects of STZ-Induced Diabetes on Na^+/Ca^{2+} Exchange

The results have so far demonstrated that the rate of decay of the Ca^{2+} transient induced by either electrical stimulation or 10 mM caffeine is significantly slower in myocytes from diabetic rat compared to control. Explanations for this might include abnormal uptake of Ca^{2+} by the SR or extrusion of Ca^{2+} by the Na^+/Ca^{2+} exchange. The Na^+/Ca^{2+} is the major mechanism by which Ca^{2+} is extruded from the cell and the exchanger can be blocked by $NiCl_2$.[32,33] Therefore, the effect of $NiCl_2$ on caffeine-induced Ca^{2+} release was investigated in age-matched control and diabetic myocytes.

FIGURE 5 shows an original chart recording of the effects of $NiCl_2$ following caffeine-evoked SR Ca^{2+} release. Following the brief exposure to caffeine, electrical stimulation was stopped and $NiCl_2$ (10 mM) was applied to cells for 10 s. Caffeine (10 mM) was then rapidly applied to cells for 10 s, before normal tyrode solution was reapplied to the cells and cell restimulated (1 Hz) until precaffeine Ca^{2+} transients were restored. The results are summarized in TABLE 2.

In the presence of $NiCl_2$, the amplitude of Ca^{2+} release measured by the percentage change versus precaffeine pulse (clarify) was not significantly ($P >$ 0.05) altered by STZ treatment. Moreover, there was no significant ($P > 0.05$) difference in the amplitude of caffeine-induced Ca^{2+} release between the pre- and postapplication of $NiCl_2$ in control and STZ-induced myocytes. The t_{pk} of

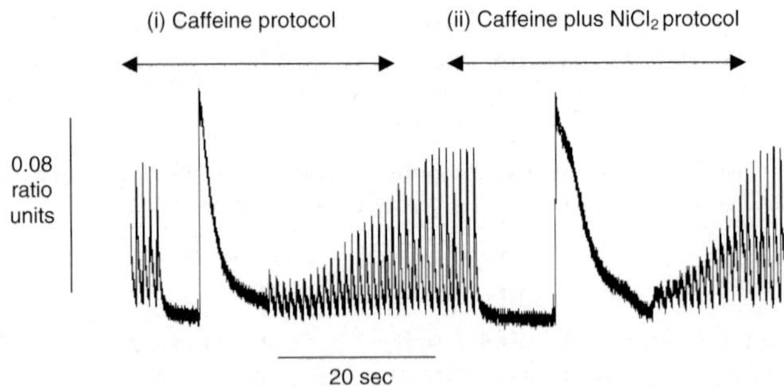

FIGURE 5. Original trace showing the time course protocol for (i) caffeine-induced Ca^{2+} release and for (ii) caffeine-induced Ca^{2+} release in the presence of $NiCl_2$ (10 mM) and recovery in age-matched control rat ventricular myocyte. Myocytes were stimulated and superfused with normal tyrode solution (1 mM Ca^{2+}) at 35–37°C. The trace is typical of 18 such myocytes from 6 rats.

TABLE 2. The effects of 8–12 weeks STZ-induced diabetes on caffeine-induced Ca^{2+} release in isolated ventricular myocytes obtained from rat heart at 35–37°C

	Age-matched control	STZ-induced (8 weeks)
Amplitude of Ca^{2+} release (% rise *vs.* basal)	25.7 ± 1.9 (18)	25.9 ± 2.2 (17)
Fractional Ca^{2+} release	89.7 ± 14.8 (18)	83.5 ± 8.8 (17)
t_{pk} of Ca^{2+} transient (ms)	250.3 ± 50.1 (18)	330.1 ± 48.2 (17)
Rate of Ca^{2+} decay (ratio units/s)	0.73 ± 0.07 (18)	0.56 ± 0.04 (17)*
$t_{1/2}$ Ca^{2+} decay (ms)	91.8 ± 4.8 (18)	156.1 ± 8.4 (17)*

Data are means ± SEM. Number in parenthesis indicates number of cells. Controls *vs.* STZ were compared using Student's independent samples *t*-test. $^*P < 0.05$.

the caffeine-induced Ca^{2+} release in the presence of $NiCl_2$ was significantly ($P < 0.05$) longer in myocytes from diabetic rat compared to control between pre- and postapplication of $NiCl_2$. The $t_{1/2}$ and rate of decay of the Ca^{2+} transient were not significantly ($P > 0.05$) altered by STZ treatment in the presence of $NiCl_2$ (TABLE 2). However, both control and STZ-induced myocytes had significantly ($P < 0.0$) longer decays in the rate of Ca^{2+} transient decline following application of $NiCl_2$.

DISCUSSION

The results of this study have shown that the STZ-induced diabetic rats were hyperglycemic and moreover, they have significantly reduced body and heart weights compared to age-matched control. In addition, the diabetic heart produced significantly less visible ventricular cardiomyocytes. These characteristics are typical of this model of DM.[16,24,34] One major long-term complication of diabetes is cardiomyopathy, in which the heart is unable to pump blood efficiently. This could be due to several factors including reduced contraction or derangement in cellular Ca^{2+} homeostasis or both.[17,18,23] In previous studies, we have shown that STZ-induced DM is not associated with reduced amplitude of contraction in electrically stimulated ventricular cardiomyocytes[34] at 1 Hz compared to age-matched control. Moreover, the time to peak contraction was significantly elevated in diabetic myocytes compared to control. These findings are in contrast to the results obtained by other workers.[17,18,35] These initial results prompted us to investigate the voltage dependency of contraction and $I_{Ca,L}$ during DM compared to control.

The results of this study have shown that STZ-induced diabetic myocytes displayed a significant reduction on the amplitude of contraction at all potentials tested compared to age-matched control myocytes. This interesting finding is in contrast to electrically stimulated myocytes in which both the force and the time to peak contraction were significantly elevated.[34] However, the present results clearly show that the process by which a voltage test causes the contraction is disrupted by the diabetic state. The reduction in contraction is most likely to be due to a decrease in the amount of Ca^{2+} entering the cell and release from the SR or a reduction in the myofilament sensitivity to Ca^{2+}. Concurrent with contraction, the results have also shown that diabetes caused a significant decrease in the amplitude of $I_{Ca,L}$ at all potential tested. This would therefore imply that a reduction of Ca^{2+} influx into the cell is decreased and this in turn results in a reduction of the amount of trigger Ca^{2+} and a subsequent decrease in SR Ca^{2+} release. These findings are consistent with other reports.[13,14]

Ca^{2+} homeostasis in the heart of STZ-induced diabetic rats is still not fully understood. This study not only measured the voltage dependence of contraction and $I_{Ca,L}$, but also changes in $[Ca^{2+}]_i$ and the mechanism of its release from the SR and its efflux from the cell. The results show that the amplitude of t_{pk} of Ca^{2+} transient was not significantly altered in 6–8 week STZ-induced diabetic myocytes compared to control. However, the basal $[Ca^{2+}]_i$ was significantly elevated in diabetic hearts compared to age-matched control. The increase in basal Ca^{2+} may be due to reduced sequestration of Ca^{2+} by the SR or reduced activity of the Na^+/Ca^{2+} exchange.[17,18] The present results have also shown that the rate of Ca^{2+} transient decay was also significantly slower in the diabetic hearts compared to control. Together, these results strongly indicate that diabetes is associated with elevated cytosolic Ca^{2+}.

The next logical approach was to investigate the mechanism of Ca^{2+} release and uptake by the SR. The amount of Ca^{2+} released by the SR is dependent on the SR Ca^{2+} content and the magnitude and duration of the trigger stimulus.[35] A rapid application of caffeine activates the SR RyR channels to open and initiate a total release of Ca^{2+} from the SR.[36] In this study, the amplitude of the caffeine-induced Ca^{2+} release was not significantly altered in control and diabetic myocytes. In contrast, it has been reported that, following a caffeine-evoked Ca^{2+} transient that amount of Ca^{2+} released from the SR is reduced in the diabetic heart.[18,37] The reported changes in caffeine-induced SR Ca^{2+} release may be attributable to the rest period preceding an application of caffeine. In this study, stimulation was abbreviated to 10 s, prior to a rapid caffeine pulse, but in other reports there were 30 s[18] and 40 s[38] quiescent phases. Longer rest periods may be associated with alterations in SR loading abilities and may contribute to a change in releasable SR Ca^{2+}. Increasingly Choi *et al.*[18] reported that the decrease in caffeine-induced Ca^{2+} release was mirrored by a decrease in the amplitude of contraction. In contrast, previous work undertaken by the authors has shown that the amplitude of contraction was significantly larger in the diabetic heart compared to age-matched controls.[33] It seems likely that alterations in Ca^{2+} release and myofilament sensitivity may contribute to changes in contractile dysfunction. Fractional Ca^{2+} release was not significantly different in STZ-induced diabetic myocytes compared to control. This suggests that the triggered response and release of Ca^{2+} from the SR is similar in the diabetic heart. It has been shown that the gain of CICR is dependent on the $I_{Ca,L}$ and subsequent influx of Ca^{2+} to trigger Ca^{2+} release from the SR. This study has shown that stimulated Ca^{2+} release and caffeine-induced Ca^{2+} release are similar, therefore any changes in $I_{Ca,L}$ may be indicative of changes in the gain in the diabetic heart. The t_{pk} of a Ca^{2+} transient following a rapid application of caffeine is an indication of RyR release sensitivity/activity. In this study, it has been reported that the t_{pk} of a caffeine-evoked Ca^{2+} transient was increased in the STZ-induced diabetic myocytes but not to a significant level. It has, however, been reported that the time course of the caffeine-induced Ca^{2+} transient decay was significantly prolonged in the diabetic myocytes. [18] Similarly, in this study it has also been shown that the $t_{1/2}$ decay of the caffeine-induced Ca^{2+} was significantly longer in the diabetic myocytes compared to control. This is in agreement with other workers who have also reported longer rates of Ca^{2+} transient decay in 8 weeks STZ-induced diabetic myocytes.[18]

In order to isolate the mechanism responsible for the delay in $[Ca^{2+}]_i$ efflux, following an application of caffeine, it is useful to use a pharmacological tool to block Ca^{2+} pathways. The main transport mechanisms involved in Ca^{2+} efflux are the Na^+/Ca^{2+}-exchanger and the PMCA pump. The Na^+/Ca^{2+}-exchanger accounts for between 68% and 87% of Ca^{2+}efflux, while the PMCA pump and mitochondria, collectively, accounts for between 13% and 32%.[32]

From the results, it can be seen that, in the presence of $NiCl_2$ the amplitude of Ca^{2+} released from the SR, in control myocytes following an application of caffeine was not significantly different than in STZ-induced myocytes. Therefore, it would seem that the total available amount of Ca^{2+} is similar in the normal and diabetic heart and that the Na^+/Ca^{2+}-exchanger does not contribute to changes in caffeine-induced Ca^{2+} release in ventricular myocytes. However, it has been reported that in the diabetic heart caffeine-induced Ca^{2+} release is significantly diminished.[18] In the presence of $NiCl_2$, the t_{pk} of the caffeine-induced Ca^{2+} transient is longer in both control and diabetic myocytes (compared to caffeine-induced Ca^{2+} release without $NiCl_2$) but is significantly increased in the STZ-induced myocyte compared to control. This would suggest that either $NiCl_2$ itself or the action of $NiCl_2$ on the Na^+/Ca^{2+}-exchanger changes the t_{pk} of the caffeine-induced Ca^{2+} release in STZ myocytes significantly more than control myocytes. Because the speed of Ca^{2+} release of the SR is indicative of RyR sensitivity, it is suggested that in the diabetic heart, the sensitivity of RyR release channels is altered though the action of $NiCl_2$ itself or through changes in $[Ca^{2+}]_i$ through the Na^+/Ca^{2+}-exchanger blockade. The rate of decay of the caffeine-induced Ca^{2+} transient is longer in diabetic myocytes versus control, but in the presence of $NiCl_2$, the rate of decay is not significantly altered. Because $NiCl_2$ blocks the Na^+/Ca^{2+}-exchanger, the rate of decay during caffeine-induced Ca^{2+} release in the presence of $NiCl_2$ is a rate of efflux from the PMCA and uptake into the mitochondria. Therefore, it is tempting to suggest that in this series of experiments, the sustained elevation in $[Ca^{2+}]_i$ following caffeine treatment is directly associated with the

Na^+/Ca^{2+}-exchanger, but not the changes PMCA Ca^{2+} efflux or mitochondrial Ca^{2+} uptake.

In conclusion, the results of this study have clearly shown that chronic diabetes is associated with concurrent decreases in voltage dependency of contraction and $I_{Ca^{2+}}$ and a delay in the decay of the Ca^{2+} transient. Together these results suggest that Ca^{2+} homeostasis is deranged during diabetes and this in turn may lead to a weak heart.

ACKNOWLEDGMENTS

The authors would like to thank the BHF for financial support, Roxy Afzal for typing the manuscript, and Ashley Matchett for technical assistance.

REFERENCES

1. KUMAR, P. & M. CLARK. 2002. Diabetes mellitus and other disorders of metabolism. *In* Clinical Medicine. P. Kumar & M. Clark, Eds.: 1069–1121. WB Saunders. London.
2. KANNEL, W.B. & D.L. MCGEE. 1979. Diabetes and cardiovascular disease. The Framingham Study. JAMA **241:** 2035–2039
3. MIETTENEN, H., S. LEHTO, V. SALOMAA, *et al.* 1998. Impact of diabetes on mortality after the first myocardial infarction. The FINMONICA Myocardial Infarction Register Study Group. Diabetes Care **21:** 69–75.
4. FALLOW, G.D. & J. SINGH. 2004. The prevalence, type and severity of cardiovascular disease in diabetic and non-diabetic patients: a matched-paired retrospective analysis using coronary angiography and the diagnostic tool. Mol. Cell. Biochem. **261:** 263–269.
5. GROSSMAN, E. & F.H. MESSERLI. 1996. Diabetic and hypertensive heart disease. Ann. Intern. Med. **125:** 304–310.
6. STANDL, E. & O. SCHNELL. 2000. A new look at the heart diabetes mellitus: from ailing to failing. Diabetologia **43:** 1455–1469.
7. CURRIE, C.J. 1997. NHS acute sector expenditure for diabetes: the present, future, and in excess in-patient cost of care. Diabetic Med. **14:** 686–692.
8. AMOS, A., D. MCCARTY & P. ZIMMET. 1997. The rising global burden of diabetes and its complications; estimates and projections to the year. Diabetic Med. **14:** S1–S85.
9. HOWARTH, F.C., M. JACOBSON, O. NASEER, *et al.* 2005. Short-term effects of streptozotocin-induced diabetes on the electrocardiogram, physical activity and body temperature. Exp. Physiol. 90: 237–245.
10. SHIMONI, Y., L. FIREK, D. SEVERSON & W. GIILES. 1994. Short-term diabetes alters K^+ currents in rat ventricular myocytes. Circ. Res. **74:** 620–628.
11. MAGYAR, J., Z. RUSZNAK, P. SZENTESI, *et al.* 1992. Action potentials and potassium currents in rat ventricular muscle during experimental diabetes. J. Mol. Cell. Cardiol. **24:** 841–853.

12. PACHER, P., Z. UNGVARI, P.P. NANASI, *et al.* 1999. Electrophysiological changes in rat ventricular and atrial myocardium at different stages of experimental diabetes. Acta Physiol. Scand. **166:** 7–13.
13. WANG, D.W., T. KIYOSUE, S. SHIGEMATSU, *et al.* 1995. Abnormalities of K^+ and Ca^{2+} currents in ventricular myocytes from rats with chronic diabetes. Am. J. Physiol. **269:** H1288–H1296.
14. CHATTOU, S., J. DIACONO & D. FEUVARY. 1993. Decrease in sodium-calcium exchange and calcium currents in diabetic rat ventricular myocytes. Acta Physiol. Scand. **166:** 137–144.
15. JOURDAN, P. & D. FEUVRAY. 1993. Calcium and potassium currents in ventricular myocytes isolated from diabetic rats. J. Physiol. **420:** 411–429.
16. BRACKEN, N.K., A.J. WOODALL, F.C. HOWARTH, *et al.* 2004. Voltage dependence of contraction in streptozotocin-induced diabetic myocytes. Mol. Cell. Biochem. **261:** 235–243.
17. HATTORI, Y., N. MATSUDA, J. KIMURA, *et al.* 2000. Diminished function and expression of the cardiac Na^+ -Ca^{2+} exchanger in diabetic rats: implication in Ca^{2+} overload. J. Physiol. **527:** 85–94.
18. CHOI, K.M., Y. ZHONG, B.D. HOIT, *et al.* 2002. Defective intracellular Ca^{2+} signalling contributes to cardiomyopathy in type 1 in diabetic rats. Am. J. Physiol. **283:** H1398–H1408.
19. GANGULY, P.K., G.N. PIERCE, K.S. DHALLA, *et al.* 1983. Defective sarcoplasmic reticular calcium transport in diabetic cardiomyopathy. Am. J. Physiol. **244:** E528–E535.
20. NETTICADAN, T., R.M. TEMSAH, A. KENT, *et al.* 2001. Depressed levels of Ca^{2+}-cycling proteins may underlie sarcoplasmic reticulum dysfunction in the diabetic heart. Diabetes **50:** 2133–2138.
21. MAKINO, N., K.S. DHALLA, V. ELIMBAN, *et al.* 1987. Sarcolemmal Ca^{2+} transport in streptozotocin-induced diabetic cardiomyopathy in rats. Am. J. Physiol. **253:** E202–E207.
22. HEYLIGER, C.E., A. PRAKASH & J.H. MCNEILL. 1987. Alterations in cardiac sarcolemmal Ca^{2+} pump activity during diabetes mellitus. Am. J. Physiol. **252:** H540–H544.
23. BRACKEN, N.K., J. SINGH, W. WINLOW, *et al.* 2003. Mechanism underlying contractile dysfunction in streptozotocin-induced type 1 and type 2 diabetic cardiomyopathy. *In* Athersclerosis, Hypertension and Diabetes. G.N. Pierce, M. Nagano, P. Zahradka & N.S. Dhalla, Eds.: 387–408. Kluwer Academic Publishers. Boston.
24. HOWARTH, F.C., M.A. QURESHI & E. WHITE. 2002. Effects of hyperosmotic shrinking on ventricular myocyte shortening and intracellular Ca^{2+} in streptozotocin-induced diabetic rats. Pflugers Arch. **444:** 446–451.
25. FRAMPTON, J.E., C.H. ORCHARD & M.R. BOYETT. 1991. Diastolic, systolic and sarcoplasmic reticulum $[Ca^{2+}]_i$ during inotropic interventions in isolated rat myocytes. J. Physiol. **437:** 351–375.
26. HOWARTH, F.C., S.C. CALAGHAN & M.R. BOYETT. 1999. Effect of the microtubule polymerizing agent taxol on contraction, Ca^{2+} transient and L-type Ca^{2+} current in rat ventricular myocytes. J. Physiol. **516:** 409–419.
27. BROWN, A.M., K.S. LEE & T. POWELL. 1981. Sodium current in single rat heart muscle cells. J. Physiol. **318:** 479–500.
28. HOWARTH, F.C. & A.J. LEVI. 1998. Internal free magnesium modulates the voltage dependence of contraction and Ca^{2+} transient in rabbit ventricular myocytes. Pflugers Arch. **435:** 687–698.

29. Vornanen, M., N. Shepherd & G. Isenberg. 1994. Tension-voltage relations of single myocytes reflect Ca release triggered by Na/Ca exchange at 35 degrees C but not 23 degrees C. Am. J. Physiol. **267:** C623–C632.
30. London, B. & J.W. Krueger. 1986. Contraction in voltage-clamped, internally perfused single heart cells. J. Gen. Physiol. **88:** 475–505.
31. Woodall, A.J., N. Bracken, A. Qureshi, *et al.* 2004. Halothane alters contractility and Ca^{2+} transport in ventricular myocytes from streptozotocin-induced diabetic rats. Mol. Cell. Biochem. **261:** 251–261.
32. Choi, H.S. & D.A. Eisner. 1999. The effects of inhibition of the sarcolemmal Ca-ATPase on systolic calcium fluxes and intracellular calcium concentration in rat ventricular myocytes. Pflugers Arch. **437:** 966–971.
33. Hobai, I.A., J.A. Bates, F.C. Howarth, *et al.* 1997. Inhibition by external Cd2+ of Na/Ca exchange and L-type Ca channel in rabbit ventricular myocytes. Am. J. Physiol. **272:** H2164–H2172.
34. Qureshi, M.A., N.K. Bracken, W. Winlow, *et al.* 2001. Time dependent effects of streptozotocin-induced diabetes on contraction in rat ventricular myocytes. Emirates J. **19:** 35–41.
35. Baartscheer, A., C.A. Schumacher & J.W. Fiolet. 2000. SR calcium depletion following reversal of the Na+/Ca^{2+}-exchanger in rat ventricular myocytes. J. Mol. Cell. Cardiol. **32:** 1035–1037.
36. O'Neil, S.C. & D.A. Eisner. 1990. A mechanism for the effects of caffeine on Ca^{2+} release during diastole and systole in isolated rat ventricular myocytes. J. Physiol. **430:** 519–536.
37. Yu, Y.Z., G.A. Quamme & J.H. Neill. 1995. Altered Ca^{2+}handling in diabetic cardiomyocytes: responses to caffeine, KCl, Quabain and ATP. Diabetes Res. Clin. Pract. **30:** 9–20.
38. Lagadic-Grossman, D. & D. Feuvray. 1991. Intracellular sodium activity in papillary muscle from diabetic rats. Exp. Physiol. **76:** 147–149.

Alterations in Atrial Natriuretic Peptide and Its Receptor Levels in Long-Term, Streptozotocin-Induced, Diabetes in Rats

ENYIOMA OBINECHE,[a] IRWIN CHANDRANATH,[b]
ERNEST ADEGHATE,[c] SHEELA BENEDICT,[a] MOHAMED FAHIM,[d]
AND ABDU ADEM[b]

[a]*Department of Medicine, Faculty of Medicine and Health Sciences, Al Ain, UAE*

[b]*Department of Pharmacology, Faculty of Medicine and Health Sciences, Al Ain, UAE*

[c]*Department of Anatomy, Faculty of Medicine and Health Sciences, Al Ain, UAE*

[d]*Department of Physiology, Faculty of Medicine and Health Sciences, Al Ain, UAE*

ABSTRACT: Diabetes mellitus (DM) shows a markedly increased incidence of cardiovascular pathology that leads to hypertension, endothelial macro- and microangiopathy, diabetic nephropathy, and myocardial infarction. Atrial natriuretic peptide (ANP), is a 28 amino acid peptide hormone synthesized mainly by the heart atria and ventricles. It has potent diuretic and natriuretic properties. In this article the effect of long-term DM on blood plasma, kidney, and heart atrial and ventricular ANP concentrations were evaluated in streptozotocin (STZ)-induced 8-month diabetic and control rats by using radioimmunoassay (RIA). Moreover, ANP receptors in STZ-induced, 8-month diabetic rat kidneys were studied by receptor autoradiography. In addition, the expression of ANP concentrations in the kidney of diabetic and control rats was evaluated by means of immunohistochemistry. Body weight loss and increased blood glucose levels were used as indices of DM in the STZ-induced diabetic rats. Our results showed significantly higher ANP concentrations in diabetic plasma ($P < 0.05$), kidney ($P < 0.01$), heart atria ($P < 0.05$), and ventricles ($P < 0.01$) compared to controls. We also demonstrated a significant decrease in ANP receptors in the outer cortex ($P < 0.05$), juxtaglomerular medulla ($P < 0.05$), and papilla ($P < 0.05$) of 8-month diabetic rat kidneys compared to controls. The observed increase in ANP levels in plasma and kidney could play a role in the development of diabetic nephropathy: probably by reducing the levels of ANP receptors in diabetic kidney. Furthermore, the role of ANP in the STZ-induced diabetic heart merits additional study.

Address for correspondence: Prof. Abdu Adem, Department of Pharmacology, Faculty of Medicine and Health Sciences, United Arab Emirates University, P.O. Box 17666, Al Ain, UAE. Voice: 00-9713-7137522; fax: 00-9713-7672033.
e-mail: abdu.adem@uaeu.ac.ae

Ann. N.Y. Acad. Sci. 1084: 223–234 (2006).
doi: 10.1196/annals.1372.025

KEYWORDS: atrial natriuretic peptide; rat; streptozotocin; kidney; heart; diabetes

INTRODUCTION

Atrial natriuretic peptide (ANP), a 28 amino acid peptide hormone, is mainly synthesized by the atrial and heart ventricles and is released in response to acute and chronic extracellular volume expansion. ANP facilitates the expression of water and sodium and has a vasodilator effect on the blood vessels.[1,2] The synthesis, storage, and release of ANP in the heart are intimately linked to changes in intravascular volume and blood pressure.[3] Diabetes mellitus (DM) may lead to abnormalities in fluid and electrolyte balance and consequently affect blood volume and blood pressure.[4] Diabetes also shows a markedly increased incidence of cardiovascular pathology that leads to hypertension, endothelial macro- and microangiopathy, renal failure, and myocardial dysfunction.[5] Alterations in renin-angiotensin-aldosterone system and arginine vasopressin (AVP) secretion, the two well-known mechanisms for controlling extracellular volume homeostasis, have been observed both in humans with DM and in rats treated with alloxan.[6] ANP also plays an important role in body fluid and electrolyte balance and in regulating blood pressure.[1,2] Plasma ANP concentrations have been reported to be either increased[6] or normal[7] in type 1 diabetic patients compared with normal subjects. The concentrations in chronic streptozotocin (STZ)-diabetic rats have also been shown to increase[8–11] though unaltered plasma ANP concentrations have been reported.[12,13] It is still not clear whether the increase in plasma concentration is due to increase in cardiac ANP secretion. Plasma ANP is of prognostic value in congestive heart failure (CHF) and reflects the effective control of volemia in renal failure so that its assay as well as that of plasma guanosine 3′, 5′-cyclic monophosphate (cyclic GMP) is of interest in these diseases. The early course of diabetic renal disease is characterized by distinct alterations in the glomerular filtration rate (GFR), which is often increased, and in many patients the amount of albumin excreted in urine is also increased.[14,15] Such an increase in protein excretion is suggestive of structural glomerular abnormalities and is usually followed by progressive derangement of glomerular barrier function, ultimately leading to end-stage renal failure.

ANP belong to a family consisting of at least three endogenous peptides: ANP; brain natriuretic peptide (BNP); and C-type natriuretic peptide (C-type NP).[16] Most ANP actions are mediated by attachment to a specific receptor on the cell membrane. Three distinct receptors have been identified.[17] Two of these contain guanylate cyclase on the intracellular domain (ANP-A and ANP-B receptor) but one receptor lacks guanylate cyclase and participates in the clearance of natriuretic peptides from the extracellular environment (ANP-C receptor).[17] This study, therefore, was designed to investigate the role of ANP in the pathogenesis of diabetic renal disease in long-term (8-month) diabetic rats. We evaluated the ANP levels in blood plasma, heart atrial and ventricular muscles in these diabetic rats compared to controls using radioimmunoassay (RIA). We also investigated the effect of STZ-induced diabetes on the distribution of ANP receptors in the kidneys in comparison to controls.

MATERIALS AND METHODS

Chemicals

The following drugs were used: ANP (Sigma, St. Louis, MO), STZ (Sigma), Na_2 EDTA (Sigma), trifluoroacetic acid, acetonitrile, biotynylated anti-rabbit IgG, streptavidin peroxidase conjugate, 3,3-diaminobenzidine tetrahydrochloride, RIA Kit (Peninsula Laboratories, Belmont, CA), and $[^{125}I]$-ANP (Amersham Pharmacia, Buckinghamshire, UK).

Animals

Wistar rats weighing between 220 and 250 g had diabetes induced (n = 10) by a single intraperitoneal injection of STZ (60 mg/kg body weight) dissolved in citrate buffer (pH 4.5). Age-matched control rats (n = 10) received an equivalent volume of citrate buffer alone. Diabetes was confirmed on the third day by checking fasting blood sugar level using a glucometer (One touch II glucometer; Life Scan Inc., Milpitas, CA). The animals were kept in separate cages in the animal house under 12 h light–12 h dark cycle, where the temperature was maintained at 22 ± 2°C and food and water were given *ad libitum* until the day of the experiment. The rats were weighed and then killed by decapitation 8 months after the induction of diabetes. Trunk blood was collected in disodium EDTA tubes, and the kidneys removed and weighed. Both normal and diabetic kidneys were preserved in Zamboni's fixative for light microscopic, morphological, and immunohistochemical studies or frozen in isopentane kept in liquid nitrogen for autoradiographic studies.

Measurement of Plasma, Heart, and Kidney ANP Levels by RIA

Blood samples were collected in disodium EDTA vacutainers with added aprotinin (500 KIU/mL of blood) and centrifuged at 1600 *g* for 15 min at 4°C. Plasma samples were stored at –80°C until assayed for ANP. Kidney and heart tissues (auricles and ventricles separately) were homogenized on ice using the Ultra turrax in 2 mL PBS. The homogenates were centrifuged at 20,000 *g* and supernatants stored at –80°C. Concentrations of ANP were determined in plasma and tissue supernatants after extraction on a Sep-Pak C18 column [(length: 300 mm, ID: 3.9 cm, 5 micron) Supelco, Bellefonte,

PA] pre-equilibrated with 1% trifluoroacetic acid. After elution with 60% acetonitrile in 1% trifluoroacetic acid and evaporation to dryness, the residue was reconstituted in assay buffer and measured for ANP immunoreactivity with a specific RIA Kit (Peninsula Laboratories). Protein levels were measured using the Bradford dye-binding procedure.[18] ANP levels in tissues were expressed in pg/mg protein.

Immunohistochemistry

Rat kidneys were trimmed free of adherent fat and connective tissue and cut into small pieces (2 mm^3) and fixed overnight in freshly prepared Zamboni's fixative. The specimens were later dehydrated in graded concentrations of ethanol, cleared in xylene, and embedded in paraffin wax. Sections of 6 μm thickness were cut and deparaffinized in xylene. The sections were then incubated for 30 min in 0.3% hydrogen peroxide solution in methanol to block endogenous peroxidase activity. The sections were washed three times (5 min each) in Tris-buffered saline (TBS) and incubated in the blocking reagent for 30 min. The samples were later incubated with polyclonal antibodies against ANP (1:1000 dilutions) for 24 h at 4°C followed by 30-min incubation in prediluted biotinylated anti-rabbit IgG. After washing in TBS, the specimens were incubated in streptavidin peroxidase conjugate for 45 min and treated with 3,3-diaminobenzidine tetra-hydrochloride to reveal sites of immunoreactivity. The slides were counter-stained with hematoxylin for 30 s, dehydrated in ascending grades of ethanol, cleared in xylene, and mounted in Cytoseal 60 (Stephens Scientific, Riverdale, NJ).

Receptor Autoradiography

Cryostatic sections of frozen kidneys from control and diabetic rats were mounted on glass slides coated with 2% 3 aminopropyl-3-ethoxysilane in acetone. The slides were preincubated at 4°C in 50 mM Tris-HCl buffer (pH = 7.4) for 10 min. The sections were then incubated with 40 pM [^{125}I]-ANP ([^{125}I]-ANP, Specific activity 2000 Ci/mmol, Amersham Pharmacia) in Tris-HCl buffer for 1 h at 4°C. Some sections were incubated with the ligand in the presence of unlabelled ANP (10^{-6}M). Later, the sections were rinsed first in 50 mM Tris-HCl buffer for 15 min, and then dipped in cold distilled water to remove the buffer salts. The sections were dried in cold dry air. The dried sections were mounted on film cassettes and ^{3}H-Ultra films (Amersham Pharmacia) were placed against the sections along with calibrated radioactive standards (iodine microscales, Amersham Pharmacia) and incubated in –20°C for 3 days. The microscales were exposed to the same film to permit conversion of the mean gray densities to molar concentrations of receptor bound ligand. The film was developed at room temperature and the areas of the medulla and cortex of the kidneys were quantified by computerized densitometry (Bio-Rad Molecular Imager System, GS-525; Hercules, CA). The readings were further converted to actual radioactivity (nCi/mg kidney tissue) using the calibrated radioactive standards. Specific binding was calculated after subtracting nonspecific binding from total binding and expressed as femto moles/mg wet weight.

Statistical Analysis

All data were expressed as means ± standard error of the mean (SEM). Data were analyzed using one-way ANOVA and P values < 0.05 were considered statistically significant.

RESULTS

Plasma ANP Levels

The body weights of 8-month diabetic animals were significantly ($P < 0.001$) lower than control animals [391.5 ± 5.69 g ($n = 9$) versus 179.33 ± 9.70 g ($n = 6$)] (FIG. 1).

The blood glucose levels for control and diabetic rats were 97.20 ± 2.60 mg/dL ($n = 6$) and 347.88 ± 24.72 mg/dL ($n = 16$), respectively, which are significantly ($P < 0.001$) different. In contrast to body weight, the mean

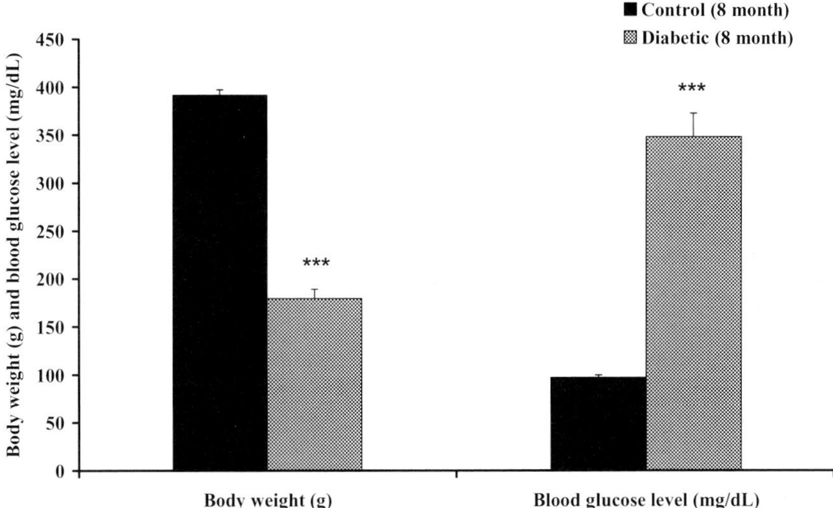

FIGURE 1. Histograms showing body weight and blood glucose of STZ induced 8-month diabetic rats compared to age-matched controls. Diabetic rats showed significant (***$P < 0.001$) difference from their respective controls. Data are expressed as mean ± SEM.

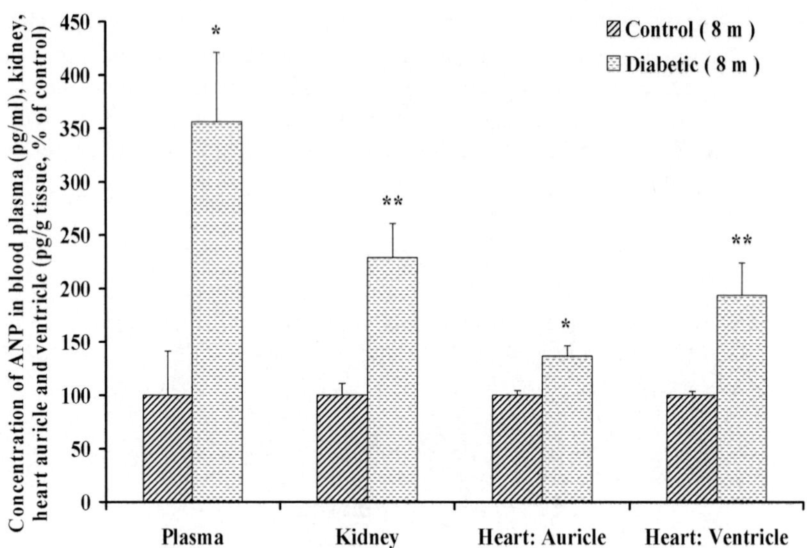

FIGURE 2. ANP levels in plasma, kidney, heart auricle, and ventricle of STZ-induced 8-month diabetic rats compared to age-matched controls. Diabetic rats show significantly higher levels of ANP ($^{*}P < 0.05$, $^{**}P < 0.01$) than their respective controls. Data are expressed as mean ± SEM.

kidney weight per 100 g body weight was significantly ($P < 0.001$) lower [0.67 ± 0.03 g ($n = 8$)] in control versus diabetic rats [0.93 ± 0.07 g ($n = 6$), data not shown]. The ANP levels in plasma, kidney, heart auricle, and heart ventricle from diabetic rats were significantly higher ($P < 0.05$) compared to controls (FIG. 2).

Immunohistochemistry

FIGURE 3 shows the immunohistochemical localization of ANP in control and diabetic kidney sections. ANP-immunoreactive cells were observed in the cortex of the kidneys of both normal and diabetic rats. These ANP-immunopositive cells were observed among the cells lining the proximal convoluted tubules (PCT). There was a significant increase in the number of ANP-positive cells in the PCT of diabetic rats compared to age- and sex-matched controls.

Receptor Autoradiography

The number of ANP receptors in different areas of the kidneys was quantified. Significantly fewer ANP receptors were found in the outer cortex ($P < 0.05$), juxtaglomerular medulla ($P < 0.05$), and the papilla ($P < 0.05$) in diabetic rats compared to controls (FIG. 4).

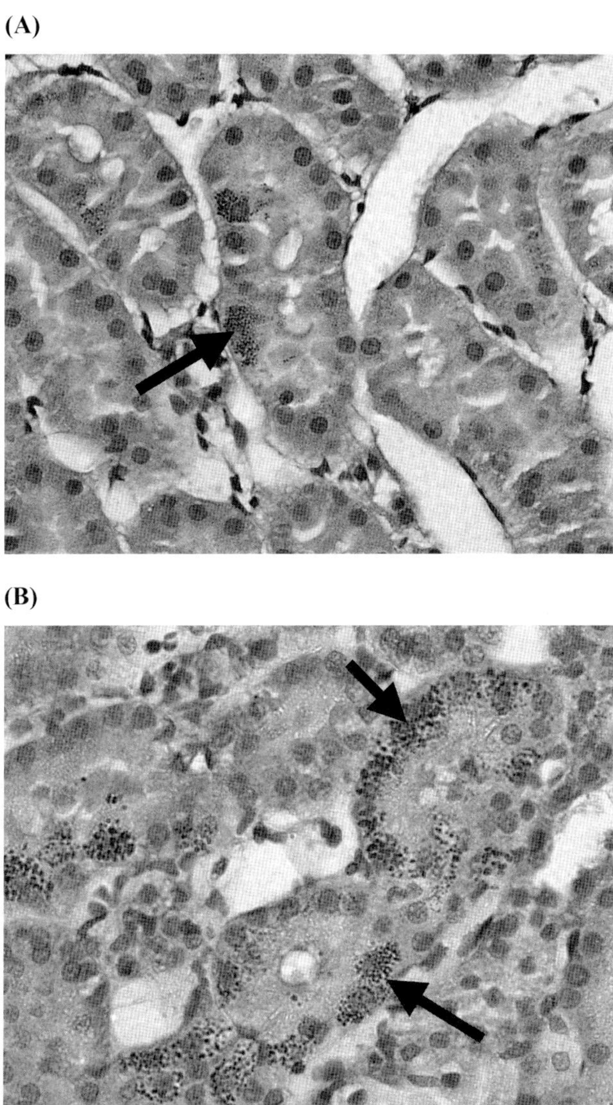

FIGURE 3. Immunohistochemical localization of ANP on (**A**) control and (**B**) diabetic rat kidney sections. Note the increase in number of ANP-positive cells (*arrow*) in the PCT of diabetic rats compared to controls. ×400.

DISCUSSION

The levels of ANP in plasma, kidney, and cardiac muscle as well as ANP receptor density in the kidneys of long-term (8 months) STZ-induced diabetic and control rats using receptor autoradiography were studied. Moreover,

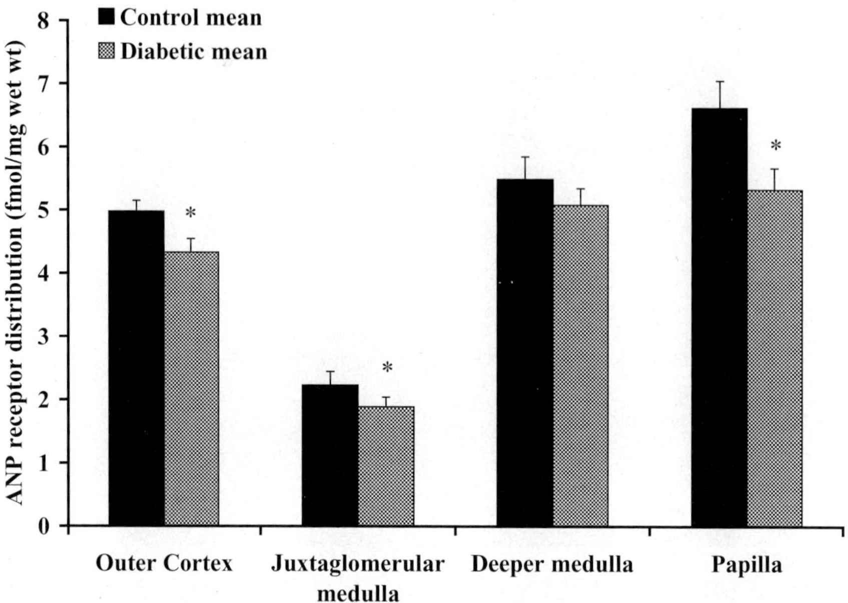

FIGURE 4. Histogram showing ANP receptor levels (femto mol/mg wet wt of tissue) in different areas of 8-month diabetic and age-matched control kidneys. Diabetic rats show significant ($^*P < 0.05$) decrease in ANP receptor density in different areas of the kidney. Data are expressed as mean ± SEM. Asterisks indicate significant difference compared to control values.

expression of ANP in the kidneys of diabetic and control rats was evaluated using immunohistochemistry.

Our results showed significantly elevated mean plasma glucose levels and also significantly reduced mean body weight but increased kidney weight in 8-month diabetic versus control rats. These findings were similar to previous studies.[8–10] The generalized muscle wasting and increased GFR previously described[19] in the diabetic rats could account in part, for the observed increase in kidney weights.

DM results in fluid and electrolyte imbalance, which in turn affects blood volume.[10] Our results have shown that ANP concentration in blood plasma was significantly increased in STZ-treated rats. These findings are in line with previous studies, which showed increases in ANP concentrations after different periods of STZ treatment ranging from 1 week to 8 months.[10–13,20–24] Plasma ANP concentrations have been shown to rise with acute hyperglycemia in human type 1 and type 2 diabetes.[7,25] We also showed that the concentrations of ANP in atrial and ventricular muscles after STZ treatment were significantly increased compared to controls, which is in line with results from other works.[26]

Significant high levels of kidney ANP were observed in STZ-treated rats compared to controls. Our immunohistochemical results indicate localization of ANP in the cells of the PCT in the renal cortex of both control and diabetic rats. However, a significant increase in ANP-positive cells was observed in the diabetic rats compared to controls. It remains to be determined what stimulates the increase in immunoreactive ANP in the proximal tubules of the diabetic rats and whether this abnormality contributes to the numerous functional and renal changes associated with DM. It is, however, tempting to suggest that their location in this section of the nephron enables them to play a direct role in sodium exchange. PCTs are more involved in the reabsorption of sodium ions compared to other parts of the nephron. This increase in the number of ANP-positive cells in the PCT of diabetic rats may also contribute to the high plasma levels of ANP.[27]

Receptor autoradiography demonstrated that the number of ANP receptors in the kidneys of 8-month diabetic rats was significantly reduced compared to controls. This was especially evident in the areas of the outer cortex, juxtaglomerular medulla, and the regions of the renal papilla. These findings are in line with earlier reports indicating significant enhancement of ANP mRNA and ANP immunoreactive staining in the proximal tubules, medullary thick ascending limbs, medullary collecting ducts, and renal cortex.[24,28] Circulating levels of peptide hormones regulate target tissue receptor numbers,[29] hence it could be argued that high plasma and kidney levels of ANP could contribute to the downregulation of ANP receptors in diabetic kidneys, this in turn may lead to a reduction in the natriuretic response to ANP reported by some workers.[30]

Elevated circulating and renal ANP levels might also contribute to other functional abnormalities, such as (early) rise in GFR, proteinuria, and suppression of renal release in the diabetic kidney.[30] It has also been reported that diabetic rat kidney cells showed biochemical features characteristic of classical apoptosis, such as processing and activation of caspase-3, cytochrome C release, poly (ADP-ribose) polymerase cleavage, and DNA fragmentation as early as 1 month following induction of diabetes.[31] Hence apoptotic mechanisms taking place in the kidney may partly explain the reduction in ANP receptors observed in this study.

The definitive function of ANP in the causation of diabetic renal disease in the long-term diabetic rat is not yet fully understood. It is speculated that abnormalities in fluid homeostasis and alterations in ANP binding and action due to decreased number of biologically active ANP receptors could be contributory to the damage observed in the kidneys of long-term diabetic rats.

In conclusion, our results show significant increases in ANP levels in blood plasma, kidney, heart atrial and ventricular muscles of 8-month diabetic rats compared to age-matched controls. We also found a significantly decreased number of biologically active ANP receptors in these kidneys compared to controls. The observed increase in ANP levels in plasma and kidney could be contributory to the development of diabetic nephropathy: probably by reducing the levels of ANP receptors in the diabetic kidney. Further studies could provide important information on the development and treatment of diabetic renal disease.

ACKNOWLEDGMENTS

This research was supported by a grant from the Faculty of Medicine and Health Sciences and Individual grant from the United Arab Emirates University.

REFERENCES

1. ANAND-SRIVASTAVA, M.B. & G.J. TRACHTE. 1993. Atrial natriuretic factor receptors and signal transduction mechanisms. Pharmacol. Rev. **45:** 455–497.
2. ESPINER, E.A., A.M. RICHARDS, T.G. YANDLE & M.G. NICHOLLS. 1995. Natriuretic hormones. Endocrinol. Metab. Clin. North Am. **24:** 481-509.
3. RUSKOAHO, H. 1992. Atrial natriuretic peptide: synthesis, release, and metabolism. Pharmacol. Rev. **44:** 479–602.
4. WALTHER, T., S. HERINGER-WALTHER, R. TSCHOPE, *et al.* 2000. Opposite regulation of brain and C-type natriuretic peptides in the streptozotocin-diabetic cardiopathy. J. Mol. Endocrinol. **24:** 391–395.
5. LITWIN, S.E., T.E. RAYA, P.G. ANDERSON, *et al.* 1990. Abnormal cardiac function in the streptozotocin-diabetic rat. Changes in active and passive properties of the left ventricle. J. Clin. Invest. **86:** 481–488.
6. CHRISTLIEB, A.R., R. LONG & R.H. UNDERWOOD. 1979. Renin-angiotensin-aldosterone system, electrolyte homeostasis and blood pressure in alloxan diabetes. Am. J. Med. Sci. **277:** 295–303.
7. SMOYER, W.E., B.H. BROUHARD, S.W. PONDER, *et al.* 1990. Plasma atrial natriuretic peptide concentrations in children with insulin-dependent diabetes mellitus. J. Pediatr. **116:** 108-111.
8. JIN, Y., J.X. WU, M. HONG, *et al.*1991. The effects of streptozotocin induced diabetes mellitus and fish oil compound on gene expression of atrial natriuretic peptide in rat. Comp. Biochem. Physiol. A. **100:** 221–225.
9. ORTOLA, F.V., B.J. BALLERMANN, S. ANDERSON, *et al.* 1987. Elevated plasma atrial natriuretic peptide levels in diabetic rats. Potential mediator of hyperfiltration. J. Clin. Invest. **80:** 670–674.
10. CHOI, K.C., H.C. PARK & J. LEE. 1994. Attenuated release of atrial natriuretic peptide and vasorelaxation in streptozotocin-induced diabetic rats. J. Korean Med. Sci. **9:** 101–116.
11. TODD, M.E., R.A. HEBDEN, B. GOWEN, *et al.*1990. Atrial structure and plasma ANF levels in rats with chronic diabetes mellitus. Diabetes **39:** 483–489.
12. HEBDEN, R.A. & J.H. MCNEILL. 1988. Concentration(s) of atrial natriuretic hormone in the plasma of rats with streptozotocin-induced diabetes mellitus. Life Sci. **42:** 1789–1795.
13. JACKSON, B., L. FRANZE, T.J. ALLEN, *et al.*1988. Effect of glycaemic control on glomerular filtration rate in the streptozotocin diabetic rat. Clin. Exp. Pharmacol. Physiol. **15:** 361–365.

14. McKENNA, K., D. SMITH, W. TORMEY & C.J. THOMPSON. 2000. Acute hyperglycaemia causes elevation in plasma atrial natriuretic peptide concentrations in type 1 diabetes mellitus. Diabet. Med. **17:** 512–517.
15. CLART, B.A., A. SCLATER, F.H. EPSTEIN & D. ELAHI. 1993. Effect of glucose, insulin and hypertonicity on arrial natriuretic peptide levels in man. Metabolism **42:** 224–228.
16. HUNT, P.J., T.G. YANDLE, M.G. NICHOLLS, *et al.* 1995. The amino-terminal portion of pro-brain natriuretic peptide (Pro-BNP) circulates in human plasma. Bioch. Biophys. Res. Comm. **214:** 1175–1183.
17. NAKAO, K., Y. OGAWA, S. SUGA & H. IMURA. 1992. Molecular biology and biochemistry of the natriuretic peptide system II: Natriuretic peptide receptors. J. Hypertens. **10:** 1111–1114.
18. BRADFORD, M.M. 1976. A rapid and sensitive method for the quantitation of microgram quantities of protein utilizing the principle of protein-dye binding. Anal. Biochem. **72:** 248–254.
19. ALLEN, T.J., M.E. COOPER, R.C. O'BRIEN, *et al.* 1990. Glomerular filtration rate in streptozocin-induced diabetic rats. Role of exchangeable sodium, vasoactive hormones, and insulin therapy. Diabetes **39:** 1182–1190.
20. SHIN, S.J., Y.J. LEE, M.S. TAN, *et al.* 1997. Increased atrial natriuretic peptide mRNA expression in the kidney of diabetic rats. Kidney Int. **51:** 1100–1105.
21. OBINECHE, E.N., E. ADEGHATE, I.S. CHANDRANATH, *et al.* 2004. Alterations in atrial natriuretic peptide and its receptors in streptozotocin-induced diabetic rat kidneys. Mol. Cell. Biochem. **261:** 3–8.
22. SAHAI, A. & P.K. GANGULY. 1991. Congestive heart failure in diabetes with hypertension may be due to uncoupling of the atrial natriuretic peptide receptor-effector system in the kidney basolateral membrane. Am. Heart J. **122**(1 Pt 1): 164–170.
23. SAHAI, A. & P.K. GANGULY. 1993. Observations on atrial natriuretic peptide, sympathetic activity and renal Ca2+ pump in diabetic and hypertensive rats. Clin. Auton. Res. **3:** 137–143.
24. SECHI, L.A., J.P. VALENTIN, C.A. GRIFFIN, *et al.* 1995. Receptors for atrial natriuretic peptide are decreased in the kidney of rats with streptozotocin-induced diabetes mellitus. J. Clin. Invest. **95:** 2451–2457.
25. PREDEL, H.G., O. SCHULTE-VELS, M. SORGER, *et al.* 1990. Atrial natriuretic peptide in patients with diabetes mellitus type I. Effects on systemic and renal hemodynamics and renal excretory function. Am. J. Hypertens. **3:** 674–681.
26. HOWARTH, F.C., A. ADEM, E.A. ADEGHATE, *et al.* 2005. Distribution of atrial natriuretic peptide and its effects on contraction and intracellular calcium in ventricular myocytes from streptozotocin-induced diabetic rat. Peptides **26:** 691–700.
27. BALLERMANN, B.J., K.D. BLOCH, J.G. SEIDMAN & B.M. BRENNER. 1986. Atrial natriuretic peptide transcription, secretion, and glomerular receptor activity during mineralocorticoid escape in the rat. J. Clin. Invest. **78:** 840–843.
28. BENIGNI, A., N. PERICO, J. DADAN, *et al.* 1990. Functional implications of decreased renal cortical atrial natriuretic peptide binding in experimental diabetes. Circ. Res. **66:** 1453–1460.
29. ALLEN, T.J., M.E. COOPER, R.C. O'BRIEN, *et al.* 1990. Glomerular filtration rate in streptozotocin-induced diabetic rats. Role of exchangeable sodium, vasoactive hormones, and insulin therapy. Diabetes **39:** 1182–1190.

30. VALENTIN, J.P., L.A. SECHI & M.H. HUMPHREYS. 1994. Blunted effect of ANP on hematocrit and plasma volume in streptozotocin-induced diabetes mellitus in rats. Am. J. Physiol. **266** (2 Pt 2): R584–R591.
31. ADEM, A., A.M. ALI-SALEH, E.P.K. MENSAH-BROWN, *et al.* 2002. Experimental diabetic neuropathy—evidence for multiple apoptotic pathways. The Third Annual Research Conference, UAE University, April 30-May 1, 2002 51–52.

Diabetic Neuropathy Differs in Type 1 and Type 2 Diabetes

ANDERS A.F. SIMA AND HIDEKI KAMIYA

Departments of Pathology and Neurology, Wayne State University, Detroit, Michigan 48201, USA

ABSTRACT: In this article we describe differences in early metabolic abnormalities between type 1 and type 2 diabetic polyneuropathy (DPN), and how these differences lead to milder initial functional defects in type 2 diabetes, despite the same hyperglycemic exposures. This early reversible metabolic phase is progressively overshadowed by structural degenerative changes eventually resulting in nerve fiber loss. In comparison, the late structural phase of DPN affects type 1 diabetes more severely. Progressive axonal atrophy and loss is hence expressed to a larger extent in type 1 diabetes. In addition, type 1 DPN is characterized by paranodal degenerative changes not seen in type 2 DPN. These differences can be related to the differences in insulin action and signal transduction affecting the expression of neurotrophic factors and their receptors in type 1 diabetes. Downstream effects on neuroskeletal and adhesive proteins, their posttranslational modifications, and nociceptive peptides underlie the more severe resultant pathology in type 1 DPN. These differences in underlying mechanisms should be seriously considered in the future design of interventional paradigms to combat these common conditions.

KEYWORDS: type 1 and type 2 diabetes; neuropathy; nerve conduction; neuropathology

INTRODUCTION

Diabetic neuropathy includes several distinct syndromes. Symmetric, mainly sensory polyneuropathy often accompanied by autonomic neuropathy is the most common form and is referred to as diabetic polyneuropathy (DPN). DPN is the most common late complication affecting both type 1 and type 2 diabetic patients.[1,2] Despite decades of clinical and experimental investigations, the mechanisms underlying DPN are not fully understood and are sometimes controversial.[3]

Address for correspondence: Anders A.F. Sima, Department of Pathology, Wayne State University, 540 E. Canfield Ave. Detroit, MI 48201. Voice: 313-577-1150; fax: 313-577-0057.
e-mail: asima@med.wayne.edu

Ann. N.Y. Acad. Sci. 1084: 235–249 (2006).
doi: 10.1196/annals.1372.004

The prevalence of DPN varies with an average prevalence of about 30% in the diabetic population.[4] DPN accompanying type 1 diabetes occurs more predictably and progresses more rapidly resulting in a more severe neuropathy.[1,5,6] Close to 100% of type 1 patients eventually develop DPN.[7]

Despite the common occurrence of DPN, there is no accepted or effective therapy available. In the last several decades numerous clinical trials employing various aldose reductase inhibitors,[8,9] antioxidants,[10] or substitution of nerve growth factor (NGF)[11,12] have been disappointing, whereas strict glycemic control has revealed beneficial effects.[13,14] In retrospect, the reasons for these disappointing outcomes are related to initiation of therapy too late in the natural history of the disease, suboptimal potencies of employed drugs and one may argue that the duration of treatments has been too short.[8,9] Equally important is the fact that DPN in type 1 and type 2 patients has been regarded as one and the same disease, implying the same underlying mechanisms, namely hyperglycemia.[13,14] The discrepancies in the epidemiology of DPN in type 1 and type 2 diabetes correspond to differences in underlying neuropathology as well as pathogenetic mechanisms.[15–17]

Our understanding of DPN has in general been gained from streptozotocin-induced diabetes (STZ-D) in rats, which develops within weeks of diabetes induction, nerve conduction velocity abnormalities, increased activity of the polyol pathway, and decreased endoneurial blood flow. However, despite these early functional and metabolic abnormalities, they do not develop structural deficits, such as progressive nerve fiber loss, even after prolonged duration of diabetes, which is the very hallmark of human DPN.[18,19] Part of the shortcomings with the STZ-D rat as a model of the human disorders is that although it develops severe hyperglycemia, it does not reflect other aspects of the human conditions, like lack of circulating insulin and C-peptide as in type 1 diabetes, or hyperinsulinemia and insulin resistance as in type 2 diabetes.

Our laboratory has taken a different approach utilizing rat models that mimic more closely the human conditions. The type 1 spontaneously diabetic BB/Wor-rat develops acute onset of diabetes at around 70–75 days of age, as a result of an immune-mediated destruction of pancreatic β cells, with total depletion of insulin and C-peptide. It therefore requires daily insulin injections titrated in such a way that it maintains a blood sugar level of 20.0–25.0 mmol glucose. The type 2 counterpart, the BBZDR/Wor-rat, in which the fa/fa allele is outbred on the BB background, develops spontaneous onset of hyperinsulinemic insulin-resistant hyperglycemia preceded by obesity.[20] Overt diabetes occurs at the same age as in the type 1 model and hyperglycemia is maintained at the same levels without insulin substitution (TABLE 1). It is associated with hyperlipidemia and hypercholesterolemia.[20] Employing these two models of the main types of human diabetes, several functional, metabolic, molecular, and structural differences have emerged, indicating that different treatment paradigms may apply to type 1 and type 2 DPN.[21,22]

TABLE 1. Animal data in 8-month-old diabetic rats

	Body weight (g)	Glucose (mM)	Insulin (pmol/L)	C-peptide (pmol/L)	IGF-1 (ng/mL)
Control	501 ± 10	5.0 ± 0.2	430 ± 20	733 ± 45	1188 ± 32
BB/Wor	$383 \pm 7^{**}$	$23.9 \pm 1.3^{**}$	$52 \pm 6^{**}$	$<25^{**}$	$771 \pm 85^{**}$
BBZDR/Wor	$586 \pm 31^{\#}$	$23.8 \pm 3.1^{**}$	$586 \pm 26^{*,\#}$	$810 \pm 81^{\#}$	$880 \pm 72^{**}$
BB/Wor + C-peptide	$386 \pm 12^{**}$	$24.0 \pm 1.3^{**}$	$40 \pm 7^{**}$	$710 \pm 66^{\#}$	$839 \pm 50^{**}$

$^{*}P < 0.01$, $^{**}P < 0.001$ vs. control-rats; $^{\#}P < 0.001$ vs. BB/Wor-rats.

NOTE: Decreased body weight in type 1 BB/Wor-rats and increased body weight in type 2 BBZDR/Wor-rats. Both animal models show the same magnitude of hyperglycemia. BB/Wor-rats are severely insulinopenic and C-peptidopenic, whereas insulin plasma levels are increased in the BBZDR/Wor-rats. Systemic IGF-1 is decreased in all diabetic groups.

DPN is the result of complicated sequential, interacting, and dynamic pathogenetic mechanisms (FIG. 1). Some mechanisms may be prominent at one point in its natural history, later to be replaced by other mechanisms.[2,9,22] In both diabetic subjects and in experimental diabetes there is an initial "metabolic phase" causing nerve dysfunction, which is amendable to metabolic corrections.[2,23,24] This is progressively replaced by a "structural phase," which with the duration of diabetes becomes increasingly nonresponsive to metabolic interventions.[2,9]

The Metabolic Phase of DPN

Several early metabolic abnormalities have been identified in the diabetic nerve. Shunting of excessive glucose through the activated polyol pathway leads to intracellular accumulation of sorbitol and fructose with consequent depletion of other organic osmolytes such as taurine and myo-inositol.[25,26] Depletion of the myo-inositol pool interferes with phosphoinositide turnover resulting in insufficient diacylglycerol to maintain protein kinase C necessary for activation of Na^+/K^+-ATPase (FIG. 1).[25,27] The type 1 BB/Wor-rat shows activation of the polyol pathway, with consequent impairment of neural Na^+/K^+-ATPase, which is corrected by aldose reductase inhibition.[28] In the type 2 BBZDR/Wor-rat, which shows the same magnitude of hyperglycemia (TABLE 1) and hence activation of the polyol pathway, the impairment of Na^+/K^+-ATPase activity is significantly less.[21] This difference in Na^+/K^+-ATPase activity is accounted for by impaired insulin signaling in type 1 diabetes adding to the polyol pathway-induced defect. This has been confirmed by the insulinomimetic effect of proinsulin C-peptide.[29,30] When BB/Wor-rats are substituted with C-peptide they show a dose-dependent correction of neural Na^+/K^+-ATPase activity and the acute nerve conduction defect.[31] Therefore, the more severe defect in Na^+/K^+-ATPase activity can be accounted for by insulinopenia and perturbed insulin signal transduction (FIG. 1).[32]

Endoneurial hypoxemia secondary to impaired endoneurial blood flow has been ascribed to impaired expression of eNOS and NO activity. It has been

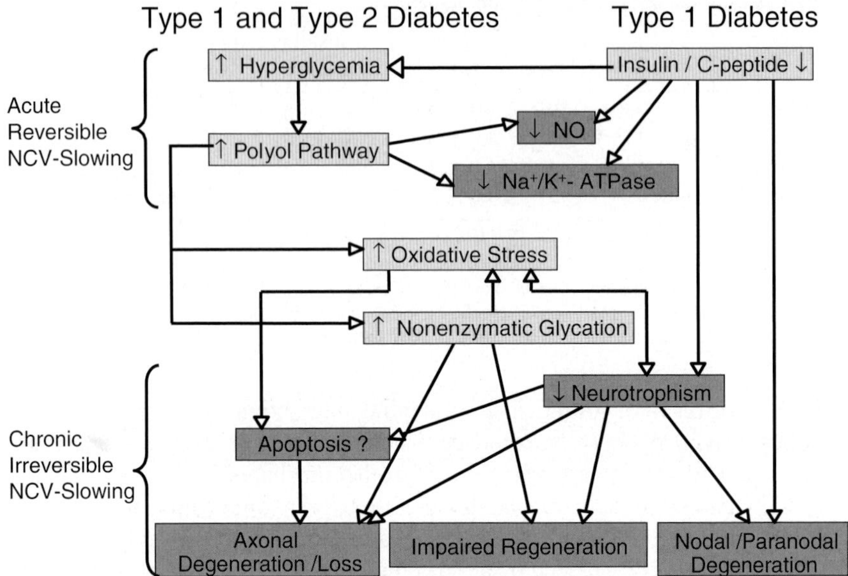

FIGURE 1. Scheme of pathogenetic mechanisms involved in DPN of type 1 and type 2 diabetes. The early metabolic abnormalities underlying the acute functional deficits are reversible. However, these become increasingly superimposed by progressive structural abnormalities, which become less reversible after metabolic corrections. For further explanation see text. (Redrawn from Sima an Kamiya.[61])

proposed that the consequences of hyperglycemia come together causing mitochondrial dysfunction, superoxide overproduction, and oxidative and nitrosative stress contributing to the depletion of NO and impaired nerve perfusion[33–35] and that these defects contribute to nerve dysfunction. In the type 1 BB/Wor-rat both endoneurial perfusion and nerve conduction are decreased and oxidative stress is increased. On the other hand, in the type 2 BBZDR/Wor-rat endoneurial nutritive blood flow and oxidative stress are similarly increased, whereas nerve conduction is not affected.[36] C-peptide substitution of type 1 rats corrects the NO-sensitive neurovascular function and nerve conduction velocity, without effecting oxidative stress or hyperglycemia.[36] These findings therefore suggest that nerve conduction deficits are not inevitably a consequence of increased oxidative stress and decreased nerve perfusion and indicate a dissociation between oxidative stress and endoneurial blood flow.

These early metabolic abnormalities are associated with functional defects (FIG. 1). In the BB/Wor-rat there is a progressive decrease in motor nerve conduction velocity (MNCV) to 70% of normal values after a 5-week duration of diabetes. The MNCV defect is significantly milder in the BBZDR/Wor-rat, which shows a 12% deficit at 5 weeks of diabetes (FIG. 2 A).[21] Sensory nerve conduction velocity (SNCV) in the type 1 BB/Wor-rat shows a 10% decrease,

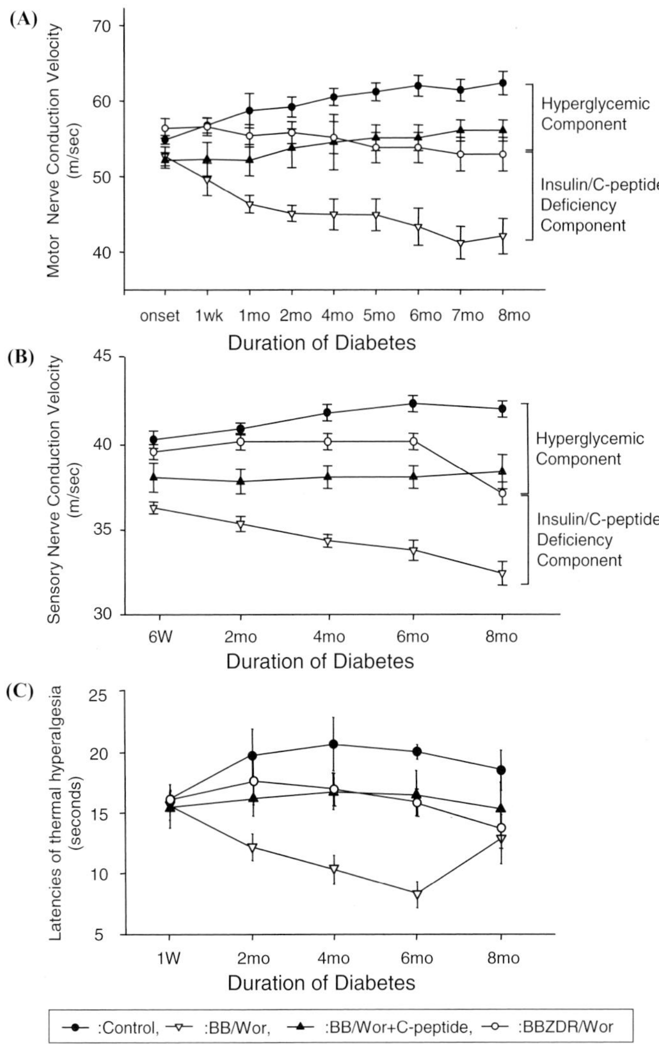

FIGURE 2. (A). Longitudinal measurements of MNCV in type 1 BB/Wor- and type 2 BBZDR/Wor-rats. Also indicated is the effect of C-peptide replacement, which does not influence hyperglycemia. Therefore the components of the nerve conduction deficits can be divided into a hyperglycemic component and an insulin/C-peptide deficiency component. **(B)**. SNCV measurements. In type 1 BB/Wor-rats this is decreased after 2 months of diabetes and decreases progressively. Type 2 BBZDR/Wor-rats show normal conduction velocity for 6 months and becomes decreased only after 8 months of diabetes. C-peptide replaced BB/Wor-rats show a pattern similar to that of BBZDR/Wor-rats. **(C)**. Latencies to withdrawal from thermal stimuli, thermal hyperalgesia, decrease progressively in the type 1 model up to 6 months duration of diabetes and then increase by 8 months. This increase correlates with profound C-fiber loss and reflects early analgesia. The defect in the type 2 model is significantly milder. Type 1 rats replaced with C-peptide show a pattern similar to that of type 2 rats.

whereas in the type 2 BBZDR/Wor-rat it is unaltered at the same duration of diabetes (FIG. 2 B).[36] These differences between type 1 and type 2 diabetes can be related to differences in neural Na^+/K^+-ATPase activities. Since the excitation of the nodal membrane underlying the impulse propagation is caused by an inward flux of Na^+, NCV velocity is related directly to nodal Na^+ permeability. In the BB/Wor-rat there is a progressive increase in the abnormal inactivation of Na^+ and a decline in the maximal peak of Na^+ permeability resulting in decreased nodal Na^+ equilibrium potentials.[37] These changes are directly associated with the decreased Na^+/K^+-ATPase activity causing intra-axonal Na^+ accumulation.[37,38] Interestingly, these biophysical abnormalities are corrected by insulin in acutely diabetic rats.[38] Nodal axonal swelling, an early structural abnormality, is more prominent in type 1 than in type 2 BB-rats.[21] It correlates with intra-axonal Na^+ accumulation and is reversed following insulin or C-peptide treatment.[29,39] However, the expression of voltage-gated α-Na^+-channels is not altered in the sciatic nerve of diabetic rats.[40] Therefore, these early metabolic dysfunctions of myelinated fibers can be directly related to the Na^+/K^+-ATPase defect, whereas the impact of impaired endoneurial blood flow is probably less as alluded to above.

Unmyelinated fiber dysfunction is reflected by thermal hyperalgesia. Again, the type 1 BB/Wor-rat shows a significantly more rapid decrease in the latencies to thermal stimuli (FIG. 2 C).[36,41] Damage to small myelinated $A\delta$ and unmyelinated C-fibers underlies hyperalgesia and allodynia.[42,43] Damage to axonal membranes of C-fibers induces increased formation of Na^+-channels and α-adrenergic receptors facilitating ectopic discharges.[44–46] The varying degree of hyperalgesia in the two models correlates with significant differences in the expression NGF and NT-3 in the sciatic nerve and of insulin receptor, IGF-1 receptor, high-affinity NGFR-TrkA, and TrkC in dorsal root ganglia (DRGs) and consequent suppression of nociceptive peptides and synthesis of neuroskeletal proteins (FIG. 3).[19,41,47] These changes eventually lead to degeneration and loss of nociceptive C-fibers.[41] The abnormalities leading up to this series of events either do not occur or are significantly milder in the type 2 BBZDR/Wor-rat.[41] Since the expression of neurotrophic factors and their receptors is intimately related to insulin signal transduction,[47–50] it is not totally surprising that insulinomimetic C-peptide significantly ameliorates these changes in type 1 diabetes (FIG. 3).[49]

To summarize, the metabolic abnormalities underlying early functional abnormalities in DPN show obvious differences between the two types of diabetes. No doubt, hyperglycemia plays an important role in the development of DPN, we would argue though, that impaired insulin availability, a potent neurotrophic agent in itself, and consequent aberrant signal transduction may play an equally important role in the pathophysiology of these changes.

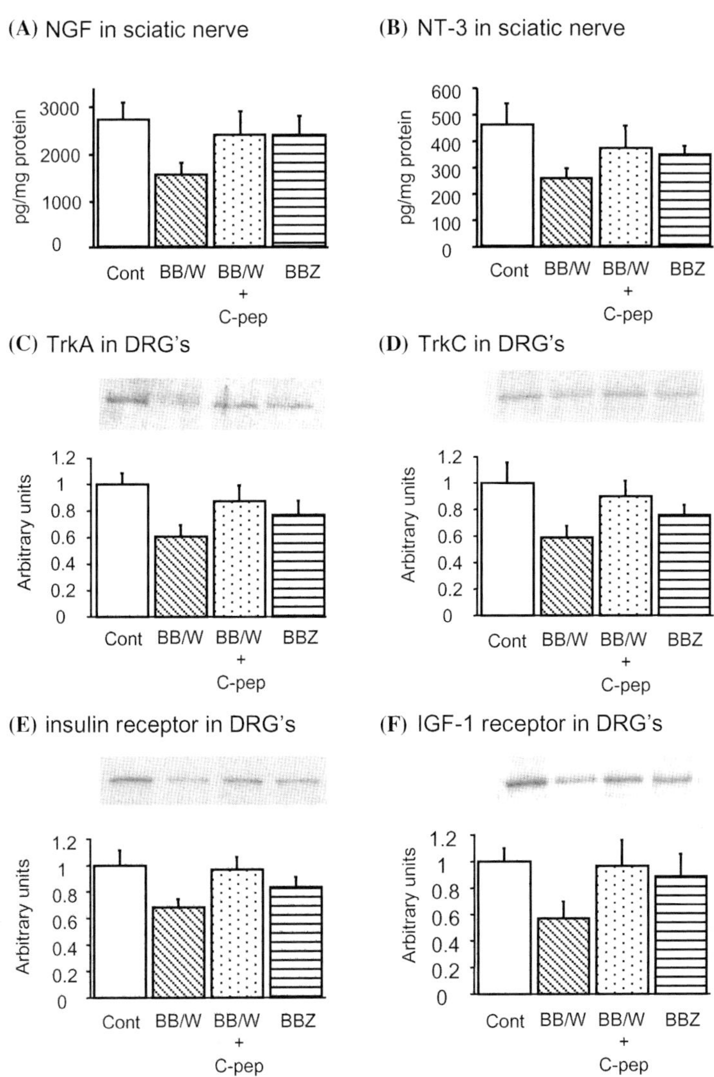

FIGURE 3. In **A** and **B**, sciatic nerve contents of NGF and NT-3 are significantly ($P < 0.005$) decreased in BB/Wor-rats of 8 months diabetes duration. In the BBZDR/Wor-rats the levels are not significantly different from controls. C-peptide replacement of BB/Wor-rat resulted in significantly increased levels of NGF and NT-3 levels (both $P < 0.05$). In **C** and **D** Western blots of their respective receptors in DRGs showed significantly decreased expression in BB/Wor-rats (both $P < 0.005$) and were not significantly altered in BBZDR/Wor-rats. The expressions were significantly increased in C-peptide-treated rats compared to untreated BB/Wor-rats (both $P < 0.05$). In **E** and **F** the expression of the insulin receptor and IGF-1R were both significantly ($P < 0.005$) decreased in DRGs from BB/Wor-rats, and not significantly different from control rats in BBZDR/Wor-rats or C-peptide replaced BB/Wor-rats.

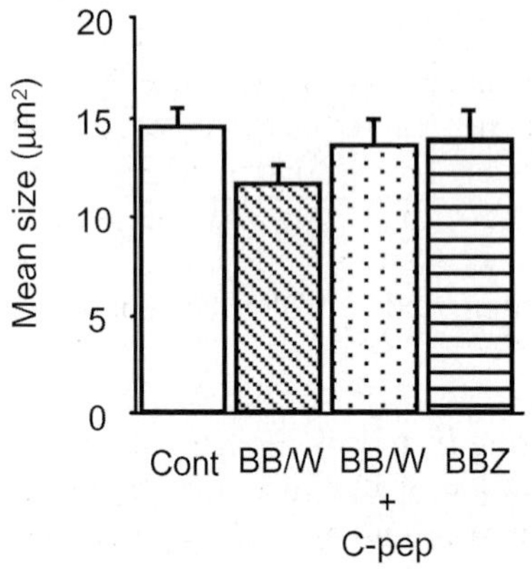

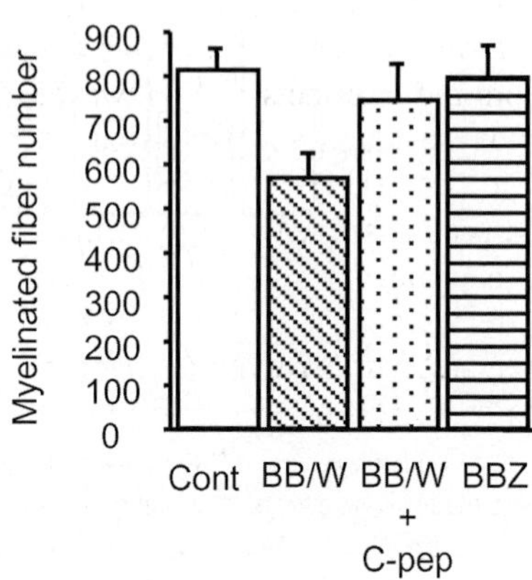

FIGURE 4. Myelinated axon area (**A**) were significantly ($P < 0.001$) decreased in 8 months diabetic BB/Wor-rats, but unaltered in type 2 BBZDR/Wor-rats and in C-peptide replaced type 1 BB/Wor-rats. Myelinated fiber numbers (**B**) in the sural nerve was significantly ($P < 0.001$) decreased in BB/Wor-rats and not significantly different from controls in type 2 BBZDR/Wor-rats or C-peptide replaced BB/Wor-rats.

The Structural Phase of DPN

From the acute metabolic abnormalities emerge progressive structural changes, which become decreasingly responsive to metabolic interventions. One of the earliest detectable changes in myelinated fibers is nodal and paranodal axonal swelling, which correlates with the early Na^+/K^+-ATPase defect and increased intra-axonal $[Na^+]^i$.[37,38] It is more expressed in type 1 BB/Wor-rats[21] and is reversible.[31,38] Other early abnormalities consist of malalignment of cytoskeletal structures[51] reflecting aberrant synthesis, phosphorylation, and assembly of neurofilaments.[52,53] These changes lead to perturbed axonal transport and progressive axonal atrophy evident in the type 1 BB/Wor-rat after 4 months of diabetes.[54–56] The axonal atrophy shows a proximal to distal gradient[54] and ultimately results in distal axonal degeneration with secondary myelin breakdown and fiber loss (FIG. 4).[54,57] Axonal degeneration has been associated with impaired neurotrophic support by insulin itself, IGF-1, and neurotrophins (FIG. 3), resulting in impaired synthesis of tubulins and neurofilament and their assembly.[52,58–61]

Significant fiber loss of 10% is already detectable in sural nerves of type 1 BB/Wor-rats after 4 months of diabetes increasing to 33% after 11 months.[54] In contrast, the type 2 BBZDR/Wor-rat exhibits significantly milder axonal atrophy and fiber loss (FIG. 4) amounting to 11% after 14 months of diabetes.[21] Primary segmental demyelination is rare in these models but is nevertheless more common in type 2 diabetic rats.[21] Differences in axonal degeneration and loss are also reflected by differences in the chronic nerve conduction defects (FIG. 2 A,B). C-peptide substitution of type 1 BB/Wor-rats prevents and improves significantly the nerve conduction defects, reflecting its insulinomimetic effects.[29,60] However, these defects are not totally prevented but show residual defects similar to the defects encountered in the type 2 model (FIG. 2A,B). This has led us to suggest that the chronic functional defects in DPN consist of a hyperglycemic component, not responsive to insulinomimetic C-peptide, and an insulin/C-peptide deficiency component not present in type 2 diabetes (FIG. 2).[61,62] It has recently been suggested that DRG cell apoptosis may be an underlying mechanism in DPN.[35,63,64] However, these findings have not been substantiated.[57,65,66]

A characteristic structural change occurring in type 1 human and experimental diabetes is the progressive degeneration of the node and paranodal apparatus.[15,67] These changes will affect nerve conduction velocity in a major way. They consist of progressive disruption of the paranodal apparatus allowing for lateralization of nodal voltage-gated Na^+-channels, thereby diminishing the initial Na^+ current of the nodal membrane. The abnormality of the paranodal ion-channel barrier is caused by decreased expression of key adhesive molecules and their insulin-mediated posttranslational modifications that underlie their protein–protein interactions.[62,68] The paranodal molecules colocalize with the insulin receptor, the expression of which is downregulated in chronically type 1 diabetic BB/Wor-rats. It is therefore not totally surprising that C-peptide replacement prevents these abnormalities.[62] These abnormalities do not occur in the type 2 model even after 14 months of diabetes.[21] Therefore, this degenerative process is specific for type 1 diabetes and contributes to the more severe conduction defect seen in type 1 diabetic rats (FIG. 2 A,B). As often misquoted, these abnormalities are not related to the Na^+/K^+-ATPase defect.

The peripheral unmyelinated fiber population represents sympathetic and nociceptive sensory fibers. This fiber population appears to be specifically sensitive to diabetic environments. Even under prediabetic conditions as in the GK-rat, which shows impaired glucose tolerance and β cell dysfunction, nociceptive neuropathy with C-fiber degeneration occurs.[69] In the type 1 BB/Wor-rat increased hyperalgesia to thermal stimulation is already present at 2 months duration of diabetes and increases progressively thereafter (FIG. 2 C).[41] This is accompanied by degenerative changes of C-fibers consisting of type 2 Schwann cell/axon relationships, whereby the mesaxon degenerates leaving the axon directly exposed to the endoneurial environment (FIG. 5). This is followed by axonal atrophy and loss, leaving behind collagen pockets and denervated Schwann cells (FIG. 5).[41] This series of events is preceded by suppressed expression of the insulin receptor in DRG cells, impaired exposure to NGF, IGF-1, NT-3, and their respective receptors NGF-RTrkA, IGF-1R, and

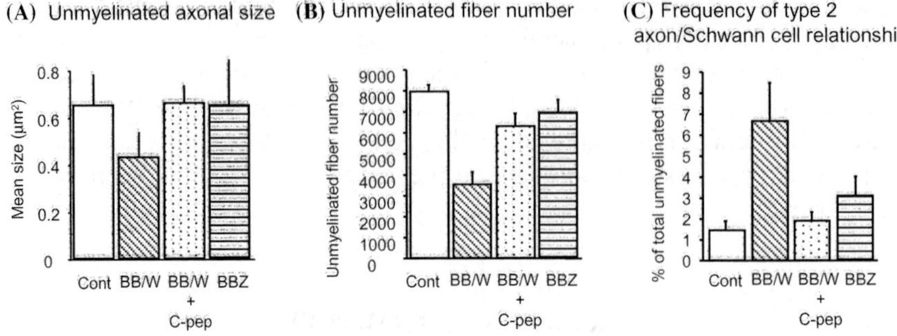

FIGURE 5. Unmyelinated fiber size (**A**) was significantly ($P < 0.05$) decreased in BB/Wor-rats but not in BBZDR/Wor-rats or in C-peptide-substituted BB/Wor-rats. Unmyelinated fiber numbers in the sural nerve (**B**) was markedly decreased ($P < 0.001$) in type 1 rats, whereas they were not significantly different from nondiabetic control rats in BBZDR/Wor-rats or in C-peptide-replenished BB/Wor-rats. The frequency of type 2 axon/Schwann cell relationship (**C**) was significantly more common in BB/Wor-rats compared to control rats ($P < 0.0001$), C-peptide replaced BB/Wor-rats ($P < 0.0001$) and to BBZDR/Wor-rats ($P < 0.005$).

TrkC (FIG. 3).[41,49] The consequences of this impairment of wide neurotrophic support are impaired synthesis of nociceptive neuropeptides, such as substance P and GRRP, axonal atrophy, and loss of their parent DRG cells.[41,49] The neuronal loss is not apoptosis-induced but correlates with progressive degeneration of the Golgi apparatus resulting in vacuolar degeneration and eventually neuronal loss (Kamiya *et al.*, unpublished data). These changes progress at a significantly slower pace in the type 2 BBZDR/Wor-rat, which correlates with an almost normal expression of neurotrophic receptors in DRG cells (FIG. 3) and milder suppression of nociceptive neuropeptides.[41] Hence, these differences between the two models can be traced to the profound differences in insulin action and its downstream regulatory effect on neurotrophic factors and their receptors.[41] This is confirmed by the beneficial effects of C-peptide replacement on nociceptive sensory neuropathy in the type 1 rat model (FIG. 3).[49]

In the type 1 diabetic BB/Wor-rat the development of sympathetic autonomic neuropathy is characterized by neuroaxonal dystrophic changes of terminal axons.[70,71] In comparison, such changes do not develop in the type 2 BBZDR/Wor-rat.[72] As to whether these changes bear any relationship to insulin action and/or neurotrophic support is not known.

In summary, this review has demonstrated marked differences in metabolic factors and their magnitudes in type 1 and type 2 experimental diabetes models, which closely mimic the human conditions. The subsequent development of structural changes relates to different sets of underlying molecular changes and differences in the severities of neurotrophic support, which can be directly related to differences in insulin action. Therefore, despite exposure to the same magnitude of hyperglycemia over prolonged periods of time the resultant outcome is markedly different. This means that apart from hyperglycemia, perturbations of insulin action and signaling play equally important roles in the development of type 1 DPN. Such differences have to be taken into account in future approaches to treating and/or preventing this common complication of diabetes.

ACKNOWLEDGMENTS

Our own studies referred to in this article were supported by the Medical Research Council of Canada, Canadian Diabetes Association, the Juvenile Diabetes Research Foundation, the National Institute of Health, the Morris Hood Diabetes Center, and the Thomas Foundation. Dr. H. Kamiya is presently a postdoctoral fellow supported by the Thomas Foundation.

REFERENCES

1. Sugimoto, K., Y. Murakawa & A.A.F. Sima. 2000. Diabetic neuropathy—a continuing enigma. Diab./Metab. Res. & Rev. **16:** 408–433.
2. Sima, A.A.F. 2003. New insights into the metabolic and molecular basis for diabetic neuropathy. Cell Mol. Life Sci. **60:** 2445–2464.
3. Sima, A.A.F. 2004. Diabetic neuropathy in type 1 and type 2 diabetes and the effects of C-peptide. Neurol. Sci. **220:** 133–136.
4. Tesfaye, S. *et al.* 1996. Prevalence of diabetic peripheral neuropathy and its relation to glycaemic control and potential risk factors: the EURODIAB IDDM complication study. Diabetologia **39:** 1377–1384.
5. Dyck, P.J. *et al.* 1999. Risk factors for severity of diabetic polyneuropathy: intensive longitudinal assessment of the Rochester Diabetic Neuropathy Study Cohort. Diabetes Care **22:** 1479–1486.
6. Sima, A.A.F. 2003. C-peptide and diabetic neuropathy. Expert Opin. Investig. Drugs **12:** 1471–1488.
7. Vinik, A.I. *et al.* 1992. Diabetic neuropathies. Diabetes Care **15:** 1926–1975.
8. Pfeifer, M.A., M.P. Shumer & D.A. Gelber. 1997. Aldose reductase inhibitors: the end of an era or the need for different trial designs? Diabetes **46**(Suppl 1)**:** 582–589.
9. Sima, A.A.F. 2001. Diabetic neuropathy; pathogenetic backgrounds, current and future therapies. Expert Rev. Neurotherapeut. **1:** 225–238.
10. Ziegler, D. *et al.* 1999. Treatment of symptomatic diabetic polyneuropathy with the anti-oxidant α-lipoic acid. Diabetes Care **22:** 1296–1301.
11. Vinik, A.I. 1999. Treatment of diabetic polyneuropathy (DPN) with recombinant human nerve growth factor (rh NGF). Diabetes **48:** A54–A55.
12. Apfel, S.C. *et al.* 2000. Efficacy and safety of recombinant human nerve growth factor in patients with diabetic polyneuropathy. JAMA **284:** 2215–2221.

13. DIABETES CONTROL AND COMPLICATIONS TRIAL RESEARCH GROUP. 1995. The effect of intensive diabetes treatment on nerve conduction in the Diabetes Control and Complications Trial (DCCT). Ann. Neurol. **38:** 869–880.
14. REICHARD, P. *et al.* 1996. Complications in IDDM are caused by elevated blood glucose level: the Stockholm Diabetes Intervention Study (SDIS) at 10-year follow up. Diabetologia **39:** 1483–1488.
15. SIMA, A.A.F. *et al.* 1988. Histopathological heterogeneity of neuropathy in insulin-dependent and non-insulin-dependent diabetes, and demonstration of axo-glial dysjunction in human diabetic neuropathy. J. Clin. Invest. **81:** 349–364.
16. SIMA, A.A.F. *et al.* 1988. Regeneration and repair of myelinated fibers in sural nerve biopsies from patients with diabetic neuropathy treated with an aldose reductase inhibitor. N. Eng. J. Med. **319:** 548–555.
17. SIMA, A.A.F., V. BRIL & D.A. GREENE. 1989. Pathogenetic heterogeneity in human diabetic neuropathy. Pediatr. Adolesc. Endocrin. **18:** 56–62.
18. YAGIHASHI, S. *et al.* 1990. Effects of long-term aldose reductase inhibition on development of experimental diabetic neuropathy. ultrastructural and morphometric studies of sural nerve in streptozotocin-induced diabetic rats. Diabetes **39:** 690–696.
19. ZOCHODNE, D.W. *et al.* 2001. Does diabetes target ganglion neurons? Progressive sensory neuron involvement in long-term experimental diabetes. Brain **124:** 2319–2334.
20. SIMA, A.A.F. *et al.* 1997. The BB/Z^{DR}-rat; A model for type II diabetic neuropathy: Exp. Clin. Endocrin. Diab. **105:** 63–64.
21. SIMA, A.A.F. *et al.* 2000. A comparison of diabetic polyneuropathy in type-2 diabetic BBZDR/Wor-rat and in type 1 diabetic BB/Wor-rat. Diabetologia **43:** 786–793.
22. SIMA, A.A.F. 2006. Pathological mechanisms involved in diabetic neuropathy. Can we slow the process? Curr. Opin. Drug Develop. **7:** 324–337.
23. TERKILDSEN, A.B. & N.J. CHRISTENSEN. 1971. Reversible nervous abnormalities in juvenile diabetics with recently diagnosed diabetes. Diabetologia **7:** 113–117.
24. FRASER, D.M. *et al.* 1977. Peripheral and autonomic nerve function in newly diagnosed diabetes mellitus. Diabetes **6:** 546–550.
25. GREENE, D.A., S.A. LATTIMER & A.A.F. SIMA. 1987. Sorbitol, phosphoinositides and sodium-potassium ATPase in the pathogenesis of diabetic complications. N. Engl. J. Med. **316:** 599–606.
26. STEVENS, M.J. *et al.* 1993. Osmotically induced nerve taurine depletion and the compatible osmolyte hypothesis in experimental diabetic neuropathy in the rat. Diabetologia **36:** 608–614.
27. ZHU, X. & J. EICHBERG. 1990. A myo-inositol pool utilized for phosphatidylinositol synthesis is depleted in sciatic nerve from rats with streptozotocin-induced diabetes. Proc. Natl. Acad. Sci. USA **87:** 9818–9822.
28. SIMA, A.A.F. *et al.* 1990. Preventive effect of long term aldose reductase inhibition (Ponalrestat) on nerve conduction and sural nerve structure in the spontaneously diabetic BB-rat. J. Clin. Invest. **85:** 1410–1420.
29. SIMA, A.A.F. *et al.* 2001. C-peptide prevents and improves chronic type 1 diabetic neuropathy in the BB/Wor-rat. Diabetologia **44:** 889–897.
30. FORST, T. *et al.* 2000. Effects of proinsulin C-peptide on nitric oxide, microvascular blood flow and erythrocyte Na^+ K^+-ATPase activity in diabetes mellitus type 1. Clin. Sci. **98:** 283–290.

31. ZHANG, W. *et al.* 2001. Human C-peptide dose dependently prevents early neuropathy in the BB/Wor-rat. Int. J. Exp. Diabetes Res. **2:** 187–194.
32. GRUNBERGER, G. *et al.* 2001. Molecular basis for the insulinomimetic effects of C-peptide. Diabetologia **44:** 1247–1257.
33. BROWNLEE, M. 2001. Biochemistry and molecular cell biology of diabetic complications. Nature **414:** 813–820.
34. CAMERON, N.E., M.A. COTTER & S. ROBERTSON. 1993. Rapid reversal of motor nerve conduction deficit in streptozotocin-diabetic rats by the angiotensin converting enzyme inhibitor lisinopril. Acta Diabetol. **30:** 46–48.
35. SCHMEICHEL, A.M., J.D. SCHMETZER & P.A. LOW. 2003. Oxidative injury and apoptosis of dorsal root ganglion neurons in chronic experimental diabetic neuropathy. Diabetes **52:** 165–171.
36. STEVENS, M.J. *et al.* 2004. C-peptide corrects endoneurial blood flow but not oxidative stress in type 1 BB/Wor-rats. Am. J. Physiol. **287:** E497–E505.
37. BRISMAR, T. & A.A.F. SIMA. 1981. Changes in nodal function in nerve fibres of the spontaneously diabetic BB-Wistar rat. Potential clamp analysis. Acta Physiol. Scand. **113:** 499–506.
38. BRISMAR, T., A.A.F. SIMA & D.A. GREENE. 1987. Reversible and irreversible nodal dysfunction in diabetic neuropathy. Ann. Neurol. **21:** 504–507.
39. SIMA, A.A.F. & T. BRISMAR. 1985. Reversible diabetic nerve dysfunction. Structural correlates to electrophysiological abnormalities. Ann. Neurol. **18:** 21–29.
40. SIMA, A.A.F. *et al.* 2004. Molecular alterations underlie nodal and paranodal degeneration in type 1 diabetic neuropathy and are prevented by C-peptide. Diabetes **53:** 1556–1563.
41. KAMIYA, H. *et al.* 2005. Unmyelinated fiber sensory neuropathy differs in type 1 and type 2 diabetes. Diabetes Metab. Res. Rev. **21:** 448–458.
42. KAPUR, D. 2003. Neuropathic pain and diabetes. Diabetes Metab. Res. Rev. **19:** S9–S15.
43. LLEWELYN, J.G. *et al.* 1991. Sural nerve morphometry in diabetic autonomic and painful sensory neuropathy: a clinicopathological study. Brain **114:** 867–892.
44. DICKENSON, A.H., E.A. MATTHEWS & R. SUZUKI. 2002. Neurobiology of neuropathic pain: mode of action of anticonvulsants. Eur. J. Pain **6:** 51–60.
45. LEE, Y.H. *et al.* 2000. Alpha-1-adreno-receptors involvement in painful diabetic neuropathy: a role in allodynia. Neuroreport **11:** 1417–1420.
46. BURCHIEL, K.J. *et al.* 1985. Spontaneous activity of primary afferent neurons in diabetic BB-Wistar rats. A possible mechanism of chronic diabetic pain. Diabetes **34:** 1210–1213.
47. REICO-PINTO, E., M.M. RECHLER & D.N. ISHII. 1986. Effects of insulin, insulin-like growth factor-II, and nerve growth factor on neurite formation and survival in cultured sympathetic and sensory neurons. J. Neurosci. **6:** 1211–1219.
48. LI, Z-G., W. ZHANG & A.A.F. SIMA. 2003. C-peptide enhances insulin-mediated cell growth and protection against high glucose induced apoptosis in SH-SY5Y cells. Diabetes Metab. Res. Rev. **19:** 375–385.
49. KAMIYA, H., W. ZHANG & A.A.F. SIMA. 2004. C-peptide prevents nociceptive sensory neuropathy in type 1 diabetes. Ann. Neurol. **56:** 827–835.
50. BRUSSEE, V., F.A. CUNNINGHAM & D.W. ZOCHODNE. 2004. Direct insulin signaling of neurons reverses diabetic neuropathy. Diabetes **53:** 1824–1830.
51. SIMA, A.A.F., A.C. LORUSSO & P. THIBERT. 1982. Distal symmetric polyneuropathy in the spontaneously diabetic BB-Wistar rat. An ultrastructural and teased fiber study. Acta Neuropathol (Berl.) **58** 39–47.

52. SCOTT, J.N., A.W. CLARK & D.W. ZOCHODNE. 1999. Neurofilament and gene expression in progressive experimental diabetes: failure of synthesis and export by sensory neurons. Brain **122:** 2109–2118.
53. XU, G.Y. *et al.* 2002. Altered ß-tubulin and neurofilament expression and impaired axonal growth in diabetic nerve regeneration. J. Neuropath. Exp. Neurol. **61:** 164–175.
54. SIMA, A.A.F., M. BOUCHIER & H. CHRISTENSEN. 1983. Axonal atrophy in sensory nerves of the diabetic BB-Wistar rat, a possible early correlate of human diabetic neuropathy. Ann. Neurol. **13:** 264–272.
55. MEDORI, R. *et al.* 1988. Experimental diabetic neuropathy: similar changes of slow axonal transport and axonal size in different animal models. J. Neurosci. **8:** 1814–1822.
56. PIERSON, C.R. *et al.* 2003. Tubulin and neurofilament expression and axonal growth differ in type 1 and type 2 diabetic polyneuropathy. J. Neuropath. Exp. Neurol. **62:** 260–271.
57. KAMIYA, H., W. ZHANG & A.A.F. SIMA. 2005. Apoptotic stress is counterbalanced by survival elements preventing programmed cell death of DRG's in subacute type 1 diabetic BB/Wor-rats. Diabetes **54:** 3288–3295.
58. ISHII, D.N. 1995. Implication of insulin-like growth factors in the pathogenesis of diabetic neuropathy. Brain Res. Rev. **20:** 47–67.
59. TOMLINSON, D.R. & P. FERNYHOUGH. 2000. Neurotrophism in diabetic neuropathy. *In* Chronic Complication in Diabetes. A.A.F. Sima, Ed.: 167–182. Harwood Acad. Publ. Amsterdam.
60. PIERSON, C.R. *et al.* 2002. Early gene responses of trophic factors differ in nerve regeneration in type 1 and type 2 diabetic neuropathy. J. Neuropathol Exp. Neurol. **61:** 857–871.
61. SIMA, A.A.F., W. ZHANG & H. KAMIYA. 2005. Metabolic-functional-structural correlations in somatic neuropathies in the spontaneously type 1 and type 2 diabetic BB-rats. *In* Clinical Management of Diabetic Neuropathy. A. Veves, Ed.: John Wiley & Sons Ltd. Chichester, UK, in press.
62. SIMA, A.A.F. & H. KAMIYA. 2004. Insulin, C-peptide and diabetic neuropathy. Science Med. **10:** 308–319.
63. RUSSEL, J.W. *et al.* 1999. Neurons undergo apoptosis in animal and cell culture models of diabetes. Neurobiol. Dis. **6:** 347–363.
64. SCRINIVASON, S., M. STEVENS & J.W. WILEY. 2000. Diabetic peripheral neuropathy: evidence for apoptosis and associated mitochondrial dysfunction. Diabetes **49:** 1932–1938.
65. CHENG, C. & D.W. ZOCHODNE. 2003. Sensory neurons with activated caspase-3 survive long-term experimental diabetes. Diabetes **52:** 2363–2371.
66. BURNAND, R.C. *et al.* 2004. Expression of axtomy inducible and apoptosis-related genes in sensory nerves with experimental diabetes. Brain Res. Mol. Brain Res. **20:** 235–240.
67. SIMA, A.A.F. *et al.* 1986. "Axo-glial dysjunction": a novel structural lesion that accounts for poorly reversible slowing of nerve conduction in the spontaneously diabetic BB-rat. J. Clin. Invest. **77:** 474–484.
68. SIMA, A.A.F. *et al.* 2004. Molecular alterations underlie nodal and paranodal degeneration in type 1 diabetic neuropathy and are prevented by C-peptide. Diabetes **53:** 1556–1563.
69. MURAKAWA, Y. *et al.* 2002. Impaired glucose tolerance and insulinopenia in the GK-rat causes peripheral neuropathy. Diabetes Metab. Res. Rev. **18:** 473–483.

70. YAGIHASHI, S. & A.A.F. SIMA. 1985. The distribution of structural changes in sympathetic nerves in the diabetic BB-rat. Am. J. Pathol. **121:** 138–147.
71. YAGIHASHI, S. & A.A.F. SIMA. 1986. Neuroaxonal and dendritic dystrophy in diabetic autonomic neuropathy. J. Neuropathol Exp. Neurol. **45:** 545–565.
72. SCHMIDT, R.E. *et al.* 2004. Experimental rat models of type 1 and type 2 diabetes differ in sympathetic neuronal dystrophy. J. Neuropathol Exp. Neurol. **63:** 450–460.

Treatment of Diabetic Polyneuropathy

Update 2006

DAN ZIEGLER

German Diabetes Clinic, German Diabetes Center, Leibniz Institute at the Heinrich Heine University, WHO Collaborating Center in Diabetes, European Training Center in Endocrinology and Metabolism, 40225 Düsseldorf, Germany

ABSTRACT: At least one of four diabetic patients is affected by distal symmetric polyneuropathy (DSP), which represents a major health problem, as it may present with partly excruciating neuropathic pain and is responsible for substantial morbidity, increased mortality, and impaired quality of life. Treatment is based on four cornerstones: (*a*) causal treatment aimed at (near)-normoglycemia, (*b*) treatment based on pathogenetic mechanisms, (*c*) symptomatic treatment, and (*d*) avoidance of risk factors and complications. Recent experimental studies suggest a multifactorial pathogenesis of diabetic neuropathy. From the clinical point of view it is important to note that, on the basis of these pathogenetic mechanisms, therapeutic approaches could be derived, some of which are currently being evaluated in clinical trials. Among these agents only α-lipoic acid is available for treatment in several countries and epalrestat in Japan. Although several novel analgesic drugs, such as duloxetine and pregabalin, have recently been introduced into clinical practice, the pharmacological treatment of chronic painful diabetic neuropathy remains a challenge for the physician. Individual tolerability remains a major aspect in any treatment decision. Epidemiological data indicate that not only increased alcohol consumption but also the traditional cardiovascular risk factors, such as hypertension, smoking, and visceral obesity, play a role in development and progression of diabetic neuropathy and, hence, need to be prevented or treated.

KEYWORDS: diabetic polyneuropathy; neuropathic pain; pathogenetic treatment; pain treatment

Address for correspondence: Prof. Dan Ziegler, FRCPE, Deutsche Diabetes-Klinik, Deutsches Diabetes-Zentrum, Leibniz-Zentrum an der Heinrich-Heine-Universität Düsseldorf, Auf'm Hennekamp 65, 40225 Düsseldorf, Germany. Voice: 0049-211-33821; fax: 0049-211-3382277.
e-mail: dan.ziegler@ddz.uni-duesseldorf.de

**Ann. N.Y. Acad. Sci. 1084: 250–266 (2006). © 2006 New York Academy of Sciences.
doi: 10.1196/annals.1372.008**

INTRODUCTION

Clinical Impact and Epidemiology

Diabetic neuropathy has been defined as a demonstrable disorder, either clinically evident or subclinical, which occurs in the setting of diabetes mellitus without other causes for peripheral neuropathy. It includes manifestations in the somatic and/or autonomic parts of the peripheral nervous system,[1] which are being classified along clinical criteria. However, due to a variety of clinical syndromes with possible overlaps there is no universally accepted classification. The most widely used classification differentiates between rapidly reversible, persistent symmetric polyneuropathies, and focal or multifocal neuropathies[2] (TABLE 1). The distal symmetric sensory or sensorimotor polyneuropathy (DSP) represents the most relevant clinical manifestation affecting approximately 30% of the hospital-based population and 25% of the community-based samples of diabetic patients.[3] The incidence of DSP is approximately 2% per year. The most important etiological factors that have been associated with DSP are age, poor glycemic control, diabetes duration, and height, with possible roles for hypertension, smoking, hypoinsulinemia, and visceral obesity.[3] There is accumulating evidence suggesting that not only surrogate markers of microangiopathy, such as albuminuria, but also those used for polyneuropathy, such as nerve conduction velocity (NCV) and vibration perception threshold (VPT), may predict mortality in diabetic patients.[4,5] Elevated VPT also predicts the development of neuropathic foot ulceration, one of the most common causes for hospital admission and lower limb amputations among diabetic patients.[6] Pain is a subjective symptom of major clinical importance as it is often this complaint that motivates patients to seek health care. Chronic neuropathic pain is present in 16-26% of diabetic patients.[7] Pain associated with diabetic neuropathy exerts a substantial impact on the quality of life, particularly by causing considerable interference in sleep and enjoyment of life.[8] Despite this significant impact, 25% and 39% of the diabetic patients, respectively, had no treatment for their pain in two surveys.[7,9]

Distal Symmetric Polyneuropathy

The term *hyperglycemic neuropathy* has been used to describe sensory symptoms in poorly controlled diabetic patients, which are rapidly reversible following institution of near-normoglycemia.[2] The most frequent form is the DSP commonly associated with autonomic involvement. The onset is insidious, and, in the absence of intervention, the course is chronic and progressive. It seems that the longer axons to the lower limbs are more vulnerable toward the nerve lesions induced by diabetes (length-related distribution). This notion is supported by the correlation found between the presence of DSP and height. DSP

TABLE 1. Classification of diabetic neuropathies (after Ref. 2)

(1) Rapidly reversible: Hyperglycemic neuropathy
(2) Persistent symmetric polyneuropathies:
  (a) Distal somatic sensory/motor polyneuropathies involving predominantly large fibers
  (b) Autonomic neuropathies
  (c) Small fiber neuropathies
(3) Focal/multifocal neuropathies:
  (a) Cranial neuropathies
  (b) Thoracoabdominal radiculopathies
  (c) Focal limb neuropathies
  (d) Proximal neuropathies
  (e) Compression and entrapment neuropathies

typically develops as a dying-back neuropathy, affecting the most distal extremities (toes) first. The neuropathic process then extends proximally up the limbs and later it may also affect the anterior abdominal wall and then spread laterally around the trunk. Occasionally are the upper limbs involved with the fingertips being affected first (glove-and-stocking distribution). Variants including painful small-fiber or pseudosyringomyelic syndromes and an atactic syndrome (diabetic pseudotabes) have been described. Small-fiber unmyelinated (C) and thinly myelinated (A-δ) fibers as well as large-fiber myelinated (A-α, A-β) neurons are typically involved. However, it is still uncertain whether the various fiber-type damages develop following a regular sequence, with small fibers being affected first, followed by larger fibers, or whether the small fiber or large fiber involvement reflects either side of a continuous spectrum of fiber damage. However, there is evidence suggesting that small fiber neuropathy may occur early, often presenting with pain and hyperalgesia before sensory deficits or nerve conduction slowing can be detected.[2] The reduction or loss of small fiber-mediated sensation results in loss of pain sensation (heat pain, pin-prick) and temperature perception to cold (A-δ) and warm (C) stimuli. Large fiber involvement leads to nerve conduction slowing and reduction or loss of touch, pressure, two-point discrimination, and vibration sensation, which may lead to sensory ataxia (atactic gait) in severe cases. Sensory fiber involvement causes "positive" sensory symptoms, such as paresthesias, dysesthesias, and pain, as well as "negative" symptoms, such as reduced sensation.

Persistent or episodic pain that typically may worsen at night and improve during walking is localized predominantly in the feet. The pain is often described as a deep-seated aching but there may be superimposed lancinating stabs or it may have a burning thermal quality. Evoked pain, such as allodynia (pain due to a stimulus that does not normally cause pain, e.g., stroking) and hyperalgesia (severe pain due to a stimulus that normally causes slight pain, e.g., pin-prick), may be present. The symptoms may be accompanied by sensory loss, but patients with severe pain may have few clinical signs. Pain may persist over several years causing considerable disability and impaired quality of life in some patients, whereas it remits partially or completely in others, despite further deterioration in small fiber function. Pain remission tends to be associated with sudden metabolic change, short duration of pain or diabetes, preceding weight loss, and less severe sensory loss.[10]

Compared to the sensory deficits, motor involvement is usually less prominent and restricted to the distal lower limbs resulting in muscle atrophy and weakness at the toes and foot. Ankle reflexes are frequently reduced or absent. At the foot level, the loss of the protective sensation (painless feet), motor dysfunction, and reduced sweat production resulting in dry and chapped skin due to autonomic involvement increase the risk of callus and foot ulcers. Thus, the neuropathic patient is a high-risk patient to develop severe and potentially life-threatening foot complications, such as ulceration, osteoarthropathy (Charcot foot), and osteomyelitis, as well as medial arterial calcification and neuropathic edema. DSP is a major contributory factor for diabetic foot ulcers, and the lower limb amputation rates in diabetic subjects are 15 times higher than in the nondiabetic population. Therefore, an early detection of DSP by screening is very important.[11] This becomes even more imperative due to the fact that many patients with DSP are asymptomatic or have only mild symptoms. In view of these causation pathways, the majority of amputations can be potentially prevented if appropriate screening and preventative measures are adopted.

Pathogenetic Mechanisms

Recently performed experimental studies suggest a multifactorial pathogenesis of diabetic neuropathy. Most data have been generated in the diabetic rat model. Two approaches have contributed to elucidate the pathogenesis of diabetic neuropathy. One approach leads to better characterization of pathophysiological, pathobiochemical, and structural abnormalities that result in experimental diabetic neuropathy and the other facilitates specific therapeutic interventions that aim to prevent the development of these alterations, to halt their progression, or to induce their regression despite concomitant hyperglycemia. At present, it is assumed that several mechanisms contribute to pathogenesis. In contrast to previous years, however, they are no longer being regarded as separate, but as resulting in a complex interplay giving rise to multiple interactions, for example, between metabolic and vascular factors.[12]

1. Increased flux through the polyol pathway that leads to accumulation of sorbitol and fructose, *myo*-inositol depletion, and reduction in Na^+-K^+-ATPase activity.
2. Disturbances in n-6 essential fatty acid and prostaglandin metabolism, which result in alterations of nerve membrane structure and microvascular and hemorrheologic abnormalities.

3. Endoneurial microvascular deficits with subsequent ischemia and hypoxia induced by generation of reactive oxygen species (oxidative stress), activation of the redox-sensitive transcription factor NF-κB, increased activity of the diacylglycerol (DAG)-protein kinase C-β (PKC-β) signal transduction pathway.
4. Deficits in neurotrophism leading to reduced expression and depletion of neurotrophic factors, such as nerve growth factor (NGF), neurotrophin-3 (NT-3), and insulin-like growth factor (IGF) as well as alterations in axonal transport.
5. Accumulation of nonenzymatic advanced glycation end products (AGEs) on nerve and/or vessel proteins.
6. Immunological processes with autoantibodies to vagal nerve, sympathetic ganglia, and adrenal medulla as well as inflammatory changes.

Diagnostic Assessment

Both the severity of symptoms and the degree of neuropathic deficits should be assessed using scores, such as the Neuropathy Symptom Score (NSS) and Neuropathy Disability or Impairment Score (NDS, NIS), that appear to be sufficiently reproducible.[13] For routine clinical and epidemiological purposes the simplified versions of NSS and NIS for assessment of DSP, which have been suggested by Young *et al.*,[14] can be used. Minimum criteria for diagnosis of neuropathy according to NSS and NDS are:

1) Moderate signs with or without symptoms (NDS $= 6–8 +$ NSS ≥ 0)
2) Mild signs with moderate symptoms (NDS $= 3–5 +$ NSS $= 5–6$).

Several other clinical scores, such as the Michigan Neuropathy Screening Instrument (MNSI), Diabetic Neuropathy Examination (DNE) Score, Clinical Neurological Examination (CNE) Score, and the Toronto Clinical Scoring System, have been proposed.[11] Unfortunately, DSP is still being underestimated and underdiagnosed in clinical practice. Only one-third or two-thirds of U.S. physicians were able to correctly diagnose mild or severe DSP, respectively.[15]

Electrodiagnostic Measures and Quantitative Sensory Testing (QST)

A sensitive detection and staging of DSP may be achieved by electrodiagnostic measures (nerve conduction, amplitudes) and QST. Electrophysiological techniques have the advantage of being the most objective, sensitive, specific, and reproducible methods, which are available in many neurophysiological laboratories worldwide, but also have limitations in as much as they measure only function in the largest, fastest conducting myelinated fibers, have relatively low specificity in detecting diabetic neuropathy, show relatively high intraindividual variability for certain parameters (amplitudes), are vulnerable to external factors, such as electrode locations or limb temperature, and provide only indirect information about symptoms and deficits.[16]

QST is the "determination of the absolute sensory threshold, defined as the minimal energy reliably detected for a particular modality."[16] It has been recommended that detection thresholds of touch-pressure, vibration, coolness, warmth, heat pain, cold pain, and mechanical pain can be used to characterize cutaneous sensation. The advantages of QST techniques are that they are highly sensitive, relatively simple, noninvasive, and nonaversive, afford precise control over stimulus intensity and testing algorithms, contribute to differentiation of the relative deficit in small versus large fibers, and are particularly valuable in screening large populations or in longitudinal trials.[16] The limitations to QST procedures include that they constitute psychophysical methods vulnerable to the effects of alertness, mood, concentration, ambient noise, etc., show a relatively high intraindividual variability, have not been adequately standardized, and may be time consuming (forced-choice methods), which may lead to a decline in concentration or boredom in the person tested, thereby resulting in diagnostic errors.

TREATMENT

Role of Intensive Diabetes Therapy in Treatment and Prevention of Diabetic Neuropathy

Seven long-term prospective studies that assessed the effects intensive diabetes therapy on the prevention and progression of chronic diabetic complications have been published[17] (TABLE 2). In type 1 diabetic patients these studies showed that intensive diabetes therapy retards but not completely prevents the development of polyneuropathy and autonomic neuropathy. In the EDIC study the benefits of 6.5 years of intensive therapy on neuropathy status extended for at least 8 years beyond the end of the DCCT despite equal HbA1c levels, similar to the findings described for diabetic retinopathy and nephropathy.[18] In contrast, in type 2 diabetic patients, who represent the vast majority of people with diabetes, the results were variable. Intensive diabetes therapy either had no effect or only partially slowed the progression of polyneuropathy. Although the Steno Type 2 study failed to show a favorable effect of multifactorial risk intervention on polyneuropathy, cardiovascular risk factors, such as visceral obesity, hypertension, and dyslipidemia, have to be treated according to the current guidelines. Despite the fact that observational studies suggested a glycemic threshold for the development and progression of the long-term complications in type 1 diabetes, the DCCT data do not support such an assumption. Thus, attempts to achieve optimal glycemic control should not aim at a certain HbA1c threshold within the diabetic range but follow "the goal of achieving normal glycemia as early as possible in as many type 1 patients as is safely possible."[19] In general, intensive diabetes therapy is associated with a moderately increased risk of weight gain and hypoglycemia.

Treatment Based on Pathogenetic Concepts

Recent experimental studies suggest a multifactorial pathogenesis of diabetic neuropathy. From the clinical point of view it is important to note that, on the basis of various pathogenetic mechanisms, therapeutic approaches could be derived, some of which have been evaluated in randomized clinical trials (TABLE 3). These drugs have been designed to favorably influence the underlying neuropathic process rather than for symptomatic pain treatment. For clinical use α-lipoic acid is licensed and used for treatment of symptomatic DSP in several countries worldwide, while epalrestat is marketed in Japan. According to a recent meta-analysis comprising 1258 patients, infusions of α-lipoic acid (600 mg i.v./day) ameliorated neuropathic symptoms and deficits after 3 weeks, while the ALADIN III Study showed that oral treatment with 600 mg t.i.d. resulted in a favorable effect on neuropathic deficits after 6 months.[20,21] Moreover, the SYDNEY 2 Trial suggests that treatment for 5 weeks using 600 mg of α-lipoic acid orally q.i.d. reduces the chief symptoms of diabetic polyneuropathy including pain, paresthesias, and numbness to a clinically meaningful degree.[22] Clinical and postmarketing surveillance studies have revealed a highly favorable safety profile of this drug. Ongoing phase III trials of the PKC-β inhibitor ruboxistaurin have to be awaited. Promising recent data from phase II studies have been reported for this compound,[23] the aldose reductase inhibitor ranirestat,[24] C-peptide,[25] and others.[26] Since in the foreseeable future normoglycemia will not be achievable in the majority of diabetic patients, the advantage of the aforementioned treatment approaches is that they may exert their effects despite prevailing hyperglycemia. Experimental studies of low-dose combined drug treatment suggest enhanced drug efficacy mediated by facilitatory interactions between drugs. In the future, combinations of drugs that produce synergistic effects could be a therapeutic option.

Symptomatic Treatment of Painful Neuropathy

Pain associated with diabetic neuropathy exerts a substantial impact on the quality of life, particularly by causing considerable interference in sleep and enjoyment of life. Pain is a subjective symptom of major clinical importance as it is often this complaint that motivates patients to seek health care. Painful symptoms in diabetic polyneuropathy may constitute a considerable management problem. The efficacy of a single therapeutic agent is not the rule, and

TABLE 2. Effects of randomized clinical trials of intensive diabetes therapy in prevention and treatment of diabetic polyneuropathy

				Neuropathy outcome			
Trial	n	Duration [years]	HbA_{1c} [%] CT vs. IT	Clinical	NCV	VPT	HRV
Type 1 diabetes							
• DCCT	1,441	up to 9	9.1 vs. 7.2	+	+	n.a.	+
• Stockholm Study	91	10	8.3 vs. 7.2	+	+	n.a.	n.a.
• Oslo Study	45	8	n.a.	n.a.	+	n.a.	n.a.
Type 2 diabetes							
• UKPDS	3,867	up to 15	7.9 vs. 7.0	–	n.a.	+ (*)	–
• Kumamoto Study	110	6	9.4 vs. 7.1	n.a.	+ (§)	+ (**)	–
• Steno Type 2 Study	160	7.8	9.0 vs. 7.7	n.a.	n.a.	–	+(§§)
• VA CSDM	153	2	9.5 vs. 7.4	–	n.a.	–	–

n.a. = not available; + = benefit; – = no effect; (*) = only $n = 217$ patients available after 15 years out of $n = 3,836$ at base line; (**) = significant difference between CT and IT for VPT on the hand but not foot; (§) = only NCV in the upper but not lower limbs available; (§§) = effects of ACE inhibitors, antioxidants, and statins not discernible from those of glycemic control; CT = conventional treatment; IT = intensive treatment; NCV = nerve conduction velocity; VPT = vibration perception threshold; HRV = heart rate variability.

TABLE 3. Treatment of diabetic neuropathy based on the putative pathogenetic mechanisms

Abnormality	Compound	Aim of treatment	Status of RCTs
Polyol pathway ↑	Aldose reductase inhibitors	Nerve sorbitol ↓	
	Sorbinil		Withdrawn (AE)
	Tolrestat		Withdrawn (AE)
	Ponalrestat		Ineffective
	Zopolrestat		Withdrawn (marginal effects)
	Zenarestat		Withdrawn (AE)
	Lidorestat		Withdrawn (AE)
	Fidarestat		Effective in phase II trials (studies halted)
	Ranirestat		Effective in phase II trial
	Epalrestat		Marketed in Japan
myo-inositol ↑	*Myo*-inositol	Nerve *myo*-inositol ↑	Equivocal
GLA synthesis ↓	γ-Linolenic acid (GLA)	EFA metabolism ↑	Withdrawn (effective: deficits)
Oxidative stress ↑	α-Lipoic acid	Oxygen free radicals ↓	Effective in RCTs (studies ongoing)
	Vitamin E	Oxygen free radicals ↓	Effective in 1 RCT
Nerve hypoxia ↑	Vasodilators	NBF ↑	
	ACE inhibitors		Effective in phase II trial
	Prostaglandin analogs		Effective in phase II trial
	$PhVEGF_{165}$ gene transfer	Angiogenesis ↑	Phase III trial ongoing
Protein kinase C ↑	PKC-β inhibitor (ruboxistaurin)	NBF ↑	Phase III trial ongoing
C-peptide ↓	C-peptide	NBF ↑	Effective in phase II trials
Neurotrophism ↓	Nerve growth factor (NGF)	Nerve regeneration, growth ↑	Ineffective
	BDNF	Nerve regeneration, growth ↑	Ineffective
LCFA metabolism ↓	Acetyl-L-carnitine	LCFA accumulation ↓	Ineffective
NEG ↑	Aminoguanidine	AGE accumulation ↓	Withdrawn

NEG = non-enzymatic glycation; AGE = advanced glycation end products; EFA = essential fatty acids; LCFA = long-chain fatty acids; AE = adverse events; NBF = nerve blood flow; RCTs = randomized clinical trials; BDNF = brain-derived neurotrophic factor.

simple analgesics are usually inadequate to control the pain. Therefore, various therapeutic schemes have been previously proposed, but none of them has been validated. Nonetheless, there is agreement that patients should be offered the available therapies in a stepwise fashion. Effective pain treatment considers a favorable balance between pain relief and side effects without implying a maximum effect. The possible treatments are summarized in TABLE 4. Prior to any decision regarding the appropriate treatment option, the diagnosis of the underlying neuropathic manifestation allowing to estimate its natural history should be established. In contrast to the agents that have been derived from the pathogenetic mechanisms of diabetic neuropathy, those used for symptomatic therapy were designed to modulate the pain, without favorably influencing the underlying neuropathy.[27]

The relative benefit of an active treatment over a control in clinical trials is usually expressed as the relative risk, the relative risk reduction, or the odds ratio. However, to estimate the extent of a therapeutic effect (i.e., pain relief) that can be translated into clinical practice, it is useful to apply a simple measure that serves the physician to select the appropriate treatment for the individual patient. Such a practical measure is the number needed to treat (NNT), that is, the number of patients that need to be treated with a particular therapy to observe a clinically relevant effect or adverse event in one patient. This measure is expressed as the reciprocal of the absolute risk reduction, that is, the difference between the proportion of events in the control group (Pc) and the proportion of events in the intervention group (Pi): NNT $= 1/(Pc{-}Pi)$. The 95% confidence interval (CI) of NNT can be obtained from the reciprocal value of the 95% CI for the absolute risk reduction. The NNT and NNH (number needed to harm) for the individual agents used in the treatment of painful diabetic neuropathy are given in TABLE 4.

Antidepressants

Recently the rate of publications of controlled clinical trials demonstrating significant pain relief with several drugs has accelerated. Nevertheless, the symptomatic pharmacological treatment of chronic painful diabetic neuropathy remains a challenge. A survey of physicians experienced in treating neuropathic pain demonstrated that only a minority would rate results of analgesic treatment as excellent or good using antidepressants (40%), anticonvulsants (35%), opioids (30%), or simple analgesics (18%).[28] For more than 30 years psychotropic agents, among which antidepressants and anticonvulsants have been evaluated most extensively, constitute an important component in the treatment of chronic pain syndromes. Several authors consider the tricyclic antidepressants (TCAs) to be the drug treatment of choice for neuropathic pain.[29] However, their use is limited due to relatively higher rates of adverse events and several contraindications. Thus, there is a need for agents that not

TABLE 4. Treatment options for painful diabetic neuropathy

Approach	Compound/measure	Dose per day	Remarks	NNT
Optimal diabetes control	Diet, OAD, insulin	Individual adaptation	Aim: $HbA_{1c} < 7.0\%$	-
Pathogenetically oriented treatment	α-Lipoic acid (thioctic acid)[§]	600 mg i.v. infusion 1,200–1,800 mg orally	Duration: 3 week Excellent safety profile	6.3*
Symptomatic treatment	*TCAs*			
	Amitriptyline	(10–)25–150 mg	NNMH: 15	2.1
	Desipramine	(10–)25–150 mg	NNMH: 24	2.2/3.2
	Imipramine	(10–)25–150 mg	CRR	1.3/2.4/3.0
	Clomipramine	(10–)25–150 mg	NNMH: 8.7	2.1
	Nortriptyline	(10–)25–150 mg	plus fluphenazine	1.2**
	SSRI			
	Citalopram	40 mg	Small sample	7.7 (ns)
	Paroxetine	40 mg	Small sample, CRR	2.9
	SSNRI			
	Venlafaxine	150–220 mg	Not licensed	6.9
	Duloxetine+	60–120 mg	NNT 120 mg, 60 mg	5.3, 4.9
	Anticonvulsants			
	Gabapentin	900–3,600 mg	High dose	3.8/4.0
	Pregabalin+	300–600 mg	NNT 600 mg, 300 mg	5.9, 4.2
	Carbamazepine	200–600 mg	Poor data quality	2.3
	Weak opioids			
	Tramadol	50–400 mg	NNMH: 7.8	3.1/4.3
	Local treatment			
	Capsaicin (0.025%) cream	q.i.d. topically	Max. duration: 8 week	8.1
	Strong opioids			
Pain resistant to standard pharmacotherapy	Oxycodone		Add-on treatment	2.6
	Electrical spinal cord stimulation (ESCS)		Invasive complications	
Physical therapy	TENS, medical gymnastics,		No AE	
	Balneotherapy, relaxation therapy		No AE	
	Acupuncture		Uncontrolled study	
	Psychological support			

[§]Available only in some countries; + licensed in US and EU; ns = not significant; *≥50% symptom relief after 3 weeks; **combined with fluphenazine; OAD = oral antidiabetic drugs; CRR = concentration-response relationship; NNMH = number needed for major harm; TENS = transcutaneous electrical nerve stimulation; AE = adverse events; SSRI = selective serotonin reuptake inhibitors; SSNRI: selective serotonin norepinephrine reuptake inhibitors.

only exert efficacy equal to or better than that achieved with TCAs, but can also have a more favorable side effect profile. Because selective serotonin reuptake inhibitors (SSRI) have been found to be less effective than TCAs, recent interest has focused on antidepressants with dual selective inhibition of serotonin and noradrenaline (SSNRI), such as duloxetine and venlafaxine. The efficacy and safety of duloxetine was evaluated in three controlled studies using a dose of 60 and 120 mg/Tag over 12 weeks.[30,31] In all three studies the average 24-h pain intensity was significantly reduced by administering both doses as compared to the placebo treatment; the difference between active and placebo meant an achievement of statistical significance after 1 week. The response rates defined as ≥50% pain reduction were 48.2% (120 mg/day), 47.2% (60 mg/day), and 27.9% (placebo), giving an NNT of 4.9 (95% CI: 3.6–7.6) for 120 mg/day and 5.3 (3.8–8.3) for 60 mg/day. The most frequent side effects of duloxetine (60/120 mg/day) include nausea (16.7/27.4%), somnolence (20.2/28.3%), dizziness (9.6/23%), constipation (14.9/10.6%), dry mouth (7.1/15%), and reduced appetite (2.6/12.4%). These adverse events are usually mild-to-moderate and transient. To minimize them, the starting dose should ideally be 30 mg/day for 4–5 days. In contrast to TCAs and some anticonvulsants duloxetine does not cause weight gain.

In a 6-week trial comprising 244 patients, the analgesic response rates were 56%, 39%, and 34% in patients given 150–225 mg venlafaxine, 75 mg venlafaxine, and placebo, respectively. As patients with depression were excluded, the effect of venlafaxin (150–225 mg) was attributed to an analgesic, rather than antidepressant, effect. The most common adverse events were tiredness and nausea.[32] Duloxetine but not venlafaxine has been licensed for the treatment of painful diabetic neuropathy.

Anticonvulsants

Gabapentin is an anticonvulsant structurally related to γ-aminobutyric acid (GABA), a neurotransmitter that plays a role in pain transmission and modulation. The exact mechanisms of action of this drug in neuropathic pain are not fully elucidated. Among others, they involve an interaction with the system L-amino acid transporter and high affinity binding to the α-2-δ subunit of voltage-activated calcium channels. In an 8-week multicenter dose-escalation trial including 165 diabetic patients with painful neuropathy, 60% of the patients on gabapentin (3600 mg/day achieved in 67%) had at least moderate pain relief compared to 33% on placebo. Dizziness and somnolence were the most frequent adverse events in about 23% of the patients each.[33] Pregabalin is a more specific α-2-δ ligand with a sixfold higher binding affinity than gabapentin. The efficacy and safety of pregabalin was reported in a pooled analysis of six studies over 5–11 weeks in 1346 diabetic patients with painful neuropathy. The response rates defined as ≥50% pain reduction were 46%

(600 mg/day), 39% (300 mg/day), 27% (150 mg/day), and 22% (placebo), giving an NNT of 4.2, 5.9, and 20.[34] The most frequent side effects for 150–600 mg/day are dizziness (22.0%), somnolence (12.1%), peripheral edema (10.0%), headache (7.2%), and weight gain (5.4%). The evidence supporting a favorable effect in painful diabetic neuropathy is more solid and dose titration is considerably easier for pregabalin than gabapentin. Although the sodium channel blocker, carbamazepine, has been widely used for treating neuropathic pain, it cannot be recommended in painful diabetic neuropathy due to very limited data. The successor drug, oxcarbazepine, has shown only marginal efficacy and, therefore, will not be marketed.

Opioids

The weak opioid tramadol is effective in painful DSP, but most severe pain requires administration of strong opioids, such as oxycodone. Although there is little data available on combination treatment, combinations of different substance classes have to be used in patients with pain resistant to monotherapy. Two trials over 4 and 6 weeks have demonstrated significant pain relief and improvement in quality of life following treatment with controlled release oxycodone, a pure μ-agonist, in a dose range of 10–100 mg (mean 40 mg/day) in patients with painful diabetic neuropathy, whose pain was not adequately controlled on standard treatment with antidepressants and anticonvulsants that were not discontinued throughout the trial.[35,36] As expected, adverse events were frequent and typical of opioid-related side effects. A recent study examined the maximum tolerable dose of a combination treatment of gabapentin and morphine as compared to monotherapy of each drug. The maximum tolerable dose was significantly lower and efficacy was better during combination therapy than monotherapy, suggesting an additive interaction between the two drugs.[37] The results of these studies suggest that opioids should be included among the therapeutic options for painful diabetic neuropathy, provided that careful selection of patients unresponsive to standard treatments, regular monitoring, appropriate dose titration, and management of side effects are ensured. Combination therapy using antidepressants and anticonvulsants may also be useful, particularly if monotherapy is not tolerated due to side effects.

Nonpharmacological Treatment

Since there is no completely satisfactory pharmacotherapy of painful diabetic neuropathy, nonpharmacological treatment options, such as psychological support, transcutaneous electrical nerve stimulation (TENS), or physical measures (e.g., cold water immersion) have been tried. So far as the pharmacological treatment is concerned, considerable efforts should also be made to develop effective nonpharmacological approaches. We recently showed a better effect of high frequency muscle stimulation (HFMS) than TENS on neuropathic symptoms after 3 days.[38] A frequency-modulated electromagnetic nerve stimulation (FREMS) applied during 10 sessions over 3 weeks resulted in a significant pain reduction as compared to placebo stimulation.[39] Monochromatic infrared energy (MIRE) has been shown to reduce neuropathic symptoms and signs in diabetic patients in uncontrolled studies.[40] However, 30 minutes of active MIRE applied 3 days per week for 4 weeks was no more effective than placebo in increasing sensation in subjects with diabetic peripheral neuropathy,[41] emphasizing the need for controlled studies in this area to allow an evidence-based treatment decision.

CONCLUSIONS

Although considerable improvement in the quality of controlled trials has recently been achieved, no major breakthrough in slowing the progression of diabetic neuropathy in the long run has been achieved with drugs used on the basis of present pathogenetic concepts. Some of the newer drugs have shown promising results in phase II trials, which require confirmation from large phase III trials. It is conceivable that drugs interfering with the pathogenesis of diabetic neuropathy may be most effective in terms of prevention, rather than intervention. Although several novel analgesic drugs have recently been introduced into clinical practice, the pharmacological treatment of chronic painful diabetic neuropathy remains a challenge for the physician. Individual tolerability remains a major aspect in any treatment decision. Almost no information is available from controlled trials on long-term analgesic efficacy and only a few studies have used drug combinations. Combination drug use or the addition of a new drug to a therapeutic regimen may lead to increased efficacy. In future, drug combinations may also include those aimed at symptomatic pain relief and quality of life on the one hand, and improvement or slowing of the progression of the underlying neuropathic process on the other.

REFERENCES

1. Consensus Statement. 1988. Report and recommendations of the San Antonio conference on diabetic neuropathy. Diabetes Care **11:** 592–597.
2. Sima, A.A.F., P.K. Thomas, D. Ishii & A. Vinik. 1997. Diabetic neuropathies. Diabetologia **40:** B74–B77.
3. Shaw, J.E., P.Z. Zimmet, F.A. Gries & D. Ziegler. 2003. Epidemiology of diabetic neuropathy. *In* Textbook of Diabetic Neuropathy. F.A. Gries, N.E. Cameron, P.A. Low, D. Ziegler, Eds.: 64–82. Thieme. Stuttgart, New York.
4. Forsblom, C.M., T. Sane, P.H. Groop, *et al.* 1998. Risk factors for mortality in type II (non-insulin-dependent) diabetes: evidence of a role for neuropathy and a protective effect of HLA-DR4. Diabetologia **4:** 1253–1262.

5. COPPINI, D.V., P.A. BOWTELL, C. WENG, *et al.* 2000. Showing neuropathy is related to increased mortality in diabetic patients—a survival analysis using an accelerated failure time model. J. Clin. Epidemiol. **53:** 519–523.
6. ABBOTT, C.A., L. VILEIKYTE, S. WILLIAMSON, *et al.* 1998. Multicenter study of the incidence of and predictive risk factors for diabetic neuropathic foot ulceration. Diabetes Care **21:** 1071–1075.
7. DAOUSI, C., I.A. MACFARLANE, A. WOODWARD, *et al.* 2004. Chronic painful peripheral neuropathy in an urban community: a controlled comparison of people with and without diabetes. Diabetic Med. **21:** 976–982.
8. GALER, B.S., A. GIANAS & M.P. JENSEN. 2000. Painful diabetic neuropathy: epidemiology, pain description, and quality of life. Diabetes Res. Clin. Pract. **47:** 123–128.
9. CHAN, A.W., I.A. MACFARLANE, D.R. BOWSHER, *et al.* 1990. Chronic pain in patients with diabetes mellitus: comparison with non-diabetic population. Pain Clinic **3:** 147–159.
10. BENBOW, S.J., A.W. CHAN, D. BOWSHER, *et al.* 1993. A prospective study of painful symptoms, small-fibre function and peripheral vascular disease in chronic painful diabetic neuropathy. Diabetic Med. **11:** 17–21.
11. BOULTON, A.J.M., R.A. MALIK, J.C. AREZZO & J.M. SOSENKO. 2004. Diabetic somatic neuropathies. Diabetes Care **27:** 1458–1486.
12. CAMERON, N.E., S.E. EATON, M.A. COTTER & S. TESFAYE. 2001. Vascular factors and metabolic interactions in the pathogenesis of diabetic neuropathy. Diabetologia **44:** 1973–1988.
13. DYCK, P.J. 1988. Detection, characterization, and staging of polyneuropathy: assessed in diabetics. Muscle Nerve **11:** 21–32.
14. YOUNG, M.J., A.J.M. BOULTON, A.F. MACLEOD, *et al.* 1993. A multicentre study of the prevalence of diabetic peripheral neuropathy in the United Kingdom hospital clinic population. Diabetologia **36:** 150–154.
15. HERMAN, W.H. & L. KENNEDY. 2005. Underdiagnosis of peripheral neuropathy in type 2 diabetes. Diabetes Care **28:** 1480–1481.
16. PROCEEDINGS OF A CONSENSUS DEVELOPMENT CONFERENCE ON STANDARDIZED MEASURES IN DIABETIC NEUROPATHY. 1992. Diabetes Care **15**(Suppl 3): 1080–1107
17. ZIEGLER, D. 2003. Glycemic control. *In* Textbook of Diabetic NeuropatyF.A. Gries, N.E. Cameron, P.A. Low, D Ziegler, Eds.: 91–96. Thieme. Stuttgart, New York.
18. MARTIN, C.L., J. ALBERS, W.H. HERMAN, *et al.* 2006. DCCT//EDIC Research Group. Neuropathy among the diabetes control and complications trial cohort 8 years after trial completion. Diabetes Care **29:** 340–344.
19. THE DIABETES CONTROL AND COMPLICATIONS TRIAL RESEARCH GROUP. 1996. The absence of a glycemic threshold for the development of long-term complications: the perspective of the Diabetes Control and Complications Trial. Diabetes **45:** 1289–1298.
20. ZIEGLER, D., H. NOWAK, P. KEMPLER, *et al.* 2004. Treatment of symptomatic diabetic polyneuropathy with the antioxidant aa-lipoic acid: a meta-analysis. Diabetic Med. **21:** 114–121.
21. ZIEGLER, D. 2004. Thioctic acid for patients with symptomatic diabetic neuropathy. a critical review. Treat. Endocrinol. **3:** 1–17.
22. ZIEGLER, D., A. AMETOV, A. BARINOV, *et al.* 2006. Oral treatment with α-lipoic acid improves symptomatic diabetic polyneuropathy. The SYDNEY 2 Trial. Diabetes Care (In press).

23. VINIK, A.I., V. BRIL, P. KEMPLER, *et al.* 2005. Treatment of symptomatic diabetic peripheral neuropathy with the protein kinase C beta-inhibitor ruboxistaurin mesylate during a 1-year, randomized, placebo-controlled, double-blind clinical trial. Clin. Ther. **27:** 1164–1180.
24. BRIL, V. & R.A. BUCHANAN. 2006. Long-term effects of ranirestat (AS-3201) on peripheral nerve function in patients with diabetic sensorimotor polyneuropathy. Diabetes Care **29:** 68–72.
25. EKBERG, K., T. BRISMAR, B.L. JOHANSSON, *et al.* 2003. Amelioration of sensory nerve dysfunction by C-Peptide in patients with type 1 diabetes. Diabetes **52:** 536–541.
26. BOULTON, A.J., A.I. VINIK, J.C. AREZZO, *et al.* 2005. Diabetic neuropathies: a statement by the American Diabetes Association. Diabetes Care **28:** 956–962.
27. ZIEGLER, D. 2003. Treatment of neuropathic pain. *In* Textbook of Diabetic Neuropathy F.A. Gries, N.E. Cameron, P.A. Low, D. Ziegler, Eds.: 211–224. Thieme. Stuttgart, New York.
28. DAVIES, H.T.O., I.K. CROMBIE, M. LONSDALE & W.A. MACRAE. 1991. Consensus and contention in the treatment of chronic nerve-damage pain. Pain **47:** 191–196.
29. FINNERUP, N.B., M. OTTO, H.J. MCQUAY, *et al.* 2005. Algorithm for neuropathic pain treatment: an evidence based proposal. Pain **118:** 289–305.
30. GOLDSTEIN, D.J., Y. LU, M.J. DETKE, *et al.* 2005. Duloxetine vs. placebo in patients with painful diabetic neuropathy. Pain **116:** 109–118.
31. RASKIN, J., Y.L. PRITCHETT, F. WANG, *et al.* 2005. A double-blind, randomized multicenter trial comparing duloxetine with placebo in the management of diabetic peripheral neuropathic pain. Pain Med. **6:** 346–356.
32. ROWBOTHAM, M.C., V. GOLI, N.R. KUNZ & D. LEI. 2004. Venlafaxine extended release in the treatment of painful diabetic neuropathy: a double-blind, placebo-controlled study. Pain **110:** 697–706.
33. BACKONJA, M., A. BEYDOUN, K.R. EDWARDS, *et al.* 1998. Gabapentin for the symptomatic treatment of painful neuropathy in patients with diabetes mellitus. JAMA **280:** 1831–1836.
34. GRIESING, T., R. FREEMAN, J. ROSENSTOCK, *et al.* 2005. Efficacy, safety, and tolerability of pregabalin treatment for diabetic peripheral neuropathy: findings from 6 randomized controlled trials [abstract]. Diabetologia **48**(Suppl 1):A351.
35. WATSON, C.P., D. MOULIN, J. WATT-WATSON, *et al.* 2003. Controlled-release oxycodone relieves neuropathic pain: a randomized controlled trial in painful diabetic neuropathy. Pain **105:** 71–78.
36. GIMBEL, J.S., P. RICHARDS, R.K. PORTENOY. 2003. Controlled-release oxycodone for pain in diabetic neuropathy: a randomized controlled trial. Neurology **60:** 927–934.
37. GILRON, I., J.M. BAILEY, D. TU, *et al.* 2005. Morphine, gabapentin, or their combination for neuropathic pain. N. Engl. J. Med. **31:** 1324–1334.
38. REICHSTEIN, L., S. LABRENZ, D. ZIEGLER & S. MARTIN. 2005. Effective treatment of symptomatic diabetic polyneuropathy by high-frequency external muscle stimulation. Diabetologia **48:** 824–828.
39. BOSI, E., M. CONTI, C. VERMIGLI, *et al.* 2005. Effectiveness of frequency-modulated electromagnetic neural stimulation in the treatment of painful diabetic neuropathy. Diabetologia **48:** 817–823.
40. POWELL, M.W., D.H. CARNEGIE & T.J. BURKE. 2006. Reversal of diabetic peripheral neuropathy with phototherapy (MIRE™) decreases falls and the fear of falling and improves activities of daily living in seniors. Age Ageing **35:** 11–16.

41. CLIFFT, J.K., R.J. KASSER, T.S. NEWTON & A.J. BUSH. 2005. The effect of monochromatic infrared energy on sensation in patients with diabetic peripheral neuropathy: a double-blind, placebo-controlled study. Diabetes Care **28:** 2896–2900.

The Effect of Streptozotocin-Induced Diabetes on the Rat Seminal Vesicle

A Possible Pathophysiological Basis for Disorders of Ejaculation

J.F.B. MORRISON,[a] S. DHANASEKARAN,[a] RAJAN SHEEN,[a] C.M. FRAMPTON,[b] AND ERIC MENSAH-BROWN[a]

[a]*Departments of Physiology, Anatomy, and Pharmacology, Faculty of Medicine and Health Sciences, UAE University, Al Ain, United Arab Emirates*

[b]*Department of Medicine, Otago University, Christchurch, New Zealand*

ABSTRACT: In the streptozotocin (STZ)-diabetic rat major increases in noradrenaline concentration and content of the seminal vesicles were evident as early as 7 weeks following induction of hyperglycemia and returned toward normal after 34 weeks of hyperglycemia. There were significant reductions in the concentration and content of dopamine at 19–42 weeks of diabetes, and small occasionally significant reductions in the content of serotonin and adrenaline, particularly around 19–26 weeks after STZ treatment. The uptake of tritiated noradrenaline in the diabetics was increased at 12 weeks compared to the controls, and decreased to control levels with increasing age. Release of tritiated noradrenline was increased in response to electrical field stimulation and high potassium solutions, and raising calcium concentration caused increased release at rest and during electrical stimulation. Immunohistochemical demonstration of tyrosine hydroxylase was increased during the period when the noradrenaline concentration and content were elevated. It is concluded that there are significant changes in the sympathetic innervation of the seminal vesicle during the course of STZ diabetes, and that alterations in the reuptake, release, and synthesis of the neurotransmitter noradrenaline may contribute to changes in the concentration of the amine in the tissue. It is possible that the changes observed are related to the remodeling and regrowth of sympathetic nerve endings damaged in the early stages of hyperglycemia. These changes may also contribute to disorders of ejaculation in diabetes.

KEYWORDS: male reproductive dysfunction; seminal vesicle; noradrenaline; catecholamines

Address for correspondence: Prof. John Morrison, Department of Physiology, Faculty of Medicine and Health Sciences, UAE University, P.O. Box 17666, Al Ain, United Arab Emirates. Voice: +971-3-7039-532; fax: +971-3-7671-966.
e-mail: john.morrison@uaeu.ac.ae

Ann. N.Y. Acad. Sci. 1084: 267–279 (2006).
doi: 10.1196/annals.1372.013

INTRODUCTION

Three types of disorder of ejaculation are reported in diabetic men: premature ejaculation, ejaculatory failure, and retrograde ejaculation. Premature ejaculation is recognized as a complication of diabetes, and occurs more commonly in patients with poor glycemic control than in those with good control.[1] Ejaculatory failure is probably a consequence of autonomic neuropathy and may be present in up to 40% of men with diabetes,[2] while retrograde ejaculation is reported as being associated with low pressure in the bladder neck in diabetic men.[3] The main smooth muscles involved in both processes are excited by the sympathetic system[4] and the innervation also includes some afferents and some parasympathetic efferents.[5] The sympathetic efferents travel through three main pathways involving neurons in the sympathetic chain, inferior mesenteric ganglia, and the pelvic ganglia.[5]

The integrity of the sympathetic innervation of the prostate gland is believed to be maintained by the presence of nerve growth factor (NGF) in the organ,[6] and there is a relationship between the levels of β-NGF mRNA and the density of the sympathetic innervation.[7,8] In streptozotocin (STZ) diabetes, the levels of NGF in the prostate gland are increased and it was of interest to see whether levels of noradrenaline in the seminal vesicle also change as they do in some other tissues (e.g., heart, tail artery, and penis) of diabetic animals.[9,10] The objective was to examine the changes in the concentrations and release of amines, particularly the sympathetic transmitter noradrenaline, in the seminal vesicles as these may shed some light on the changes in ejaculatory function found in diabetics.

METHODS

Sample Collection, Preservation, and Extraction

Experiments were performed on adult male Wistar rats that had been injected with STZ (60 mg/kg) at 10 weeks of age. The tissues of these animals were compared with those from age-matched controls. The seminal vesicles were excised up to 68 weeks later under pentobarbitone anesthesia (60 mg/kg) and blood glucose was estimated on samples of inferior vena caval blood at that time, the glucose oxidase method. All experiments were performed within the guidelines of the Animal Ethics Committee of the Faculty of Medicine and Health Sciences, United Arab Emirates University.

The tissues were removed, weighed, and samples were analyzed for amine concentration using high-performance liquid chromatography (HPLC) as has been described previously.[9,10]

Data on amine concentrations and on the amine content of the organs are presented as mean ± SEM, statistical significance was calculated using an unpaired Student's *t*-test, comparing the diabetic group with the control group of the same age.

Release and Uptake of ^{3}H-Noradrenaline

The seminal vesicles were carefully removed from four STZ-diabetic rats that had been hyperglycemic for 34 weeks and from four age-matched controls under urethane anesthesia (6 g/kg). These tissues were incubated with tritiated noradrenaline (^{3}H-NA) for 1.5 h in Tyrode solution at 37°C. The labeled tissue was transferred into tissue baths after washing off the excess ^{3}H-NA and superfused with Tyrode solution containing desipramine (10 μM). After equilibration, the resting release of ^{3}H-NA, and its release during (*a*) electrical field stimulation (EFS) [50V at 20 Hz], (*b*) depolarization with 13 mM K^+, (*c*) 5 mM Ca^{2+} at rest, and (*d*) EFS in the presence of 5 mM Ca^{2+} were examined.The superfusate was collected every 5 min and emission for the ^{3}H-NA was measured in a β-counter, and converted to counts per minute (cpm).

The rate of release was calculated and the data from all experiments were combined for the analysis comparing uptake levels between the different stimuli from diabetic and control samples. Analysis was undertaken using a general linear model with experiment and diabetic status as between sample effects and stimuli as a within-sample factor. When this analysis indicated significant stimuli or stimuli by diabetic status interactions these were further explored using Fisher's least significant difference tests in an appropriate pairwise manner. Uptake levels were $\log_e$ transformed prior to analysis and statistical significance was assumed when $P < 0.05$.

In separate experiments on animals that had been hyperglycemic for 12, 26, or 68 weeks (and their age-matched controls), the seminal vesicles were loaded with ^{3}H-NA for 1.5 h, and the tissues were washed and homogenized and the radioactivity counted. In some experiments, one of the pair of seminal vesicles was loaded with ^{3}H-NA in the presence of 10 μM desipramine, to confirm that the uptake mechanism was uptake-1. Calculations of the activity of the uptake-1 transporter were made by subtraction of the two results.

Immunohistochemistry

Six diabetic and age-matched nondiabetic rats were fixed by perfusion with 4% paraformaldehyde and the whole of the genital tract excised and kept in the fixative for a further 3 h at room temperature. The seminal vesicles of each rat was dissected out and placed in 30% sucrose and immunostained using the floating method. The tissues were transferred from 30% sucrose in 0.1 M phosphate-buffered solution (PBS) into cryomatrix frozen section-embedding medium (Shandon, Pittsburgh, PA) on metallic holders and sections frozen slowly on the cold stage of the cryostat (Shandon, Life Sciences Int., Cheshire, UK). Sections of 50–60 μm thickness were subsequently cut and after washing 3 × 5 min in 0.1 M PBS, the sections were incubated in 3% hydrogen peroxide in methanol for 30 min to block endogenous peroxidase after which they were washed with PBS. The sections were then incubated with rabbit polyclonal anti-tyrosine hydroxylase (TH) (Chemicon, Temecula, CA) diluted 1:5000 overnight at room temperature. The sections were washed 3 × 5 min with PBS and incubated with the link antibody comprising biotinylated anti-rabbit IgG diluted 1:500 for 1 h (Jackson Immuno Research Laboratories, West Baltimore Pike, PA), washed as previously described and then incubated with peroxidase labeled-extrAvidin (Sigma, St. Louis, MO) diluted 1:1000 also for 1 h. The diluent used was 0.3% triton X in 0.1 M PBS. Peroxidase activity was demonstrated with diaminobenzidene. A 1.0 mL of diaminobenzidene hydrochloride in phosphate buffer (Sigma) was diluted to 50 mL with 1 mL of 3.5% nickel chloride, 7.5 μL of 30% hydrogen peroxide, and distilled water. The sections were incubated in the diaminobenzidene for 3–5 min in a hooded incubator. The reaction was stopped with phosphate buffer and the sections mounted on gelatin-coated slides. After air drying, the sections were dehydrated, cleared in xylene, and coverslipped using Cytoseal 60 mounting medium (Stephens Scientific, Riversdale, NJ).

RESULTS

Blood Glucose

The control blood glucose concentrations were in the range 53–70 mg/dL (mean 62 mg/dL) and the diabetic levels were 189–600 mg/dL (mean 302 mg/dL). Age had no effect on blood glucose in the control group, but in the diabetic group there was a negative correlation between blood glucose and duration of diabetes; however, this was not statistically significant in this study.

Effects of Age on Amine Concentrations in the Seminal Vesicles of Control Animals

5HIAA (5-hydroxyindole-acetic acid) was not detected in any sample of the seminal vesicle, whether from a diabetic or a control animal. There was an increase in serotonin concentration in the seminal vesicles ($P = 0.028$), but there was no significant effect of age on the concentrations of noradrenaline, adrenaline, or dopamine.

EFFECTS OF STZ DIABETES

The largest change observed in the studies of the effects of STZ diabetes on the seminal vesicle was a statistically significant increase in noradrenaline whereas the other amines showed only minor changes compared with the control tissues of the same age. FIGURE 1 shows the percentage changes in

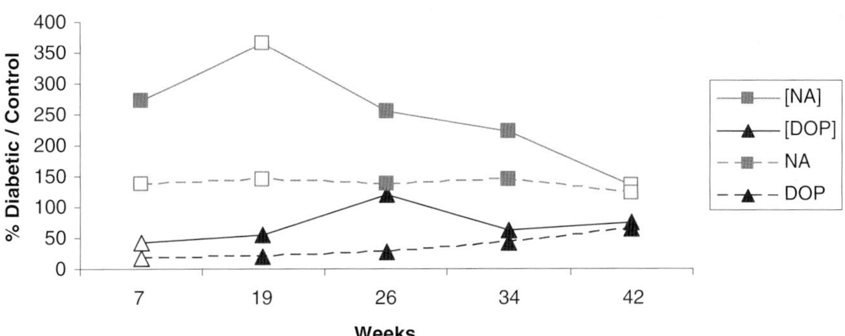

FIGURE 1. Noradrenaline and dopamine concentration and content in the seminal vesicles during STZ diabetes. Filled Symbols $P < 0.05$

concentration and total content of noradrenaline and dopamine at 17, 29, 44, and 52 weeks of age. The diabetic group were injected with STZ at the age of 10 weeks, so the duration of hyperglycemia was 7, 19, 34, and 52 weeks, respectively.

TABLE 1 shows that in the seminal vesicle, noradrenaline is markedly elevated to a highly significant P value during the first 34 weeks of hyperglycemia. During this period there are few significant changes in adrenaline or serotonin; however, both increased significantly at 26 weeks following STZ. Dopamine falls throughout the period of the experiment, and to statistically significant levels at 26, 34, and 42 weeks of hyperglycemia. TABLE 2 shows the total content of each amine per seminal vesicle and shows increases in noradrenaline, which are statistically significant at 26 and 34 weeks following STZ. There were decreases in the other amines, and the change in dopamine was significant throughout the time course studied; also the decreases in adrenaline and serotonin were significant at 26 and 34 weeks, respectively.

Release of ^{3}H-NA from the Seminal Vesicles

The release of ^{3}H-NA was used to study the release of noradrenaline from the isolated seminal vesicles. ^{3}H-NA release was measured in control and diabetic tissues in identical conditions at rest and during EFS, in a high potassium solution (13 mM [K^+]) that evoked depolarization, and in Tyrode containing 5 mM [Ca^+] to facilitate synaptic release. The release of ^{3}H-NA from control and diabetic tissues increased significantly during EFS; however, the release was greater from the diabetic tissues ($P < 0.05$).

FIGURE 2 shows that the release from diabetic tissues was also greater in 13 mM [K^+] ($P < 0.05$) and in 5 mM [Ca^{2+}] ($P < 0.05$). Field stimulation

TABLE 1. Concentrations of amines in the seminal vesicle of control and diabetic rats

	Duration of diabetes				
	7 weeks	19 weeks	26 weeks	34 weeks	42 weeks
			Noradrenaline pg/mg		
Control	551 ± 38.2 (4)	528 ± 13.5 (4)	470.1 ± 20.2 (4)	575 ± 13.5 (5)	721 ± 28.3 (5)
Diabetic	1506 ± 115.1 (4)	1931 ± 306.3 (4)	1195.9 ± 43.0 (6)	1280 ± 21.1 (5)	976 ± 40.0 (5)
P	0.006	0.055	1.24E-06	8.81E-05	NS
% Diabetic/control	273	366	254	223	135
			Adrenaline pg/mg		
Control	435 ± 32.7 (4)	481 ± 26.3 (4)	384.6 ± 15.1 (4)	430 ± 10.1 (5)	503 ± 21.4 (5)
Diabetic	640 ± 108.5 (4)	523 ± 28.1 (4)	603 ± 55 (6)	463 ± 45.4 (5)	517 ± 16.8 (5)
P	NS	NS	0.009	NS	NS
% Diabetic/control	147	109	157	108	103
			Serotonin pg/mg		
Control	280 ± 70.8 (4)	294 ± 27.1 (4)	217.6 ± 13.2 (4)	421 ± 8.8 (5)	442 ± 18.8 (5)
Diabetic	281 ± 111.5 (4)	332 ± 12.3 (4)	259.2 ± 10.6 (6)	443 ± 7.9 (5)	445 ± 8.3 (5)
P	NS	NS	0.04	NS	NS
% Diabetic/control	100	113	119	105	101
			Dopamine pg/mg		
Control	516 ± 31.9 (4)	361 ± 23.3 (4)	580.5 ± 59.9 (4)	498 ± 39.9 (5)	453 ± 12.4 (5)
Diabetic	223 ± 104.5 (4)	195 ± 14.4 (4)	282.8 ± 25.6 (6)	310 ± 22.6 (5)	338 ± 29.4 (5)
P	NS	0.01	0.009	0.02	0.049
% Diabetic/control	43	54	48	62	75

Data in pg/mg wet weight (mean ± SEM, number of animals); *P* = statistical significance.

TABLE 2. Total content of amines in the seminal vesicle of control and diabetic rats

	Duration of diabetes				
	7 weeks	19 weeks	26 weeks	34 weeks	42 weeks
			Noradrenaline pg		
Control	329160 ± 67087 (4)	417888 ± 23736 (4)	341678 ± 16545.11 (4)	354915 ± 39499 (5)	461190 ± 48439 (5)
Diabetic	453319 ± 75849 (4)	609223 ± 163646 (4)	471889 ± 11290 (4)	518563 ± 5719 (5)	562739 ± 85543 (5)
P	NS	NS	0.0013	0.05	NS
% Diabetic/control	138	146	138	146	122
			Adrenaline pg		
Control	259180 ± 54279 (4)	379152 ± 27048 (4)	280724 ± 19606 (4)	269410 ± 37795 (5)	349745 ± 78686 (5)
Diabetic	200813 ± 67097 (4)	160265.9 ± 15811 (4)	232313 ± 24931 (4)	188245 ± 23194 (5)	289819 ± 20586 (5)
P	NS	0.0009	NS	NS	NS
% Diabetic/control	77	42	83	70	83
			Serotonin pg		
Control	150921 ± 56853 (4)	237773 ± 45302 (4)	157718 ± 7512 (4)	264658 ± 41456 (5)	287669 ± 25037 (5)
Diabetic	99447 ± 67048 (4)	101643 ± 7665 (4)	105076 ± 2243 (4)	177174 ± 14134 (5)	247582 ± 10371 (5)
P	NS	NS	0.003	NS	NS
% Diabetic/control	66	43	67	67	86
			Dopamine pg		
Control	296846 ± 37581 (4)	281938 ± 11657 (4)	426617 ± 34578 (4)	311663 ± 39247 (5)	292511 ± 12361 (5)
Diabetic	54841 ± 35556 (4)	59867 ± 7556 (4)	119540 ± 8280 (4)	129667 ± 33485 (5)	190991 ± 9606 (5)
P	0.003	1.74E-05	0.003	0.007	0.0002
% Diabetic/control	18	21	28	42	65

Data in pgs per seminal vesicle (mean ± SEM, number of animals); *P* = statistical significance.

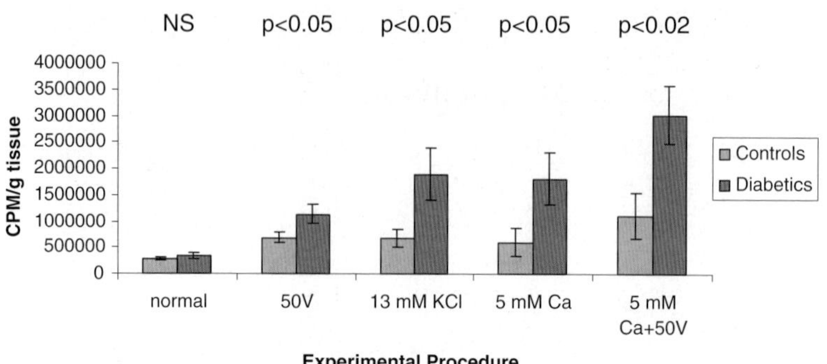

FIGURE 2. Release of ^{3}H-NA from the seminal vesicles after 34 weeks of hyperglycemia.

in the presence of 5mM [Ca^{2+}] also caused greater release from the diabetic tissues ($P < 0.02$).

Uptake of ^{3}H-NA by Diabetic and Control Seminal Vesicles

Uptake-1 was measured in the seminal vesicles of control and diabetic rats after 12, 26, and 68 weeks of hyperglycemia. At 12 weeks the activity of reuptake-1 in the diabetics was increased to 276% of the control level in animals of the same age; this figure was statistically significant ($P < 0.01$). However, there was no significant difference between the controls and diabetics at 26 and 68 weeks.

TH Immunoreactivity in the Seminal Vesicles

TH immunoreactivity was intense in nerve fibers and varicose terminals and a few neuronal cell bodies in the seminal vesicles. Immunoreactive nerve fibers and terminals were discernible mainly in the smooth muscle layer of the seminal vesicles, with a sparse distribution of immunoreactivity around the glandular epithelium. Diabetes increased both the intensity and distribution of TH-immunoreactive nerve fibers and terminals (FIG. 3).

DISCUSSION

Human and experimental diabetes is accompanied by changes in the autonomic innervation[11] of many organs,[12,13] and the changes that have been observed in both include the presence of dilated axons, engorged nerve endings, and other changes that are often described as degenerative in nature.[14]

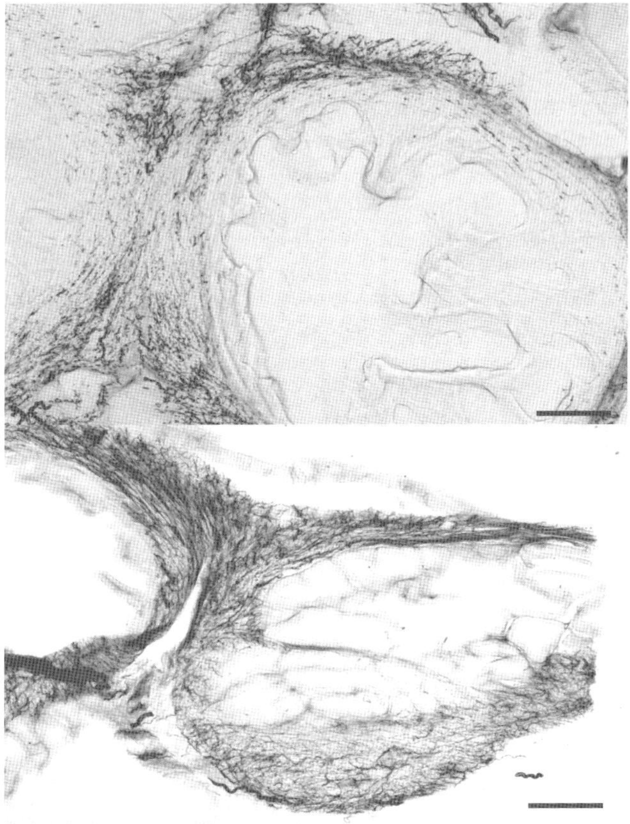

FIGURE 3. Micrographs showing nerve fibers immunoreactive to TH in the seminal vesicles of control (*top*) and diabetic rats (*bottom*). Bar = 100 μm.

However, there is also a possibility that the sympathetic nerves respond to axonal retraction by remodeling and regrowth, and there are papers in which the regeneration of unmyelinated axons has been described.[15] It may be that the exact distribution of the nerve terminals differs from normal, but a change in the number and size of axons may be accompanied by a redistribution of terminals,[16] which may have implications for the function of the target organs.

In humans, the prostate gland and seminal vesicle receive a rich sympathetic innervation,[4] which contains noradrenaline and the peptide neuropeptide Y (NPY)[17]; the latter is believed to modulate the release of noradrenaline[18] which is responsible for the initiation of ejaculation. There is evidence for an increased density and release of NPY in the diabetic seminal vesicle.[19] Dopamine β-hydroxylase was found in most of the neurons of the sympathetic chain and inferior mesenteric ganglion, mainly the former. In contrast, only two-thirds to three-quarters of the pelvic ganglia neurons contained dopamine-β-hydroxylase.[5,20] Neurons that innervate the seminal vesicles of the pig[21] contain TH and originate mainly in the ipsilateral inferior mesenteric ganglia. In the guinea pig the sympathetic innervation of the circular smooth muscle of the guinea pig seminal vesicle is mainly excitatory and using α-adrenergic mechanisms, and noradrenaline and adrenaline both increase the muscular activity of the seminal vesicle.[22] Circular smooth muscles of this species show a slow depolarization in response to release of noradrenaline, mediated through the activation of α-adrenoceptors; however, there is also evidence of corelease of ATP, which also induces excitatory junction potentials in this smooth muscle.[23] The secretory cells of the guinea pig seminal vesicle also have a sympathetic innervation from short cholinergic neurons whose preganglionic input is in the hypogastric nerve. Secretory cells are themselves inhibited by α-1 and β-2 adrenoreceptor-mediated mechanisms, but adrenergic inhibition of secretion induced by autonomic nerves is largely due to activation of inhibitory prejunctional α-2 receptors on the secretomotor terminals.[24]

The results presented here indicate that the concentration of noradrenaline increases in the seminal vesicles during the course of STZ diabetes, and peaks after about 20–30 weeks of hyperglycemia. This is in keeping with observations on other tissues, including the heart, tail artery, and penis,[9,10] and is associated with an increased presence of TH-containing nerve terminals. This enzyme is present in nerve fibers that are generally larger than normal and may have bulbous nerve endings; their density is also greater than in the controls (FIG. 3). In addition to the increase in presence of some synthetic enzymes, the sympathetic neurons innervating the seminal vesicle exhibit greater release of the amine in a variety of situations including during depolarization using electrical stimulation of high $[K^+]$. The release process involves calcium ions and there is a statistically significant increase in noradrenaline release at rest in 5 mM $[Ca^{2+}]$ and during electrical stimulation in the presence of high calcium at this stage of diabetes. This release occurs against a background of changing reuptake of noradrenaline, which is significantly increased at 12 weeks, but declines with increasing duration of diabetes. Reuptake-1 is a membrane phenomenon, and the increased activity may be related in an increased quantity of terminal membrane as may occur in sprouting and regrowth of sympathetic nerve endings, or possibly to changes in certain activity-dependent mediators, such as calcium–calmodulin as has been shown in PC12 cells.[25] However, whichever process is operative (and possibly both), it is relatively short lasting and by 6–7 months of hyperglycemia, the activity of uptake-1 is not significantly different from the control. It is clear, however, that uptake-1 may contribute to the high concentrations of noradrenaline after 12 weeks of hyperglycemia. The high concentrations and content of noradrenaline after 12 weeks may be due to increased synthesis (as suggested by the immunohistochemical data), or decreased release of metabolism.

It is of interest that dopamine levels in the seminal vesicle fall and remain low for many weeks in longer-term diabetes, which may be related to the demand for the amine by release mechanisms in the terminals, even in the presence of increased TH activity. Dopamine appears to contract the rat seminal vesicle by an indirect mechanism involving changes in the release of noradrenaline at a presynaptic site,[26] and the changes observed would therefore counteract the effects of raised noradrenaline concentrations, if dopamine were released simultaneously.

It is also known that diabetes can reduce the levels of gonadotropins[27] and therefore of testosterone, which influence the weight of the reproductive organs and also have effects on some autonomic neurons. Certain neurons in the pelvic ganglia are sensitive to testosterone[28–30] and show morphological changes associated with the presence of this hormone; however, as already stated, the major component of the sympathetic innervation originates in the sympathetic chain. It seems likely that some of the large rise in noradrenaline concentration in these tissues was related to the failure of the organs to grow at the same rate as the controls. However, there was still a substantial and statistically significant increase in the concentration of noradrenaline after corrections for the weight of the organs (TABLE 2). We cannot comment on the direct effects of changes in testosterone levels on the parameters measured in these experiments, but do acknowledge a possible role of a testosterone-sensitive mechanism in some neurons.

ACKNOWLEDGMENTS

We would like to thank the Faculty of Medicine and Health Sciences and the Sheikh Hamdan Medical Research Awards for their support of this study.

REFERENCES

1. EL SAKKA, A.I. 2003. Premature ejaculation in non-insulin-dependent diabetic patients. Int. J. Androl. **26:** 329–334.
2. DUNSMUIR, W.D. & S.A. HOLMES. 1996. The aetiology and management of erectile, ejaculatory, and fertility problems in men with diabetes mellitus. Diabet. Med. **13:** 700–708.
3. IBRAGIMOV, A.Z., T.A. ALIEV, K.I. ABDULLAEV & V.A. MIRZA-ZADE. 1990. The function of the closure apparatus of the bladder in retrograde ejaculation in diabetics. Urol. Nefrol. (Mosk.) **3:** 65–68.
4. GOSLING, J.A. 1986. The distribution of noradrenergic nerves in the human lower urinary tract. Clin. Sci. (Lond.) **70** (Suppl 14): 3s–6s.
5. DANUSER, H., J.P. SPRINGER, M.A. KATOFIASC & K.B. THOR. 1997. Extrinsic innervation of the cat prostate gland: a combined tracing and immunohistochemical study J. Urol. **157:** 1018–1024.

6. PAUL, A. & F. HABIB. 1998. Low-affinity nerve growth factor receptors (p75LNGFR) in human prostate tissue: stromal localisation. Urol. Res. **26:** 111–116.
7. MACGROGAN, D., G. DESPRES, R. ROMAND & E. DICOU. 1991. Expression of the beta-nerve growth factor gene in male sex organs of the mouse, rat, and guinea pig. J. Neurosci. Res. **28:** 567–573.
8. HELLWEG, R. & H.D. HARTUNG.1990. Endogenous levels of nerve growth factor (NGF) are altered in experimental diabetes mellitus: a possible role for NGF in the pathogenesis of diabetic neuropathy. J. Neurosci. Res. **26:** 258–267.
9. MORRISON, J.F., S. DHANASEKARAN & R. SHEEN. 2004. Effects of age and streptozotocin-induced diabetes on biogenic amines in rat tail artery. Mol. Cell. Biochem. **261:** 77–82.
10. MORRISON, J., F. HOWARTH & R. SHEEN. 2001. Catecholamines in the heart and adrenal gland of streptozotocin-treated (STZ) diabetic rats. Arch. Physiol. Biochem. **109:** 206–208.
11. SCHMIDT, R.E., S.B. PLURAD, C.A. PARVIN & K.A. ROTH. 1993. Effect of diabetes and aging on human sympathetic autonomic ganglia. Am. J. Pathol. **143:** 143–153.
12. SCHROER, J.A., S.B. PLURAD & R.E. SCHMIDT. 1992. Fine structure of presynaptic axonal terminals in sympathetic autonomic ganglia of aging and diabetic human subjects. Synapse **12:** 1–13.
13. SCHMIDT, R.E. 2002. Neuropathology and pathogenesis of diabetic autonomic neuropathy. Int. Rev. Neurobiol. **50:** 257–292.
14. TOMLINSON, D.R. & A.P. YUSOF. 1983. Autonomic neuropathy in the alloxan-diabetic rat. J. Auton. Pharmacol. **3:** 257–263.
15. BRITLAND, S.T., R.J. YOUNG, A.K. SHARMA & B.F. CLARKE. 1992. Acute and remitting painful diabetic polyneuropathy: a comparison of peripheral nerve fibre pathology Pain **48:** 361–370.
16. BEGGS, J., P.C. JOHNSON, A. OLAFSEN & C.J. WATKINS. 1992. Innervation of the vasa nervorum: changes in human diabetics. J. Neuropathol. Exp. Neurol. **51:** 612–629.
17. LANGE, W. & J. UNGER. 1990. Peptidergic innervation within the prostate gland and seminal vesicle. Urol. Res. **18:** 337–340.
18. AUMULLER, G. & A. RIVA. 1992. Morphology and functions of the human seminal vesicle. Andrologia **24:** 183–196.
19. MENSAH-BROWN E., A. ADEM, J.M. CONLON & J.F.B. MORRISON. 2005. Changes in neuropeptide Y (NPY) – nerves and in NPY binding in the seminal vesicles and prostate gland of the streptozotocin diabetic rat. Emirates Med. J. **23:** 221–227.
20. ZACHARKO, A., M.B. ARCISZEWSKI & K. WASOWICZ. 2004. Origin of the primary efferent neurons projecting to the prostate of the dog. Ann. Anat. **186:** 349–356.
21. KALECZYC, J., J.P. TIMMERMANS, M. MAJEWSKI, *et al.* 1995. Distribution and immunohistochemical characteristics of neurons in the porcine caudal mesenteric ganglion projecting to the vas deferens and seminal vesicle. Cell Tissue Res. **282:** 59–68.
22. OHKAWA, H. 1981. Evidence for adrenergic transmission in the circular smooth muscle of the guinea-pig seminal vesicle. Tohoku. J. Exp. Med. **134:** 141–158.
23. KUBOTA, Y., H. HASHITANI, H. FUKUTA, *et al.* 2003. Mechanisms of excitatory transmission in circular smooth muscles of the guinea pig seminal vesicle. J. Urol. **169:** 390–395.

24. SJOSTRAND, N.O. & M. HAMMARSTROM. 1995. Sympathetic regulation of fructose secretion in the seminal vesicle of the guinea-pig. Acta Physiol. Scand. **153:** 189–202.
25. UCHIDA, J., Y. KIUCHI, M. OHNO, *et al.* 1998. $Ca^{(2+)}$-dependent enhancement of [3H]noradrenaline uptake in PC12 cells through calmodulin-dependent kinases. Brain Res. **809:** 155–164.
26. CASTELLI, M., T. ROSSI, G. BAGGIO, *et al.* 1985. Characterization of the contractile activity of dopamine on the rat isolated seminal vesicle. Pharmacol. Res. Commun. **17:** 351–359.
27. DONG, Q., R.M. LAZARUS, L.S. WONG, *et al.* 1991. Pulsatile LH secretion in streptozotocin-induced diabetes in the rat. J. Endocrinol. **131:** 49–55.
28. KEAST, J.R. & R.J. SAUNDERS. 1998. Testosterone has potent, selective effects on the morphology of pelvic autonomic neurons which control the bladder, lower bowel and internal reproductive organs of the male rat. Neuroscience **85:** 543–556.
29. KEPPER, M. & J. KEAST. 1995. Immunohistochemical properties and spinal connections of pelvic autonomic neurons that innervate the rat prostate gland. Cell Tissue Res. **281:** 533–542.
30. WANIGASEKARA, Y., M.E. KEPPER & J.R. KEAST. 2003. Immunohistochemical characterisation of pelvic autonomic ganglia in male mice. Cell Tissue Res. **311:** 175–185.

Changes of the Different Neuropeptide-Containing Nerve Fibers and Immunocells in the Diabetic Rat's Alimentary Tract

ERZSÉBET FEHÉR,[a] BAYARCHIMEG BATBAYAR,[a] ÁGOTA VÉR,[b] AND TIVADAR ZELLES[c]

[a]*Laboratory of Oral Morphology of the Faculty of Dentistry in the Department of Anatomy, Histology, and Embryology, Semmelweis University, H-1450 Budapest, Hungary*

[b]*Department of Medical Chemistry, Molecular Biology, and Pathobiochemistry, Semmelweis University, H-1088 Budapest, Hungary*

[c]*Department of Oral Biology, Semmelweis University, H-1445 Budapest, Hungary*

ABSTRACT: **Peripheral neuropathy is a common complication of diabetes mellitus, where neuropeptides and immunocells might play important roles in the pathogenesis of the disease. In this article we have quantified the different neuropeptide-containing nerve fibers and immunocells in the streptozotocin-induced diabetic rat's alimentary tract (tongue, duodenum, colon) using immunohistochemical and immunocytochemical methods. The immunoreactive (IR) nerve fibers were found in all layers of the alimentary tract and their distribution pattern was similar in both control and diabetic groups. Mast cell–nerve fiber contacts were rarely found in the controls. However, after 4 weeks duration of diabetes the number of IR nerve fibers and the immunocompetent cells increased significantly ($P < 0.05$), and the number of mast cell–nerve fiber contacts was even more significantly increased ($P < 0.001$). The distance between nerve fibers and immunocells was about 1 μm or even less. Some of the mast cells were degranulated in the vicinity of nerve fibers. No immunocompetent cells were IR for any antisera in the control. However, after the streptozotocin treatment, a large number of the immunocompetent cells showed immunoreactivity for SP and NPY. Counting all immunocompetent cells in whole sections showed that 12.3% of them were IR for SP and 25.4% were IR for NPY. Increased number of SP-containing nerve fibers and immunocells in diabetes mellitus might be the reason for painful neuropathy and might amplify the inflammatory reaction in an**

Address for correspondence: Erzsébet Fehér, M.D., Ph.D., D.Sc., Department of Anatomy, Histology, and Embryology, Semmelweis University, Tüzoltó u. 58. Budapest, P.O. Box 95, H-1450, Hungary. Voice: +36-1215-6920-3683; fax: +36-1215-5158.

e-mail: feher@ana.sote.hu

Ann. N.Y. Acad. Sci. 1084: 280–295 (2006). © 2006 New York Academy of Sciences.
doi: 10.1196/annals.1372.023

axon reflex manner; the released histamine and leukotrienes, cytokines, and chemokines might cause inflammations and lesions of the mucosa.

KEYWORDS: neuropeptides; immunomodulation; alimentary tract; streptozotocin-induced diabetes; insulin

INTRODUCTION

Diabetes-induced alterations in axonal neuropeptide content have been reported in various organs. The levels of neuropeptides have been reported to increase, decrease, or remain unchanged, depending on the target tissue innervations. Peripheral neuropathy is a common complication of diabetes that effects the motor, sensory, and autonomic components of the nervous system,[1–3] resulting in peripheral loss of sensation, dysthesia, hyposalivation and impairments of taste, gastroparesis, diabetic diarrhea and constipation, delayed small intestinal transit,[4] and abdominal pain.[5–8] The mechanisms underlying diabetic neuropathy have been explained by biochemical, vascular, and inflammatory processes. Patients with diabetic neuropathy usually show nerve fiber loss to some degree, whereas diabetic animals, especially streptozotocin induced, do not have any significant degree of nerve fiber loss.[9–11] It has been suggested that in the early stage of diabetes mellitus both unmyelinated and myelinated nerve fibers are altered due to neurogenic inflammation.[12,13] Changes of the different neuropeptide contents were also demonstrated in various organs.[14–20] It was also shown that the diabetes of 4 and 32 weeks duration induced an increase in the tissue content of neuronal nitric oxide synthase (nNOS) in the gastroduodenum of rat.[21] It was suggested that the development of nociceptive dysfunction in diabetes was induced by the decreasing content of neuropeptides mainly the substance P (SP) and calcitonin gene-related peptide (CGRP).[22,23] Significantly reduced SP and CGRP contents were demonstrated in the trigeminal ganglion of rats with short-term diabetes, which has been followed by an increase in the expression of both peptides.[24]

The sensory nervous system is thought to be involved in the etiology of neurogenic inflammation in diabetes mellitus.[25] Some peptides in the primary sensory afferents, such as neuropeptide Y (NPY) and galanin (GAL) have been investigated to a limited extent during the different phases of inflammation. All these alterations might be the consequence of the chronic inflammation as well as changes in the innervation. Vasoactive intestinal polypeptide (VIP) and NPY can stimulate insulin secretion significantly while the SP inhibits it in the pancreas of diabetic rats.[26]

Neuropeptides have been shown to stimulate and activate mast cells isolated from different tissue sites in different animal species[27,28] suggesting the role of nerves fibers in the modulation of mast cell activity. In oral lichen planus, the number of mast cells as well as the mast cell–nerve interactions increased suggesting a controlling role over the lesioned cell populations and a secondary role in the immune response.[29] There are a lot of studies suggesting that SP,

VIP, and mast cells play a role in inflammatory processes of the gastrointestinal tract.[30–33] It is now clear that mast cells can synthesize and release a large number of biologically active substances including arachidonic acid metabolites, biogenic amines, cytokines, enzymes, and glycosaminoglycans.[34] Though the existence of a bidirectional relationship between mast cells and nerve fibers is supported by several previous studies, none of these studies provided quantitative data about the number of mast cell–nerve contacts and their ultrastructure in the diabetic alimentary tract.

Therefore, the aim of this article was to investigate the quantity of different neuropeptide-containing nerve elements and immunocytes at different stages of streptozotocin-induced diabetes mellitus of the rat (after 1, 2 and 4 weeks duration of disease) to give evidence of the imbalance in the neuroimmunomodulation in the gastrointestinal tract.

MATERIALS AND METHODS

Albino Wistar male rats (weight 120 to 150 g; $n = 40$) were used in this experiment. Animals ($n = 25$) received a single dose of streptozotocin (65 mg kg^{-1}, Zanosar; Upjohn Company, Kalamazoo MI) injected into the tail vein. Blood was withdrawn from the tail vein and glucose was measured by the glucose oxidase method (kit from Reanal Pharmaceutical Co, Budapest Hungary). Rats displaying glucose levels >16 mmol/L were considered diabetic. The diabetic animals of the insulin replacement study received injection of Ultralente insulin (Lilly, Fegersheim, France) two times daily. One group ($n = 5$) of insulin-treated animals received the treatment immediately on the morning when hyperglycemia was first identified, the others ($n = 5$) were treated only 1 week later, when the diabetes was manifested. Insulin was given intramuscularly in an individual dose to keep blood glucose level between 4.5–12.5 mmol/L. The blood glucose level of untreated diabetic rats fluctuated between 18.5–25.9 mmol/L. All groups were maintained under identical conditions. Controls ($n = 15$) were treated alike, except that streptozotocin treatment was omitted. At the end of the protocol (after 1, 2 and 4 weeks duration of diabetes as well as after 3 weeks of insulin treatment) the animals were terminally anesthetized with intraperitoneal injections of sodium pentobarbitone (60 mg/kg; Sanofi Phylaxia, Budapest, Hungary) and perfused via the aorta with saline, followed by a fixative containing 2.5% paraformaldehyde and 1% glutaraldehyde in 0.1 M phosphate-buffer (pH 7.3). Procedures conformed to the "principles of laboratory animal care" (NIH publication No. 86-23, revised 1985) just as well to a specific national law (e.g., the current version of the Hungarian Law on the Protection of Animals, No. 243/1998), and were followed in all experiments.

Small pieces of the root of the tongue, pylorus, duodenum, and colon were placed overnight in glutaraldehyde-free fixative containing 20% sucrose (at 4°C). Sections (40 μM thick) were treated for 1 h with 1% Triton-X 100 to

TABLE 1. Primary antisera used for immunohistochemistry

Antisera	Abbreviation	Species	Dilution	Source
Substance P	SP	Rabbit	1:10,000	Daifuku
Vasoactive intestinal polypeptide	VIP	Rabbit	1:10,000	Kindly provided by T. Görcs (Budapest, Hungary)
Neuropeptide Y	NPY	Rabbit	1:10,000	T. Görcs
Somatostatin	SOM	Rabbit	1:2,000	Peninsula
Galanin	GAL	Rabbit	1:8,000	Peninsula
Tyrosine β-hydroxylase	TH	Rabbit	1:1,000	Incstar

increase the membrane permeability and 15 min with 3% hydrogen peroxide in order to remove endogenous peroxidase activity. Specificity, working dilution, and sources of the primary antibodies used in this work are summarized in TABLE 1. The primary antibodies were used for 48 h at 4°C. Avidin–biotin immunoperoxidase technique was employed using a commercially available kit (Vectastain Elite ABC; Vector Laboratories, Peterborough, UK) for the immunostaining. All manipulations were performed at room temperature. The immunoreactivity was visualized with diamino-benzidine (DAB) chromogen reaction (DAB Vector; 0.025% 3,3-diamino-benzidine, 0.0015% H_2O_2 in 0.05 M Tris-HCl buffer, pH 7.5) at room temperature for 8–10 min.

For electron microscopic investigations the sections were cut by Vibratome (Technical Products International Inc., St. Louis, MO) and plunged rapidly into liquid nitrogen (without Triton) before the incubation with primary antibodies. After the DAB reaction the sections were postfixed in osmium and embedded in Epon. Ultrathin sections were cut and stained with uranyl acetate and lead citrate, then examined and photographed in a Jeol 100 electron microscope (Jeol Ltd., Tokyo, Japan) (All morphological examinations were done by the same investigator, E.F.).

Using quantitative analysis the number of immunoreactive (IR) nerve fibers, perikarya, and the immunocompetent cells were counted in a 15–20 mm^2 tissue area and calculated for 1 mm^2 tissue area. For analysis 40× magnifications were used with a graduated eyepiece graticule and the entire section was assessed. Microphotographs were also taken (n = 15–25 per animal), digitalized, and then analyzed using a PC-based image analyzing software IMAN (beta) 2.0 (MFA, Budapest, Hungary). These studies were carried out by two investigators as a double-blind trial and the obtained data were averaged. The figures and the inserts were taken by an Olympus system consisting of a BX51 microscope equipped with a DP50 digital camera (Olympus Europa Holding GmbH, Hamburg, Deutschland).

Control Experiments

Specificity of the immunoreactivities was controlled by omission of the primary antiserum or replacing the antisera with normal rabbit serum, or with sections incubated in antisera preabsorbed with excess antigen; where no immunostaining appeared.

Statistical Analysis

Statistical analysis was performed using analysis of variance (ANOVA). *Post hoc* pairwise comparisons were made with the Bonferroni test. A P value of less than 0.05 was considered to be statistically significant. Data are presented as mean ± SD.

RESULTS

In the alimentary tract IR nerve fibers were found with different varieties in all layers. There was no statistical difference in the number of IR nerve fibers between the different parts of the alimentary tract (tongue, pylorus, duodenum, and colon). The quantitative analysis of the density of neuropeptide-containing nerve fibers in different layers and tissue areas of the gastrointestinal tract is demonstrated in TABLE 2. NPY and tyrosine β-hydroxylase (TH) IR nerve terminals were mainly observed around the blood vessels. A large number of VIP IR nerve fibers and some SP IR, NPY IR nerve fibers were also distributed in the mucosa beneath the epithelial lining. The density of TH and GAL IR nerve fibers was the lowest in all experiments. The SP IR, NPY IR, and VIP IR cell bodies were mainly located in both plexuses; however, some IR neurons were also located in the connective tissue beneath the epithelium in the root of the tongue and in the pylorus. These cells were large (30–50 μM in diameter) and medium (20–30 μM in diameter) in size with round and ovoid shape, and had large nuclei and long neuronal processes.

After 1 week of the streptozotocin treatment, the total number of IR nerve fibers was decreased. However, after 4 weeks duration of diabetes the number of IR nerve fibers increased significantly ($P < 0.05$) (FIG. 1) compared to the control (FIG. 2). A large number of SP IR nerve processes were observed mainly

TABLE 2. Distribution of IR nerve fibers in the gastrointestinal tract

Antibody	Epithelium	Subepithelial tissue	Glands	Blood vessels
SP	0	++	+	+
VIP	0	++	++++	++
NPY	0	++	++	++++
SOM	0	+	+	+
GAL	+	+	+	+
TH	0	+	+	++++

The distribution of histochemically defined nerve fibers (n. f.) is summarized in 1 mm^2, with the scale of 0 to ++++ indicating density. ++++ very dense (50–100 n. f.); +++ numerous (20–49 n. f.); ++ moderate (5–19 n. f.); + few (1–4 n. f.); 0, where no nerve fibers were observed.

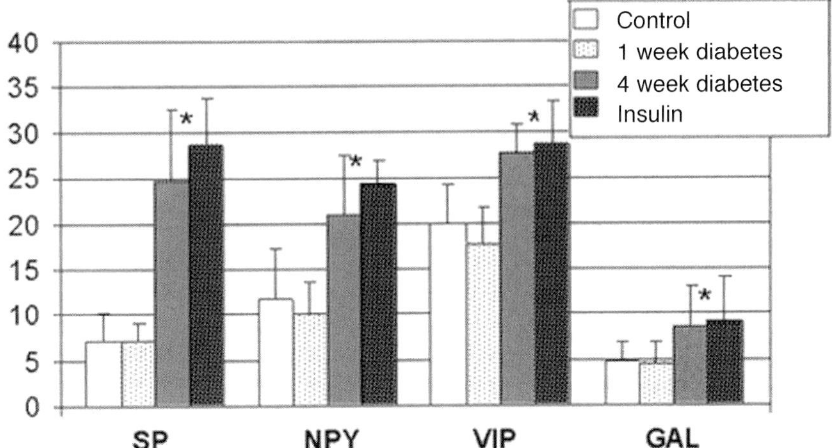

FIGURE 1. Changes in the density of different neuropeptide-containing nerve fibers/1 mm^2 in the tunica mucosa of the diabetic rat's gastrointestinal tract ($n = 75$ sections from control; $n = 25$ sections from each diabetic groups). Data are mean ± SD. Asterisks indicate significant differences between the two compared groups: $^*P < 0.05$.

in and below the epithelium (FIG. 3), especially around the blood vessels. The diameter of SP, NPY, and TH IR nerve fibers has also been markedly increased. The electron microscopic investigations showed that in the early stages of diabetes some of the nerve fibers started to degenerate.

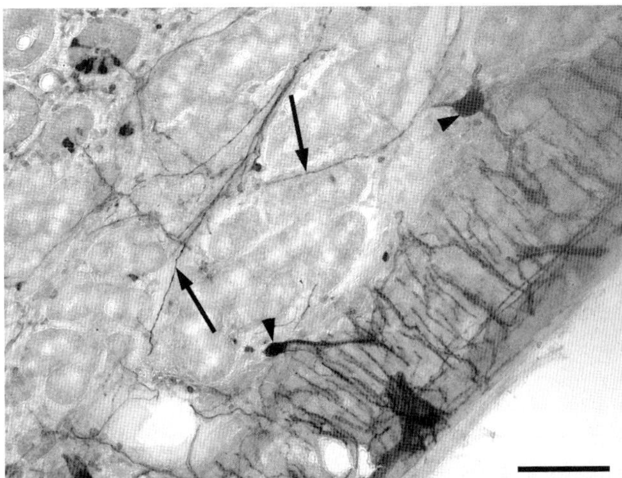

FIGURE 2. The SP IR nerve fibers (*arrows*) and IR neurons in the wall of the duodenum from the control rat. The *arrowheads* point to the IR neurons in the submucous plexus. Bar scale = 100 μM.

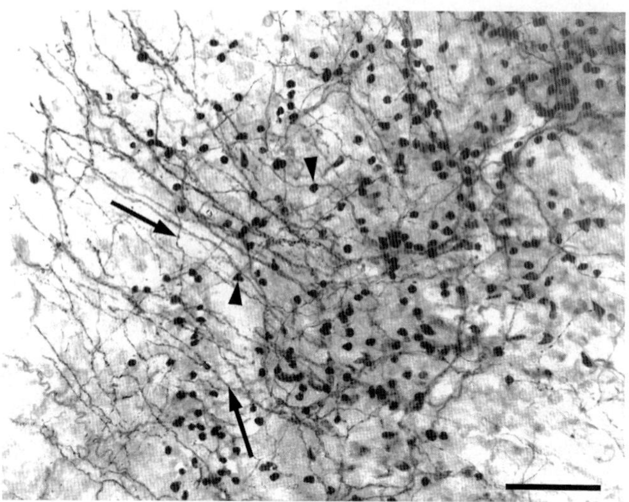

FIGURE 3. Increased NPY IR nerve fibers (*arrows*) beneath of the epithelium of the pylorus (*arrows*) from diabetic rat after 4 weeks of treatment. The *arrowheads* point to the IR immunocompetent cells. Bar scale = 100 μM .

No immunocompetent cells were IR for any antisera in the control. However, after the streptozotocin treatment, a large number of the immunocompetent cells showed immunoreactivity for SP (FIG. 4) and NPY (FIG. 5). Some of them were small, round cells (6–10 μM in diameter) being lymphocytes and

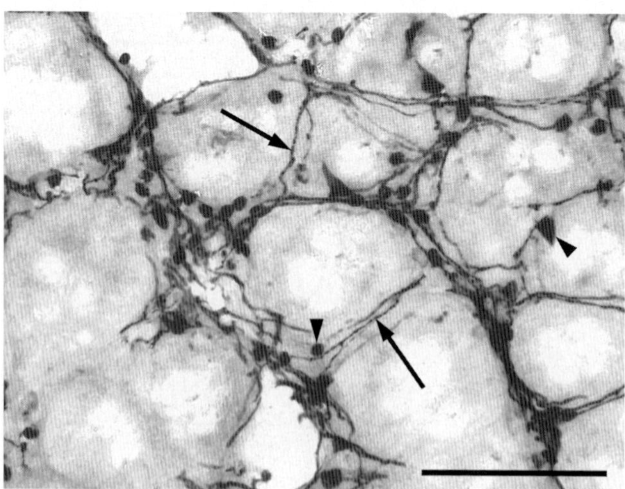

FIGURE 4. A part of the tunica mucosa of the duodenum from diabetic rat. The *arrows* indicate the SP IR nerve fibers among the Lieberkühn crypts. The *arrowheads* show the SP IR immunocompetent cells. Bar scale = 100 μM.

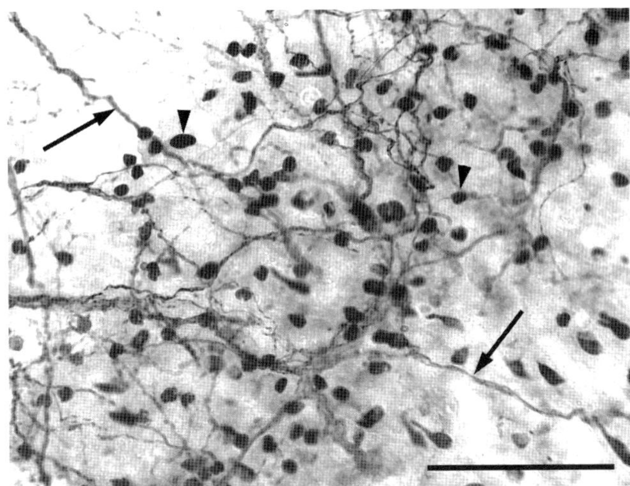

FIGURE 5. A part of the tunica mucosa of the duodenum from diabetic rat. The *arrows* indicate the NPY IR nerve fibers. The *arrowheads* show the NPY IR immunocompetent cells. Bar scale = 100 μM.

the others were larger oval cells being plasma cells and mast cells (15–20 μM in diameter) (FIGS. 4 and 5). Counting of all immunocompetent cells in whole sections showed that 12.3% of them were IR for SP and 25.4% were IR for NPY in the tongue and 32.6% for SP and 16.4% for NPY in the upper parts of the gastrointestinal tract. Only a few IR immunocytes were observed in the colon. The highest magnifications of light microscopy and the electron microscopic investigation have proved that these cells are lymphocytes, plasma cells, and mast cells (FIG. 6). The reaction end-products were distributed in the cytoplasm and at the membranes of these cells. Sometimes the SP IR nerve fibers were also located in the vicinity of the degranulated mast cells (FIG. 7), where the gap between the IR nerve fibers and mast cells was just 20–200 nm.

After immediate insulin treatment the decrease of the IR nerve fibers has been prevented (the quantity of IR nerve fibers was the same as control data). However, after the late administration of insulin the number of IR nerve terminals was further enhanced significantly ($P < 0.05$) in all portions of the alimentary tract compared to untreated diabetic rats (FIG. 1). In particular, the number of SP, VIP, and GAL IR nerve fibers increased significantly. The density of SP and VIP IR perikarya was also enhanced in the average tissue areas in the insulin-treated animals compared to that of untreated controls. The number of SP and NPY IR immunocompetent cells was reduced in all insulin-treated animals.

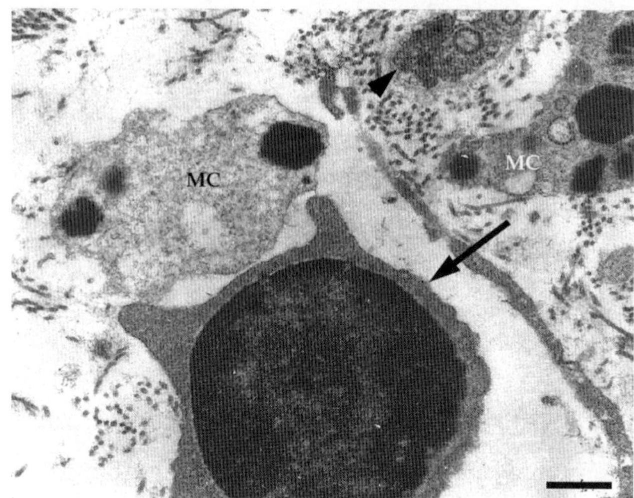

FIGURE 6. Electron micrograph of a portion of lamina propria mucosae of the diabetic rat's duodenum. The *arrow* shows a SP IR lymphocyte. The *arrowhead* shows a SP IR nerve fiber close to the mast cell (MC). Bar scale = 1 μM.

DISCUSSION

In our study a significant increase in the number of SP, VIP, and NPY IR nerve fibers was shown in the alimentary tract of rat at early stages of

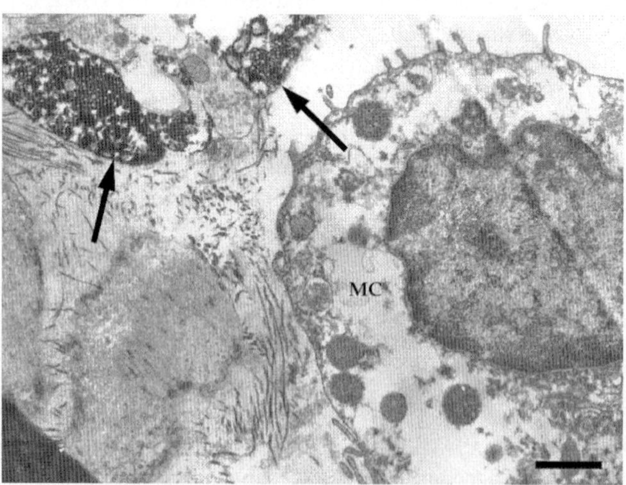

FIGURE 7. Electron micrograph of a part of the lamina propria mucosae of diabetic rat's pylorus. The *arrow* points a NPY IR nerve fiber in a close vicinity to the degranulated mast cell (MC). Bar scale = 1 μM.

experimental diabetes suggesting increased synthesis and/or regeneration of these nerve fibers to restore a diabetes-associated depletion of these neuropeptides. A marked increase in the number of CGRP and VIP IR was also observed in diabetic skin[35] and in the small intestine,[36] while no differences were detected in nerves IR for SP and NPY in contrast to our data. In the different inflamed tissues increased number of SP, CGRP, and NPY IR fibers has also been observed.[37] Similarly, elevated neuropeptide levels were found in healing bones by other investigators.[38] During inflammation, there are also marked changes in the expression of peptides in the dorsal horn neurons[39–41] suggesting that nerve regeneration coexists with degeneration and contributes to nerve function as well as nerve pathology in diabetes mellitus.[42] Plasticity of the sensory nerve fibers containing SP and CGRP was demonstrated in the trigeminal ganglion[43] and in the tongue.[44]

Nerve growth factor (NGF) is thought to be necessary for the survival and the maintenance of the neuropeptide-containing nerve fibers and in the regeneration of the peripheral nervous system, which is impaired in the diabetic state.[45–47] NGF has been shown to prevent or delay the development of sensory neuropathy in streptozotocin-induced diabetes.[48] A variety of cell types are capable of producing NGF. NGF can be synthesized by immunocompetent cells (lymphocytes, macrophages, and mast cells), fibroblasts, and smooth muscle cells as well as Schwann cells.[49,50] Elevated NGF levels have been found in inflammatory exudates, inflamed skin, and in the nerves innervating inflamed tissue.[51] In our opinion in the early stage of diabetic inflammation synthesis of different neuropeptides can be stimulated by the elevated release of NGF from inflammatory cells resulting in the increase of the number of IR nerve fibers.[52,53] SP can stimulate the release of tumor necrosis factor-α (TNF-α) and IL-β from inflammatory cells, which in turn increases NGF levels in inflamed tissues. Thus, it is conceivable that a positive feedback mechanism exists in which SP induces synthesis of NGF by cytokines leading to increased production of SP in the immunocytes and in the nerves.[53] The presumed degeneration and regeneration of the mucosal innervation can be temporally related to the recognized inflammatory changes during diabetes mellitus.[42]

It has been reported by many authors that neuropeptides play an important role in the regulation of the mucosal immune and inflammatory response.[54,55] In our study we demonstrated that some of the immunocytes showed immunoreactivity for SP and NPY in the early stages of diabetes mellitus in the alimentary tract. It was demonstrated that some neuropeptides are produced not only by neurons but also by many immunocells, such as activated lymphocytes and macrophages,[56–58] where the receptors for these neuropeptides are also present. To date, at least 27 different neuroendocrine mediators are said to be produced by cells of the lymphoid organs. These neuropeptides might stimulate further leukocyte recruitment, thereby amplifying the inflammatory response.

SP-induced release of inflammatory mediators, such as cytokines, oxygen radicals, arachidonic acid derivates, and histamine, potentiates tissue injury and stimulates further leukocyte recruitment, enhancing the inflammatory response.[59] It has been suggested that mast cells, as well as SP may be involved in the axon reflex responsible for the flare reaction (vasodilatation, neurogenic inflammation) to noxious stimuli.[60] Direct evidence for a close contact between mast cells and nerves has been obtained. A large proportion of intestinal mucosal mast cells are in direct contact with nerves some of which contain SP or CGRP.[54,61,62] We have demonstrated previously that the number of mast cell–nerve contacts and inflammatory cells was increased significantly after 4 weeks duration of diabetes mellitus.[63] Stimulation of mast cells with SP activates TNF-α gene expression and induces TNF-α secretion. Blockade of SP with either SP antibodies, or with the NK-1R antagonist CP 96,345, reduced inflammation in the jejunum.[64] Studies with neurokinin receptor antagonists suggest that blocking the binding of SP to the NK-1R interrupts the inflammatory cascade that triggers and maintains intestinal lesions.[65,66] In our previous studies it was shown that insulin treatment prevented the activation of the immunocompetent cells (being immunonegative for neuropeptides) supposing the decrease of inflammation in the oral cavity.[44]

The results of our study have revealed that after the delayed insulin treatment the number of SP, VIP, and GAL IR nerve terminals showed a further increase in the alimentary tract.[44] There are conflicting literature data about the effect of insulin on the nerve elements and their content. Some of them demonstrated that the deficit of SP and CGRP in streptozotocin-induced diabetes was prevented completely in different tissues[67,68] while others documented no alterations in the enteric SP IR nerve elements.[69] The significantly reduced tissue concentrations of VIP in the ileum was improved with insulin treatment.[70] The exact role of insulin in the regulation of the activity of the nerve elements is unclear. There has been a line of evidence indicating a functional role for insulin as a neurotrophic agent with direct actions on neurite outgrowth in culture and nerve regeneration *in vivo*.[71–73] Our results suggest that in the inflamed area insulin has further enhanced the synthesis of neuropeptides and increased the proliferation of nerve elements.

Our present results clearly prove that neuropeptide-containing nerves participate in the development of inflammation of the gastrointestinal tract in short-term diabetes. These data suggest that neuropeptides released from peripheral nerve endings in association with tissue injury may not only affect vasodilation and the inflammatory response but may also stimulate proliferation and sprouting of nerve fibers as well as other tissues where insulin treatment further increased the neuropeptide content in the nerve terminals. The demonstration that some of the immunocytes produce SP and NPY led to the hypothesis that SP and NPY act not only as a mediator of the cross-talk between the nervous and immune systems but they are also biologically involved in the direct interaction between immune cells in a paracrine and/or autocrine way, independent of sensory nerves or neurogenic inflammation. The breakup in the balance of neuropeptides, disproportionate changes of nerve fibers, and increased number of inflammatory cells (mast cells) as well as their contacts resulting enhanced secretion of inflammatory substances might cause different pathological changes in the alimentary tract, which in turn might be associated with the development of disorders in diabetes. Therefore, it can be concluded that better treatment/control of disease activity and of pain can be achieved by blocking the cascade leading to initiation and/or amplification of inflammatory process. We therefore propose, that neuropeptides in diabetes act as endogenous factors that regulate immune homeostasis. The physiological consequence of this action is that the immune microenvironment depends on the timing of neuropeptide release and the activation stage of neighboring immune cells. Inflammatory mediators in this tissue can further facilitate or modulate the release of neurotransmitters from both the nerve fibers and immunocytes. Finally, the locally released neuropeptides from nerve endings and immunocompetent cells act directly on epithelial cells, blood vessels as well as on mast cells prompting their release of histamine and other mediators increasing the inflammatory response, which results in apoptosis and necrosis.

ACKNOWLEDGMENT

The authors would like to thank Ms. E. Burka for assisting with the manuscript.

REFERENCES

1. Casamassimo, R.S. & J.E. Tucker-Lammertse. 1988. Diabetic polyradiculopathy with trigeminal nerve involvement. Oral Surg. Oral Med. Oral Pathol. **66:** 315–317.
2. Rodella, L., R. Rezzani, G. Corsetti & R. Bianchi. 2000. Nitric oxide involvement in the trigeminal hyperalgesia in diabetic rats. Brain Res. **865:** 112–115.
3. Barkai, L., P. Kempler, I. Vámosi, *et al.* 1998. Peripheral sensory nerve dysfunction in children and adolescents with type I diabetes mellitus. Diab. Med. **15:** 28–33.
4. Scott, L.C. & T.M. Ellis. 1980. Small intestinal transit and myoelectric activity in diabetic rats. *In* Gastrointestinal Motility. J. Christensen, Ed.: 395–399. Raven Press. New York.
5. Koch, K.L. 1999. Diabetic gastropathy: gastric neuromuscular dysfunction in diabetes mellitus: a review of symptoms, pathophysiology, and treatment. Dig. Dis. Sci. **44:** 1061–1075.
6. Ricci, J.A., R. Siddique, W.F. Stewart, *et al.* 2000. Upper gastrointestinal symptoms in a U.S. national sample of adults with diabetes. Scand. J. Gastroenterol. **35:** 152–159.
7. Spangeus, A., M. El-Shalhy, O. Suhr, *et al.* 1999. Prevalence of gastrointestinal symptoms in young and middle-aged diabetic patients. Scand. J. Gastroenterol. **34:** 1196–1202.
8. Verne, G.N. & C.A. Sninsky. 1998. Diabetes and the gastrointestinal tract. Gastroenterol. Clin. North Am. **27:** 861–874.

9. YASUDA, H., M. SONOBE, M. YAMASHITA, *et al.* 1989. Effect of prostaglandin E1 analogue TFC612 on diabetic neuropathy in streptozotocin induced diabetic rats. Diabetes **38:** 832–838.
10. YASUDA, H., Y. TANIGUCHI, Z. HUITIAN, *et al.* 1989. Chronically streptozotocin – diabetic monkey does not mimic human diabetic neuropathy. Exp. Neurol. **104:** 133–137.
11. ZOCHODNE, D.W., V.M.K. VERGE, C. CHENG, *et al.* 2001. Does diabetes target ganglion neurones? Progressive sensory neurone involvement in long-term experimental diabetes. Brain **12:** 2319–2334.
12. FEHÉR, E., A. GYŐRFFI & Á. FAZEKAS. 2001. Neurogenic inflammation of gingivomucosal tissue in streptozotocin-diabetic rat. Arch. Physiol. Biochem. **109:** 230–233.
13. GYŐRFFI, A., Á. FAZEKAS, E. FEHÉR, *et al.* 1996. Effects of streptozotocin induced diabetes on neurogenic inflammation of gingivomucosal tissue in rat. J. Periodont. Res. **31:** 249–255.
14. ADEGHATE, E., A.S. PONERY, A.K. SHARMA, *et al.* 2001. Diabetes mellitus is associated with a decrease in vasoactive intestinal polypeptide content of gastrointestinal tract of rat. Arch. Physiol. Biochem. **109:** 246–251.
15. BALLMANN, M. & J.M. CONLON. 1985. Changes in the somatostatin, substance P and vasoactive intestinal polypeptide content of the gastrointestinal tract following streptozotocin-induced diabetes in the rat. Diabetologia **28:** 355–358.
16. EL-SALHY, M. 1998. Neuroendocrine peptides of the gastrointestinal tract of an animal model of human type 2 diabetes mellitus. Acta Diabetol. **35:** 194–198.
17. EL-SALHY, M. 1999. Neuroendocrine peptides in stomach and colon of an animal model for human diabetes type I. Diabetes Comp. **13:** 170–173.
18. GORIO, A., A.M. DI GIULIO, L. DONADONI, *et al.* 1992. Early neurochemical changes in the autonomic neuropathy of the gut in experimental diabetes. Int. J. Clin. Pharmacol. Res. **12:** 217–224.
19. SPANGEUS, A. & M. EL-SHALHY. 2001. Myenteric plexus of obese diabetic mice (an animal model of human type 2 diabetes). Histol. Histopathol. **16:** 159–165.
20. SPANGEUS, A., S. FORSGREN & M. EL-SHALHY. 2001. Effect of diabetic stage on co-localization of substance P and serotonin in the gut in animal models. Histol. Histopathol. **16:** 393–398.
21. ADEGHATE, E., B. AL-RAMADI, A.M. SALCH, *et al.* 2003. Increase in neuronal nitric oxide synthase content of the gastroduodenal tract of diabetic rats. Cell. Mol. Life Sci. **60:** 1172–1179.
22. JIANG, Y., J.R. NYENGAARD, J.S. ZHANG, *et al.* 2004. Selective loss of calcitonin gene-related peptide-expressing primary sensory neurons of the a-cell phenotype in early experimental diabetes. Diabetes **53:** 2669–2675.
23. YOREK, M.A., L.J. COPPEY, J.S. GELLETT, *et al.* 2004. Sensory nerve innervations of epineurial arterioles of the sciatic nerve containing calcitonin gene-related peptide: effect of streptozotocin induced diabetes. Exp. Diabesity Res. **5:** 187–193.
24. TROGER, J., C. HUMPEL, B. KREMSER, *et al.* 1999. The effect of streptozotocin-induced diabetes mellitus on substance P and calcitonin gene-related peptide expression in the rat trigeminal ganglion. Brain Res. **842:** 84–91.
25. GARRETT, N.E., B.L. KIDD, S.C. CRUWYS, *et al.* 1996. Effect of streptozotocin-diabetes on knee joint inflammation-induced changes in substance P and nerve growth factor in the rat. Brain Res. Mol. Brain Res. **42:** 272–278.

26. Adeghate, E., A.S. Ponery, D.J. Pallot, *et al.* 2001. Distribution of vasoactive intestinal polypeptide, neuropeptide-Y and substance P and their effects on insulin secretion from the *in vivo* pancreas of normal and diabetic rats. Peptides **22:** 99–107.
27. Stead, R.H., M.H. Perdue, M.G. Blennerhassett, *et al.* 1990. The innervations of mast cells. *In* The Neuroendocrine-Immune Network. S. Freier, Ed.: 19–37. CRC Press. Boca Raton, FL.
28. Ebertz, J.M., C.A. Hirshman, N.S. Kettelkamp, *et al.* 1987. Substance P-induced histamine release in human cutaneous mast cells. J. Invest. Dermatol. **88:** 682–685.
29. Zhao, Z.Z., N.W. Savage, Z. Pujic, *et al.* 1997. Immunohistochemical localization of mast cells and mast cell-nerve interactions in oral lichen planus. Oral Dis. **3:** 71–76.
30. Matsson, L., L.I. Norevall & S. Forsgren. 1995. Anatomic relationship between substance P- and CGRP-immunoreactive nerve fibres and mast cells in the palatal mucosa of the rat. Eur. J. Oral Sci. **103:** 70–76.
31. Ottaway, C.A. & A.M. Stanisz. 1995. Neural-immune interactions in the intestine: implications for inflammatory bowel disease. *In* Inflammatory Bowel Disease. J.B. Karger & R.G. Shorter, Eds.: 281–300. Williams and Wilkins. Baltimore, MD.
32. Kulkari-Narla, A., A.J. Beitz & D.R. Brown. 1999. Catecholaminergic, cholinergic and peptidergic innervations of gut-associated lymphatic tissue in porcine jejunum and ileum. Cell Tissue Res. **298:** 275–286.
33. Fehér, E., K. Altdorfer, G. Bagaméri, *et al.* 2001. Neuroimmune interactions in experimental colitis. Neuroimmunomodulation **9:** 247–256.
34. Williams, R.M., J. Bienenstock & R.H. Stead. 1995. Mast cells: the neuroimmune connection. *In* Human Basophils and Mast Cells. Biological Aspects, Vol. 61. G. Marone, Ed.: 208–235. Karger. Basel.
35. Karanth, S.S., D.R. Spingall, S. Francavilla, *et al.* 1990. Early increase in CGRP- and VIP-immunoreactive nerves in the skin of streptozotocin-induced diabetic rats. Histochemistry **94:** 659–666.
36. Belai, A. & G. Burnstock. 1990. Changes in adrenergic and peptidergic nerves in the submucous plexus of streptozocin-diabetic rat ileum. Gastroenterology **98:** 1427–1436.
37. Gronblad, M., O. Korkala, Y. Konttinen, *et al.* 1991. Immunoreactive neuropeptides in nerves in ligamentous tissue: an experimental neuroimmunohistochemical study. Clin. Orthoped. Relat. Res. **265:** 291–296.
38. Aoki, M., K. Tamai & K. Saotome. 1994. Substance P- and calcitonin gene-related peptide-immunofluorescent nerves in the repair of experimental bone defects. Int. Orthop. **18:** 317–324.
39. Minami, Y., Y. Kurishi, M. Kawamura, *et al.* 1989. Enhancement of preprotachykinin A gene expression by adjuvant-induced inflammation in the rat spinal-cord: possible involvement of substance P-containing spinal neurons in nociception. Neurosci. Lett. **98:** 105–110.
40. Dubner, R. & M.A. Ruda. 1992. Activity-dependent neuronal plasticity following tissue injury and inflammation. Trends Neurosci. **15:** 96–103.
41. Weihe, E., M.K.H. Schäffer, D. Nohr, *et al.* 1994. Expression of neuropeptides, neuropeptide receptors and neuropeptide processing enzymes in spinal neurons and peripheral non-neural cells and plasticity in models of inflammatory pain.

In Neuropeptides. Nociception and Pain. T. Hökfelt, H.G. Schaible & R.F. Schmidt, Eds.: 43–69. Chapman and Hall. London.
42. YASUDA, H., M. TERADA, K. MAEDA, *et al.* 2003. Diabetic neuropathy and nerve regeneration. Prog. Neurobiol. **169:** 229–285.
43. TROGER, J., C. HUMPEL, B. KREMSER, *et al.* 1999. The effect of streptozotocin-induced diabetes mellitus on substance P and calcitonin gene-related peptide expression in the rat trigeminal ganglion. Brain Res. **842:** 84–91.
44. BATBAYAR, B., T. ZELLES, Á. VÉR, *et al.* 2004. Plasticity of the different neuropeptide-containing nerve fibres in the tongue of the diabetic rat. J. Periph. Nerv. Syst. **9:** 215–223.
45. FERNYHOUGH, P., W.J. BREWSTER, K. FERNANDES, *et al.* 1998. Stimulation of nerve growth factor and substance P expression in the iris-trigeminal axis of diabetic rats-involvement of oxidative stress and effects of aldose reductase inhibition. Brain Res. **802:** 247–253.
46. SCHMIDT, R.E., S.B. PLURAD, J.E. SAFFITZ, *et al.* 1985. Retrograde axonal transport of ^{125}I nerve growth factor in rat ileal mesenteric nerves. Effect of streptozotocin. Diabetes **34:** 1230–1240.
47. TOMLINSON, D.R., P. FERNYHOUGH & L.T. DIEMEL. 1997. Role of neurotrophins in diabetic neuropathy and treatment with nerve growth factor. Diabetes **46:** S43–S49.
48. APFEL, S.C., J.C. AREZZO, M. BROWNLEE, *et al.* 1994. Nerve growth factor administration protects against experimental diabetic sensory neuropathy. Brain Res. **634:** 7–12.
49. NOGA, O., C. ENGLMANN, G. HAUF, *et al.* 2003. The production, storage, and release of the neurotrophins NGF, BDNF and NT-3 by human peripheral eosinophils in allergics and non-allergics. Clin. Exp. Allergy **33:** 649–654.
50. TORCIA, M., L. BRACCI-LAUDIERO, M. LUCIBELLO, *et al.* 1996. Nerve growth factor is an autocrine survival factor for memory B lymphocytes. Cell **85:** 345–356.
51. DONNERER, J., R. SCHULIGOI & C. STEIN. 1992. Increased content and transport of substance P and calcitonin gene-related peptide in sensory nerves innervating inflamed tissue: evidence for a regulatory function of nerve growth factor *in vivo*. Neuroscience **49:** 693–698.
52. BREWSTER, W.J., P. FERNYHOUGH, L.T. DIEMEL, *et al.* 1995. Changes in nerve growth factor and preprotachykinin messenger RNA levels in the iris and trigeminal ganglion in diabetic rats: effects of treatment with insulin on nerve growth factor. Brain Res. Mol. Brain Res. **29:** 131–139.
53. SCHÄFFER, M., T. BREITER, H.D. BECKER, *et al.* 1998. Neuropeptides: mediators of inflammation and tissue repair? Arch. Surg. **133:** 1107–1116.
54. FEHÉR, E., K. GALLATZ & FEHÉR, J. 1999. Neuroimmunomodulation made by different neuropeptides in the human colonic mucosa. *In* Falk Symposium 112. Neurogastroenterology. From Basis to the Clinics. H.J. Krammer & M.V. Singer, Eds.: 634–644. Kluver Academic. Dordrecht.
55. SHANAHAN, F. & P.A. ANTON. 1994. Role of peptides in the regulation of the mucosal immune and inflammatory response. *In* Gut Peptides. J.H. Walsh & G.J. Dockray. Eds.: 851–868. Raven Press. New York.
56. BRACCI-LAUDIERO, L., L. ALOE, C. STENFORS, *et al.* 1996. Nerve growth factor stimulates production of neuropeptide Y in human lymphocytes. Neuroreport **7:** 485–488.

57. LECETA, J., C. MARTINEZ, M. DELGADO, *et al.* 1996. Expression of vasoactive intestinal peptide in lymphocytes: a possible endogenous role in the regulation of the immune system. Adv. Neuroimmunol. **6:** 29–36.
58. LAI, J.P., S.D. DOUGLAS, F. SHAHEEN, *et al.* 2002. Quantification of substance P mRNA in human immune cells by real time reverse transcriptase PCR assay. Clin. Diagn. Lab. Immun. **9:** 138–143.
59. HOLZER, P. & U. HOLZER-PETSCHE. 1997. Tachykinins in the gut. Part II. Roles in neural excitation, secretion, and inflammation. Pharmacol. Ther. **73:** 219–263.
60. LEMBECK, F. & P. HOLZER. 1979. Substance P as neurogenic mediator of antidromic vasodilation and neurogenic plasma extravasation. Arch. Pharmacol. **310:** 175–183.
61. STEAD, R.H., M. TOMIOKA, G. QUINONEZ, *et al.* 1987. Intestinal mucosal mast cells in normal and nematode-infected rat intestines are in intimate contact with peptidergic nerves. Proc. Natl. Acad. Sci. USA **84:** 2975–2979.
62. STEAD, R.H., M.F. DIXON, N.H. BRAMWELL, *et al.* 1989. Mast cells are closely apposed to nerves in the human gastrointestinal mucosa. Gastroenterology **97:** 575–585.
63. BATBAYAR, B., J. SOMOGYI, T. ZELLES, *et al.* 2003. Immunohistochemical analysis of substance P containing nerve fibres and their contacts with mast cells in the diabetic rat's tongue. Acta Biol. Hung. **54:** 275–283.
64. KATAEVA, G., A. AGRO & A.M. STANISZ. 1994. Substance-P–mediated intestinal inflammation: inhibitory effects of CP 96,345 and SMS 201-295. Neuroimmunomodulation **1:** 350–356.
65. O'CONNOR, T.M., J. O'CONNELL, D.I. O'BRIEN, *et al.* 2004. The role of substance P in inflammatory disease. J. Cell. Physiol. **201:** 167–180.
66. SONEA, I.M., M.V. PALMER, D. AKILI, *et al.* 2002. Treatment with neurokinin-1 receptor antagonist reduces severity of inflammatory bowel disease induced by *Cryptosporidium parvum*. Clin. Diagn. Lab. Immunol. **9:** 333–340.
67. DIEMEL, L.T., E.J. STEVENS, G.B. BREWSTER, *et al.* 1992. Depletion of substance P and calcitonin gene-related peptide in sciatic nerve of rats with experimental diabetes: effects of insulin and aldose reductase inhibition. Neurosci. Lett. **137:** 253–256.
68. MARKLE, R.A. & D.K. WALKER. 1996. Effects of streptozotocin-induced diabetes and insulin treatment on substance P of the rat arterial wall. Life Sci. **58:** 1123–1129.
69. BELAI, A., N.A. CALCUTT, A.L. CARRINGTON, *et al.* 1996. Enteric neuropeptides in streptozotocin-diabetic rats; effects of insulin and aldose reductase inhibition. J. Autonom. Nerv. Syst. **58:** 163–169.
70. NOWAK, T.V., W.W. CHEY, T.M. CHANG, *et al.* 1995. Effect of streptozotocin-induced diabetes mellitus on release of vasoactive intestinal polypeptide from rodent small intestine. Dig. Dis. Sci. **40:** 828–836.
71. RECIO-PINTO, E., M.M. RECHLER & D.N. ISHII. 1986. Effects of insulin, insulin like growth factor on neurite formation and survival in cultured sympathetic and sensory neurons. J. Neurosci. **6:** 1211–1219.
72. RECIO-PINTO, E. & D.N. ISHII. 1988. Insulin and related growth factors: effects on the nervous system and mechanism for neurite growth and regeneration. Neurochem. Int. **12:** 397–414.
73. SJÖBERG, J. & M. KANJE. 1989. Insulin like growth factor as a stimulator of regeneration in the freeze-injured rat sciatic nerve. Brain Res. **485:** 102–108.

Pattern of Distribution of Calcitonin Gene–Related Peptide in the Dorsal Root Ganglion of Animal Models of Diabetes Mellitus

ERNEST ADEGHATE,[a] HAMEED RASHED,[a] SATYAN RAJBANDARI,[b] AND JAIPAUL SINGH[c]

[a]*Department of Anatomy, Faculty of Medicine and Health Sciences, UAE University, Al Ain, United Arab Emirates*

[b]*Lancashire Teaching Hospital at Chorley and South Ribble, Chorley, PR7 1PP, England, UK*

[c]*Department of Biological Sciences, University of Central Lancashire, Preston, PR1 2HE, England UK*

ABSTRACT: This article examined the pattern of distribution of calcitonin gene–related peptide (CGRP) in the dorsal root ganglion (DRG) of normal and diabetic Wistar, Zucker lean, and Goto-Kakizaki (GK) rats to determine whether there are changes in the number and pattern of distribution of CGRP-positive neurons after the onset of latent or overt diabetes. Type 1 diabetes mellitus was induced in Wistar rats by a single dose of streptozotocin (STZ) given intraperitoneally (60 mg/kg body weight). Four weeks after the induction of diabetes mellitus, diabetic ($n = 6$) and normal ($n = 6$), Zucker lean ($n = 6$), and GK ($n = 6$) rats were anesthetized with chloral hydrate and their DRGs were removed and processed for immunohistochemistry. CGRP-positive neurons were observed in the DRG of normal and diabetic Wistar, Zucker lean (non-diabetic), and GK (animal model of type 2 diabetes) rats. CGRP was present in small-, medium-, and large-sized neurons of the DRG in these three animal models. Only a small percentage of large-sized neurons contains CGRP. The number of CGRP-positive neurons was significantly ($P < 0.05$) reduced in STZ-induced diabetic Wistar and GK rats compared to normal Wistar and Zucker lean rats. Moreover, the quantity of CGRP-containing varicose nerves was less in diabetic Wistar and GK rats compared to control Wistar and Zucker lean rats. The reduced number of CGRP-positive neurons in the DRG of GK rats indicated that subjects with latent diabetes may already have dysfunctional CGRP metabolism and thus diabetic neuropathy.

Address for correspondence: Ernest Adeghate, M.D., M.F.M., Ph.D., Department of Anatomy, Faculty of Medicine and Health Sciences, UAE University, PO Box 17666, Al Ain, United Arab Emirates. Voice: 971-3-7137496; fax: 971-3-7672033.
e-mail: eadeghate@uaeu.ac.ae

Ann. N.Y. Acad. Sci. 1084: 296–303 (2006).
doi: 10.1196/annals.1372.030

KEYWORDS: **CGRP; spinal ganglion; Wistar; Zucker; Goto-Kakizaki; immunohistochemistry; diabetes mellitus; rat**

INTRODUCTION

Diabetes is a common endocrine disorder affecting millions of people worldwide. In addition, diabetic neuropathy is a common late chronic complication in both type I and type II diabetes. Previous studies have shown that the central nervous system is involved in diabetic neuropathy.[1] Established peripheral neuropathy is irreversible, whereas it can be postulated that early correction of biochemical and functional abnormalities in the nerve could delay or prevent the onset of clinical neuropathy. There have been several studies on early neuropathy, and in one experimental study, the peripheral nerves of streptozotocin (STZ)-induced diabetic rats failed to show any structural abnormalities, but there was significant biochemical abnormalities and reduction in the nerve conduction velocity and pain threshold.[2] The prominent sensory involvement in early diabetic polyneuropathy may suggest that the disease particularly targets the dorsal root ganglion (DRG). DRGs have features that might suggest they would be vulnerable to changes known to occur in diabetes, that is, microangiopathy, excessive polyol flux, and protein glycosylation.[3,4]

Abnormalities of axonal transport are believed to be present in metabolic neuropathies even before the development of nerve fiber pathology and clinical signs of neuropathy.[5] Axonal transport is dependent on number of factors, such as sodium potassium pump, calcium, and various other ions. It has been suggested that calcitonin gene–related-peptide (CGRP) can be used as a marker for a subpopulation of nociceptive primary afferents. [6] The aim of this article was to examine the pattern of distribution of CGRP (a marker of sensory neurons) in three different animals species used for the study of diabetes. In addition, the study investigates the presence of CGRP in the subpopulation of neurons in the DRG.

Ethics

The experiment was conducted in accordance with the guidelines set by the Animal Ethics Committee of the Faculty of Medicine & Health Sciences, UAE University.

MATERIALS AND METHODS

Animals and Induction of Diabetes Mellitus

Twelve week-old male Wistar rats weighing approximately 250 g were used throughout this study. Rats were obtained from the United Arab Emirates University breeding colony. The rats were divided into two groups, STZ-induced diabetics and age-matched controls. Diabetes was induced by a single intraperitoneal injection of STZ (Sigma, Poole, UK) at 60 mg/kg prepared in 5-mM citrate buffer pH 4.50.[7] The animals were kept in plastic cages and maintained on standard laboratory animal diet with food and water *ad libitum*. One-Touch II® Glucometer (LifeScan, Johnson and Johnson, Milpitas, CA) was used to measure the blood glucose for each individual animal. The animals were considered diabetic if the random blood glucose levels were equal to or more than 300 mg/dL. After 4 weeks from the date of induction of diabetes all of the animals from both groups were sacrificed humanely after cervical dislocation. A mid-line incision on the back was made, and a deep dissection of the back region was made to isolate the DRG. The DRG of Zucker lean and Goto-Kakizaki (GK) rats were also removed and processed for immunohistochemistry.

Immunohistochemistry

The isolated DRG of control and diabetic Wistar rats, Zucker lean, and GK rats was trimmed free of adherent fat and fixed overnight in freshly prepared Zamboni's fixative.[8] The DRGs were later dehydrated in graded concentrations of ethanol, cleared in xylene, and subsequently embedded in paraffin wax at 55°C. Sections of 6 μm thickness were cut on a microtome (AS325, Shandon, Pittsburgh, PA), and placed in waterbath at 48°C. Thereafter, they were transferred onto prewashed microscopic slides, which were dried in an oven at 55°C for 30 min to enhance attachment of sections.

Sections were deparaffinized with xylene, transferred into absolute ethanol and then incubated for 30 min in 0.3% hydrogen peroxide solution in methanol to block endogenous peroxidase activity. The sections were hydrated in decreasing concentration of ethanol and brought to Tris buffered saline (TBS). The sections were washed three times (5 min each) in TBS and processed for immunohistochemistry using a previously described method.[7] Briefly, after 30 min incubation in the blocking reagent antibodies (at 1:1500 dilution) against CGRP were applied for 24 h at 4°C. The slides were then washed and incubated for 30 min with prediluted biotinylated anti-rabbit IgG. After washing in TBS the sections were incubated in streptavidin peroxidase conjugate for 45 min. The sections were incubated for 3 min in 3, 3-diaminobenzidine tetrahydrochloride containing 0.03% hydrogen peroxide in TBS. The slides were later washed, counter-stained with hematoxylin, dehydrated in ethanol, and cleared in xylene. The tissues were subsequently mounted in Cytoseal 60 (Stephens Scientific, Riverdale, NJ). Slides were examined under Zeiss Axiophot microscope (Jena, Germany) and immunopositive areas of the tissue sections were photographed.

The antisera to CGRP were purchased from Affiniti Laboratories (Exeter, UK). No specific immunostaining was observed in pancreatic tissue when primary antisera were omitted.

Statistical Analysis

All values were expressed as mean ± standard deviation (SD). Statistical significance was assessed using Students' *t*-test. Values with $P < 0.05$ were accepted as significant.

RESULTS

Distribution of CGRP in the Spinal Ganglion of Normal and Diabetic Wistar Rats, GK, and Zucker Rats

CGRP was observed in the neurons of the DRG of normal (FIG. 1 A) and diabetic (FIG. 1 B) Wistar and also in Zucker lean (nondiabetic) (FIG. 1 C) and in GK (FIG. 1 D) rats. However, the number of CGRP-immunoreactive neurons in the DRG of diabetic Wistar rats was significantly smaller compared to normal control. Similarly, CGRP-containing neurons of the DRG of GK rats were fewer compared to Zucker lean and normal Wistar rats that do not have diabetes (FIG. 1).

CGRP in the DRG of Normal and Diabetic Wistar Rats

FIGURE 2 shows the pattern of distribution of CGRP-positive cells in the DRG of normal and diabetic Wistar rats. CGRP-immunoreactive neurons were observed in the DRG of both normal and diabetic Wistar rats. Although, CGRP was present in the medium-sized neurons of the DRG of Wistar rats, it was most common in the subpopulation of small-sized neurons. The pattern of distribution of CGRP changed after the onset of STZ-induced diabetes (a model of type 1 diabetes). There was a significant ($P < 0.05$) loss of CGRP in many neurons and in fine varicose nerve fibres after the onset of diabetes.

CGRP in the DRG of Zucker Rats

The pattern of distribution of CGRP in the neuronal profiles of the DRG of Zucker lean rats is similar to that observed in the DRG of normal Wistar rats. Small-sized neurons were the largest subpopulation of neurons followed by the medium sized. Most of the small- and medium-sized neurons were immunopositive for CGRP while majority of the large neurons were not (FIGS. 3 A and B).

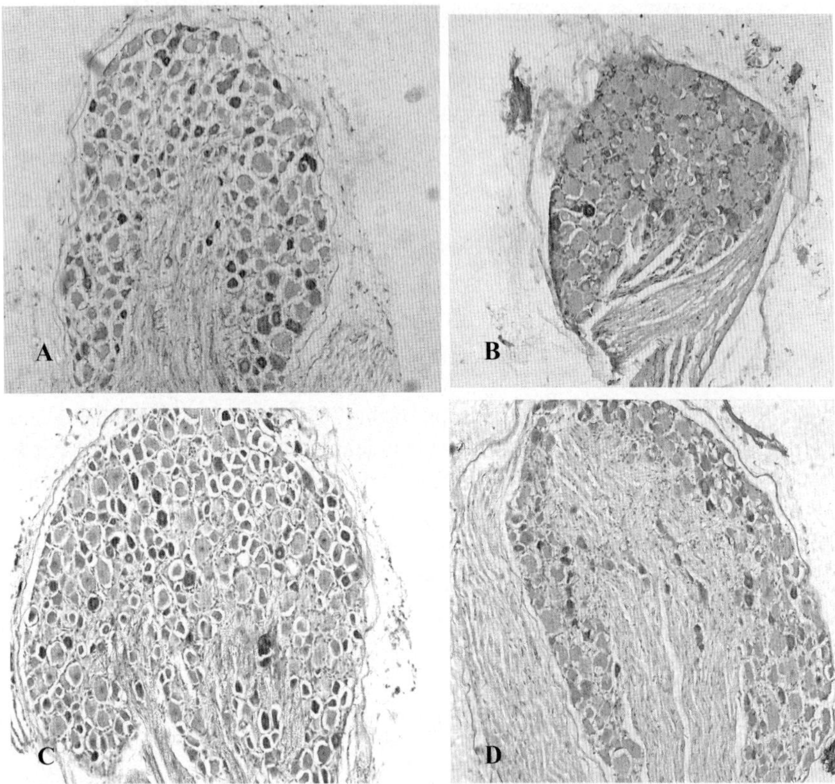

FIGURE 1. CGRP-immunoreactive neurons (*black profiles*) in the dorsal root ganglion of normal Wistar (**A**), diabetic (**B**), Zucker lean rat. (**C**), and GK (**D**) rats Note that, CGRP-positive neurons are fewer in Wistar diabetic and GK rats compared to controls. Magnification: 100×.

CGRP in the DRG of GK Rats

The GK rats are used as models of type 2 diabetes. The DRG of this animal species is similar to that of Wistar and Zucker rats. However, the number of CGRP-immunoreactive neurons was significantly ($P < 0.05$) lower compared to normal Wistar and Zucker lean rats. In addition, fewer varicose nerves of the DRG of GK rats contain CGRP when compared to normal Wistar and Zucker lean rats (Figs. 3 C and D).

DISCUSSION

The results of this study showed that the DRGs of Wistar, GK, and Zucker rats are similar in morphology with distinct subpopulations of small-, medium-, and large-sized neurons. In addition, the pattern of distribution of CGRP in

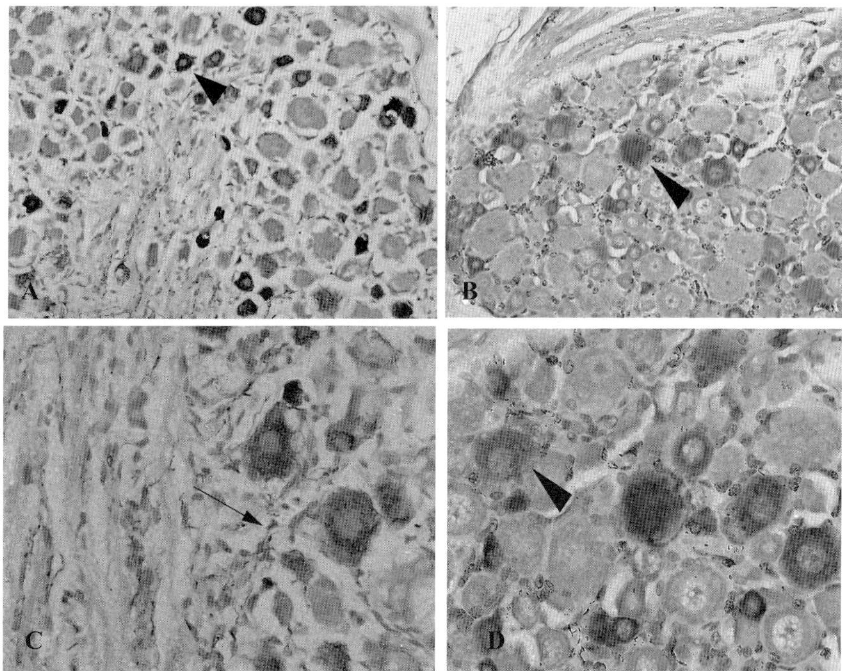

FIGURE 2. CGRP-immunopositive neurons (*arrow head*) in the dorsal root ganglion of normal Wistar (**A, C**) and diabetic (**B, D**) rats. Note that, CGRP-positive neurons are fewer in diabetic Wistar rat compared to controls. The number of CGRP-containing varicose nerves (*arrow*) are also fewer in the DRG of diabetic rats. Magnification: A, B—200×; C, D—400×.

the DRG of all of these three rat species is not different. What appears to be different is the number of cells that are positive for CGRP. There is a significant loss of CGRP-immunoreactivity after the onset of overt and latent diabetes. CGRP is important in the maintenance of important structures and cells within our system and a loss of this important neuropeptide could have severe repercussion. For example, CGRP has trophic effect on several structures including myotubules,[9] motoneuron[10] and peripheral nerves,[11] it is therefore expected that the loss of CGRP in the neurons of the DRG will affect the way it functions. The decrease in the quantity of neuropeptides after the onset of diabetes is not new. It has been shown that the quantity of vasoactive intestinal polypeptide is decreased in the gastrointestinal tract of STZ-induced diabetic rat.[12] In addition, peptides, such as insulin, also decrease in diabetes.[13] Some investigators have also reported that experimental diabetes in the mouse model is associated with loss of immunoreactive CGRP primary sensory neurons of the A-cell phenotype.[14] They concluded that this loss could play a role for the touch-evoked nociception in the model, and that the neuronal immunoreactive CGRP abnormality possibly is mediated by activation of the p75 neurotrophin

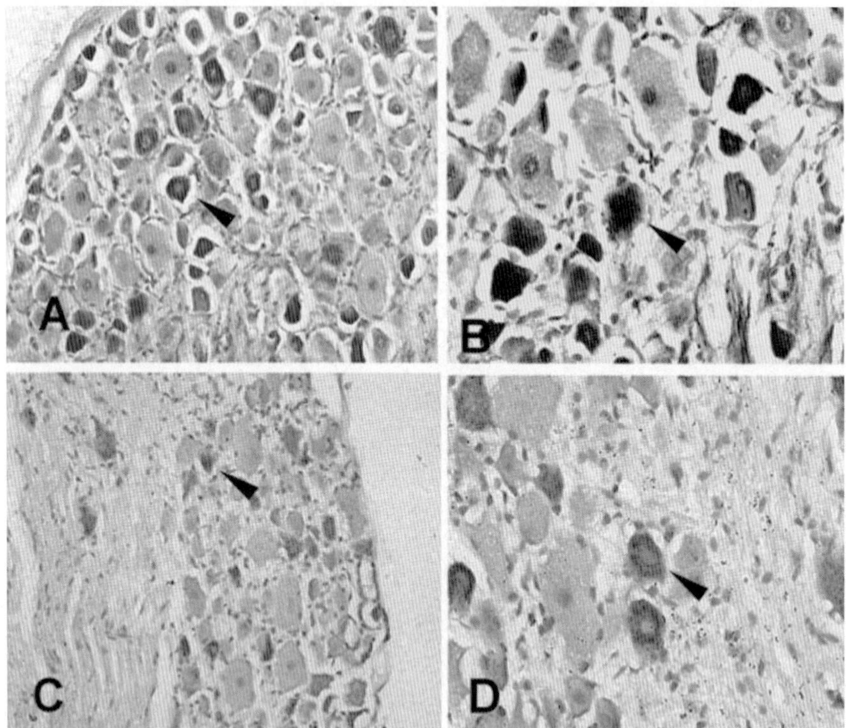

FIGURE 3. CGRP-immunopositive neurons (*arrow head*) in the dorsal root ganglion of Zucker lean (**A, B**) and GK (**C, D**) rats. Note that, CGRP-positive neurons are fewer in GK rat compared to Zucker lean rats. The number of CGRP-containing varicose nerves are also fewer in the DRG of GK rats compared to Zucker lean rats. Magnification: A, C—200×; B, D—400×.

receptor. Other investigators showed a decrease in the cell diameter of CGRP-positive cells.[15]

Another striking observation in this study is the decrease in the number of CGRP-containing varicosities in the DRG of diabetic rats. Since CGRP have been shown to modulate pain responses transmitted by primary sensory afferents, a decrease in the number of CGRP-positive neurons and nerve varicosites could be a contributory factor in the pathogenesis of neuropathic pain./p>

In conclusion, this study demonstrates a decrease in the number of CGRP-containing neurons in the DRG of diabetic Wistar and GK rats coupled with a decrease in the number of CGRP-positive varicose nerves. The reduced number of CGRP-positive neurons in the DRG of GK rats indicates that subjects with latent diabetes may already have loss of CGRP and thus diabetic neuropathy.

ACKNOWLEDGMENT

This study was supported by a Research Grant from the FMHS, United Arab Emirates University.

REFERENCES

1. EATON, S.E., N.D. HARRIS, S.M. RAJBHANDARI, *et al.* 2001. Spinal-cord involvement in diabetic peripheral neuropathy. Lancet **358:** 35–36.
2. WALKER, D., A. CARRINGTON, S.A. CANNAN, *et al.* 1999. Structural abnormalities do not explain the early functional abnormalities in the peripheral nerves of the streptozotocin diabetic rat. J. Anat. **195:** 419–427.
3. ZOCHODNE, D.W. 1996. Is early diabetic neuropathy a disorder of the dorsal root ganglion? A hypothesis and critique of some current ideas on the etiology of diabetic neuropathy. J. Peripher. Nerv. Syst. **1:** 119–130.
4. HIRADE, M., H. YASUDA, M. OMATSU-KANBE, *et al.* 1999. Tetrodotoxin-resistant sodium channels of dorsal root ganglion neurons are readily activated in diabetic rats. Neuroscience **90:** 933–939.
5. SIDENIUS, P. & J. JAKOBSEN. 1987. Anterograde fast component of axonal transport during insulin-induced hypoglycemia in nondiabetic and diabetic rats. Diabetes **36:** 853–858.
6. TRAUB, R.J., B. ALLEN, E. HUMPHREY & M.A. Ruda. 1990. Analysis of calcitonin gene-related peptide-like immunoreactivity in the cat dorsal spinal cord and dorsal root ganglia provide evidence for a multisegmental projection of nociceptive C-fiber primary afferents. J. Comp. Neurol. **302:** 562–574.
7. ADEGHATE, E. & A.S. PONERY. 2004. Diabetes mellitus influences the degree of co-localization of calcitonin-gene-related-peptide with insulin and somatostatin in the rat pancreas. Pancreas **29:** 311–319.
8. ZAMBONI, L. & C. DE MARTINO. 1967. Buffered picric acid-formaldehyde: a new rapid fixation for electron microscopy. J. Cell Biol. **35:** 148A.
9. CHANGEUX, J.P., A. DUCLERT & S. SEKINE. 1992. Calcitonin gene-related peptides and neuromuscular interactions. Ann. N. Y. Acad. Sci. **657:** 361–378.
10. BAR, P.R. & P. SODAAR. 1992. The effect of culture conditions and alpha-MSH on CGRP in motoneurons in culture. Ann. N. Y. Acad. Sci. **657:** 555–557.
11. DUMOULIN, F.L., G. RAIVICH, C.A. HAAS, *et al.* 1992. Calcitonin gene-related peptide and peripheral nerve regeneration. Ann. N. Y. Acad. Sci. **657:** 351–360.
12. ADEGHATE, E., A.S. PONERY, A.K. SHARMA, *et al.* 2001. Diabetes mellitus is associated with a decrease in vasoactive intestinal polypeptide content of gastrointestinal tract of rat. Arch. Physiol. Biochem. **109:** 246–251.
13. ADEGHATE, E. & A.S. PONERY. 2003. Pancreatic peptides, neuropeptides and neurotransmitters in diabetes mellitus: a review. Int. J. Diabetes Metab. **11:** 1–6.
14. JIANG, Y., J.R. NYENGAARD, J.S. ZHANG & J. JAKOBSEN. 2004. Selective loss of calcitonin gene-related peptide-expressing primary sensory neurons of the a-cell phenotype in early experimental diabetes. Diabetes **53:** 2669–2675.
15. TERENGHI, G., S. CHEN, A.L. CARRINGTON, *et al.* 1994. Changes in sensory neuropeptides in dorsal root ganglion and spinal cord of spontaneously diabetic BB rats. A quantitative immunohistochemical study. Acta Diabetol. **31:** 198–204.

Cardiovascular Risk Factors Predicting the Development of Distal Symmetrical Polyneuropathy in People with Type 1 Diabetes

A 9-Year Follow-up Study

LATIKA SIBAL, HUONG NAI LAW, JANICE GEBBIE, AND PHILIP HOME

Newcastle Diabetes Centre, Newcastle upon Tyne, NE4 6BE United Kingdom

Newcastle University, Newcastle upon Tyne, NE2 4HH United Kingdom

ABSTRACT: The aim of the article was to use prospectively collected data on people with type 1 diabetes to examine which routinely collected clinical measures predict the development of peripheral neuropathy in people with type 1 diabetes. Within the Newcastle Diabetes Services, structured data collection at an annual review has been collected since 1985. This includes metabolic measures, cardiovascular risk factors, and markers of complications. From 1990 data collection was standardized and computerized. For this study, all people with type 1 diabetes in the database in both 1992 and 2001 were ascertained. Data were extracted for a diagnosis of peripheral neuropathy (based on neuropathic symptoms, absence of pinprick sensation, and abnormal biothesiometer measurements and/or monofilament sensation) and for the other metabolic and cardiovascular risk measures, as well as markers of other microvascular complications. Associations with the development of neuropathy were sought. Eighteen of 404 people already had peripheral neuropathy in 1992, and 38 others developed neuropathy during follow-up. People who developed neuropathy were older (47 ± 14 [SD] versus 36 ± 11 years; $P = 0.000$), had longer-duration of diabetes (27 ± 13 versus 18 ± 10 years; $P = 0.001$), higher baseline serum cholesterol (5.8 ± 1.3 versus 5.2 ± 1.2 mmol/L, $P = 0.017$), and higher systolic (139 ± 18 versus 129 ± 20 mmHg; $P = 0.003$) and diastolic BP (82 ± 12 versus 76 ± 11 mmHg; $P = 0.009$) than those who remained free of neuropathy. We found no significant difference for BMI and glycated hemoglobin. The multivariate model showed that diastolic BP, duration of diabetes, serum

Address for correspondence: Latika Sibal, SCMS-Diabetes, The Medical School, Framlington Place, Newcastle upon Tyne, NE2 4HH, UK. Voice: 44-191-256-3365; fax: 44-191-256-3212.
e-mail: latika.sibal@ncl.ac.uk

Ann. N.Y. Acad. Sci. 1084: 304–318 (2006).
doi: 10.1196/annals.1372.036

cholesterol, and history of callus/ulcers on the feet predicted the development of peripheral neuropathy. Neuropathy developed in 11.4% of people with type 1 diabetes over a 9-year follow-up, and was predicted by factors normally associated with cardiovascular rather than microvascular disease.

KEYWORDS: **type 1 diabetes; neuropathy; risk factors**

INTRODUCTION

Peripheral neuropathy is an important microvascular complication of diabetes, resulting in substantial morbidity. In people with type 1 diabetes the prevalence approaches 50% after 20 years of diabetes. The associated morbidity coupled with the risk of foot ulcers and amputations results in not just an impairment of the quality of life, but also constitutes a huge economic burden.[1] The annual costs of diabetic peripheral neuropathy and its complications in the United States were $0.8 billion for type 1 diabetes for 2001.[2]

Previous studies have demonstrated that poor glycemic control is a risk factor for the development of peripheral neuropathy and the duration of exposure to hyperglycemia influences the severity of neuropathy.[3–7] The Diabetes Control and Complications Trial (DCCT) demonstrated that intensive insulin therapy reduced the occurrence of neuropathy by 60% compared with conventional insulin therapy.[5] The Epidemiology of Diabetes Intervention and Complications (EDIC) study which followed-up the DCCT cohort showed that the beneficial effect of prior intensive therapy on neuropathy status persisted despite similar glycemic control between the two groups during the subsequent 8-year follow-up.[8]

Factors other than hyperglycemia which predispose to the development of peripheral neuropathy have been suggested.[3,9] More recently, analysis of the EURODIAB study suggested that a higher serum cholesterol, LDL cholesterol, serum triglyceride, body mass index (BMI), hypertension, smoking, urinary albumin excretion rate, and von Willebrand factor level are all associated with the incidence of neuropathy, after adjusting for the duration of diabetes and glycated hemoglobin.[10] Other studies have suggested that other factors normally associated with a risk of cardiovascular events, namely hypertension and the presence of peripheral vascular disease, are associated with the development of neuropathy.[11,12]

We therefore hypothesized that the presence of cardiovascular risk factors, detected in routine clinical practice, might help identify those at risk of developing distal peripheral neuropathy (DPN) in people with type 1 diabetes. To test this hypothesis, we evaluated baseline predictors of DPN in people with type 1 diabetes attending the Newcastle Diabetes Services in the Northeast of England using data collected prospectively over 9 years.

METHODS

Study Design and Population

Study design was a retrospective analysis of data collected prospectively in structured format over a 9-year period. Ethics approval for data review was obtained from the local research ethics committee. A total of 404 people (54% male, mean age 40.5 ± 13.5 [SD], range 17–81 years) with type 1 diabetes attended the diabetes services in Newcastle upon Tyne for structured annual outpatient review in 1992, and had follow-up information available in 2001, or had died. Of these, 18 people had DPN (defined below) at base line and were excluded from the analysis. Of the remaining 386 people, 52 died during the follow-up and the remaining 334 people had attended the diabetes services again in 2001.

Definition of Peripheral Neuropathy

DPN was defined by presence of two of three measures performed as part of structured annual review: neuropathic symptoms, absence of pinprick sensation, and abnormal biothesiometer measurements and/or abnormal 10-g monofilament sensation. A history of neuropathic symptoms was taken to include positive symptoms, such as aching, burning or prickling sensation in the legs, and negative symptoms, such as numbness or a "dead" feeling in the feet. Pinprick sensation was assessed using Neurotips (Owen Mumford, Chipping Norton, UK) at the hallux bilaterally; neuropathy was considered if a unilateral abnormality was detected.

Vibration perception was measured using a biothesiometer (Horwell, Wilford, UK) with the average of three readings taken bilaterally on the hallux and medial malleolus measured for the purpose of the analysis as described previously. In 1997 the biothesiometer measurement was replaced by use of a 10-g monofilament used on plantar surfaces including the hallux.

Biochemical Measures and Other Microvascular Complications

Baseline glycated hemoglobin was DCCT-aligned by formal regression between the methods used in 1992–2001 (nondiabetic reference <6.1%). Microalbuminuria measured by nephelometry was defined as urine albumin:creatinine ratio ≥2.5 mg/mmol creatinine for men and ≥3.5 mg/mmol creatinine for women in people without proteinuria. We estimated glomerular filtration rate (GFR) by the modification of diet in renal disease (MDRD) equation.[13,14] The following baseline predictors of cardiovascular risk were assessed: serum total cholesterol and triglycerides, smoking, BMI, and systolic and diastolic blood pressure (BP) (standard sphygmomanometer, sitting); all were formal parts of the annual review process. Diabetic retinopathy was defined as nonproliferative, preproliferative, or proliferative classified on the basis of retinal photographs, initially taken using Polaroid film and later by digital cameras.

Definition of Cardiovascular Disease (CVD)

CVD was defined as ischemic heart disease, cerebrovascular disease, or peripheral vascular disease. Ischemic heart disease was defined as a history of myocardial infarction, angina, or revascularization including coronary angioplasty or coronary artery bypass grafting (CABG). Cerebrovascular disease was defined as stroke or transient ischemic attack (TIA). Peripheral vascular disease was defined as absent peripheral pulses (dorsalis pedis and posterior tibial) along with a history of claudication, peripheral ischemia, or a revascularization procedure in the legs.

Normotension was defined as systolic/diastolic BP less than 140/90 mmHg without antihypertensive therapy. Patients were classified as being hypertensive if they were on antihypertensive therapy or had a BP greater than this.

Statistical Analysis

Statistical analyses were performed using Minitab14 (Minitab, Coventry, UK) and SPSS 11 (SPSS, Chicago, IL). Univariate analysis was performed using Student's t-test or the Mann-Whitney U-test where appropriate. Factors which were significant on univariate analysis at $P \leq 0.100$ were assessed using logistic regression.

RESULTS

Eighteen of 404 (4.5%) people had DPN at the index visit in 1992. The remaining 386 people free of neuropathy at base line had a mean age of 39 ± 13 (SD) years and a mean duration of diabetes 20 ± 11 (range 1–56) years. Fifty-two people died during the follow-up and were thus excluded from further analysis. Thirty-eight people (11.4%) developed DPN during the follow-up period. The incidence of neuropathy increased with increasing age of the patients. The 9-year incidence in people of age <20, 20–40, 40–60, and >60 years was 0.0, 6.9, 14.2, and 42.9%, respectively. In addition, the incidence of neuropathy increased from 4% in people who had diabetes for <10 years compared with 50% in people with duration of diabetes >40 years (FIG. 1). Biothesiometer

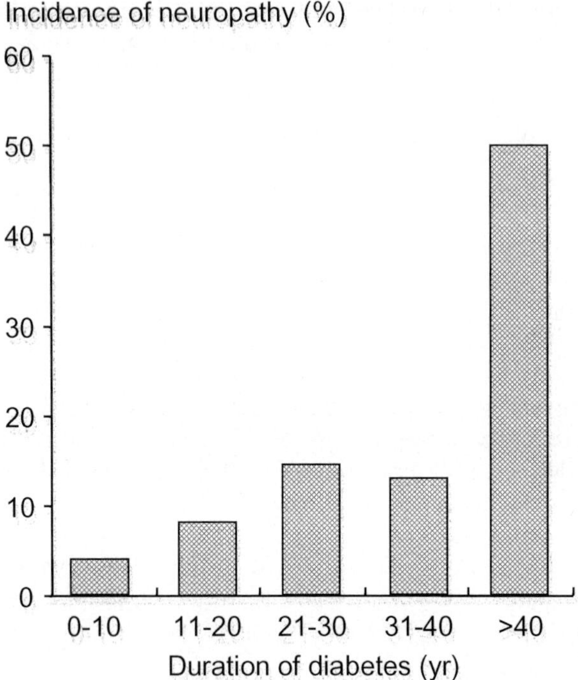

FIGURE 1. Incidence of neuropathy in relation to duration of diabetes in people with type 1 diabetes.

measurements became impaired in 54 out of 334 (16.2%) people during the follow-up when analyzed according to age-adjusted values, of whom 38 met the study criteria of peripheral neuropathy. Neuropathic symptoms were reported by 24 of the 38 (63%), pinprick sensation was impaired in 24 (63%), and impaired vibration/monofilament sensation was observed in 31 (82%).

Univariate Analysis

People who developed neuropathy were older (47 ± 14 versus 36 ± 11 years; $P = 0.000$) and had longer duration of diabetes (27 ± 13 versus 18 ± 10 years; $P = 0.001$) than those who remained free of neuropathy. Systolic and diastolic BP, serum creatinine, serum cholesterol, and triglyceride were higher than the group who remained free of peripheral neuropathy (TABLE 1).

We found no significant difference in BMI, height, and glycated hemoglobin at base line between the two groups. In addition, updated average glycated hemoglobin calculated by taking the average of four readings from 1992, 1996, 1998, and 2001, respectively, was no different between the two groups.

TABLE 1. Baseline markers of development of peripheral neuropathy during follow-up

	Neuropathy	No neuropathy	*P*
N	38	296	
Age (years)	47.1 ± 14.1	36.4 ± 11.3	0.000
Sex (% male)	55	57	NS
Duration of diabetes (years)	27 ± 13	18 ± 10	0.001
Height (m)	1.65 ± 0.29	1.68 ± 0.14	NS
BMI (kg/m^2)	25.8 ± 4.1	25.6 ± 3.5	NS
Systolic BP (mmHg)	139 ± 18	129 ± 20	0.003
Diastolic BP (mmHg)	82 ± 12	76 ± 11	0.009
Serum cholesterol (mmol/L)	5.8 ± 1.3	5.2 ± 1.2	0.017
Serum triglyceride (mmol/L)	1.5 (1.1–2.4)	1.1 (0.8–1.7)	0.018
Serum HDL (mmol/L)	1.5 ± 0.7	1.9 ± 1.5	0.062
Serum LDL (mmol/L)	3.5 ± 1.1	3.0 ± 0.8	NS
HbA$_{1c}$ (%) in 1992	9.7 ± 2.5	9.4 ± 2.2	NS
HbA$_{1c}$ (%) in 2001	8.7 ± 1.8	8.7 ± 1.5	NS
Average updated HbA$_{1c}$ (%)	8.9 ± 1.4	8.9 ± 1.3	NS
Serum creatinine (μmol/L)	92 ± 16	85 ± 17	0.030
Microalbuminuria 1992 (*n* (%))	10/30 (33)	71/244 (29)	NS
Microalbuminuria 2001 (*n* (%))	13/38 (34)	46/ 270 (17)	0.012
Alcohol excess (*n* (%))	2/38 (5)	14/296 (5)	NS
Current alcohol intake	21/38 (55)	200/296 (68)	NS
Smoking (*n* (%))	10 (26)	52 (18)	NS
CVD (*n* (%))	8 (21)	28 (9)	0.027
eGFR (mL/min/1.73 m^2)	76 ± 18	87 ± 19	0.001
Hypertension (*n* (%))	16 (42)	54 (18)	0.001
ACE inhibitors (*n* (%))	3 (8)	33 (11)	NS
Statins (*n* (%))	5 (13)	50 (17)	NS

Number (%), or mean ± SD.
HDL data in 1992 available in 147 (44%).

Analysis of quarters of baseline glycated hemoglobin showed the incidence of neuropathy increased with poorer glycemic control. The values of the quarters of glycated hemoglobin were $<$8.1, 8.2–9.0, 9.1–10.5, and $>$10.6% and the corresponding incidence was 8.7, 8.3, 15.2, and 16.4%, respectively. On combining the two upper and two lower quarters, neuropathy was noted to be present in a greater proportion of people with baseline glycated hemoglobin of $>$9.0% compared with people with a baseline glycated hemoglobin $\leq$9.0% (FIG. 2).

Smoking and Alcohol Use

Current or past cigarette use was not significantly different between the neuropathy developers and nondevelopers. Alcohol excess, defined as intake of greater than 21 units per week for men and 14 units per week for women, and moderate alcohol intake, defined as intake of recommended units of alcohol, was comparable in the two groups.

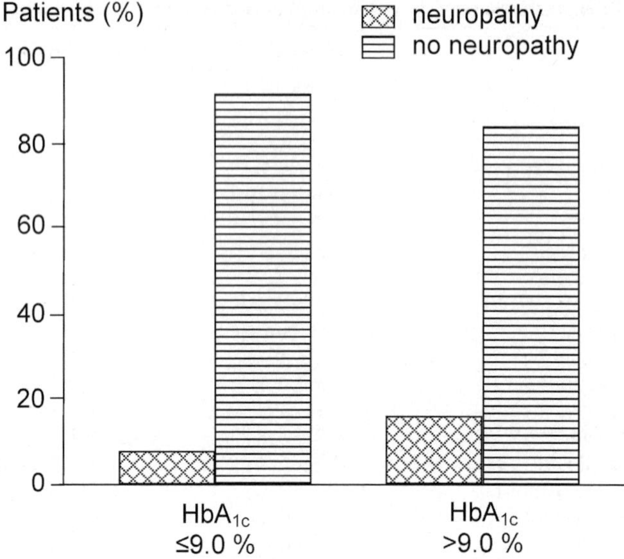

FIGURE 2. The incidence of neuropathy in people with type 1 diabetes divided by baseline glycated hemoglobin of 9.0%. Neuropathy = cross-hatch, no neuropathy = horizontal shading.

Microvascular Complications

A higher proportion of people who developed peripheral neuropathy had diabetic retinopathy at base line. Overall, there was no significant difference in the presence of nonproliferative retinopathy either at base line or during the follow-up. However, proliferative retinopathy was noted to be present in a greater proportion of people later developing neuropathy (11 versus 2%; $P = 0.001$) at base line and at follow-up (13 versus 3%; $P = 0.003$), though the numbers were small (TABLE 2).

Development of microalbuminuria during the follow-up predicted the development of peripheral neuropathy. Estimated GFR was significantly lower in the group that developed neuropathy compared with the group that remained free of neuropathy (TABLE 1).

Feet

Of the people who developed neuropathy, dry skin or callus was present in a greater proportion of people during the follow-up (18 versus 4%; $P = 0.000$), as was a history of ulcers (13 versus 1%; $P = 0.000$). In addition, absent peripheral pulses were noted in a greater number of people developing neuropathy both at base line and during the follow-up period (TABLE 3).

TABLE 2. Retinopathy in relation to incident neuropathy

Retinopathy		Neuropathy (n (%))	No neuropathy (n (%))	P
N		38	296	
Any	baseline	19 (50)	93 (31)	0.019
	follow-up	25 (66)	155 (52)	0.100
Nonproliferative	baseline	16 (42)	88 (29)	NS
	follow-up	21 (55)	146 (49)	NS
Proliferative	baseline	4 (11)	5 (2)	0.001
	follow-up	5 (13)	9 (3)	0.003

Logistic Regression

The multivariate model showed that estimated GFR inversely correlated with the development of neuropathy. Diastolic BP, duration of diabetes, serum cholesterol, and history of callus/ulcers on the feet predicted the later development of neuropathy (TABLE 4).

DISCUSSION

This study reports a lower prevalence and incidence of diabetic peripheral neuropathy in people with type 1 diabetes compared with the published literature,[3,10,15] while being consistent with other studies reporting a prevalence of 14 and 11%.[16,17] However, with increasing age of our patients, the incidence of neuropathy increased from 7% in people below the age of 40 years compared with 43% in people >60 years, in keeping with a study which demonstrated an increase in prevalence of clinical diabetic polyneuropathy from <5% in the 15–19 year to 30% in the 70–74 year age group. Furthermore, we found that as the duration of diabetes increased from <10 to >40 years, so did the

TABLE 3. Foot manifestations in association with neuropathy

		Neuropathy (n (%))	No neuropathy (n (%))	P
N		38	296	
Amputation	baseline	1 (3)	10 (3)	NS
	follow-up	2 (5)	2 (<1)	0.053
Dry skin/callus	baseline	3 (8)	30 (10)	NS
	follow-up	7 (18)	11 (4)	0.000
Ulcer	baseline	0 (0)	0 (0)	–
	follow-up	5 (13)	4 (1)	0.000
PAD	baseline	6 (16)	12 (4)	0.002
	follow-up	13 (34)	17 (6)	0.000

PAD = peripheral arterial disease.

TABLE 4. Predictors of neuropathy development on logistic regression

	P	Odds ratio	95% CI
Duration of diabetes (years)	0.025	1.050	0.99–1.09
Systolic BP (mmHg)	NS	0.985	0.96–1.02
Diastolic BP (mmHg)	0.012	1.080	1.11–1.15
Total serum cholesterol (mmol/L)	0.006	2.386	1.28–4.45
eGFR (mL/min/1.73 m^2)	0.022	0.968	0.91 to $<$1.00
Serum triglyceride (mmol/L)	NS	0.944	0.66–1.35
Smoking (*n* (%))	NS	1.107	0.32–3.81
Microalbuminuria (*n* (%))	NS	0.930	0.32–2.74
Retinopathy (*n* (%))	NS	2.013	0.68–5.99
Foot complications (*n* (%))	0.000	5.574	2.15–14.43

eGFR = estimated glomerular filtration rate by the MDRD method.

incidence of neuropathy from 4 to 50%.[18] A deficiency of our study is that tendon reflexes were not assessed, not having been found useful in clinical practice.

A strength of the study lies in the longitudinal collection of a wide range of structured data in cohort of reasonable size. The neuropathy assessments used were rapid but have been shown by others to be reliable, valid, and reproducible in detecting DPN.[19]

Other studies have confirmed that age of the patient, increasing duration of diabetes, and height are nonmodifiable risk factors of DPN,[10,11,17,20–27] factors consistent with our understanding of the pathogenesis of diabetic neuropathy (TABLE 5). Equally to be expected is that other microvascular complications, and here notably retinopathy at base line and proliferative retinopathy during follow-up, were associated with the development of neuropathy,[3,10,21,22] speculatively regarded as having similar pathogenetic origins, perhaps on the basis of similar pathways of biochemical damage. Similarly, the findings that markers of foot damage commonly associated with neuropathic abnormalities, such as callus and ulceration predict the development of neuropathy, only serve to reinforce the validity of the information collected.

However, on univariate analysis the most striking feature of the data is that it is a range of cardiovascular risk factors, including total serum cholesterol, serum triglycerides, and systolic and diastolic BP, as well as baseline CVD and hypertension, that are strongly predictive of neuropathy rather than as might perhaps be expected HbA_{1c} and excessive alcohol intake. Hypertension has been identified as a possible risk factor for neuropathy in the EDIC study.[11] Many of these variables are related, some as features of the metabolic syndrome, so it is to be expected that some drop out on multivariate analysis, and it is not safe to conclude from our data, for example, that diastolic BP is more important than systolic, or total serum cholesterol than serum triglycerides. BP is, however, a known risk factor for microvascular as well as macrovascular

TABLE 5. Summary of studies showing predictors for the development of neuropathy in diabetes mellitus

Reference	Diabetes type (1/2)	n	Follow-up (years)	Definition	Neuropathy predictors
Diabetes control and complications trial[5]	1	1,441	6.5	Clinical tests/nerve conduction/autonomic function	Conventional glucose management
Epidemiology of diabetes complications study[11]	1	453	5.3	Symptoms and clinical tests	Duration of diabetes, height, HbA_{1c}, smoking, hypertension
Rochester diabetic neuropathy study[3]	1/2/other	264	7	Clinical score and tests	Retinopathy, foot-vessel calcification (for type 1 diabetes; also proteinuria, duration of diabetes for all diabetes)
Nordwall *et al.*[41]	1	80	7–22	Nerve conduction	GHb
EURODIAB[10]	1	1,172	7.3	Symptoms/clinical tests	UAE, retinopathy, CVD, duration of diabetes, GHb, triglycerides, total cholesterol, BMI, smoking, hypertension
Young *et al.*[27]	1/2	6,487	Cross-sectional	Clinical test score; symptom score	Age, diabetes duration
Klein *et al.*[42]	1/2	1,210	10	Clinical history	GHb
EDIC study[8]	1	1,257	8 years after end of DCCT	Neuropathy score/questionnaire	Conventional blood glucose control

disease, and indeed its reduction is known to protect against progression of retinopathy.[28] Whatever the pathogenetic basis of this, it would appear that peripheral microvascular damage affecting the nerves is prone to exacerbation by the same process. The dominance of these factors in our study, compared with earlier studies, may be a function of the longer follow-up period.

Interestingly neuropathy was also associated with peripheral vascular disease during follow-up (TABLE 4), a finding also noted in the MONICA/KORA Augsburg surveys,[12] so the possibility that poor arterial supply exacerbates the process of microvascular damage in distal sensory nerves seems real. This may have clinical consequences, for drugs, such as cilostazol (a phosphodiesterase type 3 inhibitor) that causes vasodilatation, inhibits platelet aggregation, and improves peripheral circulation. This might then have a double action in the prevention of foot ulceration, as well as its known promotion of ulcer healing.[29,30] Standard antihypertensive therapy might be expected to have the same effect. These speculations would need further examination in formal trials.

Previous studies have shown that the angiotensin-converting enzyme (ACE) inhibitor lisinopril improves nerve conduction velocity and quantitative sensory testing after 12 weeks of therapy,[31] while trandolapril improved peroneal and sural nerve function at 12 months.[32] Although systolic BP at 12 months was significantly lower in the trandolapril treated group, the improvement in neuropathy was not considered to be related to the reduction in the BP. There was too little use of these drugs in people with type 1 diabetes at the time of study to give reliable information on any protective value in the current study.

The people in the neuropathy group had a lower eGFR and serum creatinine compared with the group that remained free of neuropathy during the follow-up period, and microalbuminuria during that time was also associated with incident neuropathy. Such associations have been noted previously.[33,34] Neither of these findings is helpful in understanding whether it is microvascular or major vessel disease (or both) that is predisposing to the neuropathy, for microalbuminuria is a known cardiovascular risk factor even in the absence of diabetes, while reduced glomerular function can be secondary to renal arterial disease as well as diabetic glomerulopathy.

Our study differs from other studies in that there was no difference in the base line or average glycated hemoglobin in the people who developed neuropathy compared with the group that remained free of it. This does not mean that glucose control is unimportant, if only because nearly everyone studied had higher HbA_{1c} levels than would be desired, but it may mean that hyperglycemia is permissive in its effect, and that factors related to the other predictive variables then determine rate of progression. However, when our patients were classified into two groups based on $HbA_{1c} \leq 9.0$ and $>9.0\%$, as expected a greater proportion of people with poorer control had developed neuropathy (16 versus 8%; $P = 0.034$).

In a randomized trial of clofibrate in patients with diabetic neuropathy, an improvement in neuropathic symptoms was noted with no change in nerve conduction.[35] In the Fenofibrate Intervention in Event Lowering in Diabetes (FIELD) study in people with type 2 diabetes, fenofibrate reduced the rate of progression to albuminuria with 2.6% more patients allocated fenofibrate than placebo regressing or not progressing ($P = 0.002$). In addition, laser treatment for retinopathy was reduced by 30% in the patients treated with fenofibrate compared with the placebo group. Its benefits on neuropathy require further confirmation.

Studies of rosuvastatin in diabetic rat models have shown an improvement in nerve conduction velocity, thermal hyperalgesia, and deficits in sciatic nerve and superior cervical ganglion blood flow.[36] Furthermore, in a randomized, placebo-controlled trial of simvastatin/diet versus diet-alone in type 1 diabetic patients without nephropathy, a trend for slower progression of vibratory threshold was demonstrated without any effect on the development of symptoms in the statin-treated group.[37] The mechanism underlying the benefits of statins in relation to neuropathy could be due to the lipid-lowering effect as well as the lipid-independent pleiotropic effects.[38]

Inflammatory markers associated with CVD have also been found to be raised in patients with type 1 diabetes complicated with retinopathy, nephropathy,[39] and neuropathy[40] which could potentially explain the link between cardiovascular risk factors and neuropathy.

In conclusion, the present study adds strength to the existing literature that suggests that well-recognized and modifiable cardiovascular risk factors predict the development of neuropathy in people with type 1 diabetes. Randomized clinical trials would seem indicated to investigate whether control of these modifiable risk factors does indeed lower the risk of developing peripheral neuropathy.

REFERENCES

1. THOMAS, P.K. 1994. Diabetic peripheral neuropathies: their cost to patient and society and the value of knowledge of risk factors for development of interventions. Eur. Neurol. **41**(Suppl 1): 35–43.
2. GORDOIS, A., P. SCUFFHAM, A. SHEARER, *et al.* 2003. The health care costs of diabetic peripheral neuropathy in the US. Diabetes Care **26:** 1790–1795.
3. DYCK, P.J., J.L. DAVIES, D.M. WILSON, *et al.* 1999. Risk factors for severity of diabetic polyneuropathy: intensive longitudinal assessment of the Rochester Diabetic Neuropathy Study cohort. Diabetes Care **22:** 1479–1486.
4. UK PROSPECTIVE DIABETES STUDY (UKPDS) GROUP. 1998. Intensive blood-glucose control with sulphonylureas or insulin compared with conventional treatment and risk of complications in patients with type 2 diabetes (UKPDS 33). Lancet **352:** 837–853.
5. THE DIABETES CONTROL AND COMPLICATIONS TRIAL RESEARCH GROUP. 1993. The effect of intensive treatment of diabetes on the development and progression of

long-term complications in insulin-dependent diabetes mellitus. N. Engl. J. Med. **329:** 977–986.

6. PIRART, J. 1978. Diabetes mellitus and its degenerative complications: a prospective study of 4,400 patients observed between 1947 and 1973 (part 2). Diabetes Care **1:** 252–263.
7. PIRART, J. 1978. Diabetes mellitus and its degenerative complications: a prospective study of 4,400 patients observed between 1947 and 1973 (part 1). Diabetes Care **1:** 168–188.
8. MARTIN, C.L., J. ALBERS, W.H. HERMAN, *et al.* & DCCT/EDIC Research Group. 2006. Neuropathy among the diabetes control and complications trial cohort 8 years after trial completion. Diabetes Care **29:** 340–344.
9. DYCK, P.J., W.J. LITCHY, K.A. LEHMAN, *et al.* 1995. Variables influencing neuropathic endpoints: the Rochester diabetic neuropathy study of healthy subjects. Neurology **45:** 1115–1121.
10. TESFAYE, S., N. CHATURVEDI, S.E. EATON, *et al.* 2005. Vascular risk factors and diabetic neuropathy. N. Engl. J. Med. **352:** 341–350.
11. FORREST, K.Y., R.E. MASER, G. PAMBIANCO, *et al.* 1997. Hypertension as a risk factor for diabetic neuropathy: a prospective study. Diabetes **46:** 665–670.
12. ZIEGLER, D., W. RATHMANN, B. HAASTERT, *et al.* 2005. Prevalence of polyneuropathy in impaired glucose tolerance and diabetes. The MONICA/KORA Augsburg Surveys and Myocardial Infarction Registry (KORA-A Study). Diabetologia **48**(Suppl. 1): A364, Abstract 1008.
13. LEVEY, A.S., J.P. BOSCH, J.B. LEWIS, *et al.* 1999. A more accurate method to estimate glomerular filtration rate from serum creatinine: a new prediction equation. Modification of diet in renal disease study group. Ann. Intern. Med. **130:** 461–470.
14. LEVEY, A., T. GREENE, J. KUSEK & G. BECK. 2000. A simplified equation to predict glomerular filtration rate from serum creatinine [abstract]. J. Am. Soc. Nephrol. **11:** 155A.
15. FLYNN, M.D., I.A. O'BRIEN & R.J. CORRALL. 1995. The prevalence of autonomic and peripheral neuropathy in insulin-treated diabetic subjects. Diabet. Med. **12:** 310–313.
16. BOULTON, A.J., G. KNIGHT, J. DRURY & J.D. WARD. 1985. The prevalence of symptomatic, diabetic neuropathy in an insulin-treated population. Diabetes Care **8:** 125–128.
17. KNUIMAN, M.W., T.A. WELBORN, V.J. MCCANN, *et al.* 1986. Prevalence of diabetic complications in relation to risk factors. Diabetes **35:** 1332–1339.
18. CABEZAS-CERRATO, J. 1998. The prevalence of clinical diabetic polyneuropathy in Spain: a study in primary care and hospital clinic groups. Neuropathy Spanish study group of the Spanish Diabetes Society (SDS). Diabetologia **41:** 1263–1269.
19. PERKINS, B.A., D. OLALEYE, B. ZINMAN & V. BRIL. 2001. Simple screening tests for peripheral neuropathy in the diabetes clinic. Diabetes Care **24:** 250–256.
20. ADLER, A.I., E.J. BOYKO, J.H. AHRONI, *et al.* 1997. Risk factors for diabetic peripheral sensory neuropathy. results of the Seattle prospective diabetic foot study. Diabetes Care **20:** 1162–1167.
21. FRANKLIN, G.M., S.M. SHETTERLY, J.A. COHEN, *et al.* 1994. Risk factors for distal symmetric neuropathy in NIDDM. The San Luis Valley diabetes study. Diabetes Care **17:** 1172–1177.

22. MASER, R.E., A.R. STEENKISTE, J.S. DORMAN, *et al.* 1989. Epidemiological correlates of diabetic neuropathy. Report from Pittsburgh epidemiology of diabetes complications study. Diabetes **38:** 1456–1461.
23. BARBOSA, A.P., J.L. MEDINA, E.P. RAMOS & H.P. BARROS. 2001. Prevalence and risk factors of clinical diabetic polyneuropathy in a Portuguese primary health care population. Diabet. Metab. **27:** 496–502.
24. SOSENKO, J.M., M.T. GADIA, A.M. FOURNIER, *et al.* 1986. Body stature as a risk factor for diabetic sensory neuropathy. Am. J. Med. **80:** 1031–1034.
25. BOOYA, F., F. BANDARIAN, B. LARIJANI, *et al.* 2005. Potential risk factors for diabetic neuropathy: a case control study. BMC Neurol. **5:** 24.
26. BIHAN, H., S. LAURENT, C. SASS, *et al.* 2005. Association among individual deprivation, glycemic control, and diabetes complications: the EPICES score. Diabetes Care **28:** 2680–2685.
27. YOUNG, M.J., A.J. BOULTON, A.F. MACLEOD, *et al.* 1993. A multicentre study of the prevalence of diabetic peripheral neuropathy in the United Kingdom hospital clinic population. Diabetologia **36:** 150–154.
28. ADLER, A.I., I.M. STRATTON, H.A. NEIL, *et al.* 2000. Association of systolic blood pressure with macrovascular and microvascular complications of type 2 diabetes (UKPDS 36): prospective observational study. BMJ **321:** 412–419.
29. ZOLLI, A. 2004. Foot ulceration due to arterial insufficiency: role of cilostazol. J. Wound Care **13:** 45–47.
30. WANG, T., M.B. ELAM, W.P. FORBES, *et al.* 2003. Reduction of remnant lipoprotein cholesterol concentrations by cilostazol in patients with intermittent claudication. Atherosclerosis **171:** 337–342.
31. REJA, A., S. TESFAYE, N.D. HARRIS & J.D. WARD. 1995. Is ACE inhibition with lisinopril helpful in diabetic neuropathy? Diabet. Med. **12:** 307–309.
32. MALIK, R.A., S. WILLIAMSON, C. ABBOTT, *et al.* 1998. Effect of angiotensin-converting-enzyme (ACE) inhibitor trandolapril on human diabetic neuropathy: randomised double-blind controlled trial. Lancet **352:** 1978–1981.
33. NIELSEN, V.K. 1973. The peripheral nerve function in chronic renal failure. VI. The relationship between sensory and motor nerve conduction and kidney function, azotemia, age, sex, and clinical neuropathy. Acta Med. Scand. **194:** 455–462.
34. DI PAOLO, B., P. CAPPELLI, C. SPISNI, *et al.* 1982. New electrophysiological assessments for the early diagnosis of encephalopathy and peripheral neuropathy in chronic uraemia. Int. J. Tissue React. **4:** 301–307.
35. BERENYI, M.R., B. STRAUS & O.E. MIGLIETTA. 1971. Treatment of diabetic neuropathy with clofibrate. J. Am. Geriatr. Soc. **19:** 763–772.
36. CAMERON, N., M. COTTER, M. INKSTER & M. NANGLE. 2003. Looking to the future: diabetic neuropathy and effects of rosuvastatin on neurovascular function in diabetes models. Diabetes Res. Clin. Pract. **61**(Suppl 1): S35–S39.
37. FRIED, L.F., K.Y. FORREST, D. ELLIS, *et al.* 2001. Lipid modulation in insulin-dependent diabetes mellitus: effect on microvascular outcomes. J. Diabetes Complications **15:** 113–119.
38. LIAO, J.K. 2002. Beyond lipid lowering: the role of statins in vascular protection. Int. J. Cardiol. **86:** 5–18.
39. SCHRAM, M.T., N. CHATURVEDI, C.G. SCHALKWIJK, *et al.* 2005. Markers of inflammation are cross-sectionally associated with microvascular complications and cardiovascular disease in type 1 diabetes—the EURODIAB prospective complications study. Diabetologia **48:** 370–378.

40. GONZALEZ-CLEMENTE, J.M., D. MAURICIO, C. RICHART, *et al.* 2005. Diabetic neuropathy is associated with activation of the TNF-alpha system in subjects with type 1 diabetes mellitus. Clin. Endo. **63:** 525–529.
41. NORDWALL, M., L. HYLLIENMARK & J. LUDVIGSSON. 2006. Early diabetic complications in a population of young patients with type 1 diabetes mellitus despite intensive treatment. J. Pediatr. Endocrinol. Metab. **19:** 45–54.
42. KLEIN, R., B.E. KLEIN & S.E. MOSS. 1996. Relation of glycemic control to diabetic microvascular complications in diabetes mellitus. Ann. Intern. Med. **124:** 90–96.

Audit of a Diabetes Clinic at Tawam Hospital, United Arab Emirates, 2004–2005

B. AFANDI,[a] S. AHMAD,[b] H. SAADI,[c] S. ELKHUMAIDI,[d] M.A. KARKOUKLI,[b] B. KELLY,[b] H. ASSAF,[e] AND D. MATEAR[f]

[a]*Department of Internal Medicine, Tawam Hospital, Al Ain, United Arab Emirates*

[b]*Quality Department, General Authority for Health Services for Abu Dhabi, Abu Dhabi, United Arab Emirates*

[c]*Department of Internal Medicine, Faculty of Medicine and Health Sciences, United Arab Emirates University, Al Ain, United Arab Emirates*

[d]*Department of Nursing , Tawam Hospital, Al Ain, United Arab Emirates*

[e]*Department of Quality Management, Tawam Hospital, Al Ain, United Arab Emirates*

[f]*Department of Dentistry, Tawam Hospital, Al Ain, United Arab Emirates*

ABSTRACT: The aim of this audit was to determine the current management of patients with diabetes compared to international standards and to benchmark the results against current international standards. A retrospective audit of medical records of diabetic patients attending Tawam Hospital, a tertiary healthcare facility in the Al Ain region in the Emirate of Abu Dhabi, United Arab Emirates was performed. A random sample of 30 patients (5% of the target group) was selected from the total number of 600 patients who visited the diabetes clinics in August 2005. An audit form was developed based on the priority aims and measures contained in the Institute for Clinical Systems Improvement (ICSI) Guidelines for the management of type 2 diabetes mellitus. Data analysis was carried out based on measurement specifications in the ICSI Guidelines. All patients had their blood pressure checked at their most recent appointment. All except one patient had an HbA1c test and a lipid profile performed during the study period. Although 75% of patients were referred for a dilated eye examination, only 47% complied. Approximately two-thirds of all patients had evidence of self-monitoring of blood glucose. Less than half of the patients were referred to the nutritionist and only a relatively small proportion of patients had advice on diet and exercise documented in their medical record. There was also lack of documentation, particularly for smoking status, foot examination, and body mass index (BMI).

Address for correspondence: Dr. Bachar Afandi, Department of Internal Medicine, Tawam Hospital, P.O. Box 15258, Al Ain, UAE. Voice: 00971-3-7677-444; fax: 00971-3-7677-634.
e-mail: bafandi@tawam-hosp.gov.ae

Ann. N.Y. Acad. Sci. 1084: 319–324 (2006).
doi: 10.1196/annals.1372.017

All patients received aspirin (ASA) treatment. The majority had a systolic blood pressure of 130 mmHg or less; just under half of patients had HbA1c of less than 7%. In comparison to the Center for Diseases Control (CDC) targets, we exceeded targets in three areas in relation to HbA1c testing, ASA treatment, and self-report monitoring blood glucose. We did not meet the stated target of 75% for patients having a dilated eye exam due to lack of patient compliance (more than three-quarters of all patients were referred but did not attend for appointment). Documentation of a comprehensive foot examination was present for only one-quarter of all patients compared to the recommended target of three-quarters of patients. Documentation of advice on diet and exercise was present for 40%, which did not meet the CDC target of 60%. Overall, the audit highlighted that Tawam Hospital is providing a good level of care to diabetic patients and compares favorably with international targets; however, key recommended actions have been identified for implementation to improve patient care and maintain a continuous improvement process through effective monitoring with prioritization to those related to preventative care.

KEYWORDS: **audit; diabetes; quality indicators**

INTRODUCTION

The high incidence of diabetes among the United Arab Emirates population (25% among UAE citizens and 17% among expatriates)[1] makes the management of diabetes an important area for monitoring and improvement. Also, the significant morbidity and mortality associated with diabetes indicate the clear need to monitor and improve the level of management and preventative measures provided to patients diagnosed with this disease.[2]

The aim of this audit was to determine the current management of patients with diabetes compared to international standards and to benchmark the results against current international standards. The priority aims and measures were derived from Institute for Clinical Systems Improvement (ICSI) guidelines for management of type 2 diabetes mellitus.[3] The study team agreed on 12 clinical indicators, which were to be included in the audit for diabetes management at Tawam Hospital, tertiary healthcare facility in the Emirate of Abu Dhabi, United Arab Emirates. The results were benchmarked against the targets set by the Center for Diseases Control Healthy People 2010 targets for Diabetes.[4]

METHODS

This was a retrospective audit of the medical records of diabetic patients who attended for outpatient clinic appointment in the target month of August 2005. A sample of 30 patients (standard sampling size of 5% or 30, whichever was higher, for the targeted population as per JCIA approved sampling process) was selected from the total number of patients (600) who attended the outpatient clinic in August 2005.

The inclusion criteria were similar to those of ICSI[3] and included patients 18 years and older with a primary, secondary, or tertiary diagnosis of type 1 or type 2 diabetes. Only established patients with diabetes (which requires both a visit in the target month and a diabetic visit in a window of 12–24 months before the target month) were included.

A draft audit tool was developed, based on the priority aims and measures of ICSI, and finalized by the audit team taking into account the local setting. An audit form was completed for each patient using the agreed data definitions. Data analysis was carried out based on measurement specifications in the ICSI Guideline.[3]

RESULTS

Of the total of 30 patients who were included in the audit, 18 (60%) were women and 12 (40%) were men. The average age was 48.6 years. Twenty-nine (97%) patients had type 2 diabetes. The average number of visits within the last 12 months was four outpatient visits. All patients had their blood pressure checked at their most recent appointment. All except one patient had an HbA1c test and a lipid profile performed during the study period. Although

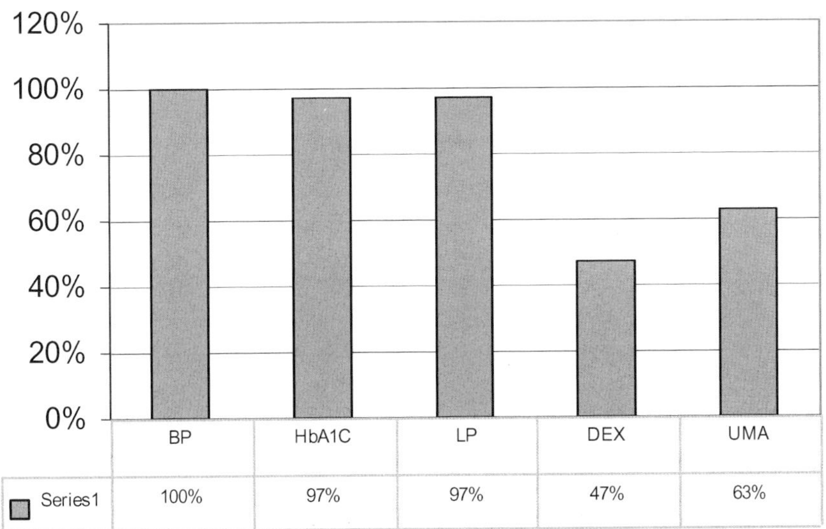

FIGURE 1. Diabetes indicators (BP, HbA1c, lipid profile (LP), dilated eye examination (DEX), urine microalbumin (UMA) checked within the previous 12 months).

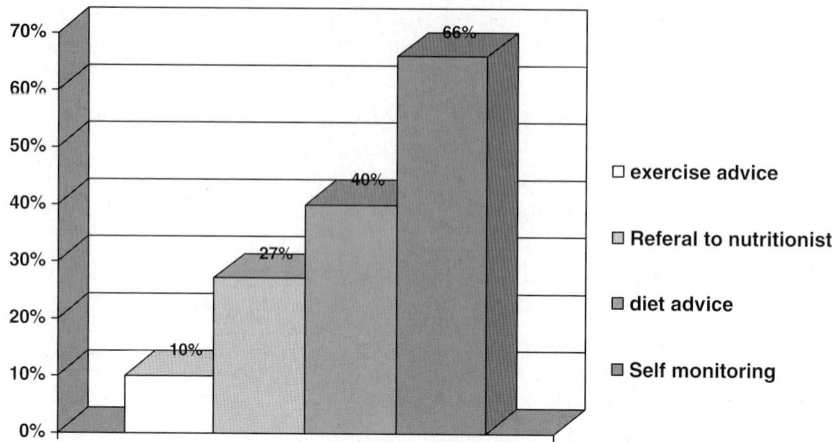

FIGURE 2. Diabetes indicators (exercise advice, referral to nutritionist, diet advice, self-monitoring).

75% of patients were referred for a dilated eye examination, only 47% complied (FIG. 1).

Approximately two-thirds of all patients had evidence of self-monitoring of blood glucose. Less that half of the patients were referred to the nutritionist and only a relatively small proportion of patients had advice on diet and exercise documented in their medical record (FIG. 2). There was also a lack of

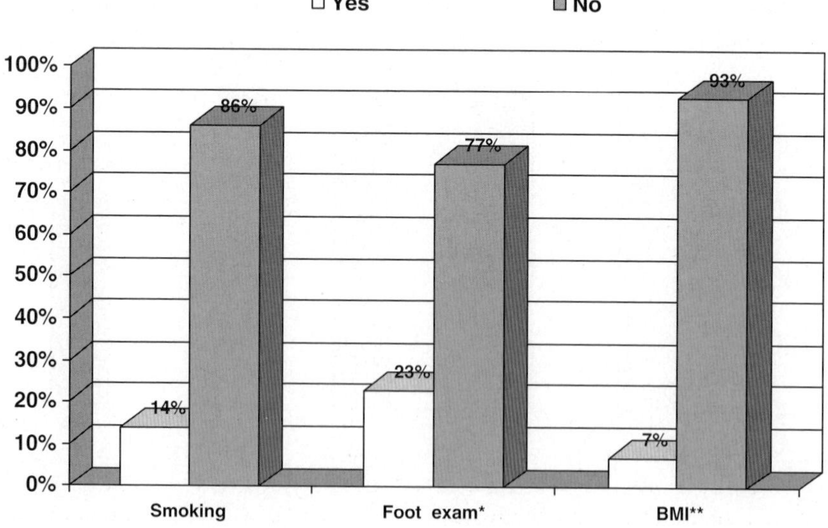

FIGURE 3. Diabetes indicators (smoking, foot examination, and BMI within the previous 12 months). *Few notes in the medical record documented normal extremities or extremities checked. **Few patients are reported as morbidly obese.

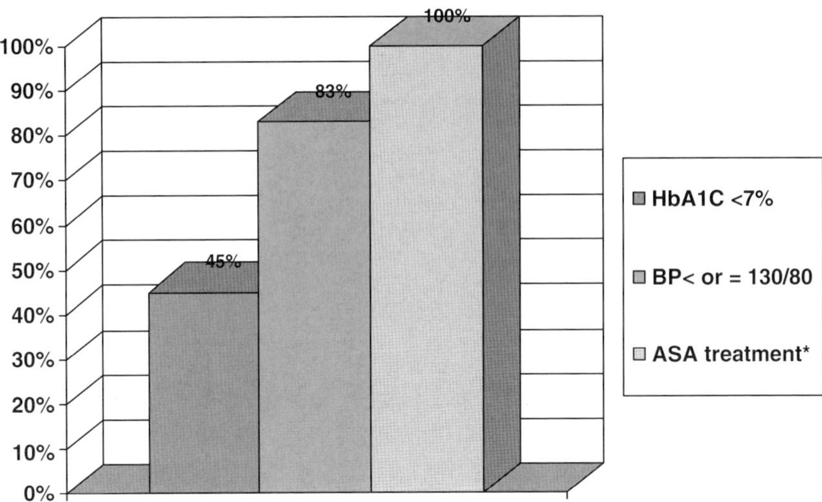

FIGURE 4. Diabetes indicators (HbA1c < 7%, BP ≤ 130, ASA (*aspirin use) checked within the previous 12 months).

documentation, particularly for smoking status, foot examination, and body mass index (BMI) (FIG. 3). All patients received aspirin (ASA) treatment. The majority had a systolic blood pressure of 130 mmHg or less; just under half of patients had HbA1c of less than 7% (FIG. 4).

We compared our results with the Center for Diseases Control (CDC) targets[4] (when applicable). We exceeded targets in three areas in relation to HbA1c testing, ASA treatment, and self-report monitoring blood glucose. We did not meet the stated target of 75% for patients having a dilated eye exam due to lack of patient compliance (more than three-quarters of all patients were referred but did not attend for appointment).

Documentation of a comprehensive foot examination was present for only one-quarter of all patients compared to the recommended target of three-quarters of patients. Documentation of advice on diet and exercise was present for 40%, which did not meet the CDC target of 60% (TABLE 1).

DISCUSSION

Overall, the audit has highlighted that the staff are highly committed to the provision of optimal level of care to diabetes patients; however, key recommended actions have been identified for implementation to further improve patient care, especially in relation to uptake of dilated eye examination; referral to clinical nutrition; and documentation of comprehensive foot examination, smoking status, BMI, and advice on diet and exercise.

TABLE 1. Documentation of the following selected indicators within 12 months compared to the Center for Diseases Control (CDC) targets[4] (when applicable)

Clinical indicators	Tawam (%)	CDC target (%)
HbA1c test	97	50
Comprehensive foot exam	23	75
Dilated eye examination	47	75
Advice on diet and exercise	40	60
Patients > 40 years prescribed aspirin unless contraindicated	100	30
Self-report monitoring blood glucose	66	60

Many initiatives have already been introduced by the local team to address the areas identified by the audit, for example, introduction of a diabetes flow sheet; however, patient education, implementation of clinical guidelines, effective communication, dietician involvement, and effective referral system are some issues that need further attention. An action plan has been agreed upon and the re-audit visit, which assesses the impact of the changes on the management of diabetes patients was scheduled after 6 months following the starting point of the implementation of the agreed corrective measures.

REFERENCES

1. MALIK M., A. BAKIR, B. ABI SAAB, *et al.* 2005. Glucose intolerance and associated factors in the multi-ethnic population of the United Arab Emirates: results of a national survey. Diabetes Res. Clin. Pract. **69:** 188–195.
2. THE WORLD HEALTH REPORT. 1997. Conquering Suffering, Enriching Humanity. World Health Organization. Geneva.
3. INSTITUTE FOR CLINICAL SYSTEMS IMPROVEMENT (ICSI). 2004. Management of Type 2 Diabetes Mellitus, 9th ed. Bloomington, MN. Available at www.icsi.org/knowledge
4. U.S. DEPARTMENT OF HEALTH AND HUMAN SERVICES. 2000. Healthy People 2010. Understanding and Improving Health 2000, 2nd ed. Washington, DC: US Government Printing Office, November 2000. Available at http://www.healthypeople.gov/Document/pdf/Volume1/05Diabetes.pdf

A Controlled Study of Psychosocial Factors in Young People with Diabetes in the United Arab Emirates

VALSAMMA EAPEN,[a] ABDEL AZIM MABROUK,[b] SUFIAN SABRI,[a] AND SALEM BIN-OTHMAN[b]

[a]*Faculty of Medicine and Health Sciences, UAE University, UAE*

[b]*School Health Services, Al Ain, UAE*

ABSTRACT: Psychosocial factors were studied in 30 young people with diabetes and 30 control subjects in the UAE. Patients perceived themselves more negatively than their parents on several domains. Also, they had lower scores in the areas of physical appearance and athletic competence when compared to control subjects. There were significant gender differences, with girls perceiving themselves more negatively. Better maternal education and availability of social support were associated with a positive self-image in the child. Parents of children exhibiting behavioral/emotional problems had a higher score on the parental General Health Questionnaire. Awareness and understanding of these psychosocial variables can help healthcare providers to target these issues as part of comprehensive diabetes management.

KEYWORDS: childhood diabetes; United Arab Emirates; diabetes care; psychosocial factors; self-perceptions; self-esteem; gender differences

INTRODUCTION

Psychological well-being and coping in the context of chronic physical illness is a challenge for children as well as their families. However, in the era of increasingly sophisticated and high technological medicine and surgery, it is all too easy to overlook the emotional needs of the child and the family. Behavioral science research in the last few decades has significantly advanced our understanding of the psychosocial issues in the context of pediatric diabetes.[1] However, these issues vary from one culture to another, and hence the need to study these factors locally in each community.

Address for correspondence: V. Eapen, Ph.D., FRCPsych, Professor of Child Psychiatry, Faculty of Medicine and Health Sciences, PO Box 17666, Al Ain, UAE. Voice: +971-3-713-7441; fax: +971-3-767-2995.

e-mail: veapen@uaeu.ac.ae

Ann. N.Y. Acad. Sci. 1084: 325–328 (2006). © 2006 New York Academy of Sciences.
doi: 10.1196/annals.1372.020

SUBJECTS AND METHODS

Parental attitudes, child's self-perceptions, and family variables were studied in 30 young people with type 1 diabetes mellitus (T1DM) and 30 control subjects ascertained through the Central School Health Clinic in Al Ain, United Arab Emirates (UAE). The patients consisted of 10 male and 20 female in the age range 7–18 years (mean age = 12.27; SD = 3.2). The control subjects were matched for age and gender and were selected at random from peers attending the same class as the patient. They were evaluated using Harter's Self Perception Profile for Children (SPPC) and the parallel parent version.[2] SPPC is a self-report inventory for measuring perceived competence in children, and the Arabic version has been validated for use in the UAE.[3] The instrument contains six separate subscales that assess the child's sense of competence and attitudes across five specific domains, namely, Scholastic Competence, Social Acceptance, Athletic Competence, Physical Appearance, and Behavioral Conduct, as well as a sixth subscale of Global Self-Worth indicating the general sense of self-esteem. A semistructured interview schedule was used to gather information on other relevant individual, family, and psychosocial variables.

RESULTS

On SPPC, patients scored themselves more negatively than their parents on all the subscales (Social Acceptance, Athletic Competence, Physical Appearance, and Behavioral Conduct) except Scholastic Competence. On the subscales, patients showed significantly lower scores in the areas of Physical Appearance ($P = 0.022$) and Athletic Competence ($P = 0.023$) when compared to control subjects. Age was significant only for the Behavioral Conduct subscale, with the older children scoring themselves more negatively than their younger counterparts ($P = 0.037$). There were significant differences between girls and boys in their scores in the areas of Global Self-Worth ($P = 0.007$), Athletic Competence ($P = 0.005$), Physical Appearance ($P = 0.002$), and Behavioral Conduct ($P = 0.023$), with girls perceiving themselves more negatively than the boys. With regard to family variables, we found that better maternal education ($P = 0.000$) and availability of social support ($P = 0.05$) were the most important determinants for the young person with diabetes in maintaining a positive self-image and global self-worth. Furthermore, there was a significant association ($P = 0.000$) between children exhibiting behavioral/emotional problems and a higher score on the parental General Health Questionnaire (GHQ) indicating possible psychiatric disturbance in the parent. Family income was found to be a significant factor for having a positive score on the Social Acceptance domain ($P = 0.04$) but this was not important for the other domains.

DISCUSSION

Our results suggest that Physical Appearance and Athletic Competence are particularly affected in young people with diabetes. It may be that some of these children are also obese and hence have a direct link to poor perception about their own physical appearance and an indirect link to their athletic competence. In this regard, Arif and Rohrer[4] suggested that being overweight may have an indirect effect via self-esteem domain on the health-related quality of life in pediatric diabetes patients. Also, our study found that girls are more vulnerable to poor self-perception than boys, which is in keeping with the observation by Grey *et al.*[5] that girls worried more about diabetes than did boys. Since female patients with diabetes are more prone to depression,[6] healthcare providers may need to pay closer attention to girls with poor self-perception and they may need additional support. The poor agreement in perception between children and their parents in all the domains except Scholastic Performance is also noteworthy. While the children had a more negative view of themselves than the parents in all the other domains, there was an agreement between parents and children with regard to the domain of scholastic performance, which may be due to the fact that this is a relatively more objective construct than the other domains. Possible explanations for the discrepancy between parental and child perceptions include the fact that parents may be avoiding socially undesirable responses and hence underreporting the problems, or it may be that parents are unaware of their children's negative experiences and perceptions. Indeed, self-esteem and self-worth are important determinants in the psychosocial adaptation and coping in young people with diabetes, and other studies have suggested that psychosocial adjustment in these situations may be enhanced through social skills training and other behavioral methods.[7]

Our finding that better maternal education and social support contributed to better self-esteem in young people with diabetes is in keeping with the finding of an earlier study[8] that observed that support from family and friends was predictive of better self-care and well-being, and that this relationship was mediated by personal model beliefs, such as the effectiveness of diabetes treatment regimen to control diabetes. Our finding of a link with better maternal education may be mediated through a similar mechanism whereby educated mothers instill such beliefs in the young person, thus influencing the child's personal belief model. On a similar vein, educated mothers may be more involved in their children's health issues, and other studies have noted the potential value of a parent–child partnership in diabetes management.[9] Another finding that would merit further exploration is the association between behavioral and emotional problems in children and the higher parental GHQ score. This may suggest a two-way interactive influence between mental health problems in children with diabetes and their parents. This finding has potential implication for management given the findings from a recent study that showed a relationship between maternal depression and child psychopathology with suggestions that remission of maternal depression with treatment improves the behavioral problems in the child.[10] Thus, it would seem that these families would benefit from identification and appropriate intervention. Parental participation seem to be a key factor in achieving treatment goals, and it has been demonstrated that such involvement can be strengthened through a low-intensity intervention integrated into routine follow-up diabetic care.[9]

CONCLUSION

Psychosocial problems are common among young people with diabetes in the UAE, just as it is the case worldwide. Parental involvement as well as understanding the domains of self-competence and self-worth, which are vulnerable in children with diabetes, can help health care providers to target these issues and offer appropriate psychosocial intervention as part of comprehensive diabetes management.

REFERENCES

1. WYSOCKI, T., L.M. BUCKLOH, A.S. LOCHRIE & H. ANTAL. 2005. The psychologic context of pediatric diabetes. Pediatr. Clin. North Am. **52:** 1755–1778.
2. HARTER, S. 1985. Manual of the Self-perception Profile for Children. University of Denver. Denver.
3. EAPEN, V., A. NAQVI & A.S. AL-DHAHERI. 2000. Cross cultural validation of Harter's Self Perception Profile in the United Arab Emirates. Ann. Saudi Med. **20:** 8–11.
4. ARIF, A.A. & J.E. ROHRER. 2006. The relationship between obesity, hyperglycemia symptoms and health-related quality of life among Hispanic and non-Hispanic white children and adolescents. BMC Fam. Pract. **7:** 3.doi: 10.1186/1471-2296-7-3.
5. GREY, M., M. DAVIDSON, E.A. BOLAND & W.V. TAMBORLANE. 1998. Clinical and psychosocial factors associated with achievements of treatment goals in adolescents with diabetes mellitus. J. Adolesc. Health **28:** 377–385.
6. KOVACS, M., D.S. OBROSKY, D. GOLDSTON & A. DRASH. 1997. Major depressive disorder in youths with IDDM: a controlled prospective study of course and outcome. Diabetes Care **20:** 45–51.
7. WYSOCKI, T. 2006. Behavioral assessment and intervention in pediatric diabetes. Behav. Modif. **30:** 72–92.
8. SKINNER, T.C., M. JOHN & S.E. HAMPSON. 2000. Social support and personal models of diabetes as predictors of self-care and well-being: a longitudinal study of adolescents with diabetes. J. Pediatr. Psychol. **25:** 257–267.
9. ANDERSON, B.A., H.O. JOYCE, J. BRACKETT & L.M.B. LAFFEL. 1999. An office-based intervention to maintain parent-adolescent teamwork in diabetes management. Diabetes Care **22:** 713–721.
10. WEISSMAN, M.M., D.J. PILOWSKY & P.J. WICKRAMARATNE. 2006. Remissions in maternal depression and child psychopathology: a STAR* D-child report. JAMA **295:** 1389–1398.

Diabetic Patients

Psychological Aspects

FATEMEH ADILI,[a] BAGHER LARIJANI,[a] AND MOHAMMADREZA HAGHIGHATPANAH[b]

[a]*Endocrinology and Metabolism Research Centre of Tehran University of Medical Sciences, Tehran 14114, Iran*

[b]*Shiraz University of Medical Sciences, Shiraz 71348-45794, Iran*

ABSTRACT: This study was undertaken to consider the psychological aspect of diabetes with regard to improving clinical outcomes. The review was limited to literature reports on the causes, solutions, and treatments of some common psychological problems known to complicate diabetes management. A literature search was undertaken using Pub-Med, CINAHL, Proquest, Elsevier, Blackwell Synergy, Ovid, Ebsco, Rose net, and Google websites, including studies published in English journals between 1995 and 2006. Therefore about 88 articles were selected based on the inclusion criteria. In earlier studies, relatively little empirical research was found to substantiate the effect of psychological counseling in complicated diabetes. The greatest deficits were seen in areas of mental health, self-esteem parent impact, and family cohesion. There were some different factors, which influence the psychological aspect of diabetic patients, such as age, gender, place of living, familial and social support, motivation, energy, life satisfaction, and lifestyle. There are various types of solutions for coping with the psychological problems in diabetic clients. The most essential solution lies in educating the patients and healthcare providers on the subject. Before initiating each educational intervention, a thorough assessment would be crucial. Treatment plans may benefit from cognitive behavior therapy (CBT), behavior family therapy, improving family communication, problem-solving skills, and providing motivation for diabetic patients. Moreover, it seems that the close collaboration between diabetologists and psychologists would be fruitful.

KEYWORDS: diabetes mellitus; psychological problems; intervention

Address for correspondence: Fatemeh Adili, Endocrinology and Metabolism Research Centre of Tehran University of Medical Sciences, 5th Floor, Dr. Shariati Hospital, North Kargar Ave., Tehran 14114, Iran. Voice: +98-912-2721993; fax: +98-21-88029399.
e-mail: adilsfat@sina.tums.ac.ir

Ann. N.Y. Acad. Sci. 1084: 329–349 (2006).
doi: 10.1196/annals.1372.016

INTRODUCTION

In the past decades, clinicians have increasingly recognized the importance of psychological support for people with diabetes and their families, and many have recommended integrating psychological counseling into routine diabetes care. Psychological issues may exert substantial influence on glycemic control in diabetic patients. Psychological factors have been shown to increase the risks of poor glycemic control, "brittle diabetes," and diabetic ketoacidosis (DKA).[1,2]

To enhance the patients' diabetes self-management skills and their quality of life, a biopsychological treatment model has been proposed, addressing both the medical and the psychological needs of people with diabetes and their families.[3–5]

Therefore, the main aim of this article is to consider the psychological aspect of diabetes with regard to improving clinical outcomes.

In the recent Diabetes Attitudes, Wishes, and Needs (DAWN) Study, which surveyed over 5000 people with diabetes in 13 countries, people with diabetes reported poor well-being, anxiety, and stress.[6]

It has been established that psychosocial issue is a clearly identifiable factor, which has a significant impact on people with diabetes, and influences their ability to manage their condition. As with the physical complications of diabetes, people with the condition face different types and degrees of psychological problems.[7–9]

It is important to note that only about a quarter of the studies reviewed were in fact psychological in nature, classified by the authors as social learning/behavior modification, relaxation training, and counseling. In 2002, Jovanovic[10] examined the literature on sex and the woman with diabetes, and concluded: "Finally there is an emerging literature that is devoted to the sexuality of women with diabetes" (p. 34). This literature has found that up to 30–40% of women with diabetes have problems with sexual function.

Recently, Ramachandran *et al.*[11] found that the number of people with diabetes in the Indian subcontinent has been increasing dramatically: approximately 30–33 million people have diabetes in India and this number could double by the year 2025. However, the impact of psychosocial factors related to diabetes care has also contributed to the growing pandemic.

Studies with an explicit theoretical basis were found to be more efficacious than studies without a clear theoretical basis.

In the most recently published systematic review of self-management training in type 2 diabetes, Norris *et al.*[12] concluded that the evidence supports the effectiveness in the short term. However, the long-term benefits of self-management training on glycemic control, cardiovascular disease factors, complications, and quality of life have yet to be demonstrated.

According to the German experience in 2004,[13] the conviction that people of middle age are able and willing to change the central areas of their lifestyle is empirically unfounded. Stable behavioral change involves a highly complex psychological process. Besides, in 2002, Daneman and Rodin[14] performed a large multicenter study on over 350 girls with diabetes and over 1000 school girls without diabetes. They revealed that eating disorders together with subclinical abnormalities of eating behavior are common.

In the findings of DAWN Study, people with diabetes reported the need for improved emotional support and communication with their care providers. Therefore, Funnell and Siminerio[15] in 2004 emphasized on the important role of educators in screening for depression and severe emotional distress among diabetic patients and helping them to find the necessary resources to cope with diabetes on a daily basis.

Although, two large clinical trials, the Diabetes Control and Complications Trial (DCCT) in the United States and the United Kingdom Prospective Study (UKPDS), demonstrated the importance of maintaining improved blood glucose control in the prevention of the complications of both type 1 and type 2 diabetes, Siminerio[16] in 2001 in her paper mentioned: "Without educational attention to the psychological needs of the individual person, efforts to improve diabetes outcomes are futile" (p. 21).

Based on the studies of Power[17] in 2002, it is important to note that individuals vary widely in their psychological responses to emotions at diagnosis, which may include shock, denial, sadness, frustration, guilt, fear, anxiety, anger, or even relief.

Reviews so far suggest that psychosocial interventions in diabetes overall are moderately effective in improving both metabolic outcomes and psychological well-being, and, importantly, no mention has been made to any adverse effects. However, the number of studies reviewed is limited, and the majority of them could be classified as educational rather than psychological, although the distinction between the two is not clear. In the past years, diabetes education has shifted toward a more behavioral approach, building on psychological theories of counseling and behavior change.[18] There is clearly an increasing need for behavioral oriented self-management programs in diabetes,[19–21] but such programs are not designed to help patients overcome serious psychological barriers or psychological disturbances.

The focus of this article is on literature pertaining to the major psychological problems, such as depression, stress and anxiety, sexual problems, eating disorders, self-destructive behaviors, and interpersonal/family conflicts, common among people with diabetes and warranting professional psychological help. There is a growing evidence that medical treatments of diabetes and the behavioral medicine approach can enhance both psychological and physiological outcomes.[22,23]

In particular, cognitive behavior therapy (CBT) appears to be effective.[24–27]

METHODS

A literature search of this review was performed using computerized databases, such as Pub-Med, CINAHL, Proquest, Elsevier, Blackwell Synergy, Ovid, Ebsco, Rose net, and Google websites. The search was limited to English language articles published in peer-reviewed journals from 1995 to 2006, cross-indexing by: diabetes mellitus, psychological intervention, counseling, psychotherapy, psychological complications (depression, anxiety, stress, sexual problems, eating disorders, brittle diabetes, poor control, family conflicts), and treatments.

In addition, literature was listed and grouped according to the main psychological problems of diabetic patients through the review and original studies, after checking for double citations. Case studies were excluded.

Studies were first classified according to the psychological problem, type of intervention, and target population. Then studies were further analyzed for design, sample size, patient characteristics, and outcome measures (psychosocial and physiological). The benefits of the interventions, psychological and medical, were then determined.

RESULTS

Depression

Depression has been found to be more prevalent among people with diabetes than in the general population. While estimates of the prevalence of depression vary, it likely affects at least one of every five people with diabetes.[28–30] There is also evidence that the course of depression may be more chronic and severe in the people with diabetes.[31] The etiology of depression in diabetes is still poorly understood, with both physiological and psychological factors likely to play a role and interact with each other.[32,33] It is noteworthy that depressive symptoms are more prevalent in other medical illnesses, for example, rheumatoid arthritis and cardiovascular disease.[34] Depression in diabetes is associated with poor treatment adherence, hyperglycemia, and subsequently an increased risk of developing diabetes-related complications, particularly cardiovascular disease and retinopathy.[8,35,36] Overlap between symptoms of depression and diabetes dysregulation may complicate the diagnosis (e.g., fatigue, sleep disturbances, sexual dysfunction), although screening was found to be feasible in diabetes patient using a general depression screener, such as Beck's Depression Inventory (BDI).[37]

Given the magnitude of the problem of depression in diabetes and its clinical ramifications, it is surprising to find only one controlled study to evaluate the benefits of psychotherapy in depressed diabetic patients. This is of course not to suggest that depressed diabetic patients are not offered psychotherapy, but research into the effects has evidently received little attention.

Some studies suggest that approximately 40% of people with diabetes have significantly elevated levels of depressive symptomatology, although they are not all diagnosed as clinically depressed.[38] In a study of 634 people with diabetes, higher rates of depression were found in women, those who were unmarried, and those with lower levels of education and in people who had three or more diabetes-related complications. In this study, age, type of diabetes, and duration of diabetes were not significantly associated with depression, and the association between depression and HbA1c levels did not reach statistically significant level, although there was a tendency for higher levels of depression to be associated with higher levels of HbA1c.[38] Other studies[39–41] have found that HbA1c levels were significantly higher in patients with depression than in those who were not depressed. Levels of diagnosable depression among people with diabetes are about three times the estimated prevalence in the population at large.[41] Depression has also been associated with increased rates of smoking and substance abuse. Even subclinical depression (i.e., persistent depression symptoms that fall short of the criteria for diagnosing depression) appears to be associated with diminished functioning and increased medical morbidity.[42] Some studies[43–47] strongly suggest that effective treatment of depression in people with diabetes can prevent or delay the onset of diabetes complications, both macrovascular and microvascular.

Interpersonal therapy (IPT) and CBT are both proven treatment for depression in people who have no other medical conditions.[30] According to the model from which IPT is derived, stressful and conflicted relationships cause, maintain, and exacerbate depression. IPT helps patients to develop and refine specific skills in communication and social interaction, and it may be particularly useful for those with diabetes, because so many stressful treatment-related situations involve interactions with other people. CBT is based on the observation that depressed people tend to think in negative ways. Negative, self-defeating thoughts and actions are identified and efforts are made to replace them with more accurate and constructive thoughts and behaviors.[1,25,30,48–50] Both ITP and CBT help patients build skills for coping better with stressful life circumstances. This may provide these patients some advantage over treatment with antidepressant medication in terms of more lasting relief from depression, a significant advantage given to the recurrent feature of depression in diabetes.[48]

So far, research on the effectiveness of CBT in diabetes care is meager. Two research projects are currently testing the usefulness of short and structured group meetings based on CBT principles for people with type 1 diabetes who present long-term poor glycemic control, using a scientifically rigorous, randomized controlled design.[26,51] In both studies, the effects of group CBT are compared to a control group attending meetings, which are similar in structure and intensity to the CBT ones, but, which are not based on CBT. The effects on glycemic control, self-care behavior, emotional well-being, and patient appreciation of the various groups are being evaluated and compared. The group meetings take place 6 to 8 times a week, and are delivered to small groups of 6 to 8 people by a trained psychologist alone,[26] or by a psychologist and a diabetes educator.[51] The meetings have a clear structure: the homework previously assigned is reviewed, a new topic is introduced and discussed, and new homework assignments are given. Modest improvements in glycemic control have been registered. The collaboration of a psychologist and a diabetes educator is also proving to be successful.

Stress and Anxiety

Diabetes is a complex and demanding disease that can induce serious psychological stress, in addition to other life stresses (e.g., major life events, occupational stress).[1]

In people diagnosed with type 2 diabetes, stress can affect blood glucose level. The mechanism behind these effects is related to the so-called "stress hormones." These hormones, which include adrenaline and cortisol, have as one of their primary effects, the mobilization of stored energy including glucose and fatty acids. Direct effects of stress on the nerves controlling the pancreas can also inhibit insulin release. Energy mobilization is part of the "fight or flight" response and is useful to prepare individuals to deal with stressors. In individuals who do not have diabetes, these energy sources can be quickly used. However, in people with diabetes, the lack of insulin or the presence of significant insulin insensitivity causes the newly released glucose to build up in the bloodstream.[1,30,52] Surwit[52] in 2002, examined 60 patients who were given five weekly group sessions of stress management training, while 48 were assigned to a control condition in which they received five weekly group sessions of diabetes education. All were followed up for 1 year. At the end of the 1-year follow-up period, people receiving stress management training showed a significant reduction of blood glucose control. This improvement would be large enough to impact on the long-term development of microvascular complications of diabetes and possibly other complications as well.

While little is known about the rate of anxiety disorder among people with diabetes, one study[38] suggests that people who have diabetes may suffer from this disorder as frequently as they do from depression, and at much higher rates than people who do not have diabetes. This study of over 600 people with diabetes found that women, African American, and those with less education were more likely to report symptoms consistent with a clinically significant anxiety disorder. The only diabetes-related predictor of significant anxiety disorder symptoms was the presence of two or more long-term diabetes complications. Type of diabetes, duration of diabetes, and glycohemoglobin level were not associated with and increased risk for anxiety symptomatology. Prevalence studies, using structured diagnostic interviews have reported an increased incidence of anxiety disorders, especially generalized anxiety disorder and simple phobia, in people with diabetes.[30,53]

Some of the symptoms of anxiety disorder overlap with those of clinical depression. This is because some psychological problems share similar symptoms and because some people suffer from more than one clinical psychological disorder.[30] Anxiety disorders are an exaggerated emotional response to the normal fears most people have, and people with diabetes often live with sources and levels of fear greater than those most people experience. Fear of hypoglycemia, complications, and the effects of diabetes on day-to-day life are some of the more common fears reported by people who have diabetes.[30] In addition, little is known about the effects of anxiety on the metabolic control in people with diabetes. It is reasonable to assume that severe anxiety affects quality of life and may affect metabolic control indirectly by interfering with diabetes self-care.

Stenstrom *et al.*[54] in 2003, evaluated the relationship between stress management and relaxation-training program, glycemic control (HbA1c) and mood in two randomized groups of 31 persons with type 1 diabetes. The program involved group education 2 h a week for 14 weeks. Whereas one group received the program, the other acted as a control group and received the program later. HbA1c was measured and subjects filled out a mood adjective checklist before the start of intervention and 1 month and 1 year after completing it. In both groups, significant positive mood changes were obtained, but no significant changes in mood. For those attending the group sessions less frequently, the HbA1c values were significantly worse on each of the three measurement occasions than the values of those attending more frequently. The effectiveness of the program, with its failure to improve glycemic control but enhancing the mood of participants, is discussed in terms of characteristics of the sample and various methodological issues as well as in comparison with results of similar studies involving type 1 and type 2 diabetes. Similarly, Attari *et al.*,[55] most recently, performed the effect of stress management training on glycemic control in type 1 diabetic patients. The participants were 60 type 1 diabetes patients (aged 16–30 years). Thirty of the subjects attended a 3-month stress management training class during which the prescribed insulin remained constant in contrast to the control. HbA1c from all patients were measured before and after the intervention. Besides, in order to assess the ways of coping, every patient completed a questionnaire and the scores were compared between two groups. Trained patients showed significantly improved ways of coping. HbA1c changed from 11.7 ± 2.9 and 10.9 ± 2.1 before training to 8.5 ± 1.7 and 10.3 ± 2.1 after intervention in the trained and control groups, respectively and the changes were significant in the study group ($P < 0.001$). In addition, the difference between means of HbA1c in the two groups was statistically significant at the end of the study ($P < 0.001$). Results show a clinically significant beneficial effect of stress management training on glycemic control among type 1 diabetes patients.

Moreover, very little information is available on the use of drugs in people with diabetes. Lustman *et al.*,[56] reported improved glycemic control in patients treated with alprazolam (Xanax), regardless of whether or not they had a formal diagnosis of anxiety disorder. Moreover, in the general population, CBT, including techniques, such as systematic desensitization (exposure) and cognitive restructuring, can reduce anxiety and associated avoidance behaviors,[57] no studies were found applying CBT in diabetic patients fearful of hypoglycemia. However, an intensive, well-researched psychoeducational program, Blood Glucose Awareness Training (BGAT), can help patients to lower their fear of hypoglycemia.[58] While (long lasting) fear of self-injecting and self-testing appears to be relatively rare in insulin-treated diabetic patients, they can often be accompanied by serious psychological comorbidity and poor metabolic control.[59] No controlled studies were found on treatment of needle phobia in diabetes patients.

Sexual Problems

Patients with diabetes experience chronic vascular complications, which lead to a wide range of medical problems. Genitourinary problems are included among these complications, which are related to both neuropathy and vasculopathy. The most important clinical features relating to genitourinary involvement in patients with diabetes include erectile dysfunction (ED) and retrograde ejaculation in men, and bladder dysfunction[60,61] and female sexual dysfunction or FSD is more difficult to define and specific studies in diabetics are limited. Problems with arousal, lubrication, and orgasmic dysfunction occur, but the fatigue of diabetes may be influencing these complaints, and in general, psychological issues appear to predominate.[61]

Jovanovic[10] performed a study to evaluate the association of sexual function and diabetes in women. This literature has found that up to 30–40 % of women with diabetes have problems with sexual function. Women with diabetic nerve and blood vessel complications have more sexual problems than those without diabetic complications, indicating that vessel damage was the underlying cause. No relationship was found between HbA1c and sexual dysfunction.

However, the main sexual problem of women with diabetes is related to arousal.[10,61–63] If a woman does not feel in the mood for a sexual encounter, she cannot function properly during sex. Arousal includes the psychological state and the resulting physical responses of vaginal changes, including the secretion of lubricating moisture, the relaxation of the pelvic floor muscles, and the engorgement of the labia and clitoris. If psychological arousal does not occur, the physical response can be elicited with physical manipulation. However, until proper moisturizing occurs, and relaxation and engorgement take place, trauma may occur and impede intercourse. Therefore, the mood of women with diabetes is the key to the whole process of sexual enjoyment. The problem is women's heads, starting with their state of well-being. It is therefore best treated by addressing the cause of our mental distress.

In women with and without diabetes,[10,64] libido is a function of response to the partner, the immediate atmosphere, distraction, stress, fatigue, and hormonal status. Fear of conception or contracting a sexually transmitted disease can impede spontaneity. Women with diabetes must feel confident with their healthcare provider and ask advice on the best means of birth control. Women suffer from depression twice as frequently as men. The libido in most women is so fragile that even minor episodes of depression can result in problems of arousal. The diagnosis and treatment of depression are also crucial in the assessment of the diabetic women with sexual dysfunction. Antidepressive medications are beneficial. Psychiatric conclusion as a means to choose the optimal antidepressive medication can be helpful. However, these medications have side effects, such as loss of libido, so care has to be taken in the choice of drug. Arousal, foreplay, intercourse, and orgasm are all activities of energy expenditure.[10,65,66] Depending on the duration and repetition of response and climax, 0 to 600 kcal can be used. If the blood glucose level is normal at the time of initiation of sexual behavior and the stomach does not have enough extra calories in reserve, strenuous sexual activity may trigger hypoglycemia. Leaving a bite to eat or a midnight snack on the night, may be just what the doctor ordered after a magnificent encounter.

Moreover, Bancroft and Gutierrez in 1996[67] assessed that the etiology of ED in men with diabetes remains unclear and is likely to be multifactorial. To explore clinical factors of possible etiological relevance, 59 men with diabetes and ED, referred to a sexual problem clinic, were compared with an age-matched group of nondiabetic clinic attenders with ED. Sexual interest was both higher and correlated negatively with age in the diabetic groups. There were differences in the sexual problems experienced by partners in the two groups. Both groups had received nocturnal penile tumescence (NPT) monitoring and the majority had received intracavernosal injections of prostaglandin E1 (PGE1) to assess capacity for erectile response. Twenty-nine percent of the diabetic men had satisfactory NPT, and most of the men had other evidence of psychogenic causation. The men with diabetes were more likely to have a satisfactory response to intracavernosal injections of PGE1, and this was particularly the case among those with impaired NPTs. This difference requires explanation and may be of etiological relevance.

Eating Disorders

The problem of eating disorders in people with diabetes has received increased attention in the past few years. Eating disorders appear to be more common in people who have diabetes than they are in the general population.[30] In contrast, a publication[68] reported that in a German multicenter study, prevalence rates for clinical eating disorders (anorexia nervosa and bulimia nervosa) were not considerably higher for patients with either type of diabetes than they were for the general population.

Eating disorders come in two forms.[1,14,30] One, anorexia nervosa, involves a severe self-imposed restriction of caloric intake, often combined with extremely high levels of exercise. The other bulimia nervosa, involves binge eating followed by purging, usually by means of vomiting or the use of diuretic medications or laxatives. While some young men suffer from eating disorders, the condition is about 10 times more common among young women. This is probably because of the far more intense pressure on young women to remain thin.

Although there is no clear agreement in the literature concerning the prevalence of eating disorders in those who have diabetes, a meta-analysis of the existing data suggests a prevalence of 1 to 1.5 times compared to that found in the general population of those from the same gender with similar age and educational level.[69] Women who have type 1 diabetes are about 10 times more likely than men with the same diagnosis to have an eating disorder.

Moreover, a recent cross-sectional study,[70] indicates the prevalence of eating disorders and subthreshold eating disorders in adolescent females with type 1 diabetes in twice as common as in nondiabetic girls. Rydall *et al.* in 1997,[71] concluded that between one-third and one-half of all young women with type 1 diabetes frequently take less insulin than they need for good glycemic control in order to control their weight. Eating disorders have especially devastating consequences for a person with diabetes. Eating disordered behavior, including manipulation of insulin dosage to control weight, can severely compromise diabetes self-care, glycemic control, and medical management. Eating disorders in people with diabetes are often unrecognized and untreated.[1,14,30,72] Differentiating between normal concerns with food and body image and pathological ones can be difficult in patients with diabetes. Those suffering from eating disorders are often resistant to acknowledging the problem. For many of these patients controlling eating feels crucially important, and they are terrified at the prospect of giving up the control, which they feel they will be pressured to do if they acknowledge their disorder. For these reasons, the healthcare provider must be alert about the signs of eating disorders, such as frequent DKA, elevated glycohemoglobin levels in a knowledgeable patient, anxiety about or avoidance of being weighed, frequent and severe hypoglycemia, beginning with alcohol, or severe stress in the family.[30]

Eating disorders may be responsive to psychotherapy.[30] Psychotherapeutic interventions should address the complex of underlying issues, which often cause and sustain eating disorders behavior. Given the tremendous difficulties inherent in treating established eating disorders in people with diabetes, healthcare providers should be familiar with strategies for primary prevention for young female patients who have diabetes. Pharmacotherapy may benefit some patients with eating disorders. Since many patients suffering from eating disorders are also depressed, treatment with any of the antidepressant may be of help.

Based on the study of Daneman and Rodin,[14] a large multicenter study performed by their group on over 350 girls with diabetes and over 1,000 school girls without diabetes revealed that eating disorders together with subclinical abnormalities of eating behavior are about twice as common in teenage girls with diabetes compared to their peers without diabetes. The types of eating disorders found in excess in this group were bulimia nervosa and eating disorder not otherwise specified. There were no cases of the less common and more concerning anorexia nervosa. Ten percent of girls with diabetes aged between 12 and 18 years met the criteria for a full blown clinical eating disorder and 14% for a subthreshold disorder, compared to 4% and 8%, respectively, of the nondiabetic controls. These findings suggest that about one in four girls with type 1 diabetes will manifest worrisome evidence of an eating disturbance at some time during their teenage years. A similar association has not been found in teenage boys with diabetes. The data underline the magnitude of the problem and the need for strategies to deal with it.

Self-Destructive Behaviors

The term "self-destructive behaviors" is used to describe chronic or periodic serious mismanagement of the diabetes, resulting in extremely high HbA1cs, frequent DKAs, and/or recurrent severe hypoglycemia.[1] Such behaviors have been most commonly observed in adolescent patients with diabetes.[73] Self-care is a critical issue in diabetes because more than 99% of diabetes care is self-care. The vast majority of diabetes care takes place not 2–4 times a year in the healthcare provider's office, but literally countless times each day in the places where people with diabetes live, work, eat, and play.[30] The levels of self-care and glycemic control among people with diabetes in the United States are not good. The average HbA1c of a person with type 2 diabetes is 9.5%, representing an average blood glucose level of about 250 mg/dL or about 14 mmol/L. It is apparent that one essential goal of diabetes care is to improve diabetes-related coping skills and CBT among people with diabetes and, as a consequence, to improve self-care behavior, metabolic outcomes, and quality of life as well. Quality of life is affected by improved coping skills and CBT.

In a descriptive outcome study, Geffken *et al.*[74] reported that residential treatment included individual, group, and family psychotherapy, diabetes education, and close medical supervision. Treatment was associated with a significant reduction in diabetes-related hospitalizations, improved school attendance and (nonsignificant) decreased glycosylated hemoglobin levels.

In a randomized controlled trial, Fosburry *et al.*[75] compared the effect of individual outpatient cognitive analytic therapy (CAT), a focused time-limited psychotherapy delivered by a psychotherapist, and individual diabetes education provided by a diabetes nurse specialist, in 26 chronically poorly controlled type 1 patients (10 CAT, 16 education). Of the 26 patients, 18 were female, mean age was 31 years (range 19–52 years), and baseline HbA1c 11.9 ± 1.7%. Interestingly, glycemic control improved significantly in the control group at 3 months follow-up, with a mean fall of 1.3% in HbA1c; by the 9-month follow-up the fall in HbA1c had reduced to 0.9%. Three months after completing CAT, the mean HbA1c had dropped to 1.5%, to decrease further by

2% at 9-month follow-up. Although not statistically different from education, glycemic control showed prolonged improvement after CAT. In contrast to education, self-reported interpersonal functioning improved after CAT. Most recently, Snoek and colleagues[51] reported on the effect of a short, four-session, cognitive behavioral group training (CBGT) program for persistent poorly controlled type 1 diabetes patients. CBGT is delivered in small groups by a team of psychologists and diabetes nurse specialists. This study, including 24 patients (15 female; mean age 35 ± 11 years; mean HbA1c 9.3 ± 1.2%) showed the mean HbA1c drop by 0.8% at 6 months from base line. Improvement in daily self-care did not negatively affect the patients' emotional well-being. Moreover, in 1995, Chiari *et al.*[76] introduced a 24-h 7-day-a-week toll-free telephone service and specific guidelines to help the patients at home to reduce the risk of DKA progression during intercurrent illnesses. Five years later they analyzed the calls received at this emergency telephone hotline service (ETHS). From 1 January 1996 to 31 December 2001 a total of 9125 calls were recorded (5.1 ± 4.2 calls per day), but only 24% of them were veritable hotline calls and were received from 767 patients or parents resulting in a mean of 2.5 ± 0.8 calls per patient or parent. Fifty-nine percent of these users called from outside Parma's area. Their mean age (7.8 ± 4.2 years) and duration of diabetes (2.8 ± 1.2 years) were significantly lower ($P < 0.001$) and shorter ($P < 0.001$) compared to those (12.8 ± 2.9 and 4.9 ± 3.2 years, respectively) found in the population, which called for nonemergency reasons. Twenty-two percent of the veritable hotline calls were received on Saturdays and Sundays or holidays, in the morning (25%), in the evening (59%), or during the night (16%). Telephone care has been finally demonstrated to be a useful way to provide a continuous support for patients and their families in the management of diabetes in some critical situations. ETHS helps them to achieve and maintain a better metabolic control and to avoid DKA during acute intercurrent illness and consequently hospital admissions. Besides, Cox and colleagues[77] in 2001, demonstrated that blood glucose awareness training (BGAT) has been shown to improve awareness of blood glucose (BG) fluctuations among adults with type 1 diabetes. This study investigates the long-term (12-month) benefits of BGAT-2. A total of 73 adults with type 1 diabetes participated in a 6-month repeated baseline design with a 12-month follow-up. At 6 months and 1 month before BGAT-2 and at 1, 6, and 12 months after BGAT-2, subjects used a handheld computer for 50 trials and completed psychological tests. In the assessment, subjects completed diaries, recording occurrences of DKA, severe hypoglycemia, and motor vehicle violations. During follow-up, 50% of the subjects received booster training. During the first and last halves of both the baseline period and the follow-up period, dependent variables were generally stable. However, from base line to follow-up, BGAT-2 led to (*a*) improved detection of hypoglycemia and hyperglycemia; (*b*) improved judgment regarding when to lower high BG, raise low BG, and not drive while hypoglycemic; (*c*) reduction in the occurrence of DKA, severe hypoglycemia, and motor vehicle violations; and (*d*) improvement in terms of worry about hypoglycemia, quality of life, and diabetes knowledge. Reduction in severe hypoglycemia was not associated with a worsening of metabolic control (HbA1c). The presence or absence of booster training did not differentially affect these benefits. In conclusion, BGAT has sustained broad-ranging benefits, independent of booster intervention. Grey *et al.*[78] performed a study to determine whether initial effects on metabolic control and quality of life associated with a behavioral intervention combined with intensive diabetes management (IDM) can be sustained over 1-year period in youths implementing intensive therapy regimens. Therefore, 77 patients (43 females, 95% white) 12 to 20 years (mean $= 14.2 \pm 1.9$; duration, 8.7 ± 3.9) electing to initiate IDM were randomly assigned to one of two groups: with or without coping skills training (CST), which consists of six small group sessions and monthly follow-up to help youths cope with their lives in the context of diabetes management—skills included social problem solving, cognitive behavior modification, and conflict resolution. Data were collected before the intervention and at 3, 6, and 12 months after the intervention by using the Self-Efficacy for Diabetes Scale, Children's Depression Inventory, Issues in Coping with IDDM, and the Diabetes Quality of Life: Youth scales. Clinical data (glycosylated hemoglobin level, height, weight, adverse effects) were collected monthly. The CST and IDM groups were comparable at base line. CST subjects had lower glycosylated hemoglobin ($P = 0.001$) and better diabetes ($P = 0.002$) and medical ($P = 0.04$) self-efficacy, and less impact of diabetes on their quality of life ($P = 0.005$) than youths receiving IDM alone after 1 year. In males, CST did not affect adverse outcomes of IDM hypoglycemia, DKA, and weight gain, but CST decreased the incidence of weight gain ($P = 0.05$) and hypoglycemia in females ($P = 0.03$). However, the addition of behavioral intervention to IDM in adolescence results in improved metabolic control and quality of life over 1 year.

The counseling process by means of which the healthcare provider facilitates the development of diabetes-related coping skills in people with diabetes involves a number of specific techniques. These techniques are designed to help patients identify problematic diabetes-related issues, identify thoughts and feelings associated with these issues, identify attitudes and beliefs underlying the problem and establish self-care goals, and develop and commit to a plan for achieving the goal. These CST techniques, designed to facilitate patients' self-awareness about the cognitive, emotional, social, and spiritual components of their lives as they relate to the daily decisions about diabetes care, are described below, and more fully elsewhere.[30]

Interpersonal Conflicts

Research strongly emphasizes that better family functioning (e.g., cohesiveness, less conflicts) is associated with less deterioration in glycemic control and severe acute complications, such as DKA and severe hypoglycemia.[79] Dumont *et al.*[80] determined whether individual and family psychosocial functioning predicts the risk for recurrent acute diabetic complications. An onset cohort of 61 children and adolescents with type 1 diabetes received conventional diabetes care. Episodes of ketoacidosis and of severe hypoglycemia were recorded for 8 years, and glycemic control was measured by glycohemoglobin. Measures of psychosocial functioning of the patient and their parents were obtained during the first year. Over a period of 8 years, 28% of subjects had at least one episode of ketoacidosis, and 21% had at least one episode of hypoglycemia. The odds of observing recurrent hypoglycemia versus recurrent ketoacidosis was 14 times greater in boys than in girls (Fisher's exact test $P < 0.05$). Girls with recurrent ketoacidosis had more behavioral problems and lower social competence, higher levels of family conflict, lower levels of family cohesion, expressiveness, and organization in year 1 compared to controls. These relationships were independent of any association with poor glycemic control. Recurrent hypoglycemia in boys was generally unrelated to individual and family functioning or glycohemoglobin. In 2006, Wysocki *et al.*[81] developed a group behavior modification program, which, was related to the background behavioral family system therapy (BFST) for adolescents with diabetes. This system has improved family relationships and communication, but effects on adherence and metabolic control are weak. They evaluated a revised intervention, BFST for diabetes (BFST-D) among 104 families who were randomized to standard care (SC) or to 12 sessions of either an educational support group (ES) or a BFST-D over 6 months. Family relationships, adherence, glycosylated hemoglobin (HbA1c), and healthcare utilization were measured at base line and after treatment. Based on the results, BFST-D significantly improved family conflict and adherence compared to SC and ES, especially among those with baseline HbA1c $\geq$ 9.0%. BFST-D and ES significantly improved HbA1c compared to SC among those with baseline HbA1c $\geq$ 9.0%. Therefore, the revised intervention (BFST-D) improved family conflict and treatment adherence significantly, while both ES and BFST-D reduced HbA1c significantly, particularly among adolescents with poor metabolic control. Recurrent severe hypoglycemias, are known to be a major cause of interpersonal conflicts and marital discord.[82]

Zoffmann *et al.*[83] conducted the interactions between healthcare providers and 11 diabetes patients with poor glycemic control in a grounded theory study at a Danish university hospital. Keeping Life and Disease Apart was identified as a core category. It involved a pattern of conflicts both between and within patients and health professionals, which disempowered them in problem solving. Three approaches to problem solving were identified: A compliance-expecting approach kept the pattern unchanged, a failure-expecting approach deadlocked the pattern, and a mutuality-expecting approach appeared to neutralize the conflict. Moreover, in a randomized controlled trial, Sundelin and colleagues[84] studied the psychological effects of a family-oriented support intervention provided after diagnosis of diabetes in children and adolescents aged 3–15 years. The aim of this study was to see whether psychological support from diagnosis, compared with conventional treatment, and whether in the longer term it will result in better family climate and diabetes control. A total of 38 families were randomly assigned to two groups and followed up for over 2 years. Tests were administered on five separate occasions to register family climate and function, but no beneficial effects were observed from this intervention as was the case in the study among adults by Spiess *et al.*[85] All in all, family support should be provided to facilitate coping with everyday management and demands of diabetes regarding prevention of further conflicts.

DISCUSSION

In line with previous reviews, we found a limited number of published psychological intervention studies in diabetes, covering the six selected problem areas. Only 10 randomized controlled trials were identified, reporting mostly on relatively small or unrepresentative samples. Therefore lack of rigor and statistical power would be a course for concern. Many studies did not include a control group or follow-up measures, so we cannot say with confidence that the intervention was effective or enduring. Studies often describe comprehensive interventions, which incorporate a variety of medical and psychological components. The effectiveness of psychological treatments specially, CBT was most convincingly demonstrated in the field of depression in diabetes,[25] while results from studies applying CBT in patients with eating and self-destructive behaviors[48] seem promising. Future controlled studies should confirm the effects of psychological interventions in different groups of diabetic patients who suffer from anxiety disorders and sexual problems with different levels of complexity. Developing CBT obviously requires skills and knowledge, but even nonpsychologists can be trained to apply CBT to individual and group consultations. This opens up new opportunities for helping people with diabetes to cope more effectively with the daily demands of diabetes self-care. If we still cannot cure diabetes, the least we can do is help those affected to live with this burden as well as possible.[25]

Over the past decades, psychological aspects of diabetes have been gaining interest from clinicians and researchers. This is well illustrated by a fast growing body of literature on emotional, cognitive, and behavioral issues related to diabetes. Indeed, most healthcare professionals need better knowledge and awareness of the psychological aspects of diabetes and how to effectively support their patients.[86]

Recent studies suggest that psychotherapy may relieve emotional distress in people with diabetes who suffer from depression and anxiety disorder, just as these treatments relieve symptoms in those who do not have diabetes.[41,53,56] Moreover, individual psychotherapy, family counseling and medical management would benefit psychological problems.[30] Although we should not underestimate the critical importance of small-scale research,[1] larger, randomized controlled trials are warranted to provide sufficient statistical power and avoid selection bias. In addition, to enhance feasibility and ensure large enough samples, multicenter studies are required.[87] Probably, most importantly, the integration of psychological services as part of diabetes care needs to be stimulated to ensure the necessary conditions for conducting controlled studies. Guidelines endorsed by the International Diabetes Federation and World Health Organization[1] state that ideally both healthcare professionals and patients would have access to a psychologist as an integrated team member or as an accessible resource to the diabetes team.

One can only hope that the growing awareness of the critical connection between diabetes and emotional distress will lead to the development of a more adequate research base than the one to which we must currently turn for guidance. Clinicians and psychological experts in a wide variety of settings can contribute of this development.[30] But not many patients will like being sent to a psychologist, feeling stigmatized as "mad" or so on. Moreover, if psychology is offered to patients only as a "last solution," that is, after every medical treatment has failed, the success of such referrals is likely to be low.[1] As we prepare for the kind of clinical trials, which are likely to provide definitive answers to our questions about the problem-specific effectiveness of various psychotherapeutic and psychoeducational interventions, small-scale research will continue to play a critical role in advancing our understanding. Healthcare providers who treat patients with diabetes might consider creating clinical databases. These databases could include information about patients, such as demographic and disease-specific characteristics and presenting problems, a description of the treatment employed, and treatment duration and outcomes. Providers could supplement this information with the results of pre- and post-treatment psychological assessments, using available standardized self-report measures. Over time, such a database could be large enough to be used for designing more effective interventions.[30]

Despite disappointing results from studies aiming to reduce diabetes onset-related distress,[84,85] the benefits of a more proactive approach to psychological issues in diabetes care deserve our attention, as indicated by a recent study evaluating the effects of systematic monitoring of psychological well-being in diabetes outpatients.[88] While in some cases patients with diabetes and psychological problems may be referred to psychologists and mental healthcare specialists outside the diabetes clinic, offering treatment that can incorporate metabolic and psychological factors is likely to be the most effective. In addition, incorporating psychological services within the diabetes team will prevent the frequent scenario of a patient being referred to mental health services, only to be bounced back because of the mental health team comments that "it is a diabetes problem." Research into the effects of psychological interventions in diabetes requires a behavioral medicine approach,[3] which involves close collaboration between psychologists, diabetologists, and other healthcare team members. Management of diabetes is teamwork. Besides, more research must be conducted in the field of diabetes to demonstrate the health and economic benefits to society of improved psychological interventions, and psychosocial and behavioral care.

REFERENCES

1. SNOEK, F.J. & T.C. SKINNER. 2002. Psychological counseling in problematic diabetes: does it help? Diabetes UK. Diabet. Med. **19:** 265–273.
2. RUGGIERO, L., R.E. GLASGOW, J.M. DRYFOOS, *et al.* 1997. Diabetes self-management. Self-reported recommendations and patterns in a large population. Diabetes Care **20:** 568–576.
3. JENKINS, C.D. 1995. An integrated behavioral medicine approach to improving care of patients with diabetes mellitus. Behav. Med. **21:** 53–65.
4. JACOBSON, A.M. 1996. The psychological care of patients with insulin dependent mellitus. N. Engl. J. Med. **334:** 1249–1253.
5. FEIFER, C. & M. TANSMAN. 1999. Promoting psychology in diabetes primary care. Prof. Psychol. Res. Pract. **30:** 14–21.
6. ALBERTI, G. 2002. The DAWN (Diabetes Attitudes, Wishes and Needs) Study. Pract. Diabet. Internat. **19:** 22a–24a.
7. COLAGIURI, R. 2004. Integrating psycho-social issues into national diabetes programmes. Diabetes Voice **49:** 31–33.
8. LUSTMAN, P.J., R.J. ANDERSON, K.E. FREEDLAND, *et al.* 2000. Depression and poor glycemic control: a meta-analytic review of the literature. Diabetes Care **23:** 934–942.
9. ANDERSON, R.J., K.E. FREEDL, R.E. CLOUSE, *et al.* 2001. The prevalence of comorbid depression in adults with diabetes. Diabetes Care **24:** 1069–1078.
10. JOVANOVIC, L. 2002. In the mood: sex and the woman with diabetes. Diabetes Voice **47:** 34–36.
11. RAMACHANDRAN, S., C. AUGUSTINE, V. VISWANATHAN, *et al.* 2005. Improving psycho-social care: the Indian experience. Diabetes Voice **50:** 19–21.
12. NORRIS, S.L., M.M. ENGELGAU & K.M.V. NARAYAN. 2001. Effectiveness of self-management training in type 2 diabetes: a systematic review of randomized controlled trials. Diabetes Care **24:** 561–587.
13. WOODS-BUGGELN, S. 2004. Enhancing health communication: the German experience. Diabetes Voice **49:** 41–44.
14. DANEMAN, D. & G. RODIN. 2002. Eating disorders and other vulnerabilities: a passing phase? Diabetes Voice **47:** 25–30.
15. FUNNELL, M. & L. SIMINERIO. 2004. Diabetes education: overcoming affective roadblocks. Diabetes Voice **49:** 22–23.
16. SIMINERIO, L. 2001. Diabetes education in the spotlight. Diabetes Voice **46:** 20–21.
17. POWER, T. 2002. Defining the role of social workers in diabetes care. Diabetes Voice **47:** 41–43.
18. COATES, V.E. & J.R.P. BOORE. 1996. Knowledge and diabetes self-management. Patient Educ. Counsel. **29:** 99–108.

19. DOHERTY, Y., P. JAMES & S. ROBERTS. 2000. Stage of change counseling. *In* Psychology in Diabetes Care. F.J. Snoek & T.C. Skinner, Eds.: 99–139. Wiley & Sons. Chichester.
20. ANDERSON, R.M., M.M. FUNNELL, P.M. BUTLER, *et al.* 1995. Patient empowerment. Results of a randomized controlled trial. Diabetes Care **7:** 943–949.
21. MENDEZ, F.J. & M. BLENDEZ. 1997. Effects of a behavioral intervention on treatment adherence and stress management in adolescents with IDDM. Diabetes Care **20:** 1370–1375.
22. MEYER, T.J. & M.M. MARK. 1995. Effects of psychosocial interventions with adult cancer patients: a meta-analysis of randomized experiments. Health Psychol. **14:** 101–108.
23. LINDEN, W., C. STOSSEL & J. MAURICE. 1996. Psychological interventions for patients with coronary artery disease. A meta-analysis. Arch. Intern. Med. **156:** 745–752.
24. WHITE, G.A. 2001. Cognitive Behavior Therapy for Chronic Medical Problems. A Guide to Assessment and Treatment in Practice. Wiley & Sons. Chichester.
25. VEN, N.V.D., K. WEINGER & F. SNOEK. 2002. Cognitive behavior therapy: how to improve diabetes self-management. Diabetes Voice **47:** 10–13.
26. WEINGER, K., E. SCHWARTZ, A. DAVIS, *et al.* 2002. Cognitive behavioral treatment in type 1 diabetes: a randomized control trial. Diabetes **51:** (Suppl. 2): A430.
27. WHITE, C.A. 2001. Cognitive behavioral principals in managing chronic disease. Western J. Med. **175:** 338–342.
28. KOVACS, M., D.S. OBROSKY, D. GOLDSTON, *et al.* 1997. Major depressive disorder in youth with IDDM: a controlled prospective study of course and outcome. Diabetes Care **20:** 45–51.
29. ANDERSON, R.J., K.E. FREEDLAND, R.E. CLOUSE, *et al.* 2001. The prevalence of comorbid depression in adults with diabetes. A meta-analysis. Diabetes Care **24:** 1069–1078.
30. RUBIN, R.R. 2000. Psychotherapy and counseling in diabetes mellitus. *In* Psychology in Diabetes Care. F.J. Snoek & T.C. Skinner, Eds.: 235–263. John Wiley & Sons. Baltimore, MD.
31. PEYROT, M. & R.R. RUBIN. 1999. Persistence of depressive symptoms in diabetic adults. Diabetes Care **22:** 448–452.
32. KARLSON, B. & C.D. AGARDH. 1997. Burden of illness, metabolic control and complications in relation to depressive symptoms in IDDM patients. Diabet. Med. **14:** 1066–1072.
33. TALBOT, F. & A. NOUWEN. 2000. A review of the relationship between depression and diabetes in adults. Is there a link? Diabetes Care **23:** 1556–1562.
34. APPELS, A., J. BAR, C. BRUGGEMAN, *et al.* 2000. Inflammation, depressive symptomatology, and coronary artery disease. Psychom. Med. **62:** 601–605.
35. KOVACS, M., P. MEKERJI, A. DRASH, *et al.* 1995. Biomedical and psychiatric risk factors for retinopathy among children with insulin-dependent diabetes mellitus. Diabetes Care **18:** 1592–1599.
36. CIECHANOWSKI, P.S., W.J. KATON & J.E. RUSSO. 2000. Depression and diabetes. Impact of depressive symptoms on adherence, function, and costs. Arch. Intern. Med. **160:** 3278–3285.
37. LUSTMAN, P.J., R.E. CLOUSE, L.S. GRIFFITH, *et al.* 1997. Screening for depression in diabetes using the Beck Depression Inventory. Psychosom. Med. **59:** 24–31.
38. PEYROT, M. & R.R. RUBIN. 1997. Levels and risk of depression and anxiety symptomatology among diabetic adults. Diabetes Care **20:** 585–590.

39. LUSTMAN, P.J., L.S. GRIFFITH & R.E. CLOUSE. 1996. Recognizing and managing depression in patients with diabetes. *In* Practical Psychology for Diabetes Clinicians: How to Deal with the Key Behavioral Issues Faced by Patients and Health Care Teams. B.J. Anderson & R.R. Rubin, Eds.: 143–154. American Diabetes Association. Alexandria, VA.
40. LUSTMAN, P.J., L.S. GRIFFITH & R.E. CLOUSE. 1997. Depression in adults with diabetes. Semin. Clin. Neuropsychiatry **2:** 15–23.
41. LUSTMAN, P.J., R.E. CLOUSE, A. ALRAKAWI, *et al.* 1997. Treatment of major depression in adults with diabetes: a primary care perspective. Clin. Diabet. **15:** 122–126.
42. FRASURE-SMITH, N., F. LESPERANCE & M. TALAJIC. 1995. Depression and 18-month prognosis after myocardial infarction. Circulation **91:** 999–1005.
43. SNOEK, F.J. & E.M.V. BALLEGOOIE. 2004. Psycho-social care for people with diabetes: what the guidelines say. Diabetes Voice **49:** 28–30.
44. VILEIKYTE, L. 2005. The psycho-social impact of diabetes foot damage. Diabetes Voice **50:** 11–13.
45. LERNMARK, B., B. PERSSON, L. FISHERT, *et al.* 1999. Symptoms of depression are important to psychological adaptation and metabolic control in children with diabetes mellitus. British Diabetic Association. Diabet. Med. **16:** 14–22.
46. KANNER, S., V. HAMRIN & M. GREY. 2003. Depression in adolescents with diabetes. J. Child Adolesc. Psychiat. Nurs. **16:** 15–24.
47. BERRY, D., R. WHITTEMORE, A. URBAN, *et al.* 2003. Management of depression in children and adolescents with type 1 diabetes [abstract]. Clin. Excell. Nurse Pract. **7:** 60–70.
48. VEN, N.V.D., M. CHATROU & F.J. SNOEK. 2000. Cognitive-behavioral group training. *In* Psychology in Diabetes Care. F.J. Snoek & T.C. Skinner, Eds.: 207–233. John Wiley & Sons. New York.
49. COSWAY, R., M.W.J. STRACHAN, A. DOUGALL, *et al.* 2001. Cognitive function and information processing in type 2 diabetes. Diabetes UK. Diabet. Med. **18:** 803–810.
50. OKUBO, Y., H. KISHIKAWA, E. ARAKI, *et al.* 1995. Intensive insulin therapy prevents the progression of diabetic microvascular complications in Japanese patients with non-insulin-dependent diabetes mellitus: a randomized prospective 6-year study. Diab. Res. Clin. Pract. **28:** 103–117.
51. SNOEK, F.J., N.C.W. VEN, C.H.C. LUBACH, *et al.* 2001. Effects of cognitive behavioral group training (CBGT) in adult patients with poorly controlled insulin-dependent (Type 1) diabetes: a pilot study. Patient Educ. Counsel. **45:** 143–148.
52. SURWIT, R. 2002. Type 2 diabetes and stress. Diabetes Voice **47:** 38–40.
53. LUSTMAN, P.J., L.S. GRIFFITH, R.E. CLOUSE, *et al.* 1997. Efficacy of cognitive therapy for depression in NIDDM: results of a controlled clinical trial [abstract]. Diabetes **46**(Suppl 1): 13A.
54. STENSTROM, U.L.F., A. GOTH, C. CARLSSON, *et al.* 2003. Stress managing training as related to glycemic control and mood in adults with type 1 diabetes mellitus. Diabetes Res. Clin. Pract. **60:** 147–152.
55. ATTARI, A., M. SARTIPPOUR, M. AMINI, *et al.* 2006. Effects of stress management training on glycemic control in patients with type 1 diabetes. Diabetes Res. Clin. Pract. **73:** 23–28.
56. LUSTMAN, P.J., L.S. GRIFFITH, R.E. CLOUSE, *et al.* 1995. Effects of alprazolam on glucose regulation in diabetes. Diabetes Care **18:** 1133–1139.

57. MARK, I. & R. DAR. 2000. Fear reduction by psychotherapies. Recent findings, future directions. Br. J. Psychol. **176:** 507–511.
58. GONDER-FREDERICK, L.A., D.J. COX, W. CLARKE, *et al.* 2000. Blood glucose awareness training. *In* Psychology in Diabetes Care. F.J. Snoek & T.C. Skinner, Eds.: 169–206. Wiley & Sons. Chichester.
59. ZAMBANINI, A., R.B. NEWSON, M. MAISEY, *et al.* 1999. Injection-related anxiety in insulin-treated diabetes. Diabetes Res. Clin. Pract. **11:** 199–202.
60. FEDELE, D. 2005. Therapy Insight: sexual and bladder dysfunction associated with diabetes mellitus [abstract]. Nat. Clin. Pract. Urol. **2:** 282–290.
61. JACKSON, G. 2004. Sexual dysfunction and diabetes [abstract]. Int. J. Clin. Pract. **58:** 358–362.
62. GUAY, A.T. 1997. The endocrinologist as the focus in a multidisciplinary approach to management of erectile dysfunction [abstract]. Endocr. Pract. **3:** 1–8.
63. RUTHERFORD, D. & A. COLLIER. 2005. Sexual dysfunction in women with diabetes mellitus. Gynecol. Endocrinol. **21:** 189–192.
64. BRONNER, G. 2006. Female sexual function and chronic disease [abstract]. Harefuah **145:** 114–116.
65. ENZLIN, P., M. CHANTAL, D. VAN, *et al.* 2002. Sexual dysfunction in women with type 1 diabetes: a controlled study. Diabetes Care **25:** 672–677.
66. JOVANOVIC, L. 1998. Sex and the diabetic women: desire versus dysfunction. Diabet. Rev. **6:** 65–72.
67. BANCROFT, J. & P. GUTIERREZ. 1996. Erectile dysfunction in men with and without diabetes mellitus: a comparative study[abstract]. Diabet. Med. **13:** 916.
68. HEPERTZ, S., C. ALBUS, R. WAGENER, *et al.* 1998. Comorbidity of diabetes and eating disorders: does diabetes control reflect disturbed eating behavior? Diabetes Care **21:** 1110–1116.
69. HALL, R.C.W. 1997. Bulimia nervosa and diabetes mellitus. Semin. Clin. Neuropsychiatry **2:** 24–30.
70. JONES, J.M., M.L. LAWSON, D. DANEMAN, *et al.* 2000. Eating disorders in adolescent females with and without type 1 diabetes: cross sectional study. Br. Med. J. **320:** 1563–1566.
71. RYDALL, A.C., G.M. RODIN, M.P. OLMSTED, *et al.* 1997. Disordered eating behavior and microvascular complications in young women with insulin-dependent diabetes mellitus. N. Engl. J. Med. **336:** 1849–1854.
72. EPEL, E., S. JIMENEZ, K. BROWNELL, *et al.* 2004. Are stress eaters at risk for the metabolic syndrome? Ann. N. Y. Acad. Sci. **1032:** 208–210.
73. MORRIS, A.D., D.I.R. BOYLE, A.D. MCMAHON, *et al.* 1997. Adherence to insulin treatment, glycaemic control, and ketoacidosis in insulin-dependent diabetes mellitus. Lancet **350:** 1505–1510.
74. GEFFKEN, G.R., C. LEWIS, S.B. JOHNSSON, *et al.* 1997. Residential treatment for youngsters with difficult-to-manage insulin dependent diabetes mellitus. J. Pediatr. Endocrinol. Metab. **10:** 517–527.
75. FOSBURRY, J.A., C.M. BOSLEY, A. RYLE, *et al.* 1997. A trial of cognitive analytic therapy in poorly controlled type 1 patients. Diabetes Care **20:** 959–964.
76. CHIARI, G., B. GHIDINI & M. VANELLI. 2003. Effectiveness of a toll-free telephone hotline for children and adolescents with type 1 diabetes. A 5-year study. Acta Biomed. Ateneo. Parmense. **74**(Suppl 1): 45–48.
77. COX, D.J., L. GONDER-FREDERICK, W. POLONSKY, *et al.* 2001. Blood glucose awareness training (BGAT-2) long-term benefits. Diabetes Care **24:** 637–642.

78. GREY, M., E.A. BOLAND, M. DAVIDSON, *et al.* 2000. Coping skills training for youth with diabetes mellitus has long-lasting effects on metabolic control and quality of life. J. Pediatr. **137:** 107–113.
79. SKINNER, T.C., S. CHANNON., L. HOWELLS, *et al.* 2000. Diabetes during adolescence. *In* Psychology in Diabetes Care. F.J. Snoek & T.C. Skinner Eds.: 25–59. Wiley & Sons. Chichester.
80. DUMONT, R.H., A.M. JACOBSON, C. COLE, *et al.* 1995. Psychosocial predictors of acute complications of diabetes in youth. Diabet. Med. **12:** 612–618.
81. WYSOCKI, T., M.A. HARRIS, L.M. BUCKLOH, *et al.* 2006. Effects of behavioral family systems therapy for diabetes on adolescents' family relationships, treatment adherence, and metabolic control. J. Pediatr. Psychol. **9:** [Epub ahead of print].
82. FISHER, L., C.A. CHESLA, K.M. CHUN, *et al.* 2004. Patient-appraised couple emotion management and disease management among Chinese American patients with type 2 diabetes. J. Fam. Psychol. **18:** 302–310.
83. ZOFFMANN, V. & M. KIRKEVOLD. 2005. Life versus disease in difficult diabetes care: conflicting perspectives disempower patients and professionals in problem solving. Qual. Health Res. **15:** 750–765.
84. SUNDELIN, J., G. FORSANDER & S.E. MATTSON. 1996. Family-oriented support at the onset of diabetes mellitus: a comparison of two group conditions during 2 years following diagnosis. Acta Paediatr. **85:** 49–55.
85. SPIESS, K., G. SACHS, P. PIETSCHMANN, *et al.* 1995. Program to reduce onset distress in unselected type 1 diabetic patients: effects on psychological variables and metabolic control. Eur. J. Endocrinol. **132:** 580–586.
86. SNOEK, F. 2002. Understanding the human side of diabetes. Diabetes Voice **47:** 37–40.
87. DELAMATER, A.M., A.M. JACOBSON, B. ANDERSON, *et al.* 2001. Psychosocial therapies in diabetes. Report of the psychosocial therapies working group. Diabetes Care **24:** 1286–1292.
88. POUWER, F., F.J. SNOEK, H.M. PLOEG, *et al.* 2001. Monitoring of psychological well-being in outpatients with diabetes mellitus. Effects on mood, HbA1c, and patients' evaluation of the quality of diabetes care: a randomized controlled trial. Diabetes Care **24:** 1929–1935.

Effect of Psychological Intervention on Exercise Adherence in Type 2 Diabetic Subjects

ROBERT MARTINUS,[a] ROD CORBAN,[b] HENNING WACKERHAGE,[c] STEVE ATKINS,[a] AND JAIPAUL SINGH[a]

[a]*Department of Biological Sciences, University of Central Lancashire, Preston, Lancashire PR1 2HE UK*

[b]*School of Sport and Exercise Science, Waikato Institute of Technology, Hamilton, NZ*

[c]*Department of Biomedical Sciences, University of Aberdeen, Aberdeen, Scotland, AB24 3FX UK*

ABSTRACT: Previous research has pointed to the efficacy of physical activity in individuals suffering from type 2 diabetes mellitus (type 2 DM). However, as with other populations, adherence to exercise programs is often problematic. This study assessed the effectiveness of a combination of exercise and psychological interventions in type 2 diabetics in terms of disease management and exercise adherence. Forty newly diagnosed type 2 diabetic subjects (54 $\pm$ 6.5 years) took part in the study. Subjects were allocated to an exercise-only intervention (EO) or a combined exercise and psychological adherence intervention (EP) group. Adherence to the program was also monitored at a 6-month follow-up. The results confirmed a significant improvement in physiological parameters (total mass, fat mass, grip strength, peak flow, flexibility, and VO_2 max) after the 12-week program in both groups ($P < 0.001$). The EP group had significant changes in body fat, grip strength, and peak flow ($P < 0.05$) in comparison to the EO group. Components of the visual analog mood scale (VAMS) were positively influenced in both groups from the therapy program ($P < 0.001$). The directed psychological intervention had a significant influence on attendance to the 12-week program ($P < 0.001$). This also resulted in significantly better adherence 6 months later ($P < 0.05$). In conclusion, the results have demonstrated that psychological intervention is of paramount importance for ensuring high adherence rates during exercise therapy for type 2 diabetic subjects.

KEYWORDS: type 2 diabetes mellitus; exercise counseling; adherence; physiological variables

Address for corresspondence: Prof. Jaipaul Singh, Department of Biological and Forensic Sciences, University of Central Lancashire, Preston, Lancashire, PR1 2HE UK. Voice: 0044-1772-893515; fax: 0044-1772-892929.

e-mail: jsingh3@uclan.ac.uk

Ann. N.Y. Acad. Sci. 1084: 350–360 (2006).
doi: 10.1196/annals.1372.024

INTRODUCTION

The prevalence of type 2 diabetes mellitus (type 2 DM) has seen a fivefold increase worldwide over the last 20 years.[1] This condition is now regarded as the most common metabolic disorder worldwide, and is increasing among adults.[2] Estimates of the prevalence of the condition in England are 3.3% for men and 2.5% for women.[3] Type 2 DM is also associated with a number of other conditions, such as nephropathy (kidney disorders), retinopathy (damage to the retina), neuropathy (damage to nerves), exocrine insufficiencies (reduced digestive enzyme secretion), and cardiomyopathy (coronary heart disease).[2]

With the everescalating prevalence of type 2 DM, the financial burden placed on society is increased, absorbing the costs of treating the disease and its complications. Estimates of the precise cost of diagnosis, treating, and caring for diabetic subjects vary. However, according to one study, diabetic subjects account for approximately £5.2 billion a year.[4] Within the UK, the prevalence of diabetes is predicted to reach 3.5–4 million by 2010.[5]

The largest contributory risk factors for type 2 DM are behavioral and lifestyle related. Around 80% of all type 2 diabetics are obese.[1] Type 2 diabetes is also more common among people who are physically inactive.[6] High levels of physical activity and cardiorespiratory fitness have been shown to confer a protective effect against the development of type 2 DM, even in a dose–response manner.[6,7] In a recent review, strong inverse relationships between components of a metabolic "syndrome," physical activity, and cardiorespiratory fitness, across a variety of demographics, were reported.[8] This meta-analysis also revealed that lifestyle interventions, including exercise, may improve insulin resistance and glucose tolerance in the obese. The role of physical activity and cardiorespiratory fitness, in mediating the development of diabetes, is less well understood.[9] However, exercise should be considered an essential "therapeutic lifestyle change" that may improve insulin resistance and the entire cluster of metabolic risk factors.[8]

In light of the spiraling National Health Services costs due to diabetes, a low cost and easily administered treatment needs to be implemented. Currently, drug therapy and dietary advice are the main treatments for type 2 DM. The proposed benefits of physical activity and exercise are largely ignored. Although recommended by Diabetes UK and the Primary Care Trust (PCT) Framework, it is usually only verbally suggested by the general practitioner. Although there are over 200 registered GP exercise referral schemes in the UK,[10] they do not particularly target type 2 DM. While exercise referral schemes offer a therapeutic form of treating these conditions, the specificity in terms of exercise prescription for the diabetic may be deemed inadequate.

The main objective of any treatment involving diabetic subjects is achieving good glycemic control. However, beneficial effects of exercise training have been observed to wane within 3 to 10 days following exercise.[11] Therefore, effective exercise therapy programs are associated with high exercise adherence, as this would ensure long-term glycemic control. However, as type 2 DM chiefly affects the middle aged and elderly, ascertaining long-term exercise adherence proves challenging. Participation and adherence to exercise programs, among older adults, are relatively low.[12] Approximately 50% of individuals who begin an exercise program will drop out within the first 6 months,[13] emphasizing the transient nature of engagement with such programs.

The time course elements of exercise adherence are poorly understood. Interventions to enhance long-term adherence to physical activity and exercise should be at an early stage in programming.[14] Importantly, it should be noted that few subjects maintained physical activity behaviors following the completion of an intervention.[15]

Studies of factors associated with exercise adherence following the completion of such interventions are rare. The use of psychological support throughout intervention schemes is rare. A recent review concluded that there was no existing UK referral program that is based on an accepted model of behavior change when assessing the effectiveness of physical activity promotion schemes in primary care.[16] It has been recommended that referral schemes incorporate an accepted theoretical model of behavior, and appropriate training, as well as specific training for exercise specialists.[16] Moreover, a recent review by the Health Development Agency, within the UK, suggested that those physical activity interventions based from within a theoretical framework were more likely to be successful.[17] It may be that these models allow a better understanding of why interventions may or may not work.[18] Also contained within this review was an analysis of effective exercise interventions within healthcare settings. Data examining such interventions suggest that those that are judged as "successful" included components, such as: advice from a health professional, education regarding the efficacy of exercise in a written form, and most importantly referral to an exercise specialist. Such specialists are most likely individuals that have knowledge of exercise physiology and exercise prescription as well as knowledge regarding motivators and barriers to physical activity.[18]

Given the obvious benefits of physical activity for individuals with type 2 DM, the main aim of this study was to investigate the role of psychological intervention in improving adherence rates to a regime of exercise for the treatment of type 2 DM. The study was designed to use newly diagnosed type 2 diabetic subjects referred from local GPs, highlighting how a recognized diabetic treatment can be implemented into the infrastructure of the PCT.

METHODS

Referral Scheme

A new pilot GP exercise referral scheme was set up to recruit newly diagnosed type 2 diabetic subjects. Approximately 30 GP practices in the Preston

Borough Area of northern England were contacted and informed of the exercise referral scheme. The scheme, and intervention study, was ethically approved by the PCT for north west England, and by the Ethics Committee of the University of Central Lancashire.

Subjects

Forty newly diagnosed type 2 diabetic subjects (23 females and 17 males; mean age 54 $\pm$ 6.5 years) were recruited to the study. Subjects gave written informed consent to take part. All subjects were not on any anti-diabetic drug therapy.

Study Design

Subjects were allocated to two groups. The exercise-only (EO) and exercise and exercise counseling intervention (EP) groups undertook a 12-week physical activity program. Physiological and psychological measurements were taken pre-intervention, immediately post-intervention, and at 6-month follow-up following the cessation of the formal program. The design of this study was to determine what influence psychological intervention had upon exercise adherence, and whether it had beneficial physiological/ psychological improvement in type 2 diabetic subjects.

Procedures

Physiological measurements: A submaximal, incremental exercise test[19] was used to predict maximal oxygen consumption (VO_2 max). Subjects were tested using a mechanically braked Monark 818 cycle ergometer (Monark, Vansbro, Sweden). Lung function was assessed using the Mini–Wright peak flow meter (Clement Clark, Harlow, UK). An Omron BF302 handheld bioelectrical impedance monitor (Omron, Bannockburn, IL) assessed body fatness. Muscular strength was measured using a Takei Grip A 5001 analog handgrip dynamometer (Cranlea, Birmingham, UK). Maximum values determined from three trails were taken as the measure of strength. Flexibility was assessed using a European standard sit-and-reach box (Bodycare, Southam, UK). The greatest score from three trails was recorded.

Psychological measurements: A visual analog mood scale (VAMS)[20] was used to assess mood states. This instrument is strongly related to the well-used Profile of Mood States.[21] The VAMS instrument consisted of six 100 mm horizontal lines, each representing one of the original mood scales (anxious, depression, angry, energetic, fatigues, and confused). Each line was anchored by the words "not at all" and "extremely." Subjects were asked to indicate the strength of their feelings by marking the line with and "X" between the two extremes. The response was measured to the nearest millimeter for each scale.

In each case, the patient was instructed to rate his/her feelings "during the past week, including the day of the measurement."

Exercise program

Exercise sessions were conducted at a local health fitness center. Subjects were instructed to sign a register on completion of the session. The results were recorded over the 12-week period and were expressed as a percentage of total sessions attended. The EO program consisted of 24 exercise sessions (12 weeks/two sessions per week) and two testing days (pre and post), a total of 26 sessions. The exercise program was developed to include both cardiovascular and resistance activities. Both exercise-only and psychological intervention groups were put on a 12-week exercise-training program. During each week of the intervention, one session was cardiovascular activity and one session resistance activity.

The cardiovascular session entailed a 10-min warm up using a cycle ergometer. The main aerobic activity was set at a moderate target heart rate of 50–70% of age-related heart rate maximum intensity.[22] The duration of activity varied depending upon initial physical fitness. The objective was to progress all the subjects to train for at least 30 min at the end of the 12-week program. The mode of activity varied, but included treadmill, cross-trainer, rower, and cycle ergometer. The session was concluded with a 5-min cool down.

The resistance sessions used the same warm up and cool down. Resistance training involved light gym-based weights, working on endurance/toning. Subjects trained large muscles groups at 15–20 repetitions using a low resistance. Throughout the 12 weeks, resistance was increased gradually and the number of sets increased from one to two. A qualified fitness instructor supervised all sessions.

Psychological Intervention

The EP group completed a 12-week exercise program with additional exercise counseling. During weeks 2, 6, and 10 of the exercise program, each participant within the EP group attended a short 10-min talk at the end of their exercise session. These educational sessions aimed to provide an understanding of diabetes mellitus and the role of exercise in the control of the disease. These sessions were clearly aimed at giving individuals information regarding the effectiveness of exercise in the treatment of their disease, and educating them on the best ways to exercise along with identifying any barriers and steps to remove these barriers. An additional aim of these sessions was to help the individual in terms of their own self-efficacy toward physical activity. Given the participants could be seen as in the early stages of behavior change, importance was placed upon consciousness raising and increasing self-efficacy.

Three weeks into the training session, all candidates in the intervention group were introduced to relaxation techniques. The progressive muscle relaxation

(PMR) technique[23] enables deep relaxation once practiced. The technique works under the principle of feeling tension in the muscles, and then learning to let go of the tension. The subjects were asked to perform PMR several times per week at home for 15 min, gradually learning so that a combination of muscle groups could be contracted at the same time.[24]

Exercise adherence: While attending exercise sessions, each patient was instructed to sign a register on completion of the session. The results were recorded over the 12-week period. The program consisted of 24 exercise sessions (12 weeks/two sessions per week) and two testing days (pre and post), a total of 26 sessions. No control was made as to additional training or physical activities engaged in by subjects.

Follow-up: Upon completion of the EO and EP programs, all subjects were contacted to ascertain the maintenance of exercise behaviors.

Statistical Analysis

All results were expressed as mean ± standard error mean (SEM). Physiological and mood differences between the EO and EP groups, pre and post the 12-week intervention, were analyzed using a 2 × 2 (analysis of variance) ANOVA. Percentage attendance to the program between the two groups was investigated by a Student's *t*-test. A chi-squared test was used to analyze frequency distribution between the two groups on the 6-month follow-up. Significance levels were set at $P < 0.05$. Data were analyzed using SPSS 12.1 statistical software.[24]

RESULTS

Physiological Variables

Changes in physiological performance, by group, are summarized in TABLE 1. The results showed that both EO and EP groups had significant reductions in body mass and body fatness following the intervention period

TABLE 1. Physiological characteristics pre- and post-intervention for the EO and EP groups

	Pre-intervention		Post-intervention	
Parameters	EO	EP	EO	EP
Body mass (kg)	85.00 ± 3.8	85.56 ± 3.8	83.90 ± 3.5*	83.50 ± 3.7*
Body fat (%)	35.84 ± 1.6	35.36 ± 1.4	35.09 ± 1.6*	33.33 ± 1.3*
VO_2 max ($l.min^{-1}$)	1.92 ± 0.14	1.93 ± 0.12	2.09 ± 0.13*	2.21 ± 0.11*
Grip strength (kgf)	29.08 ± 3.2	28.24 ± 2.6	31.54 ± 3.6*	33.12 ± 2.8*
Flexibility (cm)	9.08 ± 1.7	7.29 ± 1.6	11.31 ± 2.2*	8.82 ± 1.5*

n = 20, $^*P < 0.01$.

TABLE 2. The VAMS of EO and EP groups at the time of pre-exercise and post-exercise program.

	Pre-intervention		Post-intervention	
VAMS mood state	EO	EP	EO	EP
Anxious	28.4 ± 7.0	29.2 ± 3.6	21.5 ± 5.7**	8.3 ± 1.6**
Depressed	17.8 ± 3.5	14.5 ± 3.7	13.2 ± 3.0**	8.0 ± 2.8**
Anger	14.8 ± 3.4	16.6 ± 2.8	12.3 ± 2.2*	8.1 ± 1.9*
Energetic	34.7 ± 6.5	43.4 ± 7.2	48.2 ± 7.2**	56.6 ± 5.7**
Fatigued	36.1 ± 3.7	39.9 ± 4.0	23.9 ± 3.4**	20.5 ± 3.3**
Confused	11.6 ± 4.8	26.9 ± 5.9	6.3 ± 1.5**	7.6 ± 1.4**

Values are mean ± SE, $n = 20$ for all groups.
*Significant reduction between pre- and post-intervention measurements ($P > 0.05$).
**Significant reduction between pre- and post-intervention measurements ($P > 0.01$).

($P < 0.001$). Differences between groups were not significant ($P > 0.05$). Predicted VO_2 max and flexibility also increased significantly ($P < 0.01$), though no differences between groups were identified. Grip strength improved significantly for both groups, though the magnitude of improvement was greater for the EO group ($P < 0.01$).

Changes in Mood

The results from the VAMS study are presented in TABLE 2. The data demonstrate that subjects in the EO and EP groups showed significant improvements in all components of the VAMS ($P < 0.05$). The EP group showed a significant difference in the magnitude of improvement in anxiety than EO ($P < 0.01$). No other VAMS component differed, in magnitude of improvement, by group ($P > 0.05$).

Exercise Attendance and Adherence

Attendance on the program was 65.09 ± 11.7 ($n = 20$) for the EO and 65.09 ± 11.7 ($n = 20$) for the EP groups. There was a significant difference in program attendance between the EO and EP groups during the 12-week intervention (65.09 ± 11.7% for EO, 83.26 ± 9.3% for EP; $P < 0.001$). Analysis of these dropout figures using chi-squared tests showed dropout from exercising was significant for the EO compared to the EP group ($P < 0.03$).

DISCUSSION

This study investigated the effects of moderate exercise on selected physiological and psychological variables in type 2 diabetic subjects, using either an exercise-only, or exercise and psychological intervention. The results showed that moderate exercise of one aerobic and one resistance training session per week improved the physiological and psychological profile in type 2 diabetic subjects over a 3-month period. In addition, psychological intervention had a significant influence in program attendance and exercise adherence up to the 6-month follow-up.

The strategy chosen in this study to increase physical activity in the intervention group was developed as a suitable and cost-effective form of therapy for the clinical practice. Using a new GP exercise referral scheme, for type 2 diabetics, this study demonstrates the simplicity of an exercise therapy program, which can be implemented into the PCT infrastructure. Numerous clinical studies on diabetic subjects have demonstrated that supervised, intense training can improve physical function.[8] Such interventions are problematic due to the feasibility of such training in the long-term.[25] A large prospective study reported that only 20–30% of the diabetic subjects continued taking part in organized exercise training after 2 years.[26] These findings agreed with those from our study and show that motivation and compliance is important in ensuring that diabetic subjects continue with exercise programs. It is likely that those instructions for exercise training, which have been made for healthy subjects, are either not well suited or sufficient for diabetic subjects. Individualized instructions could be more effective to increase physical exercise in these subjects. In the clinical practice, this could mean more widespread use of exercise physiologists and psychologists.[27] Again, this is consistent with the view that any exercise intervention should consider the sociocultural contexts of the individuals.[18]

Despite the potential benefits of exercise, many subjects still do not adhere to long-term programs. Exercise adherence is a multifaceted concept, and nonadherence should be identified early on in the behavioral change process. Special attention should be given to those with depressive symptoms, more chronic diseases, and functional limitations. It is evident from this study that a reasonable level of support is needed to ensure adherence, however, the logistics of providing such support are extensive. Improving the compliance of subjects to directed interventions could be achieved through the use of adherence-enhancing interventions.[28] This study exemplifies such an intervention strategy, and shows the benefits for adherence when such an integrated approach is used. This is particularly important during the early stages of such an intervention. What is even more impressive here is that the exercise counseling session was far from comprehensive. Specifically, they involved three 10-min sessions over a 10-week period. As a consequence, the argument that one on one sessions are too expensive, both financially and logistically, are perhaps exaggerated.

This study reaffirms that exercise programs can be used as an effective form in the nonpharmacological treatment in diabetes mellitus. Moreover, if exercise is not going to be adopted as a lifestyle change, benefits may wane

3–10 days post-exercise.[11] Therefore, exercise adherence is paramount in diabetes management. The findings of this study have shown that the combined supplementary psychological intervention is extremely effective in promoting attendance to the exercise program. It is also important to note that adherence to exercise training was continued even after 6 months. This again implies that an effective combination of psychological support and exercise programming can have long-lasting consequences for the diabetic patient. The present results show that by educating subjects, increasing self-efficacy, and improving motivation, it is possible to maintain exercise compliance, which in turn can result in many physiological and psychological benefits. Interventions must concentrate on the individual and moreover, it must cater for their perceptions and barriers to exercise. Similarly, the role of a variety of other predictors are important in influencing adherence. These included previous experience, social cognitions, and perceived improvements.[28] Further studies are needed to investigate the role of these factors in improving adherence. Additionally, the role of time course changes must be addressed. Stages of change from within the transtheoretical model of behavior change have received a great deal of attention in relation to exercise adherence. The present findings support such an emphasis, suggesting that interventions (even simple ones) that address what the model tells us about behavior change are more likely to be effective. Specifically, the interventions applied here can be seen to be consistent with cognitive processes of change and, according to the model, these will be more effective for those in earlier stages of change. Ensuring that subjects retain the exercise "habit" is a challenge to the health professional. This will imply that a combination of cognitive and behavioral process is at work. This study ensured that a "self-orientated" exercise prescription was used to ensure that the "matching notion"[29] was in evidence again.

CONCLUSION

In conclusion, a combined exercise program of moderate aerobic and resistance activity is effective in inducing positive physiological and psychological changes in the newly diagnosed type 2 diabetic subjects. Psychological intervention was also found to increase exercise adherence after 6 months. The diabetic subjects who received psychological counseling intervention significantly improved more than their exercise-only counterparts in many physiological and psychological parameters. Although physical performance is not directly attributed to psychological intervention, this did not adversely affect a considerable increase in physical performance, by increasing attendance to the program. It is recommended that psychological intervention should be employed in conjunction with exercise training to obtain maximal benefit especially in type 2 diabetic subjects.

REFERENCES

1. ZIMMET, P., K.G.M.M. ALBERTI & J. SHAW. 2001. Global and societal implications of the diabetes epidemic. Nature **414:** 782–787.
2. KUMAR, P. & M. CLARK. 2002. Diabetes mellitus and other disorders of metabolism. *In* Clinical Medicine. P. Kumar and M. Clark, Eds.: 1069–1121. WB Saunders. London.
3. DEPARTMENT OF HEALTH. 2002. National Service Framework for Diabetes. The Stationary Office. London.
4. CURRIE, C.J. 1997. NHS acute sector expenditure for diabetes: the present, future, and excess in-patient cost of care. Diabetic Med. **14:** 686–692.
5. AMOS, A., D. MCCARTY & P. ZIMMET. 1997. The rising global burden of diabetes and its complications; estimates and projections to the year. Diabetic Med. **14:** S1–S85.
6. KELLEY, D.E. & B.H. GOODPASTER. 1999. Effects of physical activity on insulin action and glucose tolerance in obesity. Med. Sci. Sports Exerc. **31:** S619–S623.
7. KHOL., J. 2001. Physical activity and cardiovascular disease: evidence for a dose-response. Med. Sci. Sports Exerc. **33:** S472–S483.
8. CARROLL, S. & M. DUDFIELD. 2004. What is the relationship between exercise and metabolic abnormalities? Sports Med. **34:** 371–418.
9. LIESE, A.D., E.J. MAYER-DAVIS & S.M. HAFFNER. 1998. Development of the multiple metabolic syndrome: an epidemiological perspective. Epidemiol. Rev. **20:** 157–172.
10. DEPARTMENT OF HEALTH, UK AUTHORITY. 2001. Exercise referral systems: A National Quality Assurance Framework. Crown Copyright. Her Majesty's Government, UK.
11. IVY, J.L. 1997. Role of exercise training in the prevention and treatment of insulin resistance and non-insulin-dependent diabetes mellitus. Sports Med. **24:** 321–336.
12. MOREY, M., P.M. DUBBERT, M. DOYLE, *et al.* 2003. From supervised to unsupervised exercise: factors associated with exercise adherence. J. Aging Phys. Act. **11:** 351–368.
13. DISHMAN, R.K. 1990. Advances in Exercise Adherence. Human Kinetics. Leeds, UK.
14. MARCUS, B.H., J.S. ROSSI., V.C. SELBY, *et al.* 1992. The stages and processes of exercise adoption and maintenance in a work place sample. Health Psychol. **11:** 386–395.
15. DISHMAN, R.K. & J. BUCKWORTH. 1996. Adherence to physical activity. *In* W.P. Morgan, Ed.: 63–80. Physical Activity and Mental Health. Taylor & Francis. Washington.
16. RIDDOCH, C., A. PUIG-RIBERA & A. COOPER. 1998. Effectiveness of physical activity promotion schemes in primary care: a review. Health Promotion Effectiveness Review: Summary Bulletin 14. Health Education Authority. Her Majesty's Government, UK.
17. HEALTH DEVELOPMENT AGENCY. HER MAGESTY GOVERNMENT, UK. 2005. Effectiveness of public health interventions for increasing physical activity among adults: a review of reviews (evidence briefing second edition). Health Development Agency. Her Majesty's Government, UK.

18. MUTRIE, N. 2005. Applied Exercise Psychology: Promoting Activity & Evaluating Outcomes. Proceedings from the 11th ISSP World Congress of Sport Psychology. August 2005, Sydney, Australia.
19. ASTRAND, P.O. 1988. Work Tests With Bicycle Ergometer. Varberg. Stockholm, Sweden.
20. LITTLE, K. & E. PENMAN. 1989. Measuring subacute mood changes using the profile of moods states and visual analogue scales. Psychopathology **22:** 32–49.
21. MCNAIR, D.M., M. LORR & L.F. DROPPLEMEN. 1971. Manual for the Profile of Moods States. Educational and Industrial Testing Service. San Diego.
22. POLLOCK, M.L., G.A. GAESSER & J.D. BUTCHER. 1998. The recommended quantity and quality of exercise for developing and maintaining cardiorespiratory and muscular fitness and flexibility in healthy adults. Med. Sci. Sports Exerc. **30:** 975–991.
23. JACOBSON, E. 1930. Progressive Relaxation. Chicago University Press. Chicago.
24. SPSS. 1996. The statistical package for social sciences (SPSS/PC+). SPSS.Chicago.
25. SKARFORS, E.T., T.A. WEGENER, H. LITHELL & I. SELINUS. 1987. Physical training as treatment for type 2 DM (noninsulin-dependent) in elderly men. A feasibility study over 2 years. Diabetologia **30:** 930–933.
26. HANEFELD, M., S. FISCHER, H. SCHMECHEL, *et al.* 1991. Diabetes intervention study: multi-intervention trial in newly diagnosed NIDDM. Diabetes Care **14**: 308–317.
27. VANNINEN, E., M. UUSITUPA, O. SIITONEN, *et al.* 1992. Habitual physical activity, aerobic capacity and metabolic control in subjects with newly-diagnosed type 2 (non-insulin-dependent) diabetes mellitus: effect of 1-year diet and exercise intervention. Diabetologia **35:** 340–346.
28. MARTIN, K.A. & A.R. SINDEN. 2001. Who will stay and who will go? A review of older adults adherence to randomised controls of exercise. J. Aging Phys. Act. **9:** 91–114.
29. MARCUS, B.H., J.S. ROSSI, V.C. SELBY, *et al.* 1992. The stages and processes of exercise adoption and maintenance in a work place sample. Health Psychol. **11:** 386–395.

The Effect of a Fat-Enriched Diet on the Pattern of Distribution of Pancreatic Islet Cells in the C57BL/6J Mice

ERNEST ADEGHATE,[a] FRANK CHRISTOPHER HOWARTH,[b] HAMEED RASHED,[a] TARIQ SAEED,[a] AND AMSTRONG GBEWONYO[a]

[a]*Department of Anatomy, Faculty of Medicine and Health Sciences, United Arab Emirates University, Al Ain, UAE*

[b]*Department of Physiology, Faculty of Medicine and Health Sciences, United Arab Emirates University, Al Ain, UAE*

ABSTRACT: The C57BL/6J mice are inbred strains and develop the metabolic syndrome of obesity, hyperinsulinemia, hyperglycemia, and hypertension, when fed a high-fat diet. These features are similar to those observed in the human metabolic syndrome. This article examined the effect of fat-enriched (FE) diet on the pattern of distribution of insulin-, glucagon-, somatostatin-, and pancreatic polypeptide (PP)-positive cells in the pancreatic islets of C57BL/6J mice using immunohistochemical methods. Insulin-immunoreactive cells were observed in both the peripheral and central regions of the islets of Langerhans in both FE- and control diet-fed mice. The percentage distribution of insulin-positive cells was similar in FE (83.5 ± 6.4) compared to control diet-fed C57BL/6J mice (83.8 ± 6.5). Glucagon-containing cells were discerned in the periphery of pancreatic islets in both FE- and control diet-fed mice. The percentage distribution of glucagon was not statistically different in mice fed with FE (9.9 ± 2.7) compared to control diet (11.3 ± 4.9). Somatostatin-positive cells were seen in the outer part of the islet of Langerhans and constitute 12.1% (±6.3) and 10% (±5.5) of pancreatic islet cells in FE- and control diet-fed mice, respectively. PP-immunoreactive cells were observed in the peripheral region of the pancreatic islets of both FE- and control diet-fed mice. The percentage distribution of PP-positive cells was significantly (2.0 ± 1.2) lower compared to control (5.1 ± 2.4). In conclusion, the number of PP is significantly reduced in FE diet-fed mice and may play a role in the pathogenesis of diet-induced metabolic syndrome in C57BL/6J mice.

KEYWORDS: C57BL/6J mice; peptides; islet; pancreas; immunohistochemistry; metabolic syndrome

Address for correspondence: Prof. Ernest Adeghate, Department of Anatomy, Faculty of Medicine and Health Sciences, United Arab Emirates University, P.O. Box 17666, Al Ain, UAE. Voice: +971-3-7137496; fax: +971-3-7672033.
e-mail: eadeghate@uaeu.ac.ae

Ann. N.Y. Acad. Sci. 1084: 361–370 (2006).
doi: 10.1196/annals.1372.002

INTRODUCTION

The prevalence of obesity and the accompanying metabolic syndrome is continuing to rise among adolescents in the developed world.[1] The C57BL/6J mouse is an inbred line that develops the metabolic syndrome of obesity, hyperinsulinemia, hyperglycemia, and hypertension, when fed a fat-enriched (FE) diet.[2] This mouse strain is an appropriate model of the human metabolic syndrome because it develops the metabolic syndrome of obesity, hypertension, hyperglycemia, and hyperinsulinemia when fed an FE diet but remains lean and in good health when restricted to control diet.[2]

The development of metabolic syndrome in C57BL/6J mice is said to be similar to the progression of metabolic disease observed in humans. For example, the onset of diabetes and obesity occurs gradually in humans and is often precipitated by intake of FE diet.[3] Moreover, diet-induced diabetes and obesity in the C57BL/6J mice is characterized by selective deposition of adipose tissue in the intestinal mesentery.[4,5] This observation corroborates the idea that abdominal obesity is an independent risk factor for diabetes in humans.

In addition, FE diet-fed C57BL/6J mice may also develop immune defect[6] as well as atherosclerosis.[7]

The mechanism by which FE diets induce metabolic syndrome in C57BL/6J mice is still unclear. The FE diet obesity that develops in C57BL/6J mice is not simply due to hyperphagia[8,9] or a decrease in physical activity[10] but due to the fact that C57BL/6J mice can attain increased feed efficiency.[8,9] The processes by which C57BL/6J mice increase feed efficiency and become obese is still unclear. The purpose of this article was to investigate the pattern of distribution of hormone-containing islet cells in the pancreas of FE diet-fed C57BL/6J mice in order to shed further light on the cellular and molecular basis of FE diet-induced obesity in this mouse strain.

MATERIALS AND METHODS

Twelve C57BL/6J male mice were used for the experiment. Two groups of age-matched C57BL/6J male mice were placed on either an FE diet (TD01460, Harlan Teklad, UK) or a control diet (TD02293, Harlan Teklad, UK). The FE diet comprised 24% protein, 41% carbohydrate, and 24% fat whereas, the control diet comprised 19% protein, 67% carbohydrate, and 4% fat. For the FE diet approximately 45% of the energy is derived from fat whereas, for the control diet only 11% of calories are derived from fat. At the start of the experiment, the mean weight of the animals when they commenced the experimental diets was 19.5 ± 0.5 g, $n = 29$. The duration of the feeding program was 7 months. Body weight and blood glucose (One Touch II; Lifescan Inc., Milpitas, CA) were measured periodically. The study was approved by the Animal Ethics Committee of the Faculty of Medicine and Health Sciences, UAE University.

Immunohistochemistry

At the end of the experiment, the pancreas of the six mice from each group (FE- and control diet-fed) was removed after chloral hydrate anesthesia. The isolated pancreata were trimmed free of adherent fat and connective tissue and cut into small pieces (2 mm^3) and fixed overnight in freshly prepared Zamboni's fixative.[11] The tissue samples were later dehydrated in graded concentrations of ethanol, cleared in xylene, and subsequently embedded in paraffin wax at 55°C. Sections of 6 μm thickness were cut on a microtome (AS325; Shandon, Pittsburgh, PA). The sections were deparaffinized, transferred into absolute ethanol, and processed for immunohistochemistry using established methods.[12] Briefly, the sections were incubated for 30 min in 0.3% hydrogen peroxide solution in methanol to block endogenous peroxidase activity and later treated with a blocking reagent for 30 min before incubation in antibodies against either insulin, glucagon, somatostatin, or pancreatic polypeptide (PP) (1:2000) for 24 h at 4°C. The slides were then washed and incubated for 30 min with prediluted biotinylated anti-rabbit IgG for 30 min, before incubation in streptavidin peroxidase conjugate for 45 min. The peroxidase activity was revealed by incubating the specimens for 3 min in 3,3-diaminobenzidine tetrahydrochloride containing 0.03% hydrogen peroxide in TBS. The slides were later washed and counterstained with hematoxylin for 30 sec before mounting in Cytoseal 60 (Stephens Scientific, Riverdale, NJ).

The antisera to insulin, glucagon, somatostatin, and PP were purchased from Dako (Copenhagen, Denmark). The antisera to insulin, glucagon, and somatostatin were supplied prediluted. No specific immunostaining was observed in pancreatic tissue when primary antisera were omitted.

Morphometric Analysis of Pancreatic Islet Cells

The total number of cells in the islets of C57BL/6J mice fed on FE diet and control rats were counted using Axiovision Microimaging System® (Carl Zeiss, Jena, Germany) attached to a light microscope. In addition, insulin-, glucagon-, somatostatin-, and PP-positive cells within a given islet were also counted. A total of 10 random fields were taken from a total of 6 slides for each rat per group. The percentage of insulin, glucagon, somatostatin, and PP-positive cells was calculated for each islet. The values obtained from sections of C57BL/6J mice fed on FE diet were compared with those of control.

Electron Microscopy Studies

At the end of the experiment, C57BL/6J mice fed on FE diet and controls were anesthetized and perfused transcardially with McDowell and Trump fixative[13] for 30 min. Pancreatic tissue fragments were processed for electron microscope examination according to previously described techniques.[14] Briefly, tissue samples were washed several times with phosphate buffer (PB) and then postfixed with 0.1% osmium tetroxide in PB for 1 h. After washing several times with distilled water, the tissues were dehydrated in ascending concentrations of ethanol, treated with propylene oxide, and then placed in propylene oxide and resin (1:1) for 1 h followed by pure resin overnight. Tissue samples were embedded and polymerized at 60°C for 24 h. Sections were cut using a diatome knife (Agar Scientific, Essex, UK) then mounted on 3.05 mm, 20 mesh copper grid and contrast stained with saturated aqueous uranyl acetate for 30 min and Reynolds lead citrate for 5 min.[15] Sections were examined using a transmission electron microscope (CM10; Philips, Eindhoven, The Netherlands). Photographs were taken using Kodak (Rochester, NY) electron ester thick base 4489 film.

RESULTS

At the end of the study, the weight gain in FE diet-fed C57BL/6J mice (45.7 ± 1.3 g) was significantly higher that of controls (36.6 ± 2.0 g). Similarly, the blood glucose level was also higher in FE fed mice (166.0 ± 20.0 mg/dL) compared to controls (147.7 ± 9.4 mg/dL).

Insulin-immunoreactive cells were observed in both the peripheral and central regions of the islets of Langerhans in both the FE- and control diet-fed C57BL/6J mice (FIG. 1). The percentage distribution of insulin-positive cells

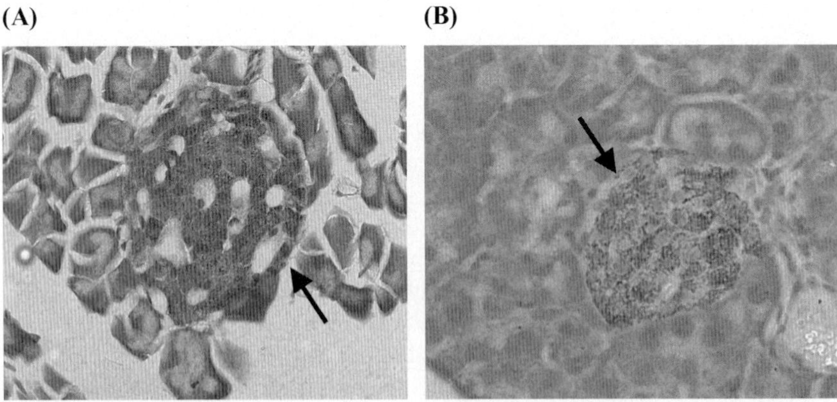

FIGURE 1. Light micrographs showing the pattern of distribution of insulin-immunoreactive cells (*arrow*) in the pancreatic islets of C57BL/6J mice fed on FE and control diet. Note that the pattern of distribution of insulin-positive cells is similar in the islets of C57BL/6J mice fed with either FE (**A**) or control (**B**) diet. Magnification: × 400.

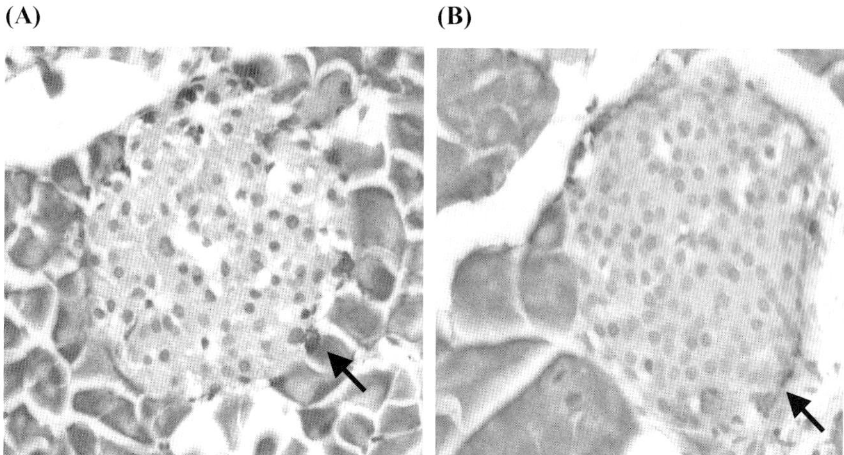

FIGURE 2. Light micrographs of the pattern of distribution of glucagon-positive cells (*arrow*) in the pancreatic islets of C57BL/6J mice fed on high-FE and control diet. The pattern of distribution of glucagon-immunoreactive cells is similar in the islets of C57BL/6J mice fed with either FE (**A**) or control (**B**) diet. Magnification: × 400.

was similar in FE diet (83.5 ± 6.4) compared to that of control diet-fed C57BL/6J mice (83.8 ± 6.5) (FIG. 5). FIGURE 3 shows glucagon-containing cells in the periphery of pancreatic islets in both FE- (FIG. 2 A) and control diet-fed (FIG. 2 B) mice, where they formed a mantle of cells. The percentage distribution of glucagon was not statistically different in mice fed with FE (9.9 ± 2.7) compared to control diet-fed mice (11.3 ± 4.9) (FIG. 5). Somatostatin-positive cells were seen in the outer part of the islet of Langerhans and constitute 12.1% (±6.3) and 10% (±5.5) of pancreatic islet cells in FE and control diet-fed mice, respectively (FIG. 3). FIGURE 4 shows PP-immunoreactive cells in the peripheral region of the pancreatic islets of both FE- and control diet-fed mice. The percentage of PP-immunoreactive cells was significantly ($P < 0.02$) lower in FE diet-fed mice compared to control (FIG. 5).

Infiltration by Lymphoid Tissue

The pancreatic islets of C57BL/6J mice are often associated with lymphatic cells, however, this lymphatic infiltration is more pronounced around the islets of FE diet-fed C57BL/6J mice (FIG. 6 A) compared to control (FIG. 6 B). In some cases, the pancreatic islets of FE diet-fed C57BL/6J mice were completely surrounded by lymphoid tissue (FIG. 6 B). Most of the cells in the infiltrate are lymphocytes.

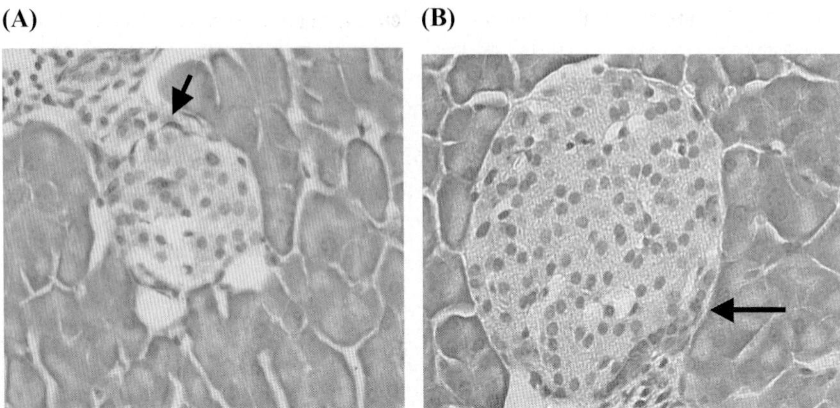

FIGURE 3. Micrographs of the pattern of distribution of somatostatin-immunoreactive cells (*arrow*) in the pancreatic islets of C57BL/6J mice fed on FE and control diet. The pattern of distribution and the number of somatostatin-positive cells are similar in the islets of C57BL/6J mice fed with either FE (**A**) or control (**B**) diet. Magnification: × 400.

Electron Microscopic Studies

The ultrastructure of the acinar cells of the FE diet-fed mice was similar to that of control mice. The structure of the cytoplasmic organelles including mitochondria, zymogen granules, and Golgi apparatus was comparable in both

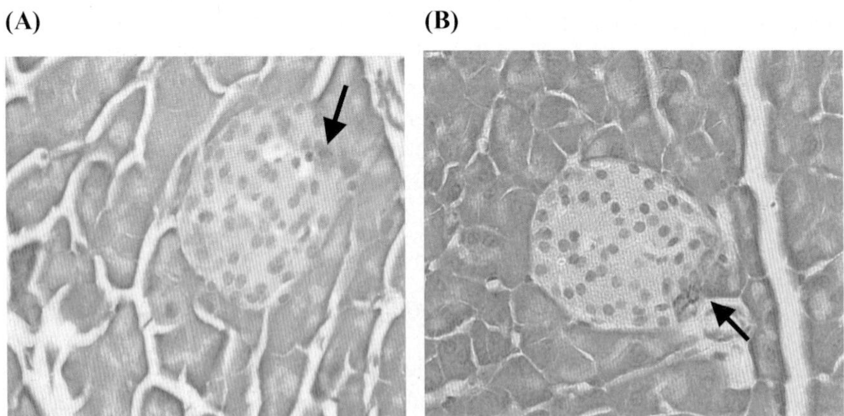

FIGURE 4. Light micrographs showing the pattern of distribution of PP-immunopositive cells (*arrow*) in the islets of C57BL/6J mice fed on FE and control diet. Although the pattern of distribution of PP-immunoreactive cells is similar in the islets of C57BL/6J mice fed with either FE (**A**) or control (**B**) diet, the number of PP-immunoreactive cells is higher in C57BL/6J mice fed on FE diet. Magnification: × 400.

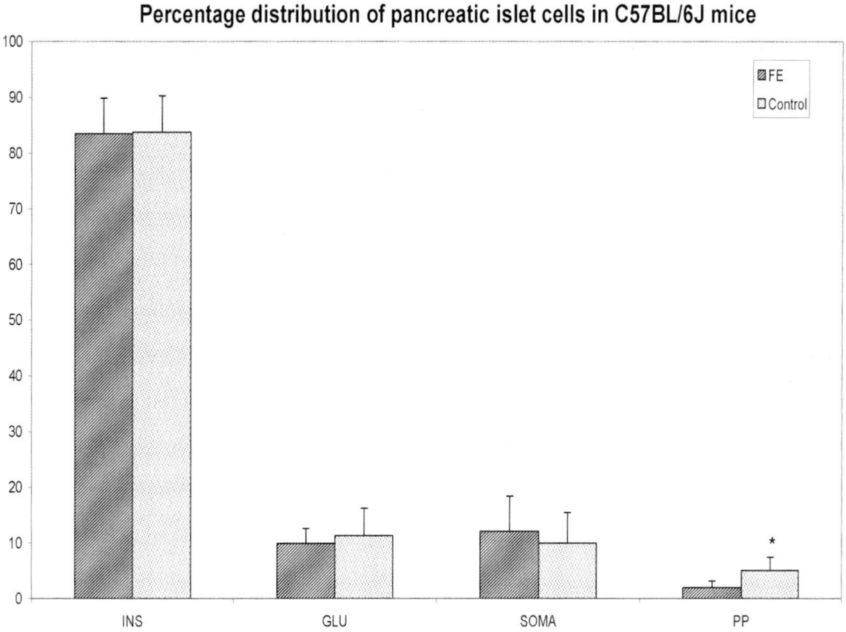

Percentage distribution of pancreatic islet cells in C57BL/6J mice

FIGURE 5. Histograms showing the percentage distribution of pancreatic islet cells in the pancreas of C57BL/6J mice fed on fat-enriched (FE) diet (*dark upward diagonal*) and control (*small confetti*). Note that the pattern of distribution of insulin (INS)-, glucagon (GLU)-, and somatostatin (SOMA)-immunoreactive cells are similar in both FE and control mice. In contrast, the percentage distribution of pancreatic polypeptide (PP)-positive cells was significantly higher ($^{*}P < 0.02$) in control compared to mice fed on FE diet.

groups of mice. However, the rough endoplasmic reticulum of C57BL/6J mice fed with FE diet is more dilated (FIG. 7).

DISCUSSION

This study shows that the pattern of distribution and the number of insulin-, glucagon-, and somatostatin-positive cells are similar in the pancreas of FE- and control diet-fed C57BL/6J mice. The pattern of distribution of these pancreatic peptides is similar to those observed in Wistar[16] and Sprague–Dawley[12] rats. However, there are disparities in the number of insulin-, glucagon-, and somatostatin-immunoreactive cells in the pancreas of both FE- and control diet-fed C57BL/6J mice compared to Wistar[16] and Sprague–Dawley[12] rats. The number of insulin-positive cells was significantly higher in C57BL/6J mice compared to Wistar and Sprague–Dawley rats. A possible reason for the relatively higher number of insulin-producing cells in C57BL/6J mice is the presence of hyperinsulinemia in this strain of mice. It thus appears that the

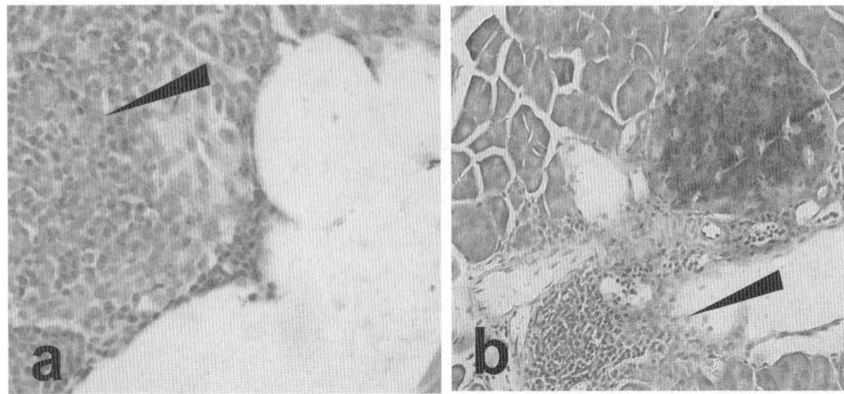

FIGURE 6. Light micrographs showing lymphatic infiltration (*arrow*) around the pancreatic islets of C57BL/6J mice fed on (a) fat-enriched (FE) and (b) control diet. That density of lymphatic infiltration is more prominent around the islets of C57BL/6J mice fed with FE diet compared to control. Magnification: × 400.

number of insulin-positive cells will have to increase to compensate for the increase in the blood level of insulin.

The number of glucagon-positive cells was smaller in C57BL/6J mice compared to Wistar[16] and Sprague–Dawley[12] rats. This observation is not

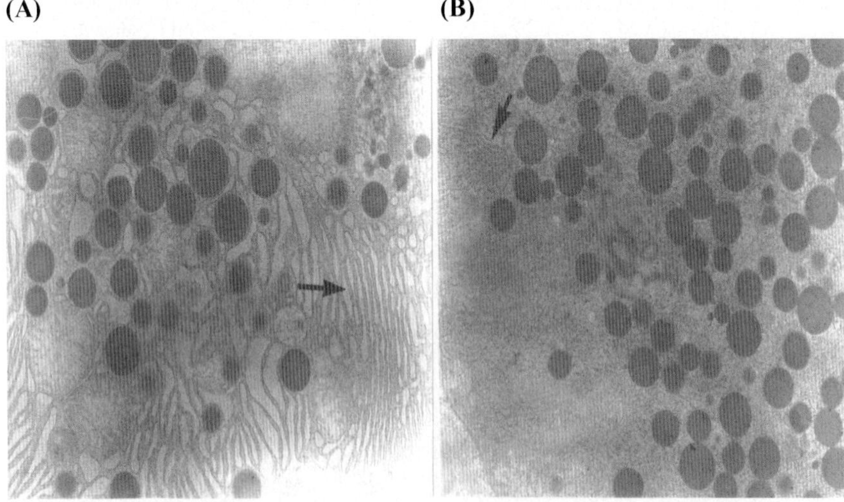

FIGURE 7. Electron micrographs of pancreatic acinar cells of C57BL/6J mice fed on FE and control diet. The ultrastructure of the acinar cells of C57BL/6J mice fed with either FE diet (**A**) is similar to that of control (**B**). However, the rough endoplasmic reticulum of C57BL/6J mice fed with FE diet is more dilated. Magnification: × 400.

surprising because it is well known that insulin inhibits glucagon release.[17] The hyperinsulinemia observed in C57BL/6J mice would therefore logically pair with a low plasma or pancreatic tissue level of glucagon. Similarly, the number of somatostatin-immunoreactive cells was significantly higher in C57BL/6J mice compared to the values in Wistar[16] and Sprague–Dawley[12] rats.

Although the number of PP-positive cells in C57BL/6J mice was comparable to that of Sprague–Dawley rats,[12] there was a significant difference between the number of PP cells in FE diet-fed C57BL/6J mice compared to control. Previous reports have shown that PP is involved in the regulation of energy balance.[18] In humans, low plasma levels of PP have been seen in obesity and people injected with pharmacological doses of PP have been shown to reduce their food intake.[19] The results of this study confirmed the role of PP in the regulation of energy balance. It also shows that FE diet may influence the metabolism of PP. The diet-induced obesity in C57BL/6J mice may thus be initiated via the PP.

The presence of lymphatic infiltration around the islets of C57BL/6J mice shows that inflammatory process may also play a role in the destruction of the islets cells, which may eventually lead to diabetes. The pancreatic islets of FE diet-fed C57BL/6J mice contained more infiltrates compared to control. In fact, FE diet-fed C57BL/6J mice have been shown previously to develop immune defect.[6] A possible reason for this observation may be that FE diet may make C57BL/6J mice more susceptible to infection because of a more sluggish metabolism compared to control.

REFERENCES

1. DAVIS, C.L., B. FLICKINGER, D. MOORE, *et al.* 2005. Prevalence of cardiovascular risk factors in schoolchildren in a rural Georgia community. Am. J. Med. Sci. **330:** 53–59.
2. SURWIT, R.S., C.M. KUHN, C. COCHRANE, *et al.* 1988. Diet-induced type II diabetes in C57BL/6J mice. Diabetes **37:** 1163–1167.
3. WEST, K.M. & J.M. KALBFLEISCH. 1971. Influence of nutritional factors on prevalence of diabetes. Diabetes **20:** 99–108.
4. REBUFFÉ-SCRIVE, M., R. SURWIT, M. FEINGLOS, *et al.* 1993. Regional fat distribution and metabolism in a new mice model (C57BL/6J) of non-insulin-dependent diabetes mellitus. Metabolism **42:** 1405–1409.
5. SURWIT, R.S., M.N. FEINGLOS, J. RODIN, *et al.* 1995. Differential effects of fat and sucrose on the development of obesity and diabetes in C57BL/6J and A/J mice. Metabolism **44:** 645–651.
6. CREVEL, R.W., J.V. FRIEND, B.F. GOODWIN & W.E. PARISH. 1992. High-fat diets and the immune response of C57Bl mice. Br. J. Nutr. **67:** 17–26.
7. PAIGEN, B. 1995. Genetics of responsiveness to high-fat and high-cholesterol diets in the mice. Am. J. Clin. Nutr. 62: 458S–462S.
8. PAREKH, P.I., A.E. PETRO, J.M. TILLER, *et al.* 1998. Reversal of diet-induced obesity and diabetes in C57BL/6J mice. Metabolism **47:** 1089–1096.

9. COLLINS, S., T.L. MARTIN, R.S. SURWIT & J. ROBIDOUX. 2004. Genetic vulnerability to diet-induced obesity in the C57BL/6J mice: physiological and molecular characteristics. Physiol. Behav. **81:** 243–248.
10. BROWNLOW, B.S., A. PETRO, M.N. FEINGLOS & R.S. SURWIT. 1996. The role of motor activity in diet-induced obesity in C57BL/6J mice. Physiol. Behav. **60:** 37–41.
11. ZAMBONI, L. & C. DE MARTINO. 1967. Buffered picric acid-formaldehyde: a new rapid fixation for electron microscopy. J. Cell. Biol. **35:** 148A.
12. ADEGHATE, E. & T. DONÁTH. 1991. Morphometric and immunohistochemical study on the endocrine cells of pancreatic transplants. Exp. Clin. Endocrinol. **98:** 193–199.
13. MCDOWELL, E.M. & B.F. TRUMP. 1976. Histologic fixatives suitable for diagnostic light and electron microscopy. Arch. Pathol. Lab. Med. **100:** 405–414.
14. DRAPER, C.E., E. ADEGHATE, P.A. LAWRENCE, *et al.* 1998. Age-related changes in morphology and secretory responses of male rat lacrimal gland. J. Auto. Nerv. Sys. **69:** 173–183.
15. REYNOLDS, E.S. 1963. The use of lead citrate at high pH as an electron-opaque staining in electron microscopy. J. Cell. Biol. **17:** 208–212.
16. AHMED, I., E. ADEGHATE, A.K. SHARMA, *et al.* 1998. Effects of Momordica charantia fruit juice on islet morphology in the pancreas of the streptozotocin-diabetic rat. Diabetes Res. Clin. Pract. **40:** 145–151.
17. GANONG, W.L. 1989. Endocrine function of the pancreas and the regulation of carbohydrate metabolism. *In* Review of Medical Physiology, 14th ed. 280–300. Prentice-Hall International. Connecticut.
18. ASAKAWA, A., A. INUI, H. YUZURIHA, *et al.* 2003. Characterization of the effects of pancreatic polypeptide in the regulation of energy balance. Gastroenterology **124:** 1325–1336.
19. KOSKA, J., A. DELPARIGI, B. DE COURTEN, *et al.* 2004. Pancreatic polypeptide is involved in the regulation of body weight in Pima Indian male subjects. Diabetes **53:** 3091–3096.

Effect of Vitamin C on Liver and Kidney Functions in Normal and Diabetic Rats

MARIAM AL SHAMSI,[a] AMR AMIN,[b] AND ERNEST ADEGHATE[a]

[a]*Department of Anatomy, Faculty of Medicine and Health Sciences, UAE University, Al Ain, United Arab Emirates*

[b]*Department of Biology, Faculty of Science, UAE University, Al Ain, United Arab Emirates*

ABSTRACT: Diabetes mellitus (DM) is recognized as one of the leading causes of morbidity and mortality in the world. About 5–6% of the world population suffers from this disease and the number of people diagnosed with diabetes is rapidly increasing. Diabetes has been demonstrated to be associated with oxidative stress and hyperglycemia, one of the most important indictors of oxidative stress. The endogenous mechanisms of enzymes and antioxidants are able to destroy the reactive species and create a balance between antioxidant and free radicals. In diabetes, the oxidative stress is increased because of the deficiency in the antioxidant defense. The intake of antioxidants, such as vitamin C, may reduce the oxidative stress associated with diabetes and hence help to restore the antioxidant defense system. The aim of this article was to investigate the effect of different doses of vitamin C on the biochemical parameters of normal and streptozotocin (STZ)-induced diabetic rats. Biochemical analysis was used to study the effect of this vitamin on the biochemical parameters of normal and diabetic rats. Liver and kidney enzymes were elevated after the onset of diabetes. Moderate doses of vitamin C significantly ($P < 0.0008$) reduced plasma gamma-glutamyl level in diabetic rats. Moreover, vitamin C significantly ($P < 0.01$) reduced the blood urea nitrogen level of diabetic rats. The plasma level of electrolytes, such as calcium and sodium, also changed significantly ($P < 0.00001$) after oral administration of vitamin C. Antioxidants, such as vitamin C, may ameliorate the biochemical parameters of diabetic rats.

KEYWORDS: diabetes mellitus; vitamin C; liver function test; kidney function test; electrolytes

Address for correspondence: Ernest Adeghate M.D., M.F.M., Ph.D., Department of Anatomy, Faculty of Medicine and Health Sciences, UAE University, PO Box 17666, Al Ain, United Arab Emirates. Voice: +971-3-7137496; fax: +971-3-7672033.

e-mail: eadeghate@uaeu.ac.ae

Ann. N.Y. Acad. Sci. 1084: 371–390 (2006).
doi: 10.1196/annals.1372.031

INTRODUCTION

Diabetes mellitus (DM) affects approximately 6% of the world population. The prevalence rate of diabetes continues to increase.[1] Hyperglycemia induces the production of superoxide by mitochondria, leading to the formation of a strong oxidant proxy nitrite, which damages DNA. The damage of the DNA activates the nuclear enzyme poly (ADP-ribose) polymerase, which depletes the intracellular concentration of NAD (+), thus slowing glycolysis, ATP formation, and ADP ribosylation of GAPDH. All of these processes contribute to the development of late degenerative complications.[2]

Vitamin C is a water-soluble antioxidant that was first isolated and characterized by Szent-Gyorgyi in 1928.[3] It is an abundant component of plants. In plants, it reaches a concentration of over 20 mM in chloroplast and occurs in the cell compartments, including the cell wall. It plays a role in photosynthesis as an enzyme cofactor and in the control of cell growth.[4] Ascorbate is synthesized by most vertebrates excluding humans, monkeys, guinea pigs, the Indian fruit bat, and in some fish it is synthesized in the liver.[5]

Vitamin C is important for many enzymatic reactions and also acts as a free-radical scavenger. Specific nonoverlapping transport protein mediate the transport of the oxidized form of vitamin C, dehydroascorbic acid, and the reduced form, L-ascorbic acid across biological membranes. Dehydroascorbic acid uptake across the membrane occurs via the facilitated diffusion through glucose transporters, Glut 1, 3, and 4, while L-ascorbic acid enters cell via Na^+ dependent system (SVCT 1 and SVCT 2).[6]

The cellular uptake of vitamin C is promoted by insulin and inhibited by hyperglycemia.[7] Ascorbic acid has been shown to have several antioxidant properties.[8] It is an essential cofactor involved in many biochemical functions, and it acts as an electron donor or reducing agent; it is said to have ascorbate oxidant activity.[9] It has greater roles in the aqueous interstitial and intracellular fluid compartments.[5] Ascorbate effectively scavenge singlet oxygen, superoxide, hydroxyl and water soluble peroxyl radical, and hypochlorous acid.[10]

MATERIALS AND METHODS

Experimental Animals

Male Wistar rats aged 7–8 weeks and weighing 200–300 g were used in this study. All rats were obtained from the Faculty of Medicine and Health Sciences, United Arab Emirates University, and were housed in a temperature (25°C) and humidity-controlled rooms and 12 h light–dark periods. The animals were fed on a standard rat chow and tap water *ad libitum*.

Induction of Experimental Diabetes

Diabetes was induced in the rats by a single intraperitoneal injection of streptozotocin (STZ) (Sigma, St. Louis, MO) at a dose of 60 mg/kg body weight.[11] The STZ was freshly dissolved in citrate buffer (0.5 M, pH 4.5). The rats were considered diabetic if the fasting blood glucose level values were more than 250 mg/dL.

Experimental Design

Rats were randomly divided into three groups according to three different doses of vitamin C (low dose 10 mg/kg, moderate dose 50 mg/kg, and high dose 100 mg/kg of vitamin C). Rats were orally treated with vitamin C by using an intubation loop. The rats were divided into five subgroups of six animals each.

1. Group I (normal untreated rats). Rats were not treated either with STZ or with vitamin C.
2. Group II (STZ-induced diabetic control rats). Rats were not treated with vitamin C.
3. Group III (vitamin C-treated diabetic rats). Rats were treated with the three different doses (low, moderate, and high) of vitamin C for 10 days prior to the induction of diabetes.
4. Group IV (vitamin C-treated diabetic rats). Rats were treated with the three different doses (low, moderate, and high) of vitamin C 10 days after the onset of diabetes.
5. Group V (normal nondiabetic-treated group). This group was treated with the three different doses of vitamin C.

Biochemical Analysis

Blood urea nitrogen (BUN), creatinine (CRE), alkaline phosphatase (ALP), alanine aminotransferase (ALT), aspartate aminotransferase (AST), lactic dehydrogenase (LDH), gamma-glutamyl transferase (γ-GT), calcium (Ca), phosphorus (PHOS), sodium (Na), potassium (K), and magnesium (Mg) were performed in Al-Qattara Veterinary Laboratory by using Beckman Coulter (Synchron LX20 PRO Clinical System, Fullerton, CA).

Statistical Analysis

Data were expressed as mean $\pm$ SD. Student's *t*-test and was used to analyze the significance of differences between mean values. Different groups were analyzed by analysis of variance using Duncan's multiple range tests. A *P* value of less than 0.05 was considered statistically significant.

RESULTS

Liver Enzymes

Plasma ALP Level

The result shows that the low dose (10 mg/kg body weight) of vitamin C significantly ($P < 0.004$) reduced the level of plasma ALP in normal rats. Moreover, the low dose of vitamin C caused a decrease in the plasma ALP level of rats treated with vitamin C before the onset of diabetes. Moderate dose (50 mg/kg body weight) of vitamin C had no significant effect on the plasma ALP level of normal rats and of rats treated before and after the onset of diabetes (FIG. 1). The oral administration of the high dose (100 mg/kg body weight) of vitamin C had no effect on the plasma ALP level (data not shown).

Plasma ALT Level

The low dose (10 mg/kg body weight) of vitamin C reduced the plasma ALT level in rats treated 10 days before the onset of diabetes without any statistical significance. In contrast, after the oral administration of a low dose of vitamin C, the plasma ALT level in rats treated 10 days after the onset of diabetes increased without any statistical significance. Moderate dose (50 mg/kg body weight) of vitamin C increased the plasma ALT level in rats treated 10 days before and after the onset of the diabetes without any statistical significance (FIG. 2). The plasma ALT level of normal rats did not change after the oral administration of moderate dose of vitamin C. Administration of high dose (100 mg/kg body weight) of vitamin C had no significant effect on plasma ALT level.

Plasma AST Level

FIGURE 3 shows that the oral administration of low dose of vitamin C had no effect on the level of plasma AST in normal rats. There was a large but not significant reduction in the plasma AST level in rats treated before and after the onset of diabetes. After the oral administration of moderate dose (50 mg/kg body weight) of vitamin C, the plasma level of AST in rats treated 10 days before the onset of diabetes increased with no statistical significance (FIG. 3). However, there was a significant reduction in the plasma AST level of normal rats after treatment with moderate dose of vitamin C. On the other hand, the high dose (100 mg/kg body weight) of vitamin C significantly increased the level of plasma AST in normal rats. The high dose of vitamin C increased the plasma AST level in rats treated before and after the onset of diabetes (data not shown).

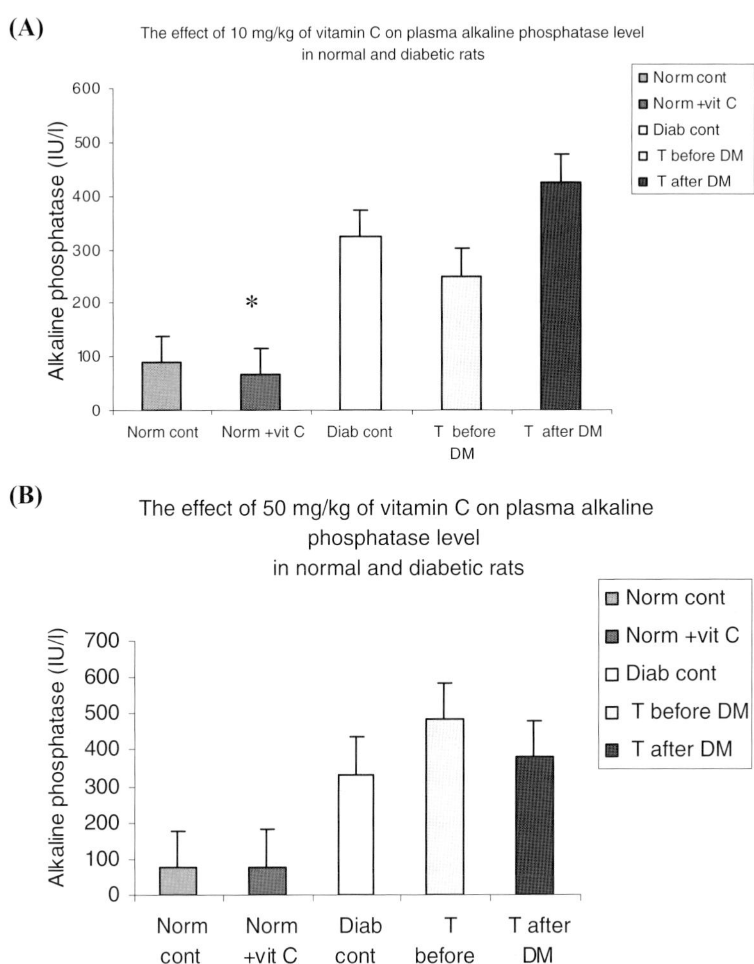

FIGURE 1. (**A**) Histograms showing the effect of 10 mg/kg of vitamin C on plasma ALP level of normal and diabetic rats. 10 mg/kg of vitamin C induced a significant decrease in the plasma ALP level in normal nondiabetic rats. $^*P < 0.05$ (norm cont versus norm + vitamin C). (Data are mean ± SD, $n = 6$.) DM = diabetes mellitus. (**B**) Histograms showing the effect of 50 mg/kg of vitamin C on plasma ALP level of normal and diabetic rats. (Data are mean ± SD, $n = 6$.) DM = diabetes mellitus.

Plasma LDH Level

Vitamin C had no significant effect on plasma LDH level of normal rats and in rats treated before the onset of diabetes. Moreover, the plasma LDH level of rats treated for 10 days after the onset of diabetes increased without any statistical significance after low-dose treatment of vitamin C. However,

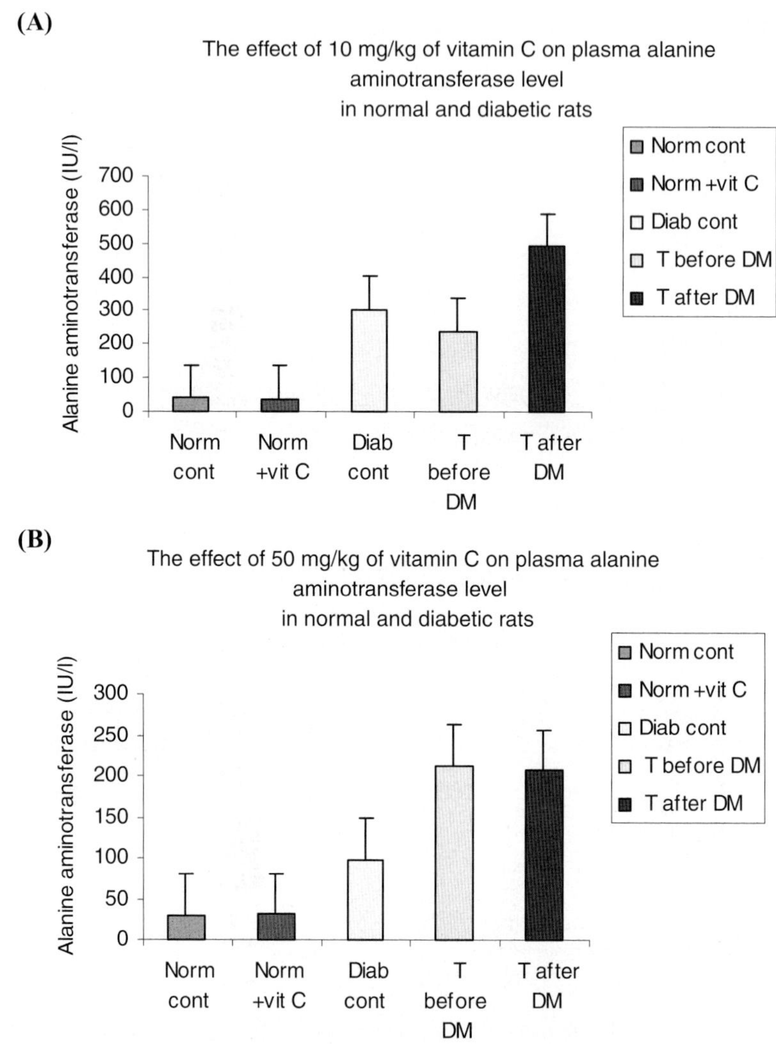

FIGURE 2. (**A**) Histograms showing the effect of 10 mg/kg of vitamin C on plasma ALT level of normal and diabetic rats. (Data are mean ± SD, $n = 6$.) DM = diabetes mellitus. (**B**) Histograms showing the effect of 50 mg/kg of vitamin C on plasma ALT level of normal and diabetic rats. (Data are mean ± SD, $n = 6$.) DM = diabetes mellitus.

the oral administration of moderate dose (50 mg/kg body weight) of vitamin C significantly ($P < 0.00005$) increased the plasma LDH level of normal rats. Moderate dose of vitamin C decreased the plasma LDH level in rats treated for 10 days before and after the onset of diabetes without any statistical significance (FIG. 4). The high dose (100 mg/kg body weight) of vitamin C

(A)

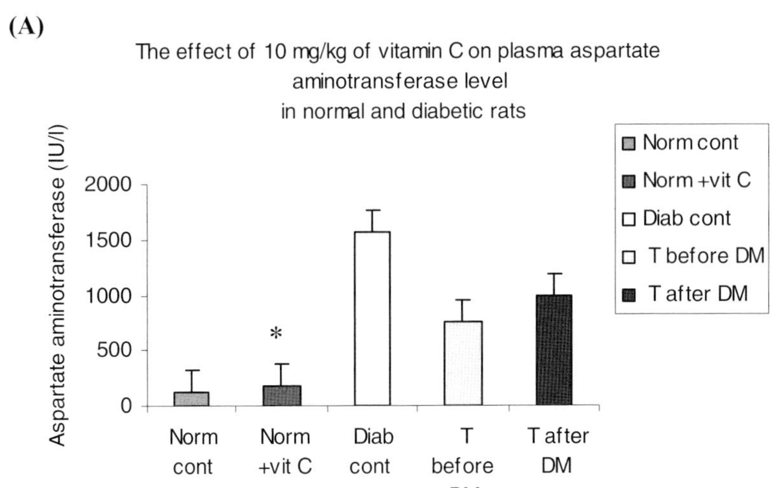

(B)

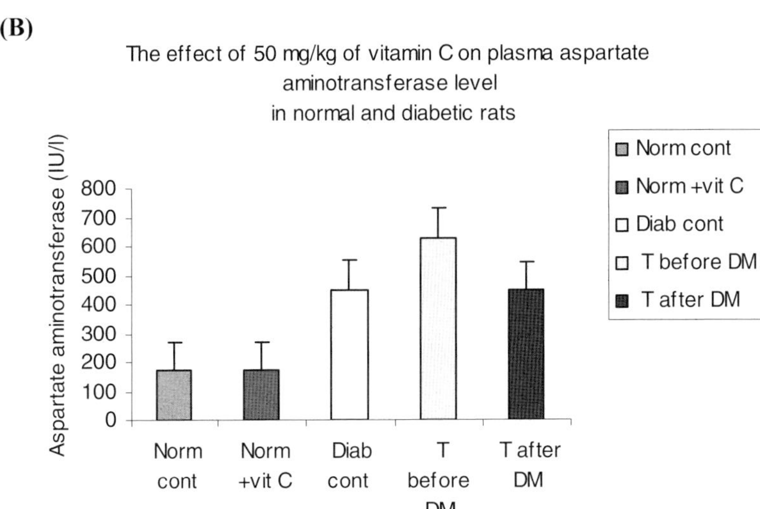

FIGURE 3. (**A**) Histograms showing the effect of 10 mg/kg of vitamin C on plasma AST level of normal and diabetic rats. 10 mg/kg of vitamin C induced a significant increase in the plasma AST level in normal nondiabetic rats. $^{*}P < 0.05$ (norm cont versus norm + vitamin C). DM = diabetes mellitus. (**B**) Histograms showing the effect of 50 mg/kg of vitamin C on plasma AST level of normal and diabetic rats. (Data are mean ± SD, $n = 6$.) DM = diabetes mellitus.

significantly ($P < 0.0001$) reduced the plasma LDH level in normal rats. On the other hand, the high dose of vitamin C elicited an increase in the plasma LDH level after the onset of diabetes. Vitamin C had no significant effect on plasma LDH level in diabetic rats (data not shown).

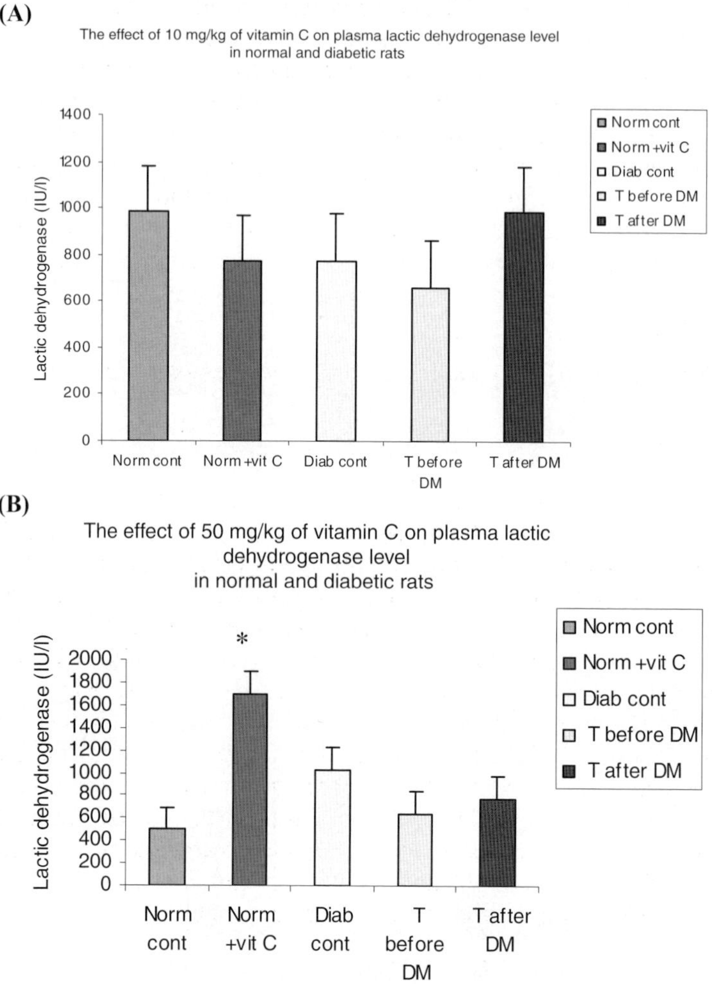

FIGURE 4. (**A**) Histograms showing the effect of 10 mg/kg of vitamin C on plasma LDH level of normal and diabetic rats. 10 mg/kg of vitamin C had no significant effect on the plasma LDH level of normal and diabetic rats. (Data are mean ± SD, $n = 6$.) DM = diabetes mellitus. (**B**) Histograms showing the effect of 50 mg/kg of vitamin C on plasma LDH level of normal and diabetic rats. 50 mg/kg of vitamin C induced a significant increase in the plasma LDH level in normal nondiabetic rats. *$P < 0.05$ (norm cont versus norm + vitamin C). (Data are mean ± SD, $n = 6$). DM = diabetes mellitus.

Plasma γ-GT Level

The oral administration of low dose (10 mg/kg body weight) of vitamin C failed to induce significant changes in plasma γ-GT level in normal rats. However, there was a decrease in the plasma γ-GT level of rats treated 10 days before and after the onset of diabetes compared to untreated diabetic rats. The treatment with moderate dose (50 mg/kg body weight) of vitamin C significantly decreased the plasma γ-GT level of rats treated with vitamin C before ($P < 0.018$) and after ($P < 0.0008$) the onset of diabetes and it had no effect on normal rats (FIG. 5). The oral administration of the high dose (100 mg/kg body weight) of vitamin C was also capable of reducing the plasma γ-GT level in rats treated before and after the onset of diabetes without any statistical significance. Also, the high doses of vitamin C had no effect on the plasma γ-GT level of normal rats compared to normal control (data not shown).

Effect of Vitamin C on Kidney Function of Normal and Diabetic Rats

BUN Level

FIGURE 6 shows that low dose (10 mg/kg body weight) of vitamin C had no effect on BUN level in both normal and diabetic rats compared to untreated rats. However, the administration of moderate dose (50 mg/kg body weight) of vitamin C significantly increased the BUN level in normal rats. On the other hand, moderate dose of vitamin C caused a decrease in the level of BUN in rats treated with vitamin C 10 days before the onset of diabetes without any statistical significance. However, a significant ($P < 0.012$) reduction in the BUN was observed in rats treated with vitamin C after the onset of diabetes (FIG. 6). The level of BUN in rats treated for 10 days before the onset of diabetes significantly ($P < 0.011$) increased after oral administration of high dose (100 mg/kg body weight) of vitamin C (data not shown), while no change was observed in the BUN of rats treated for 10 days after the onset of diabetes. Moreover, the high dose of vitamin C caused a significant increase in the BUN level of normal-treated rats compared to normal control.

Plasma CRE Level

The level of plasma CRE of nondiabetic rats was not affected by treatment with low dose of vitamin C. Moreover, the plasma CRE level of rats treated for 10 days before and after the onset of diabetes decreased but without any statistical significance. The moderate dose of vitamin C had no effect on the plasma CRE level of normal rats. However, moderate dose reduced the plasma CRE level of rats treated 10 days before and after the onset of diabetes but with no statistical significance (FIG. 7).

After the oral administration of high dose (100 mg/kg body weight) of vitamin C, the plasma CRE level of normal and rats treated 10 days before the onset of diabetes did not change (data not shown).

(A)

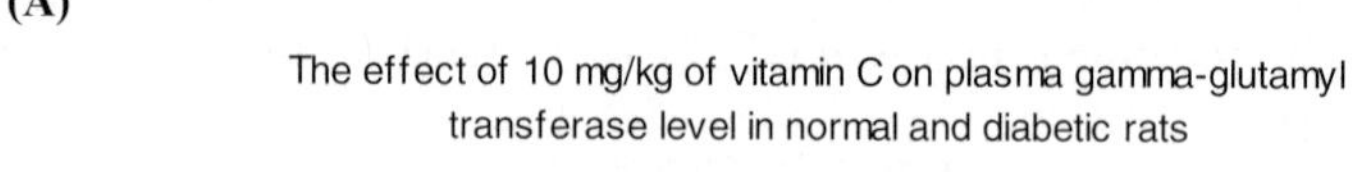

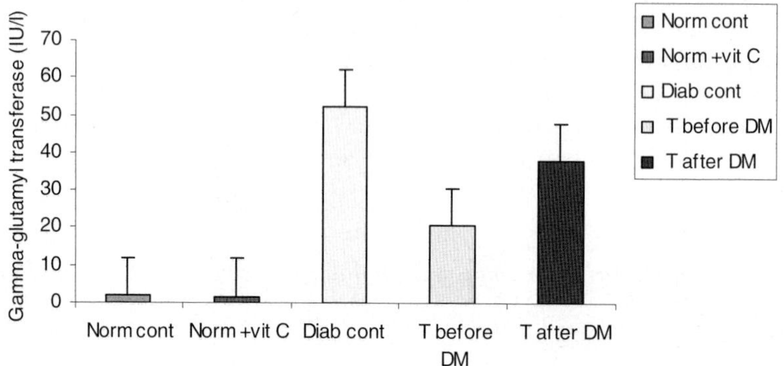

(B)

The effect of 50 mg/kg of vitamin C on plasma gamma-glutamyl transferase level in normal and diabetic rats

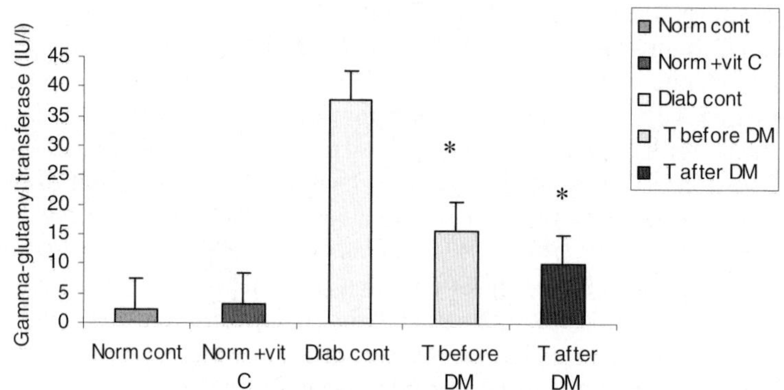

FIGURE 5. (**A**) Histograms showing the effect of 10 mg/kg of vitamin C on plasma γ-GT level of normal and diabetic rats. 10 mg/kg of vitamin C had no significant effect on the plasma γ-GT level of normal and diabetic rats. (Data are mean ± SD, $n = 6$.) DM = diabetes mellitus. (**B**) Histograms showing the effect of 50 mg/kg of vitamin C on plasma γ-GT level of normal and diabetic rats. 50 mg/kg of vitamin C induced a significant decrease in the plasma γ-GT level in rats treated before and after the onset of DM. $^*P < 0.05$ (diab cont versus treated before DM); $^*P < 0.05$ (diab cont versus treated after DM). (Data are mean ± SD, $n = 6$.) DM = diabetes.

Effect of Vitamin C on Electrolytes Level in Normal and Diabetic Rats

Plasma Ca Level

The oral administration of low dose (10 mg/kg body weight) of vitamin C had no significant effect on the plasma Ca level of normal rats. On the other hand,

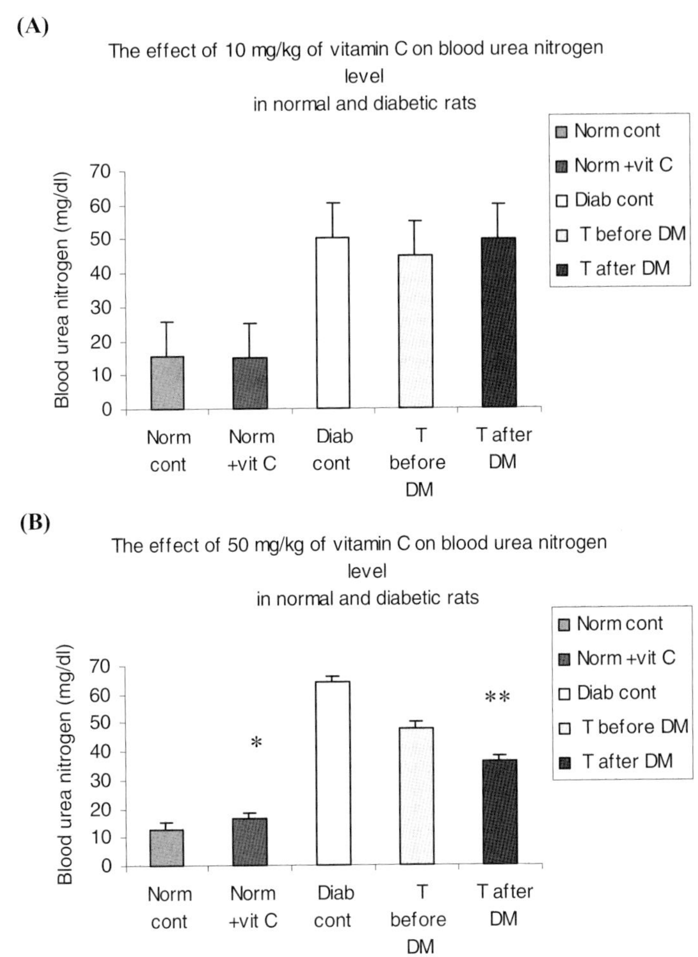

FIGURE 6. (**A**) Histograms showing the effect of 10 mg/kg of vitamin C on BUN level of normal and diabetic rats. 10 mg/kg of vitamin C had no significant effect on the BUN level of normal and diabetic rats. (Data are mean ± SD, $n = 6$.) DM = diabetes mellitus. (**B**) Histograms showing the effect of 50 mg/kg of vitamin C on BUN level of normal and diabetic rats. 50 mg/kg of vitamin C induced a significant increase in the BUN level of normal nondiabetic rats. $^{*}P < 0.05$ (norm cont versus norm + vitamin C). Also, there was a significant decrease in BUN in rats treated after the onset of DM. $^{**}P < 0.05$ (diab cont versus treated after DM). (Data are mean ± SD, $n = 6$.) DM = diabetes.

low dose caused a significant increase in rats treated for 10 days before ($P < 0.02$) and after ($P < 0.008$) the onset of diabetes compared to untreated diabetic controls. The moderate dose (50 mg/kg body weight) of vitamin C increased the plasma Ca level of normal rats but without any statistical significance. However, moderate administration of vitamin C caused significant increases

(A)

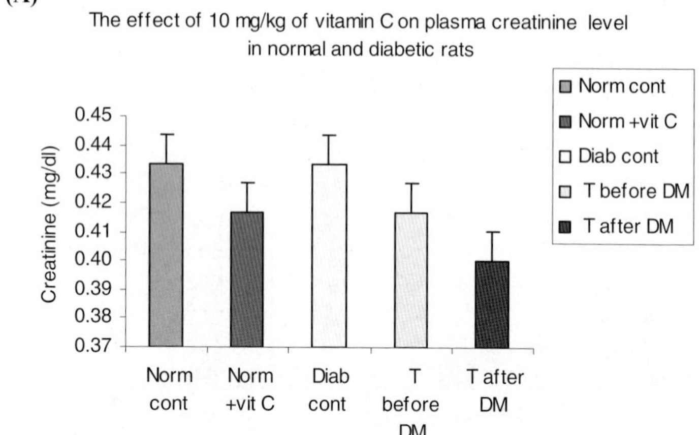

(B)

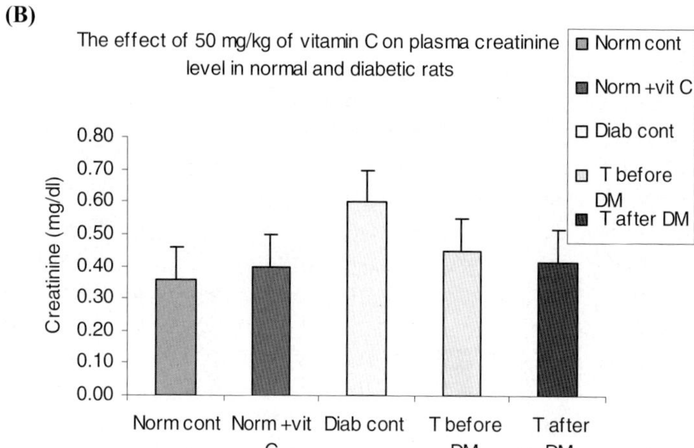

FIGURE 7. (**A**) Histograms showing the effect of 10 mg/kg of vitamin C on plasma CRE level of normal and diabetic rats. 10 mg/kg of vitamin C had no significant effect on the plasma CRE level of normal and diabetic rats. (Data are mean ± SD, $n = 6$.) DM = diabetes mellitus. (**B**) Histograms showing the effect of 50 mg/kg of vitamin C on plasma CRE level of normal and diabetic rats. 50 mg/kg of vitamin C had no significant effect on the plasma CRE level of normal and diabetic rats. (Data are mean ± SD, $n = 6$.) DM = diabetes mellitus.

in the plasma Ca level in rats treated for 10 days after the onset of the diabetes (FIG. 8). After the oral administration of high (100 mg/kg body weight) of vitamin C, a decrease in the plasma Ca level was observed in normal rats when compared to control. However, this decrease did not reach statistical significance. No significant change was observed on the plasma Ca level in rats treated 10 days before and after the onset of the diabetes (data not shown).

Plasma PHOS Level

The results presented in FIGURE 9 demonstrated the effect of low dose (10 mg/kg body weight) of vitamin C on plasma PHOS level in normal and diabetic rats. The result shows that low dose of vitamin C caused no significant change in the plasma PHOS level of normal-treated rats compared to normal controls. In diabetic rats, low dose of vitamin C caused a slight but not significant increase in plasma PHOS level when compared to diabetic controls.

The oral administration of moderate dose (50 mg/kg body weight) of vitamin C induced a significant ($P < 0.016$) increase in the level of plasma PHOS level in rats treated for 10 days before the onset of the diabetes. The moderate dose had no effect on the plasma PHOS level of normal-treated rats. High dose of vitamin C had no significant effect on the plasma PHOS level of normal and diabetic rats (data not shown).

Plasma Na Level

The oral administration of low dose vitamin C (10 mg/kg body weight) caused significant ($P < 0.00001$) increase in plasma Na level of normal rats. Also, in diabetic rats, it induced significant increases in the level of plasma Na in rats treated for 10 days before and after the onset of the diabetes compared to diabetic controls (FIG. 10). The moderate dose (50 mg/kg body weight) of vitamin C caused increases in plasma Na level without any statistical significance in normal rats when compared to normal control. In contrast, moderate dose increased the plasma Na level without any statistical significance in rats treated for 10 days before the onset of diabetes. However, moderate dose of vitamin C induced significant ($P < 0.033$) increases in plasma Na level of rats treated for 10 days after the onset of diabetes when compared to control. The oral administration of high dose (100 mg/kg body weight) of vitamin C increased the plasma Na level significantly in normal rats and in rats treated 10 days before and after the onset of the diabetes (data not shown).

Plasma K Level

FIGURE 11 shows that oral treatment with low dose of vitamin C had no significant effect on the plasma K level in normal rats when compared to normal control. The level of K was slightly increased in rats treated for 10 days before and after the onset of the diabetes when compared with untreated diabetic control. The moderate dose (50 mg/kg body weight) of vitamin C given to normal and diabetic rats had no significant effect on the plasma K level. The oral administration of high dose (100 mg/kg body weight) of vitamin C given to normal and diabetic rats had no significant effect on plasma K level (data not shown).

(A)

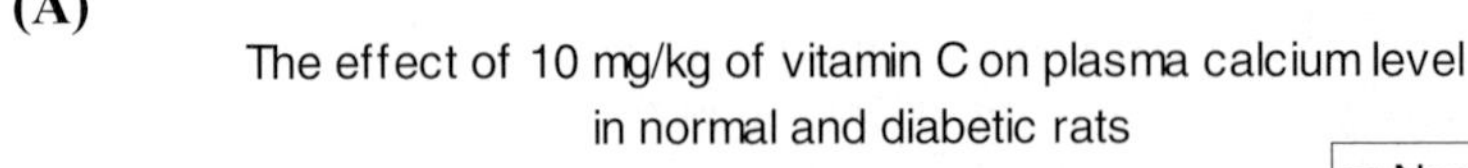

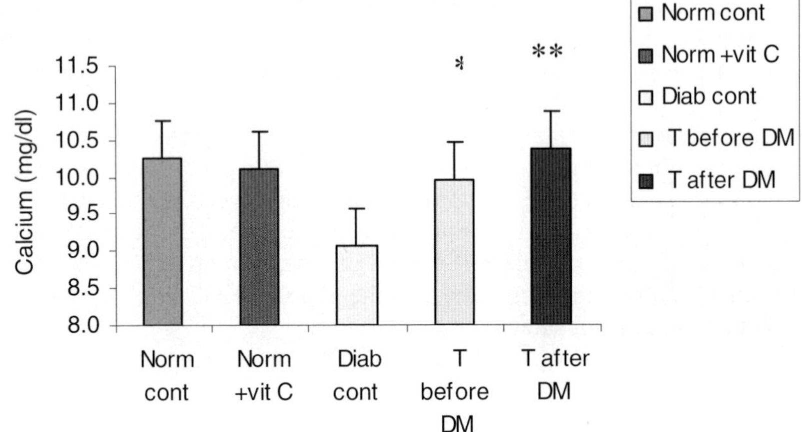

(B)

The effect of 50 mg/kg of vitamin C on plasma calcium level
in normal and diabetic rats

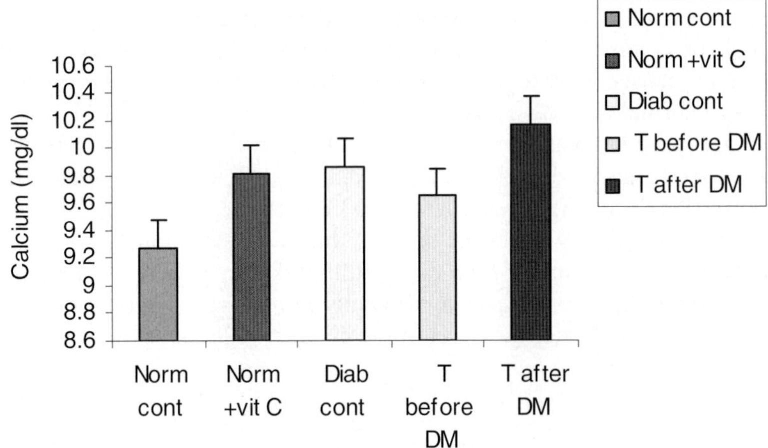

FIGURE 8. (**A**) Histograms showing the effect of 10 mg/kg of vitamin C on plasma Ca level of normal and diabetic rats. 10 mg/kg of vitamin C induced a significant decrease in the plasma Ca level in rats treated before and after the onset of DM. $^{*}P < 0.05$ (diab cont versus treated before DM); $^{**}P < 0.05$ (diab cont versus treated after DM). (Data are mean $\pm$ SD, $n = 6$.) DM = diabetes mellitus. (**B**) Histograms showing the effect of 50 mg/kg of vitamin C on plasma Ca level of normal and diabetic rats. 50 mg/kg of vitamin C had no significant effect on the plasma Ca level of normal and diabetic rats. (Data are mean $\pm$ SD, $n = 6$.) DM = diabetes mellitus.

(A)

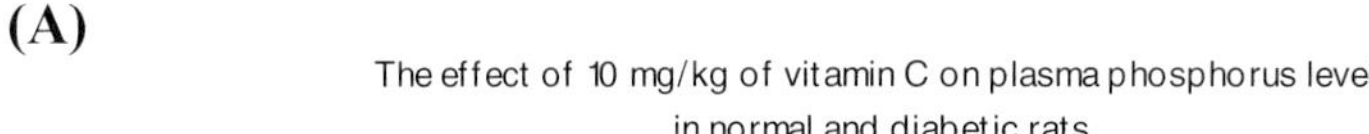

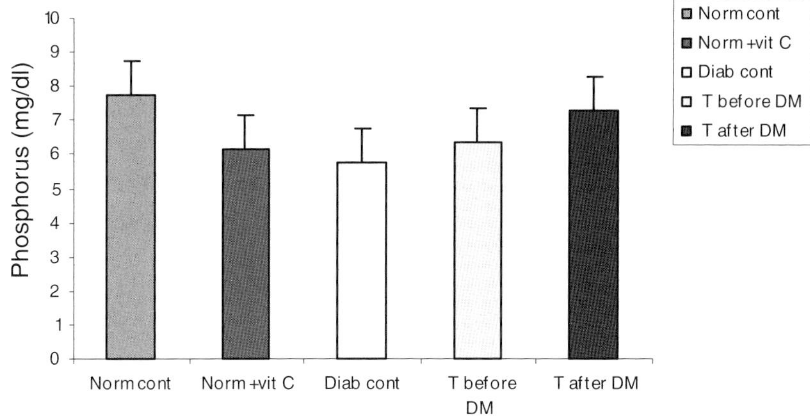

(B)

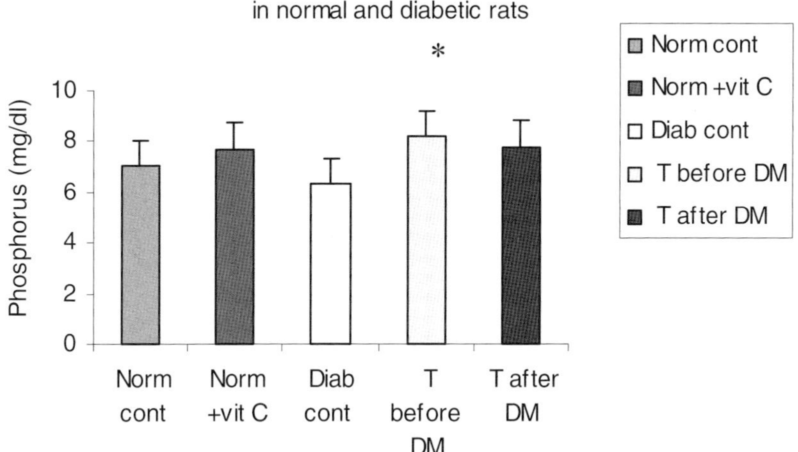

FIGURE 9. (**A**) Histograms showing the effect of 10 mg/kg of vitamin C on plasma PHOS level of normal and diabetic rats. 10 mg/kg of vitamin C had no significant effect on the plasma PHOS level of normal and diabetic rats. (Data are mean ± SD, $n = 6$.) DM = diabetes mellitus. (**B**) Histograms showing the effect of 50 mg/kg of vitamin C on plasma PHOS level of normal and diabetic rats. 50 mg/kg of vitamin C induced a significant decrease in the plasma PHOS level in rats treated before the onset of DM. $^*P < 0.05$ (diab cont versus treated before DM). (Data are mean ± SD, $n = 6$.) DM = diabetes mellitus.

(A)

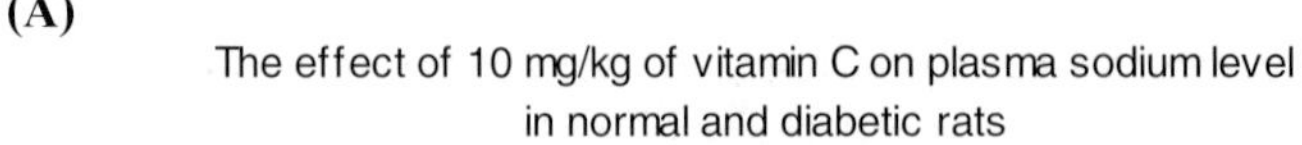

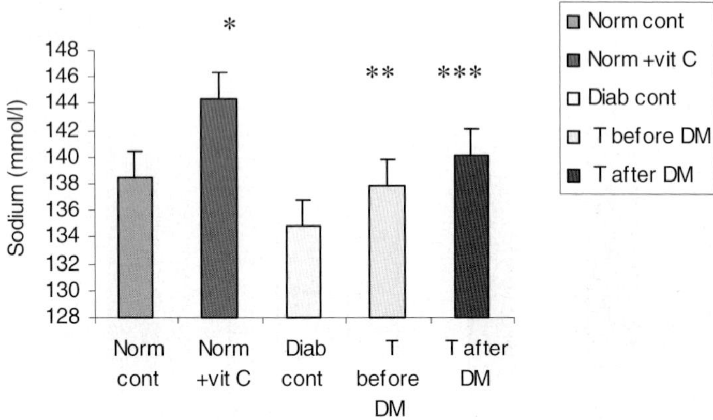

(B)

The effect of 50 mg/kg of vitamin C on plasma sodium level
in normal and diabetic rats

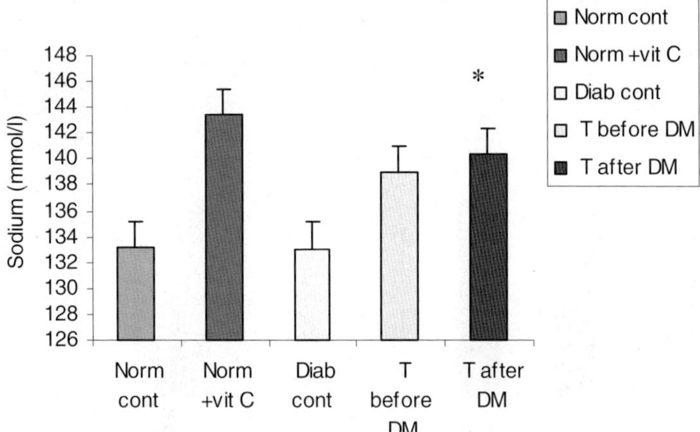

FIGURE 10. (**A**) Histograms showing the effect of 10 mg/kg of vitamin C on plasma Na level of normal and diabetic rats. 10 mg/kg of vitamin C induced a significant increase in the plasma Na level of normal nondiabetic rats. $^{*}P < 0.05$ (norm cont versus norm + vitamin C). Also, there was a significant increase in the Na level in rats treated before $^{**}P < 0.05$ (diab cont versus treated before DM) and after $^{***}P < 0.05$ (diab cont versus treated after DM) the onset of DM. (Data are mean $\pm$ SD, $n = 6$.) DM = diabetes mellitus. (**B**) Histograms showing the effect of 50 mg/kg of vitamin C on plasma Na level of normal and diabetic rats. 50 mg/kg of vitamin C induced a significant increase in the plasma Na level in rats after the onset of DM. $^{*}P < 0.05$ (diab cont versus treated after DM). (Data are mean $\pm$ SD, $n = 6$.) DM = diabetes mellitus.

(A)

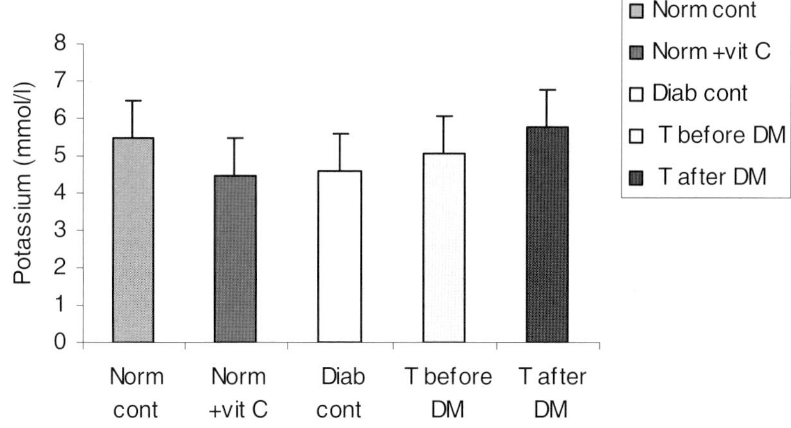

(B)

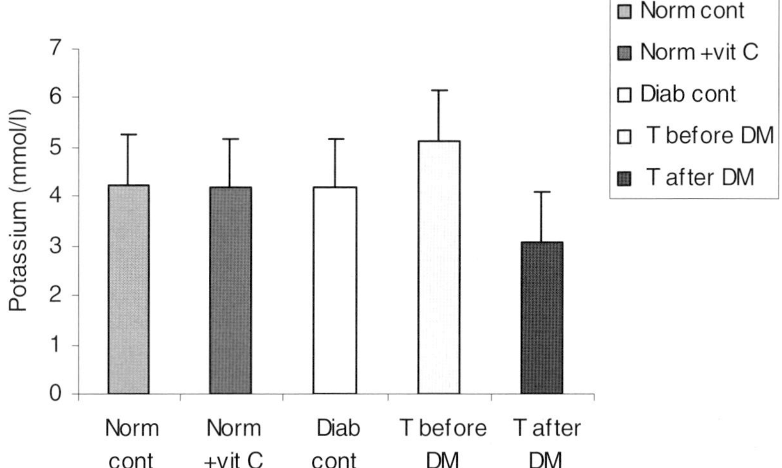

FIGURE 11. (**A**) Histograms showing the effect of 10 mg/kg of vitamin C on plasma K level of normal and diabetic rats. 10 mg/kg of vitamin C had no significant effect on the plasma K level of normal and diabetic rats. (Data are mean ± SD, $n = 6$.) DM = diabetes mellitus. (**B**) Histograms showing the effect of 50 mg/kg of vitamin C on plasma K level of normal and diabetic rats. 50 mg/kg of vitamin C had no significant effect on the plasma K level of normal and diabetic rats. (Data are mean ± SD, $n = 6$.) DM = diabetes mellitus.

Plasma Mg Level

FIGURE 12 shows the effect of low dose (10 mg/kg body weight) of vitamin C on plasma Mg level in normal and diabetic rats. These results show that normal rats treated with low dose of vitamin C had a significant ($P < 0.020$) decrease in plasma Mg level when compared to normal control. In contrast, there was no significant difference in plasma Mg level of rats treated before and after the onset of the diabetes when compared to diabetic control. The moderate dose of vitamin C increased the level of plasma Mg but without any statistical significance, and there was no effect on normal and diabetic rats either before or after the onset of diabetes when compared to control significantly. The result showed that high dose of vitamin C significantly ($P < 0.004$) increased the plasma Mg level of normal rats when compared to normal control. There was a significant ($P < 0.016$) reduction in the plasma Mg level in rats given high dose of vitamin C 10 days after the onset of diabetes when compared to diabetic control (data not shown).

DISCUSSION

Effect of Vitamin C on Biochemical Parameters of Normal and Diabetic Rats

Liver Function

Liver enzymes are used as markers of hepatotoxicity especially ALT, which is a more specific indicator for liver damage. From the demonstrated data, the plasma level of ALT increased after the onset of diabetes, and vitamin C administration had no beneficial effect in reducing ALT level. Moreover, vitamin C was unable to reduce the elevated plasma level of AST.

Serum ALP level also increased in DM. Low dose of vitamin C significantly reduced the ALP level. However, the administration of high dose of vitamin C had a negative effect on ALP level because the level of ALP was increased. There was no significant effect on plasma level of LDH in diabetic group after treatment with vitamin C but low dose significantly increase LDH level and high dose can also significantly reduce its level in normal nondiabetic rats.

Effect of Vitamin C on Kidney Function in Normal and Diabetic Rats

In the present study, all the three doses of vitamin C had no effect on CRE level in normal rats. The administration of high dose of vitamin C significantly increased blood CRE level in rats treated for 10 days after the onset of diabetes,

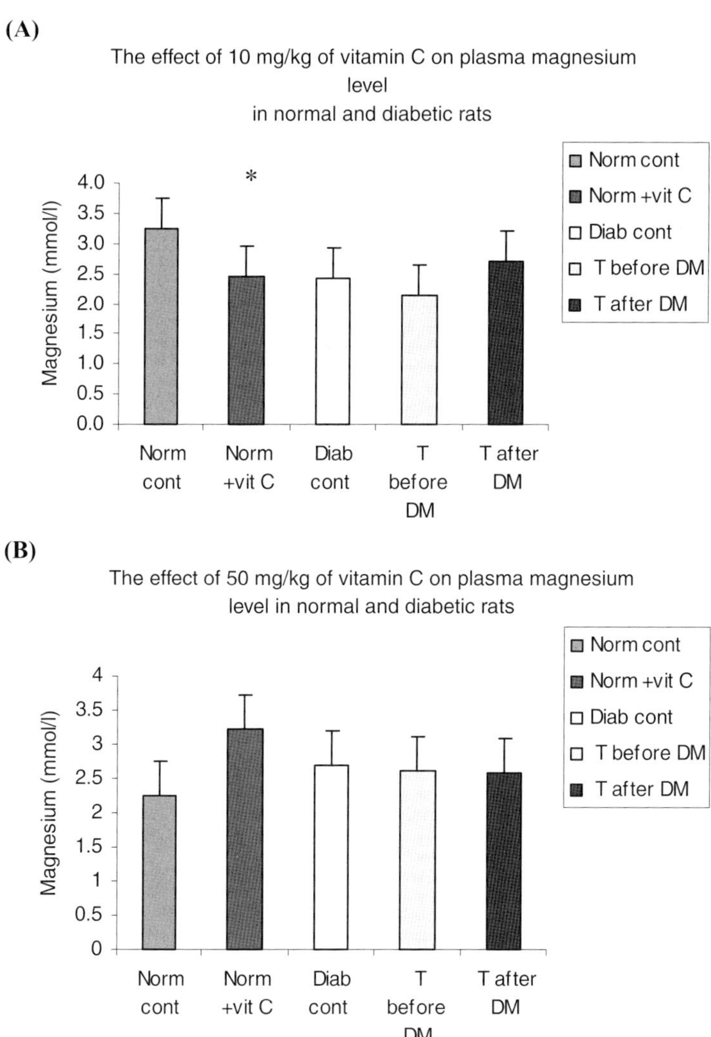

FIGURE 12. (**A**) Histograms showing the effect of 10 mg/kg of vitamin C on plasma Mg level of normal and diabetic rats. 10 mg/kg of vitamin C induced a significant decrease in the plasma magnesium level in normal nondiabetic rats. $P < 0.05$ (norm cont versus norm + vitamin C). (Data are mean ± SD, $n = 6$.) DM = diabetes mellitus. (**B**) Histograms showing the effect of 50 mg/kg of vitamin C on plasma Mg level of normal and diabetic rats. 50 mg/kg of vitamin C had no significant effect on the plasma Mg level of the normal and diabetic rats. (Data are mean ± SD, $n = 6$.) DM = diabetes mellitus.

and this may imply that high dose of vitamin C had adverse effect on kidney function. The high dose of vitamin C significantly increased BUN level in rats treated for 10 days before and after the onset of diabetes.

CONCLUSION

Vitamin C significantly affected the biochemical parameters of both normal and diabetic rats. The investigation on liver enzymes, kidney parameters, and electrolytes showed that the levels of these parameters are altered during STZ-induced diabetes. The result obtained from this study have provided insight into the hypoglycemic effect of vitamin C, and they may be a useful therapies in the management of DM.

REFERENCES

1. ADEGHATE, E. 2001. Diabetes mellitus-multifactorial in aetiology and global in prevalence. Arch. Physiol. Biochem. **109:** 197–199.
2. CERIELLO, A. 2003. New insights on oxidative stress and diabetic complications may lead to a "causal" antioxidant therapy. Diabetes Care **26:** 1589–1596.
3. SMIRNOFF, N. & G.L. WHEELER. 2000. Ascorbic acid in plants: biosynthesis and function. Crit. Rev. Biochem. Mol. Biol. **35:** 291–314.
4. MANCHESTER, K.L. 1998. Albert Szent-Györgyi and the unraveling of biological oxidation. TIBS **23:** 37–40.
5. SHAPIRO, S.S. & C. SALIOU. 2001. Role of vitamins in skin care. Nutrition **17:** 839–844.
6. CUNNINGHAM, J.J. 1998. The glucose/insulin system and vitamin C: implications in insulin-dependent diabetes mellitus. J. Am. Coll. Nutr. **17:** 105–108.
7. PADAYATTY, S.J., A. KATZ, Y. WANG, *et al.* 2003. Vitamin C as an antioxidant: evalution of its role in disease prevention. J. Am. Coll. Nutr. **22:** 18–35.
8. ADEGHATE, E., A. S. PONERY, D.J. PALLOT & J. SINGH. 2001. Distribution of vasoactive intestinal polypeptide, neuropeptide-Y and substance P and their effects on insulin secretion from the in vitro pancreas of normal and diabetic rats. Peptides **22:** 99–107.
9. DRISKO, J.A., J. CHAPMAN & V.J. HUNTER. 2003. The use of antioxidant therapies during chemotherapy. Gynecol. Oncol. **88:** 434–439.
10. RICE, M.E. 2000. Ascorbate regulation and its neuroprotective role in the brain. Trends Neurosci. **23:** 209–216.
11. ADEGHATE, E. 1999. Effect of subcutaneous pancreatic tissue transplants on streptozotocin-induced diabetes in rats. Tissue Cell **31:** 73–83.

The Protective Effect of *Tribulus terrestris* in Diabetes

AMR AMIN,[a] MOHAMED LOTFY,[a] MOHAMED SHAFIULLAH,[b] AND ERNEST ADEGHATE[c]

[a] *Biology Department, United Arab Emirates University, Al-Ain, Abu-Dhabi, UAE*

[b] *Pharmacology Department, United Arab Emirates University, Al-Ain, Abu-Dhabi, UAE*

[c] *Anatomy Department, United Arab Emirates University, Al-Ain, Abu-Dhabi, UAE*

ABSTRACT: *Tribulus terrestris* L (*TT*) is used in the Arabic folk medicine to treat various diseases. The aim of this article was to investigate the protective effects of *TT* in diabetes mellitus (DM). Diabetes is known to increase reactive oxygen species (ROS) level that subsequently contributes to the pathogenesis of diabetes. Rats were divided into six groups and treated with either saline, glibenclamide (Glib), or *TT* for 30 days. Rats in group 1 were given saline after the onset of streptozotocin (STZ)-induced diabetes; the second diabetic group was administered Glib (10 mg/kg body weight). The third diabetic group was treated with the *TT* extract (2 g/kg body weight), while the first, second, and third nondiabetic groups were treated with saline solution, Glib, and *TT* extract, respectively. At the end of the experiment, serum and liver samples were collected for biochemical and morphological analysis. Levels of serum alanine aminotransferase (ALT) and creatinine were estimated. In addition, levels of malondialdehyde (MDA) and reduced glutathione (GSH) were assayed in the liver. The tested *TT* extract significantly decreased the levels of ALT and creatinine in the serum ($P < 0.05$) in diabetic groups and lowered the MDA level in liver ($P < 0.05$) in diabetic and ($P < 0.01$) nondiabetic groups. On the other hand, levels of reduced GSH in liver were significantly increased ($P < 0.01$) in diabetic rats treated with *TT*. Histopathological examination revealed significant recovery of liver in herb-treated rats. This investigation suggests that the protective effect of *TT* for STZ-induced diabetic rats may be mediated by inhibiting oxidative stress.

KEYWORDS: diabetes; antioxidant; *Tribulus terrestris*; medicinal plants; streptozotocin; oxidative stress

Address for correspondence: Amr Amin, Biology Department, United Arab Emirates University, P.O. Box: 17551, Al-Ain, Abu-Dhabi, United Arab Emirates. Voice: 971-3-7134389, 971-3-7134227; fax: 971-3-7671291.

e-mail: a.amin@uaeu.ac.ae

Ann. N.Y. Acad. Sci. 1084: 391–401 (2006). © 2006 New York Academy of Sciences.
doi: 10.1196/annals.1372.005

INTRODUCTION

Diabetes mellitus (DM) is one of the most common endocrine diseases in the world that affects more than 6% of the world population.[1] There are an estimated 143 million people worldwide with the disease, almost five times more than estimates 10 years ago. This number will probably double by the year 2030.[2] Hyperglycemia associated with diabetes increases the glucose autoxidation and protein glycation, and the subsequent oxidative degradation of glycated proteins leads to enhanced production of reactive oxygen species (ROS).[3] ROS are through to play a major role in a variety of physiologic and pathophysiological processes in which increased oxidative stress may play an important role in disease mechanisms.[4] Lower endogenous antioxidants and elevated lipid peroxidation (LP) levels are risk factors for the development of diabetic complications, such as atherosclerosis.[5,6]

Tribulus terrestris L (*TT*) is a member of the plant family Zygophyllaceae. It is called "Qutiba" in Bedouin language and is widely distributed in the entire Mediterranean region. It flowers throughout the year and all parts of the plant are used for various purposes in folk medicine. The fruit is regarded as tonic diuretic and aphrodisiac. It is also used to treat urinary disorder, impotency, and heart diseases. The seeds are recommended in hemorrhages, kidney stone, and gout.[7] The extract of *TT* contains protodioscin (PTN), a steroidal saponin, that has been extensively used for the treatment of various ailments, such as urinary, cardiovascular,[8] and gastrointestinal disorders.[9] Administration of *TT* to humans and animals improves libido and spermatogenesis.[10] PTN has been reported to upregulate the levels of testosterone and leuteinizing hormone,[11] dehydroepiandrosterone,[12] dihydrotestosterone, and dehydroepiandrosterone sulfate.[13] *TT* has a proerectile effect.[14] Saponin from *TT* is also known for its hypoglycemic effect.[15]

The purpose of this article was to investigate the protective role of *TT* against the streptozotocin (STZ)-induced diabetes in rats.

MATERIALS AND METHODS

Chemicals

STZ was purchased from Sigma Co. (St. Louis, MO). Sodium lauryl sulfate (SDS), acetic acid, thiobarbituric acid aqueous solution (TBA), n-butanol, pyridine, 1,1,3,3-tetramethoxypropane standard, trichloroacetic acid (TCA), phosphate buffer, 5,5-dithiobis(2-nitrobenzoic acid) (DTNB), and reduced glutathione (GSH) standard, reagents, were obtained from Fluka (Taufkirchen, Germany). All the chemicals used were of analytical grade.

Extraction

TT was obtained from the local stores. The herb was grounded to a fine powder in an electrical grinder. Its dried powder was exhaustively extracted with 70% ethyl alcohol. The extracts were evaporated in a rotary evaporator at 40°C under reduced pressure. The yield was 6.8%.

Animals

Male Wistar rats (220–240 g) used in this study were raised and housed at the Animal Facility of the Faculty of Medicine and Health Sciences, UAE University. Rats were maintained at 22 ± 2°C and were subjected to 12-h light–dark cycle. Rats were housed in standard cages, fed on standard laboratory food, and had free access to water *ad libitum*. This study was conducted according to the animal ethics protocols of UAEU. Rats were fasted for 12 h before the experiments.

Induction of DM

DM was induced by a single dose of intraperitoneal (60 mg/kg body weight) injection of STZ.[16] The rats were considered diabetic if the fasting level values were more than 300 mg/dL.[16]

Experimental Design

Six rats were randomly assigned into six experimental groups. The first, second, and third (diabetic-treated) groups and the fourth, fifth, and sixth groups (normal nondiabetic groups). All rats were treated for 30 days of the experimental period. The first group (the diabetic control) has been orally receiving only 0.9% NaCl (saline) solution. The second group (the diabetic rats) was orally administered glibenclamide (Glib; 10 mg/kg body weight/day) in saline solution. The third group (the diabetic rats) was orally given 2 g/kg body weight of *TT* extract dissolved in saline. The fourth group (the normal rats) was orally receiving only 0.9% NaCl (saline) solution. The fifth group (the normal rats) was only receiving similar dose of Glib. The sixth group (the normal rats) received 2 g/kg body weight of *TT* extract dissolved in saline.

At the end of the experimental period, body weights were determined and rats were sacrificed by cervical decapitation. Blood was collected and the separated serum was used for further estimation. The liver was immediately excised, rinsed in ice-cold saline, dried, weighed, and homogenized in Tris-HCl buffer of pH 7.4 (0.1 M) using a Teflon homogenizer. The tissue homogenate was then centrifuged in a cooling centrifuge at 4000 rpm for 15 min at 4°C in order to remove the debris, and the supernatant was used for the analysis of biochemical parameters. The tissue homogenate was stored at −20°C until further use.

Biochemical Parameters

Liver and Kidney Functions

Blood samples were processed for serum alanine aminotransferase (ALT), aspartate aminotransferase (AST), urea, creatinine, and the electrolytes calcium and phosphorous were estimated following the manufacturer's instructions.

Estimation of Protein

Protein content, in all samples, was estimated by the method in Reference 17. Bovine serum albumin was used as standard. Enzymes are normalized on the basis of total protein content.

LP

LP was assayed by the method of Reference 18, in which the released malondialdehyde (MDA) serves as an index of LP. 1,1,3,3-Tetramethoxypropane was used as standard. A mixture of 0.2 mL of homogenate, 0.2 mL 8.1% SDS, 1.5 mL 20% acetic acid (pH 3.5), 1.5 mL 0.8% TBA, and 0.6 mL distilled water was made. The mixture was boiled in a tightly closed glass tube in a water bath for 60 min. Immediately, the solution was cooled in ice bath or tap water for 5 min. One milliliter of water and 5 mL of n-butanol/pyridine mixture were added and shaken vigorously. After centrifugation at 4000 rpm for 10 min at 4°C, the organic layer was taken and its absorbance was measured against reagent blank using a glass cuvette at 532 nm. The level of MDA was expressed as nmol of MDA/mg of liver tissue protein.

Reduced GSH

Reduced GSH was estimated as described in Reference 19. Briefly, 0.5 mL of homogenate was precipitated with equal volume of 5% TCA. The contents were mixed well for complete precipitation of proteins and centrifuged at 4000 rpm for 15 min at 4°C. A mixture of 0.1 mL of supernatant, 1.9 mL of 0.2 M phosphate buffer (pH 8.0), and 2 mL of 0.6 mM DTNB was made, vortexed, then the absorbance at 412 nm was read against a blank containing TCA instead of sample. A series of GSH standards treated in a similar way as the sample were also run to determine the GSH content. The amount of GSH is expressed as nmol/ mg liver tissue protein.

Histopathology

Liver tissues were fixed in a 10% neutral-buffered formalin solution, embedded in paraffin, and sectioned. Thin sections were then deparaffinized, hydrated, and stained with hematoxlin and eosin and examined using a microscope.

Statistical Analysis

Values are expressed as mean ± SD. One-way analysis of variance (ANOVA) and Student's *t*-test are applied to calculate the statistical significance between the various groups. A value of $P < 0.05$ was considered to be statistically significant.

RESULTS AND DISCUSSION

Liver and Kidney Functions

After treatment of the STZ-induced and normal rats with 10 mg/kg body weight of Glib and 2 g/kg body weight of *TT* extract, respectively, levels of ALT and AST were decreased in all treated groups compared with the nontreated ones, and the decrement in STZ-induced rats treated with *TT* was significant ($P < 0.05$) compared to the STZ-induced nontreated group (FIG. 1).

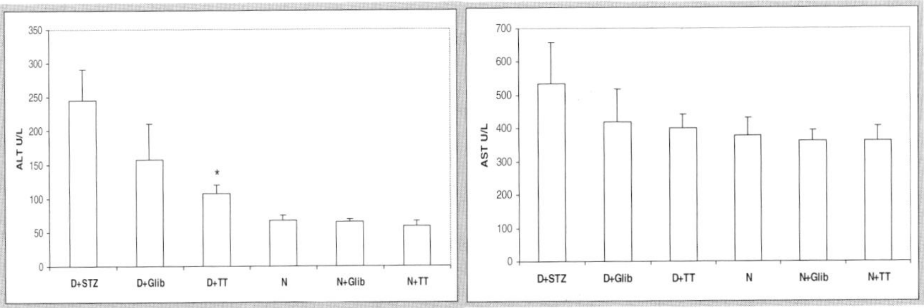

FIGURE 1. Effect of Glib and *TT* on serum ALT and AST of controls and experimental groups of diabetic (D) and nondiabetic (N) rats. Results are expressed as mean ± *SD* ($n = 6$). $^*P < 0.05$. Comparisons are made between nontreated groups and treated groups.

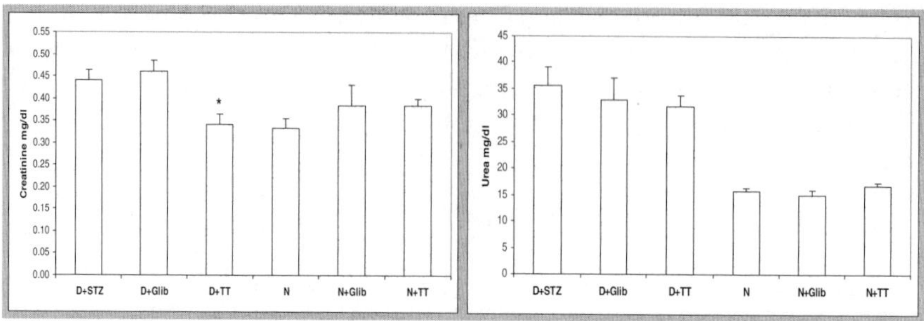

FIGURE 2. Effect of Glib and *TT* on serum creatinine and urea of controls and experimental groups of diabetic (D) and nondiabetic (N) rats. Results are expressed as mean ± *SD* ($n = 6$). *$P < 0.05$. Comparisons are made between nontreated groups and treated groups.

Oral administration of 10 mg/kg body weight of Glib and 2 g/kg body weight of *TT* extract had shown a significant decrement ($P < 0.05$) of serum creatinine levels in the STZ-induced *TT*-treated group and there were insignificant changes in between rats in the normal groups. However, there was an insignificant reduction in the levels of serum urea in the STZ-induced rats. There were no significant alterations in the levels of serum urea in all normal treated groups (FIG. 2).

In STZ-induced diabetic rats there was a significant increment ($P < 0.05$) of serum calcium under the oral administration of 10 mg/kg body weight of Glib while there was an insignificant decrement of serum calcium after the administration of 2 g/kg body weight of *TT* extract. The effect of 10 mg/kg body weight of Glib and 2 g/kg body weight of *TT* extract on normal rats leads to insignificant increment of calcium levels in all normal groups. On the other hand, treatment with Glib on both STZ-induced and normal rats increases the levels of serum phosphorous insignificantly while *TT* extracts decrease the serum levels of phosphorus (FIG. 3).

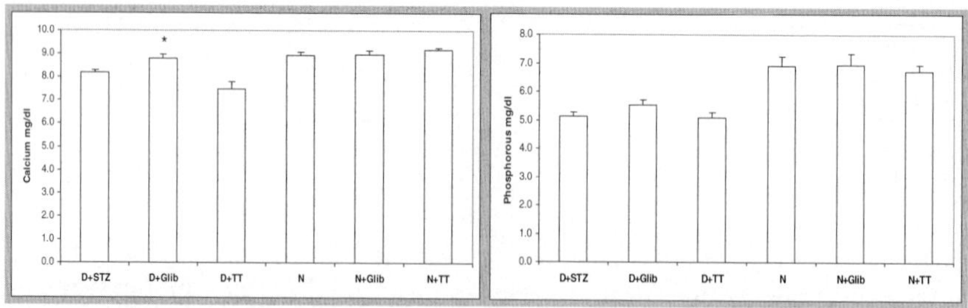

FIGURE 3. Effect of Glib and *TT* on serum calcium and phosphorous of controls and experimental groups of diabetic (D) and nondiabetic (N) rats. Results are expressed as mean ± *SD* (n = 6). *$P < 0.05$. Comparisons are made between nontreated groups and treated groups.

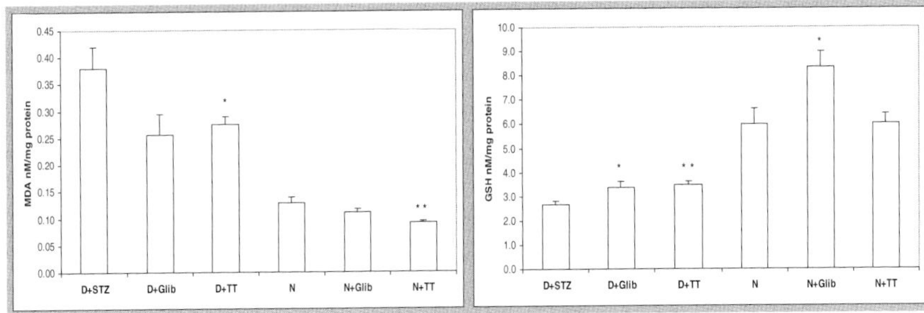

FIGURE 4. Effect of Glib and *TT*, on liver MDA and GSH of controls and experimental groups of diabetic (D) and nondiabetic (N) rats. Results are expressed as mean ± *SD* ($n = 6$). $^{*}P < 0.05$, $^{**}P < 0.01$. Comparisons are made between nontreated groups and treated groups.

Antioxidants

Effects of tested herb on STZ-induced diabetic rats and normal rats were examined by monitoring the levels of MDA. Following treatment with *TT*, levels of hepatic MDA decreased significantly both in the diabetic and non-diabetic groups [($P < 0.05$) and ($P < 0.01$) respectively]. Treatment with Glib also insignificantly decreased the levels of MDA in both STZ-induced diabetic and normal rats. Following Glib treatment, the activity of hepatic GSH was significantly increased ($P < 0.05$) in both diabetic and nondiabetic groups. However, treatment with *TT* increased GSH levels significantly ($P < 0.01$) in diabetic rats and insignificantly in nondiabetic rats (FIG. 4).

TT *Protects against Liver Damage*

In diabetic rats, hepatocytes were disrupted and severe dilatations of liver sinusoids were observed. In addition, *TT* protected against necrotic lesion in the liver. The liver appears near normal after treatment with *TT* (FIG. 5). On the other hand, the liver structure seems to be normal in all the normal rat groups (FIG. 6).

DISCUSSION

Diabetes is one of the world's fastest growing metabolic disorders. While the knowledge of the heterogeneity of this disease increases, so also is the need for more appropriate therapies.[20] Traditional medicinal plants are used throughout the world for a wide range of diabetic presentations. The study of such medicines might offer a natural key to find new antidiabetic drugs.[21]

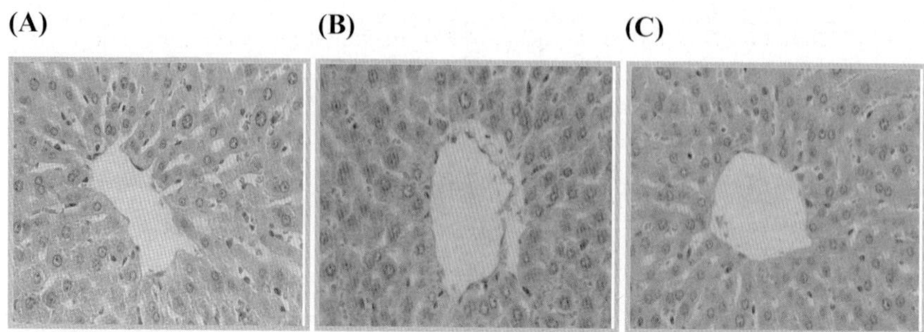

FIGURE 5. Histopathological effects of *TT* and Glib on the liver of diabetic rats. Light micrographs of liver sections. (**A**) Liver section of STZ-induced diabetic rats showing hepatocytes degeneration with dilatation of sinusoids in centrilobular area with some congestion and hemorrhage. (**B**) Liver sections of STZ-induced diabetic rats treated with 10 mg/kg B.W. of Glib showing less degrees of hepatocyte degeneration and nearly no dilated sinusoid in midzonal area. (**C**) Liver section of STZ-induced diabetic rats treated with 2g /kg B.W. of *TT* showing minor degree of degeneration of hepatocytes and dilated sinusoids. Areas with normal hepatic architecture can also be observed. H & E: Magnification: ×400.

Liver enzymes, such as ALT and AST, are used as markers for liver damage. ALT is thought to be a more specific indicator of liver damage. Serum ALT decreased after treatment of the STZ-induced diabetic rats with *TT* and this result indicates the protective effect of the herb. The same effect is shown on the decrement levels of AST. So these results show that *TT* has hepatoprotective effects.

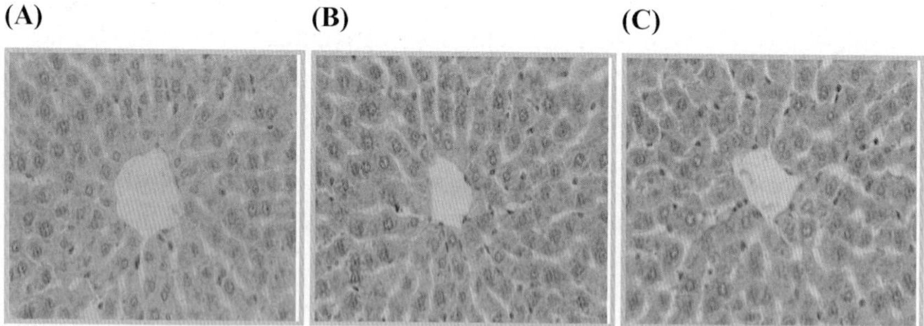

FIGURE 6. Histopathological effects of *TT* and Glib on liver of normal rats. Light micrographs of liver sections. (**A**) Liver sections showing normal hepatic architecture, where the hepatocytes are arranged around the central vein and alternate with blood sinusoids. Each hepatic cell possesses a limiting membrane, centrally placed large nucleus, and prominent nucleoli. (**B**) Liver section of normal rats treated with 10 mg/kg B.W. of Glib showing normal hepatocytes arrangement and normal dilatation of sinusoids in centrilobular area. (**C**) Liver sections of rats treated with 2 g/kg B.W. of *TT* showing similar degrees of hepatocyte architecture with normal dilated sinusoid in midzonal area. H & E: Magnification: ×400.

Increase in creatinine level is indicative of impairment of renal function.[22,23] *TT* restores the kidney functions after the treatment of the rats. Serum creatinine and urea levels decreased after the administration of the herb and this means that *TT* has a beneficial effect on kidney functions.

Hypoinsulinemia in STZ-induced diabetic rats increases the activity of the enzyme fatty acyl Coenzyme A oxidase, which initiates β-oxidation of fatty acids, resulting in LP.[24] Increased LP impairs membrane function by decreasing membrane fluidity and changing the activity of membrane-bound enzymes and receptors. Its products (lipid radical and lipid peroxide) are harmful to most cells in the body and are associated with a variety of diseases, such as atherosclerosis and brain damage.[25] In this study, the decreased level of liver MDA ($P < 0.05$) was shown in STZ-induced diabetic *TT*-treated rats compared with nontreated diabetic rats. The extract could significantly reduce ($P < 0.01$) liver MDA levels in normal rats also. Similar reductions were also observed in liver MDA levels after treatment with Glib in diabetic and normal rats but insignificantly. These findings suggest that the extract has antioxidant effects and can protect tissues from LP.

Insulin deficiency in the diabetic pair's glucose utilization, leads to an increase in oxygen-free radicals. The present results show an increased activity of hepatic antioxidant enzyme GSH in STZ-diabetic rats. GSH, as one of the important nonenzymatic antioxidants in the antioxidant defense system, is synthesized mainly in the liver.[26] It is involved in the synthesis of important macromolecules and in the protection against reactive O_2 compounds.[27] The decreased GSH concentration contributes to the pathogenesis of complications associated with the chronic diabetic state. This study has shown that liver GSH levels were significantly increased ($P < 0.01$) in STZ-induced diabetic rats treated with the extract and the increment was insignificant in case of normal rats treated with the *TT* extract, while a significant increase ($P < 0.05$) of GSH levels was observed in Glib-treated diabetic and normal rats. This investigation reports significantly increased levels of liver GSH, in extract-treated diabetic and normal rats and also reduced MDA in extract-treated diabetic and normal rats, which may be attributed to the presence of such antioxidant compounds in *TT*.

Histopathological changes in the liver STZ-induced diabetic rats show dilatation of blood vessels, congestion in the lobules, some hemorrhagic coagulative foci in hepatic parenchyma, and infiltration of mixed inflammatory cells around the necrotic hepatocytes. In this study, there was a pronounced restoration of the normal hepatic architecture after the treatment of STZ-induced diabetic rats with *TT* ethanolic extract.

CONCLUSION

From this study it can be seen that increased oxidative stress is apparent in STZ-induced diabetic rats. The ethanolic extract of *TT* exhibits a significant antioxidant activity against STZ-induced diabetes. Further studies are needed to explain the mechanism(s) of protective effects of *TT* .

ACKNOWLEDGMENTS

This work was financially supported by the Research Affairs at the UAE University under contract no. 04-04-2-11/05. The investigators acknowledge the assistance of Seeta Hamdi, Karima El-Mansory, Mr. Hameed Rashed, and Kattara Veterinary Laboratory.

REFERENCES

1. Adeghate, E. 2001. Diabetes mellitus-multifactorial in aetiology and global in prevalence. Arch. Physiol. Biochem. **109:** 197–199.
2. Harris, M.I., K.M. Flegal, C.C. Cowie, *et al.* 1998. Prevalence of diabetes, impaired fasting glucose, and impaired glucose tolerance in U.S adults. The Third National Health and Nutrition Examination Survey, 1988–1994. Diabetes Care **21:** 518–524.
3. Limaye, P.V. & S. Sivakami 2003. Evaluation of the fluidity and functionality of the renal cortical brush border membrane in experimental diabetes in rats. Int. J. Biochem. Cell. Biol. **35:** 1163–1169.
4. Halliwell, B. & J.M.C. Gutteridge. 1999. Oxidative stress and antioxidant protection: some special cases. *In* Free Radicals in Biology and Medicine, 3rd ed. B. Halliwell & J.M.C. Gutteridge, Eds.: 530–533. Clarendon Press. Oxford.
5. Doi, K., F. Sawada, G. Toda, *et al.* 2001. Alteration of antioxidants during the progression of heart disease in streptozotocin-induced diabetic rats. Free Radic. Res. **34:** 251–261.
6. Baydas, G., H. Canatan & A, Turkoglu. 2002. Comparative analysis of the protective effects of melatonin and vitamin E on streptozotocin-induced diabetes mellitus. J. Pineal Res. **32:** 225–230.
7. Shinwari, M.I. & M.A. Khan. 2000. Folk use of medicinal herbs of Margalla Hills National Park, Islamabad. J. Ethnopharmacology **69:** 45–56.
8. Wang, B., L. Ma & T. Liu. 1990. 406 cases of angina pectoris in coronary heart diseases treated with saponin of *Tribulus terrestris*. Chung His Chieh Ho Tsa Chih. **10:** 85–87.
9. Chemexcil. 1992. Selected medicinal plants of India (a monograph of identity, safety and clinical usage) *In Tribulus terrestris* Linn. N.O. Zygophyllaceae, Ed.: **100:** 323–326. Compiled by Bharatiya Vidya Bhavan's Swamy Prakashananda Ayurveda Research Centre for Chemexci, Tata Press. Bombay.
10. Tomova, M., R. Gjulemetova, S. Zarkova, *et al.* 1981. Steroidal saponins from *Tribulus terrestris* L. with a stimulating action on the sexual functions. *In* International Conference of Chemistry and Biotechnology of Biologically Active Natural Products, Varna, Bulgaria. September 21–26, **3:** 298–302.
11. Gauthaman, K. & P.G. Adaikan. 2005. Effect of *Tribulus Terrestris* on nictinamide adenine dinucleotide phosphate-diaphorase activity and androgen receptors in rat brain. J. Ethnopharmacol. **96:** 127–132.

12. ADIMOELJA, A. & P.G. ADAIKAN. 1997. Protodioscin from herbal plant *Tribulus terrestris* L. improves male sexual functions possibly via DHEA. Int. J. Impot. Res. **9:** 64.
13. GAUTHAMAN, K., P.G. ADAIKAN, R.N.V. PRASAD, *et al.* 2000. Changes in hormonal parameters secondary to intravenous administration of *Tribulus terrestris* extract in primates Int. J. Impot. Res. **12**(Suppl 2): 6.
14. ADAIKAN, P.G., K. GAUTHAMAN, R.N.V. PRASAD, & S.C. NG. 2000. Proerectile pharmacological effects of *Tribulus terrestris* extract on the rabbit corpus cavernosal smooth muscle *in vitro*. Ann. Acad. Med. Singapore **29:** 22–26.
15. MINGJUAN, L., Q. WEIJING, W. YIFEI, *et al.* 2002. Hypoglycemic effect of saponin from *Tribulus terrestris*. J. Chinese Med. Mat. **25:** 420–422.
16. ADEGHATE, E. 1999. Effect of subcutaneous pancreatic tissue transplant streptozotocin-induced diabetes in rats: I. Morphological studies on normal, diabetic and transplanted pancreatic tissues. Tissue Cell **31:** 66–72.
17. LOWRY, O.H., N.J. ROSEBROUGH, A.L. FARR & R.J. RANDALL. 1951. Protein measurement with the Folin phenol reagent. J. Biol. Chem. **193:** 265–275.
18. OKHAWA, H., N. OHISHI & K. YAGI. 1979. Assay for lipid peroxides in animal tissue by thiobarbituric acid reaction. Anal. Biochem. **95:** 351–358.
19. ELLMAN, G.L. 1959. Tissue sulphydryl groups. Arch. Biochem. Biophys. **82:** 70–77.
20. BAILY, C.J. & P.R. FLATTE. 1986. Antidiabetic drugs, new developments. Indian Biotechnol. **6:** 139–142.
21. ABDEL-BARRY, J.A., I.A. ABDEL-HASSAN & M.H. AL-HAKIIEN. 1887. Hypoglycemic and antihyperglycemic effects of Trigonella foenum-graecum leaf in normal and alloxan induced diabetic rats. J. Ethnopharmacol. **58:** 149–155.
22. BRAULICH, H., F. MARX, C. FLECH & G. STEIN. 1997. Kidney function in rats after 5/6 nephrectomy (5/6 NX): effect of treatment with vitamin E. Exp. Toxicol. Pathol. **49:** 135–139.
23. HWANG, D.F., Y.S. LAI & M.T. CHIANG. 1997. Toxic effects of grass carp, snake and chicken bile juices in rats. Toxicol. Lett. **85:** 85–92
24. HORIE, S., H. ISHII & T. SUGA. 1981. Changes in peroxisomal fatty acid oxidation in diabetic rat liver. J. Biochem. **90:** 1691–1696.
25. ACWORTH, I.N., D.R. MCCABE & T. MAHER. 1997. The analysis of free radicals, their reaction products, and antioxidants. *In* Oxidants, Antioxidants, and Free Radicals. S.I. Baskin & H. Salem, Eds.: 23–77. Taylor and Francis Publishers. Washington (DC).
26. KAPLOWITZ, N., M. OOKHTENS & T.Y. AW. 1985. The regulation of hepatic glutathione. Ann. Rev. Pharmacol. Toxicol. **25:** 715–744.
27. BURK, R.F. 1983. Glutathione-dependent protection by rat liver microsomal protein against lipid peroxidation. Biochem. Biophys. Acta **757:** 21–28.

Effect of High-Calorie Diet on the Prevalence of Diabetes Mellitus in the One-Humped Camel (*Camelus dromedarius*)

M. AL HAJ ALI,[a] FRED NYBERG,[b] S.I. CHANDRANATH,[a]
A.S. PONERY,[c] A. ADEM,[a] AND E. ADEGHATE[c]

[a]*Department of Pharmacology, Faculty of Medicine and Health Sciences, UAE University, Al Ain, United Arab Emirates*

[b]*Department of Pharmaceutical Bioscience, Uppsala University, Uppsala, SE-75124 Sweden*

[c]*Department of Anatomy, Faculty of Medicine and Health Sciences, UAE University, Al Ain, United Arab Emirates*

ABSTRACT: The one-humped camel is a typical desert animal. It has the capability of withstanding the harsh climatic changes and the scarcity of food and water, in addition to the high-ambient temperature. The prevalence of diabetes mellitus in two different groups of the one-humped camel, group (A) control ($n = 102$) camels and group (B) high-calorie diet-fed camels ($n = 103$), in Al-Ain region (UAE) was studied using biochemical and radioimmunoassay techniques. In this article, 7% of the control camels have diabetes mellitus (blood glucose level: $\geq$140 mg/dL) compared to 21% of the high-calorie-fed camels. Plasma insulin level was significantly ($P < 0.05$) lower in group B compared to group A. The low insulin level in camels consuming high-caloric diet could be a sign of exhaustion of pancreatic beta cells. The hematological parameters were nearly similar in both groups and no significant differences were seen. Liver and kidney enzymes were normal in both groups. Iron and copper were significantly ($P < 0.005$) higher in the high-calorie-fed camels compared with the control. Our study indicates that high-caloric feed consumption in camels is associated with the development of disorders in glucose metabolism leading to diabetes mellitus.

KEYWORDS: diabetes mellitus; one-humped camel; high-caloric feed; biochemical; radioimmunoassay techniques

Address for correspondence: Ernest Adeghate, M.D., M.F.M., Ph.D., Department of Anatomy, Faculty of Medicine and Health Sciences, UAE University, P.O. Box 17666, Al Ain, United Arab Emirates. Voice: 971-3-7137496; fax: 971-3-7672033.
e-mail: eadeghate@uaeu.ac.ae

Ann. N.Y. Acad. Sci. 1084: 402–410 (2006).
doi: 10.1196/annals.1372.034

INTRODUCTION

The one-humped camel is a nomadic animal, well adapted to very hot and dry climates of the desert. Its ability to withstand torrid heat and extreme desiccation is of paramount importance to its survival. The one-humped camel is a typical desert animal. It is similar to ruminants in many aspects like regurgitation of ingesta, and microbial fermentation in the stomach.[1–3] However, in comparison to the compound stomach of typical ruminants that comprises four compartments, the stomach of the camel has only three compartments. The effects of high-caloric diets on human diabetic patients have been reported,[4–6] whereas studies concerning the effects on animals have been few and concentrated on mice,[7–9] dogs,[6,10–12] and cats.[13,14] The epidemiology of diabetes in animals needs to be elaborated as the risk of diabetes mellitus in human is increasing as the result of the changes in the lifestyle of urban residents. In animals, diabetes has been diagnosed in dogs,[11] cats,[13] and other mammals. However, in the dromedaries no such studies had been done. In view of the fact that camels are herbivores, it would be expected that diabetes mellitus would be rare, but the management and feeding habit of camels have changed in this part of the world, due to the changes that affected life of the people after the discovery of petroleum in the Gulf region. Although, experiments on animals should be useful in elucidating the underlying mechanisms, it is not clear even whether there are benefits of high-caloric feed for animals. Thus the aim of the article is to determine whether high-caloric diet (honey, milk, dates, and ghee) fed to camels has any influence in triggering diabetes mellitus in this huge desert animal.

MATERIALS AND METHODS

Camels ($n = 205$) selected for this study were divided into two groups (A and B). Group A consists of 102 camels. They were kept in semiopen camps, where feed and water are provided *ad libitum* and the camels are allowed to forage for themselves on desert plants and shrubs during the daytime (8–10 h) and return back to their camps before sunset. The feed supplied to this group consists mainly of dry grass (roughage) and some wheat-bran mixed with dates. Group B consists of 103 camels. They were kept in special closed camps with well-arranged and clean fences provided with good shelters. Feed is provided to this group two times per day, in the early morning and evening, and consists of green grass, such as alfa-alfa, concentrate feed, such as barely, grain, maize, dates, honey, and ghee, and supplements of vitamins and minerals. Water is supplied daily in special troughs with restrictions especially during race events.

Blood is collected from the jugular vein with the camels at rest for hematology and chemistry analysis in evacuated blood-collecting tubes, one containing anticoagulant (EDTA) for hematological analysis and the other without anticoagulant for the biochemical analysis. Blood was collected from all camels in both groups in the early morning before feed is supplied. Camels with high glucose level ($\geq$ 140 mg/dL) were again tested on day 10, and day 20. The hematological parameters tested were hematocrit (HCT), hemoglobin (HB), leukocyte count (WBC), erythrocyte count (RBC), mean corpuscular volume (MCV), mean corpuscular hemoglobin (MCH), and mean corpuscular hemoglobin concentration (MCHC), using (CELL DYN 3700, Abbott Diagnostics, Santa Clara, CA). While, for the biochemistry analysis, serum is tested for aspartate aminotransferase (AST), gamma-glutamyl transferase (GGT), glutamate oxalacetate transaminase (GOT), alanine aminotransferase (ALT), blood urea nitrogen (BUN), creatine, lactate dehydrogenase (LDH), creatine kinase (CK), copper (Cu), iron (Fe), total protein (TP), and glucose (Glu) levels, using (Ace Alfawasser Mann, West Caldwell, NJ).

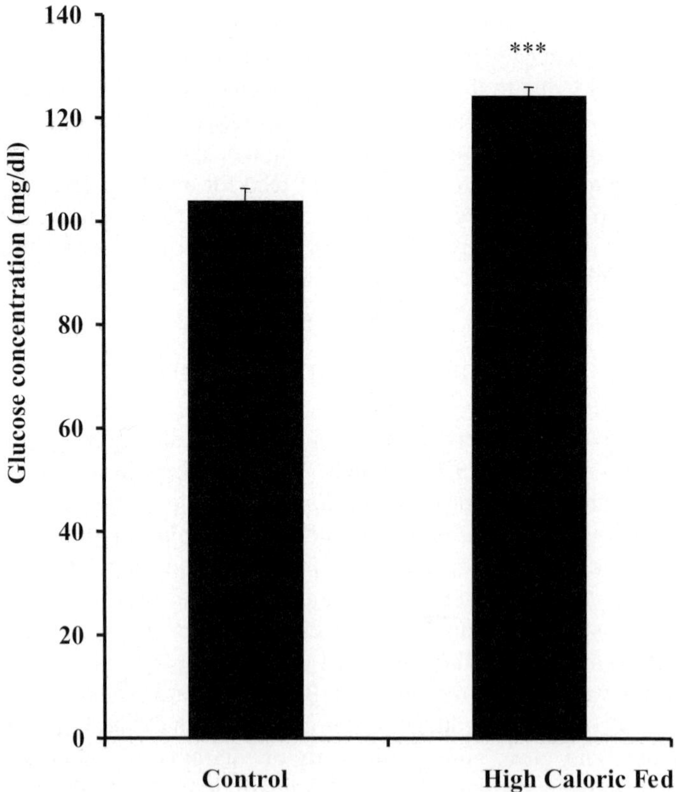

FIGURE 1. Histograms of blood glucose in control camels and in those fed on high-calorie diet. Blood glucose is significantly (***$P < 0.001$) higher in high-calorie-fed camels compared to control.

RESULTS

The blood glucose level in the high-calorie-fed camels was significantly ($P < 0.05$) higher compared with the control. The results indicated that 21% of the high-calorie-fed camels were hyperglycemic (≥140 mg/dL) compared with 7% of the control camels (FIG. 1). Radioimmunoassay of insulin was performed to determine the extent of diabetes. The plasma insulin level was significantly lower in the high-calorie-fed camels compared to control (FIG. 2).

The hematological and biochemistry results of both groups A and B was analyzed and tabulated as (mean ± SE) in TABLE 1. All the hematological parameters HCT, WBC, RBC, HB, MCV, MCH, and MCHC were nearly the same with no significant differences among the different parameters. In the biochemical analysis significant differences were observed in iron and copper (FIG. 3) and in creatinine and blood urea nitrogen levels (FIG. 4). There is also a significant difference in the LDH (FIG. 5).

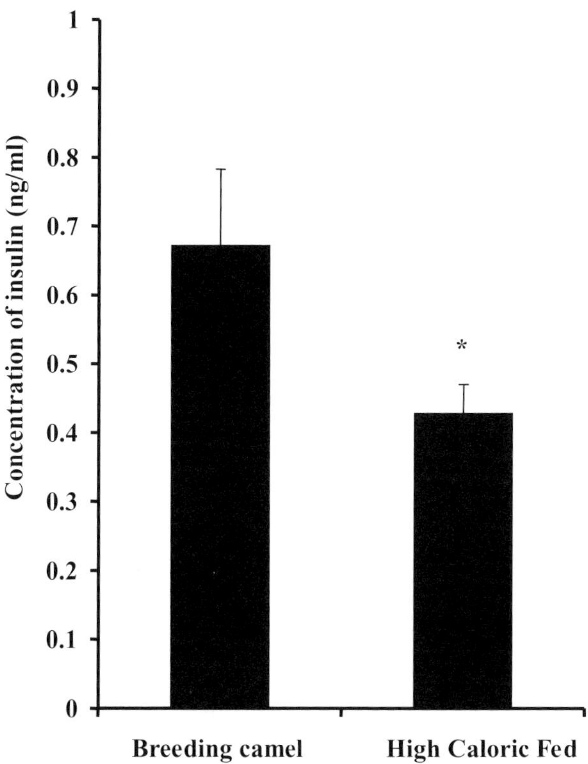

FIGURE 2. Histograms of plasma insulin level in control camels and in those fed on high-calorie diet. Plasma insulin is significantly ($^*P < 0.05$) lower in camels fed on high-calorie diet compared to control.

TABLE 1. Blood chemistry of control and camels fed on high-calorie diet

	Control (mean ± S.E.)	*n*	High-calorie diet fed (mean ± SE)	*n*
WBC ($\times 10^3 \mu$L)	10.19 ± 0.22	102	10.19 ± 0.19	103
RBC ($\times 10^6 \mu$L)	9.05 ± 0.14	102	9.29 ± 0.09	103
HB (gm/dL)	12.79 ± 0.15	102	13.05 ± 0.11	103
HCT (%)	26.36 ± 0.29	102	26.87 ± 0.2	103
MCV	29.36 ± 0.23	102	28.99 ± 0.15	103
MCH	14.2 ± 0.08	102	14.07 ± 0.06	103
MCHC	48.37 ± 0.13	102	48.53 ± 0.01	103
GGT	28.28 ± 1.23	102	31.01 ± 1.03	103
CK	61.24 ± 2.73	102	64.08 ± 3.53	103

DISCUSSION

Nutritional state of an animal is a critical determinant for its capability to survive and well-being. Camels are adapted to desert plants and shrubs with

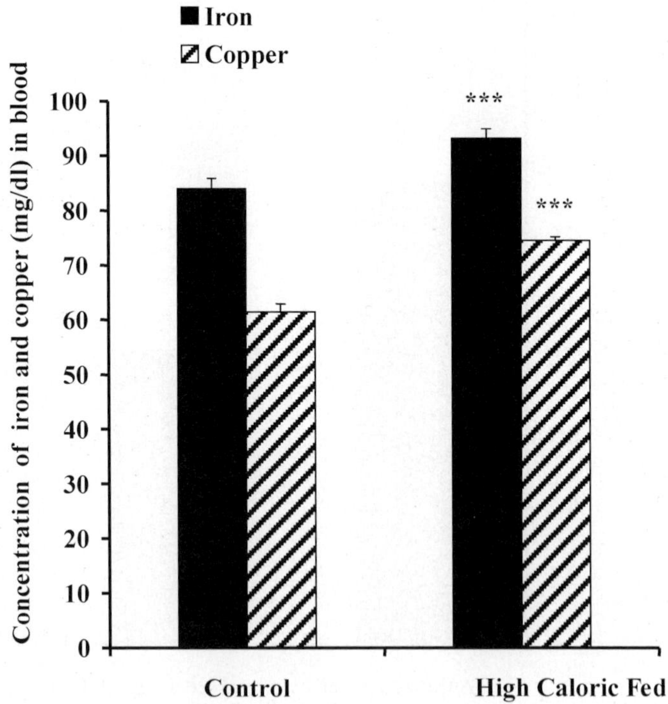

FIGURE 3. Histograms of blood iron and copper level in control camels and in those fed on high-calorie diet. The blood levels of iron and copper are significantly (***$P < 0.001$) higher in camels fed on high-calorie diet compared to control.

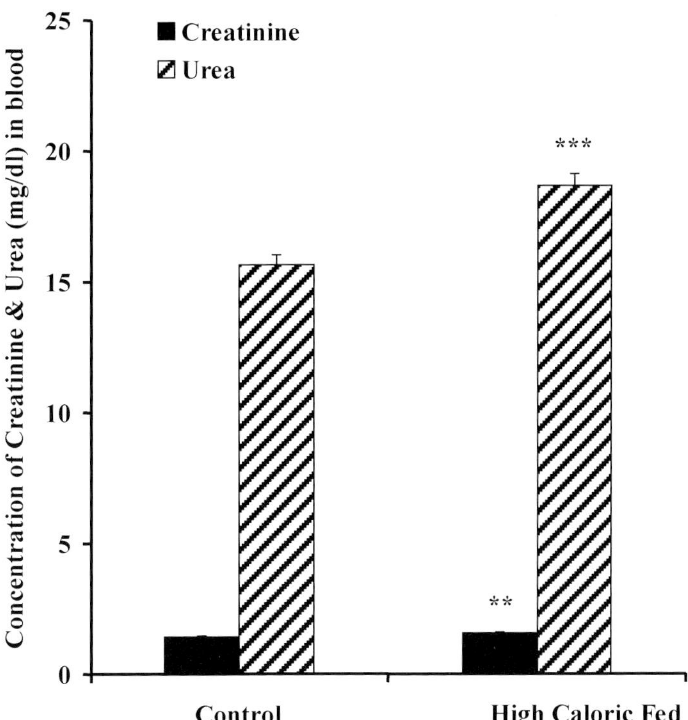

FIGURE 4. The figure shows the blood level of creatinine and urea in control camels and in those fed on high-calorie diet. The levels of creatinine and urea are significantly (**$P < 0.01$; ***$P < 0.001$) higher in camels fed on high-calorie diet compared to control.

high-fiber contents. They can forge for themselves on range vegetation and desert shrubs by moving around for long distances and rarely have stomach or gut problems. Digestive complications arise when they are stall fed with concentrate and lack access to roughage. Our objective in this study was to determine the influence of high-caloric diet (maize, barley, grain, full cream cow's milk, dates, honey, and ghee) and compare it with control camels, fed normal diet (dry grass and were allowed to forage for themselves in the desert plants and shrubs for 8–10 h daily). Studies on high-caloric diet fed to different animals indicated that this predisposes the body to obesity and diabetes mellitus.[15] It had been shown in laboratory animals that high-caloric saturated fat intake induced diabetes due to delayed insulin secretion.[16,17] Fat- and protein-enriched diet was found to be the critical stimulus for hyperglycemia and hyperinsulinemia in companion animals,[14] whereas studies done in dogs and cats revealed that certain carbohydrates, including rice, caused higher glycemic levels than others, such as nougat.[18] High consumption of cow's milk during childhood may be associated positively with diabetes mellitus.[5,19] High intake

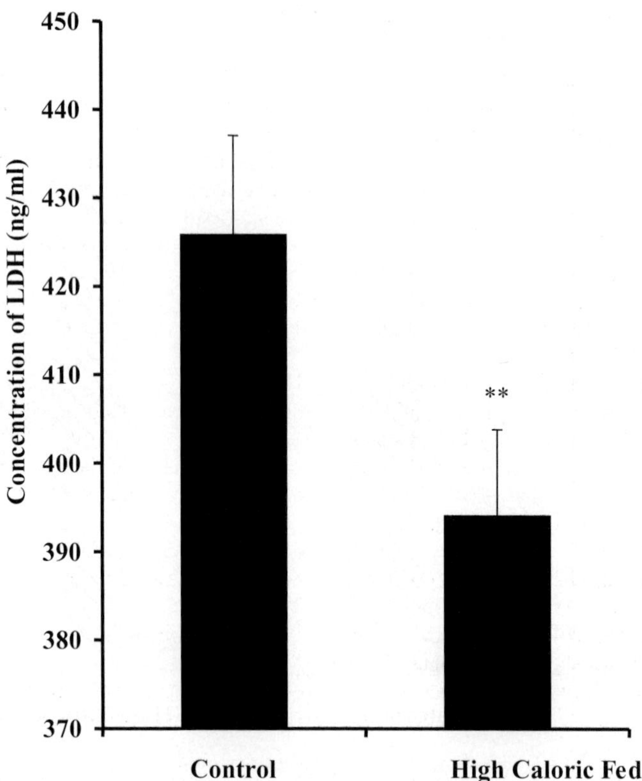

FIGURE 5. This figure shows the blood level of LDH in control camels and in those fed on high-calorie diet. The levels of LDH is significantly ($^{**}P < 0.01$) lower in camels fed on high-calorie diet compared to control.

of total dietary fat is positively related to relative fasting hyperinsulinemia in nondiabetic women; particularly those who are sedentary. In a different study, it had been shown that early exposure to cow's milk and solid foods may be associated with increased risk of diabetes mellitus.[5] Thus, high-caloric diet may enhance the onset of diabetes mellitus in these animals. No studies have been done on the prevalence of diabetes mellitus in the one-humped camels. Our data analysis showed that 7% of the control camels compared with 21% for the high-calorie diet-fed camels had higher glucose level (hyperglycemia) and lower insulin level in their serum. These results might be explained by the large differences in feed consumptions by both groups of camels. Thus, the consumptions of high-caloric diet may promote the onset of diabetes mellitus in these camels. Further studies are required to check whether the state of hyperglycemia is reversible or not.

REFERENCES

1. DOUGBAG, A.S. & R. BERG. 1980. Histological and histochemical studies on the mucosa of the initial dilated and middle long narrow part of the third compartment of the camel's stomach Anat. Histol. Embryol. **9:** 155–163.
2. DOUGBAG, A.S. & R. BERG. 1981. Histological and histochemical studies on the pyloric mucosa of the camel's stomach. Anat. Histol. Embryol. **10:** 187–192.
3. EERDUNCHAOLU, D.V., K. TAKEHANA, A. KOBAYASHI, *et al.* 1999. Morphological characterization of gland cells of the glandular sac area in the complex stomach of the Bacterian camel. Anat. Histol. Embryol. **28:** 183–191.
4. BUHLING, K.J., E. ELSNER, C. WOLF, *et al.* 2004. No influence of high and low carbohydrate diet on the oral glucose tolerance test in pregnancy. Clin. Biochem. **37:** 323–327.
5. KOSTRABA, J.N., K.J. CRUICKSHANKS, J. LAWLER-HEAVNER, *et al.* 1993. Early exposure to cow's milk and solid foods in infancy, genetic predisposition, and risk of IDDM. Diabetes **42:** 288–295.
6. NELSON, R.W., S.L. IHLE, L.D. LEWIS, *et al.* 1991. Effects of dietary fibre supplementation on glycemic control in dogs with alloxan-induced diabetes mellitus. Am. J. Vet. Res. **52:** 2060–2066.
7. KOTAKE, J., Y. TANANKA, N. UMEHARA, *et al.* 2004. Effects of a high-monounsaturated fat diet on glucose and lipid metabolism in normal and diabetic mice. J. Nutr. Sci. Vitaminol. (Tokyo) **50:** 106–113.
8. LEE, S.M. 1982. The effect of a high fibre diet on diabetic nephropathy in the Db/db mouse. Diabetologia **22:** 349–353.
9. PETRO, A.E., J. COTTER, D.A. COOPER, *et al.* 2004. Fat, carbohydrate and calories in the development of diabetes and obesity in the C57BL/6J mouse. Metabolism **53:** 454–457.
10. KEALY, R.D., D.E. LAWLER, J.M. BALLAM, *et al.* 2002. Effects of diet restriction on life span and age-related changes in dogs. J. Am. Vet. Med. Assoc. **220:** 1315–1320.
11. KIMMEL, S.E., K.E. MICHEAL, R.S. HESS & C.R. WARD. 2000. Effects of insoluble and soluble dietary fiber on glycemic control in dogs with naturally occurring insulin dependent diabetes mellitus. J. Am. Vet. Med. Assoc. **216:** 1076–1081.
12. NELSON, R.W., C.A. DUESBERG, S.L. FORD, *et al.* 1998. Effects of dietary insoluble fibre on control of glycemia in dogs with naturally acquired diabetes mellitus. J. Am. Vet. Med. Assoc. **212:** 380–386.
13. NELSON, R.W, J.C. SCOTT-MONCRIEFF, E C. FELDMAN, *et al.* 2000. Effect of dietary insoluble fiber on control of glycemia in cats with naturally acquired diabetes mellitus. J. Am. Vet. Med. Assoc. **216:** 1082–1088.
14. RAND, J.S., H.A. FARROW, L.M. FLEEMAN & D.J. APPLETON. 2003. Diet in the prevention of diabetes and obesity in companion animals [abstract]. Asia Pac. J. Clin. Nutr. **12** (Suppl): S6.
15. POPOV, D., M. SIMIONESCU & P.R. SHEPHERD. 2003. Saturated fat diet induces moderate diabetes and serve glomerulosclerosis in hamsters. Diabetologia **46:** 1408–1418.
16. SCHNEIDER, K, H. LAUBE & T. LINN. 1996. A diet enriched in protein accelerates diabetes manifestation in NOD mice. Acta Diabetol. **33:** 236–240.
17. SURWIT, R.S., M.N. FEINGLOS, J. RODIN, *et al.* 1995. Differential effects of fat and sucrose on the development of obesity and diabetes in C57BL/6J and A/J mice. Metabolism **44:** 645–651.

18. RIESTRA, A., G. CUBAS & J.A. AMADO. 1995. The effect of the ingestion of nougat on blood glucose and insulin in healthy subjects. Nutr. Hosp. **10:** 354–357.
19. VIRTANEN, S.M., E. HYPPONEN, E. LAARA, *et al.* 1998. Cow's milk consumption, disease-associated autoantibodies and type 1 diabetes mellitus: a follow-up study in sibling of diabetic children. Childhood Diabetes in Finland Study Group. Diabet. Med. **15:** 730–738.

Vitamin E Ameliorates Some Biochemical Parameters in Normal and Diabetic Rats

MARIAM AL SHAMSI,[a] AMR AMIN,[b] AND ERNEST ADEGHATE[a]

[a]*Department of Anatomy, Faculty of Medicine and Health Sciences, UAE University, Al Ain, United Arab Emirates*

[b]*Department of Biology, Faculty of Science, UAE University, Al Ain, United Arab Emirates*

ABSTRACT: Diabetes is associated with hyperglycemia, one of the most important causes of oxidative stress. Endogenous antioxidants are able to destroy the reactive species and create a balance between antioxidant and free radicals. In diabetes, the oxidative stress is increased due to the deficiency in the antioxidant defense. The intake of antioxidants, such as vitamin E, may reduce the oxidative stress associated with diabetes and hence help to restore the antioxidant defense system. The aim of this article was to investigate the effect of different doses of vitamin E on the biochemical parameters of normal and streptozotocin (STZ)-induced diabetic rats. Biochemical analysis was used to study the effect of this vitamin on the biochemical parameters of normal and diabetic rats. The plasma levels of alkaline phosphatase (ALP), alanine aminotransferase (ALT), aspartate aminotransferase (AST), lactic dehydrogenase (LDH), and gamma-glutamyl transferase (γ-GT) were significantly increased after the onset of diabetes. In addition, STZ-induced diabetes also caused an increase in the level of blood urea nitrogen (BUN) and creatinine. Oral administration of vitamin E (0.2–0.4 mg daily) significantly ($P < 0.05$) decreased the plasma level of ALT, AST, and γ-GT. In addition, there was a slight but not significant reduction in the plasma level of ALP. Parameters of kidney function, such as BUN and creatinine, were slightly reduced after the oral administration of vitamin E. The plasma level of electrolytes, such as calcium and sodium, also changed significantly ($P < 0.00001$) after the oral administration of vitamin E. Vitamin E ameliorates the metabolic and biochemical parameters of diabetic rats.

Address for correspondence: Ernest Adeghate, M.D., M.F.M., Ph.D., Department of Anatomy, Faculty of Medicine and Health Sciences, UAE University, P. O. Box 17666, Al Ain, United Arab Emirates. Voice: 971-3-7137496; fax: 971-3-7672033.
e-mail: eadeghate@uaeu.ac.ae

Ann. N.Y. Acad. Sci. 1084: 411–431 (2006).
doi: 10.1196/annals.1372.033

KEYWORDS: diabetes; antioxidant; vitamin E; streptozotocin; liver and kidney function tests

INTRODUCTION

Diabetes mellitus is a chronic disease associated with severe late complications. It affects the metabolism of carbohydrates, protein, fat, and electrolytes, which cause changes in the structure of the vascular system.[1] Recently, studies suggest that protein kinase C activation may play an important role in the development of diabetes complication, and the use of its inhibitors can reduce these complications. It is reported that an inhibitor of protein kinase C was able to reduce renal and retinal dysfunction in diabetic animals.[2] The end product of the nonenzymatic glycation increases cytokines level in vascular cells, which contributes to the development of diabetic complication.[3]

Furthermore, the products of oxidative stress derived from glucose autooxidation, advanced glycation, and mitochondrial dysfunction may damage endothelial cell function.[4] Hyperglycemia induces the production of superoxide by mitochondria, leading to the formation of a strong oxidant proxy nitrite, which damages the DNA. The damage of the DNA activates the nuclear enzyme poly (ADP-ribose) polymerase, which depletes the intracellular concentration of NAD (+), thus slowing glycolysis, ATP formation, and ADP ribosylation of GAPDH. All of these processes further contribute to the development of late degenerative complications.[5]

In the normal condition, endogenous mechanisms, enzymes, and antioxidant molecules are able to destroy reactive molecular species and reduce the harmful effect of noxious substances,[6] but in diabetes the hyperglycemia and possible free fatty acid induce the reactive molecular species and oxidative stress, which play role in causing insulin resistance and β cell dysfunction. Reactive oxygen and nitrogen species may also play a role in the pathogenesis of the late diabetes complication because they have the ability to oxidize and damage DNA, protein, and lipid.[7]

Antioxidant can be produced endogenously or provided from exogenous sources, such as vitamin E.[8] Vitamin E is a chain-breaking radical scavenger[9] characterized by low molecular weight and lipid solubility, which help it to scavenge reactive species in lipid-laden compartments like cell membrane.[10] Vitamin E has the ability to scavenge a wide spectrum of free radicals including singlet oxygen, superoxide, and hydroxyl radicals.[11] Also, it is believed that vitamin E can act as membrane stabilizer by forming complexes with the products of membrane lipid hydrolysis, such as lysophospholipids and free fatty acids.[12]

This article was set to examine the effect of vitamin E on biochemical parameters, such as liver enzymes, kidney parameters, and plasma electrolytes level in normal and diabetic rats.

MATERIALS AND METHODS

Experimental Animals

Male Wistar rats aged 7–8 weeks and weighing 200–300 g were used in this study. All rats were obtained from the Faculty of Medicine and Health Sciences, United Arab Emirates University. All rats were housed in a temperature (25°C) and humidity controlled rooms in 12-h light–dark periods. The animals were fed on a standard rat chow and tap water *ad libitum*. The experiment was performed according to the guidelines set by the Animal Ethics Committee, Faculty of Medicine and Health Sciences, United Arab Emirates University.

Induction of Experimental Diabetes

Diabetes was induced in the rats by a single intraperitoneal injection of streptozotocin (STZ) (Sigma, St. Louis, MO) at a dose of 60 mg/kg body weight.[13] The STZ was freshly dissolved in citrate buffer (0.5 M, pH4.5). The rats were considered diabetic if the fasting blood glucose level values were more than 250 mg/dL.

Experimental Design

Rats were randomly divided into three groups according to three different doses of vitamin E (low dose, 0.2 mg; moderate dose, 0.4 mg; and high dose, 0.8 mg per animal of vitamin E). Rats were treated orally with vitamin E by using an intubation loop. Each of these groups was divided into five subgroups of six animals each. *Group I* (*normal untreated rats*)—Rats were not treated either with STZ or with vitamin E. *Group II* (*STZ-induced diabetic control rats*)—Rats were not treated with vitamin E. *Group III* (*vitamin E-treated diabetic rats*)—Rats were treated with the three different doses (low, moderate, and high) of vitamin E for 10 days prior to the induction of diabetes. *Group IV* (*vitamin-treated diabetic rats*). Rats were treated with the three different doses (low, moderate, and high) of vitamin E 10 days after the onset of diabetes. *Group V* (normal *nondiabetic-treated group*). This group was treated with the three different doses of vitamin E.

Biochemical Analysis

Biochemical analysis of blood urea nitrogen (BUN), creatinine (CRE), alkaline phosphatase (ALP), alanine aminotransferase (ALT), aspartate aminotransferase (AST), lactic dehydrogenase (LDH), gamma-glutamyl transferase (γ-GT), calcium, phosphorus, sodium, potassium, and magnesium was performed in Al-Qattara Veterinary Laboratory (Al Ain, UAE) using Beckman Coulter (Synchron Lx20 PRO) clinical system.

Statistical Analysis

Data are expressed as mean ± SD. Student's *t*-test was used to analyze the significance of differences between mean values and different groups were analyzed by analysis of variance using Duncan's multiple range tests. A P value of less than 0.05 was considered statistically significant.

RESULTS

The plasma levels of ALP, ALT, AST, LDH, γ-GT were significantly increased after the onset of STZ-induced diabetes. In addition, STZ-induced diabetes also caused an increase in the level of BUN and CRE.

Plasma ALP Level

The low dose of vitamin E decreased the plasma level of ALP in rats treated with vitamin E for 10 days after the onset of diabetes. However, the plasma level of ALP was slightly increased in rats treated with vitamin E for 10 days before the onset of diabetes but without any significance. The moderate dose (0.4 mg) of vitamin E had no significant effect on the plasma ALP level of normal-treated rats.

On the other hand, the moderate dose increased the plasma ALP level in rats treated with vitamin E before the onset of diabetes. This increase was not statistically different when compared to control. No significant change was observed in the plasma ALP level of rats treated after the onset of diabetes (FIG.1). The oral administration of high dose (0.8 mg) of vitamin E had no effect on the plasma ALP level of normal- and treated-diabetic rats (data not shown).

Plasma ALT Level

The oral administration of low dose of vitamin E had no effect on normal rats when compared to controls. On the other hand, low dose (0.2 mg) of vitamin E significantly reduced the level of plasma ALT in rats treated before ($P < 0.014$) and after ($P < 0.006$) the onset of diabetes. Moderate dose (0.4 mg) of vitamin E also reduced plasma ALT level in rats treated before and after the onset of diabetes but without any significance. Moderate dose had no effect on normal-treated rats when compared with normal control (FIG. 2). No significant change was observed in the ALT level of normal rats after oral administration of high dose (0.8 mg) of vitamin E (data not shown).

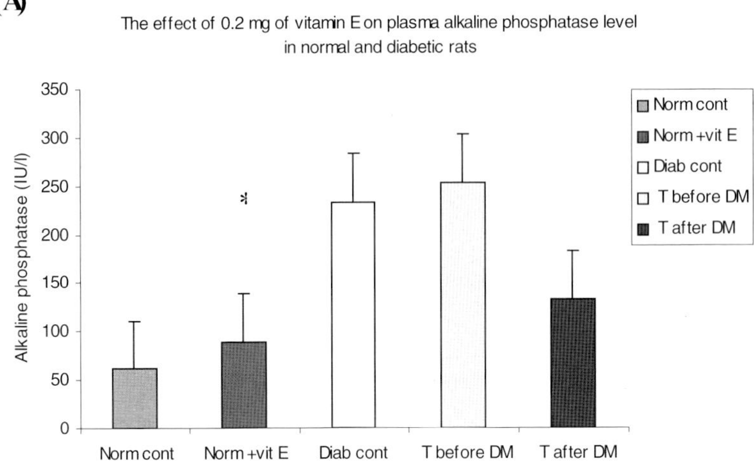

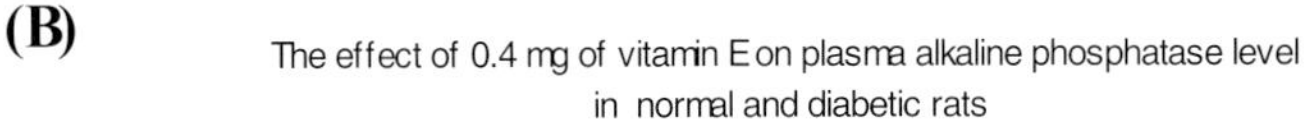

(B)
The effect of 0.4 mg of vitamin E on plasma alkaline phosphatase level in normal and diabetic rats

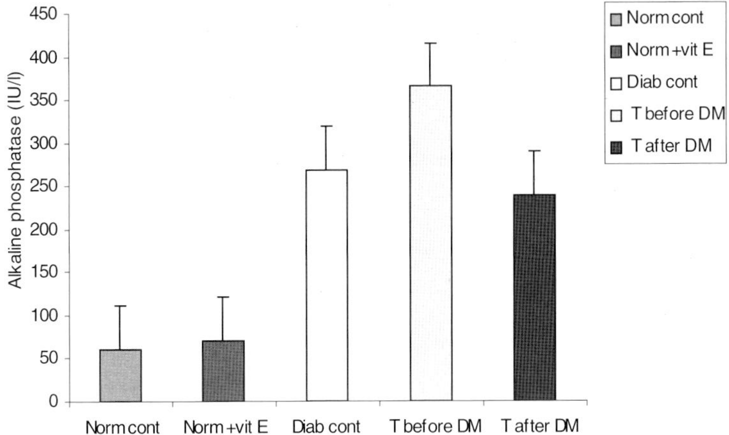

FIGURE 1. (**A**) Histograms showing the effect of 0.2 mg of vitamin E on plasma ALP level of normal and diabetic rats. Vitamin E (0.2 mg) induced significant increases in plasma ALP level in normal nondiabetic rats. $^{*}P < 0.05$ (norm cont versus norm+ vitamin E). (Data are mean $\pm$ SD, $n = 6$.) DM = diabetes mellitus. (**B**) Histograms showing the effect of 0.4 mg of vitamin E on plasma ALP level of normal and diabetic rats. (Data are mean $\pm$ SD, $n = 6$.) DM = diabetes mellitus. Note a slight but not significant reduction in the ALP level of rats treated after the onset of diabetes.

(A)

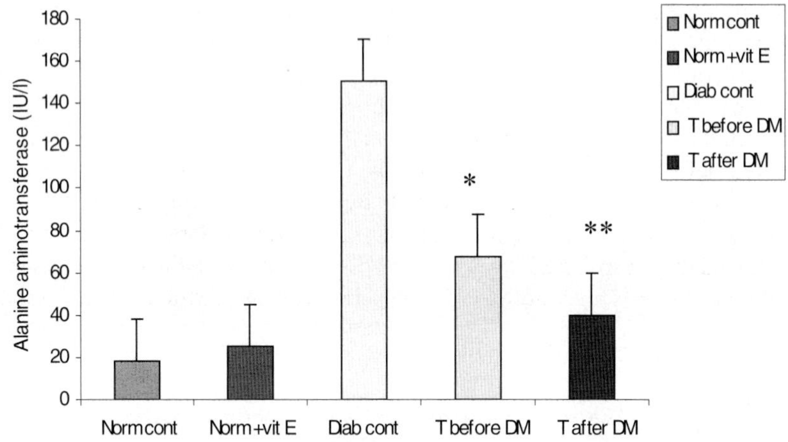

(B)

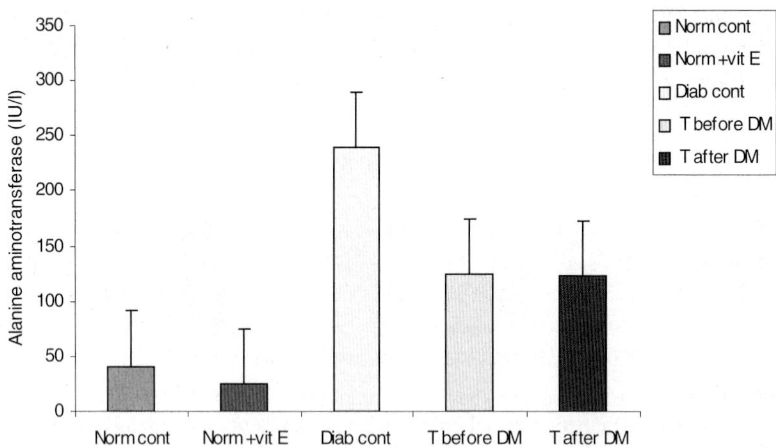

FIGURE 2. (**A**) Histograms showing the effect of 0.2 mg of vitamin E on plasma ALT level of normal and diabetic rats. Vitamin E (0.2 mg) induced significant decreases in plasma ALT level in rats treated before and after the onset of diabetes mellitus. $^*P < 0.05$ (treated before DM versus diab cont); $^{**}P < 0.01$(treated after DM versus diab cont). (Data are mean $\pm$ SD, $n = 6$.) DM = diabetes mellitus. (**B**) Histograms showing the effect of 0.4 mg of vitamin E on plasma ALT level of normal and diabetic rats. (Data are mean $\pm$ SD, $n = 6$.) DM = diabetes mellitus.

Plasma AST

FIGURE 3 shows that low dose (0.2 mg) of vitamin E had no effect on plasma AST level of normal rats when compared with normal control. In diabetic rats, the low dose significantly ($P < 0.019$) reduced the plasma AST level of rats treated for 10 days after the onset of diabetes. After the oral administration of moderate dose (0.4 mg) of vitamin E a decrease in the plasma AST level of normal-treated rats was observed but without any statistical significance. The moderate dose of vitamin E can increase the plasma AST level in rats treated before and after the onset of diabetes. This increase had no statistical significance when compared with diabetic control. The high dose (0.8 mg) of vitamin E had no effect on the plasma AST level of normal-treated rats but increased the plasma AST of rats treated before and after the onset of diabetes (data not shown). This increase has no statistical significance when compared to diabetic controls.

Plasma LDH Level

The oral administration of low dose (0.2 mg) of vitamin E significantly ($P <$ 0.033) reduced the level of plasma LDH in untreated normal rats. No change in plasma LDH level was observed in normal rats after oral administration of moderate (0.4 mg) of vitamin E (FIG. 4). The high dose (0.8 mg) of vitamin E had no effect on the level of plasma LDH level in normal rats and rats treated for 10 days before the onset of diabetes rats (data not shown).

Plasma γ-GT *Level*

The effect of low dose (0.2 mg) of vitamin E on plasma γ-GT in normal and diabetic rats is shown in FIGURE 5. Diabetic rats exhibited high plasma γ-GT level. In normal rats with low dose of vitamin E, there was a significant increase in plasma γ-GT level ($P < 0.012$). The low dose of vitamin E successfully reduced this level in rats treated before and after the onset of diabetes but without any statistical significance. However, after the oral administration of the moderate dose (0.4 mg) of vitamin E, diabetic rats exhibited high plasma γ-GT level. The result showed that high dose of vitamin E had no significant effect on the plasma γ-GT level of normal and diabetic rats (data not shown).

BUN Level

The level of BUN of normal rats was found to be significantly increased after the administration of low dose (0.2 mg) of vitamin E ($P < 0.03$). The treatment

(A)

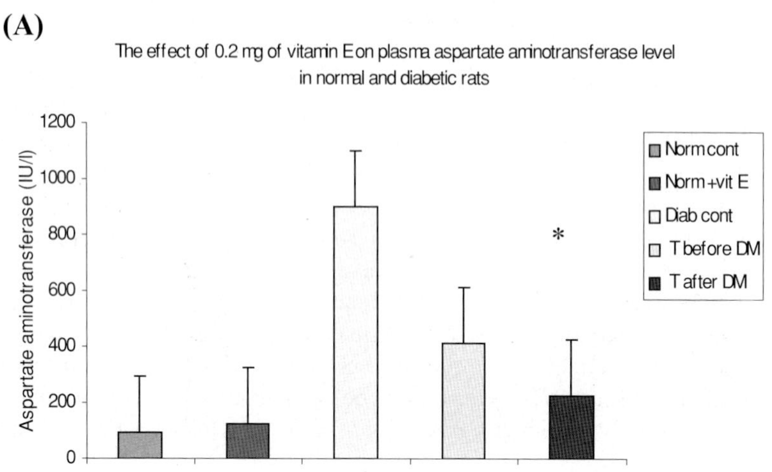

(B)

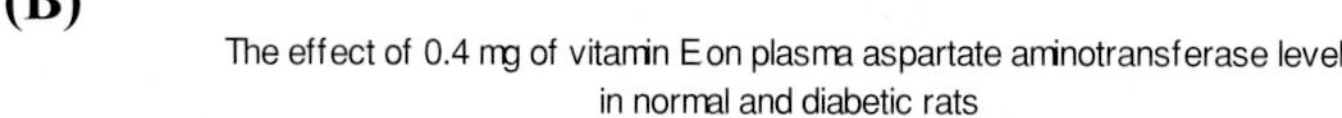

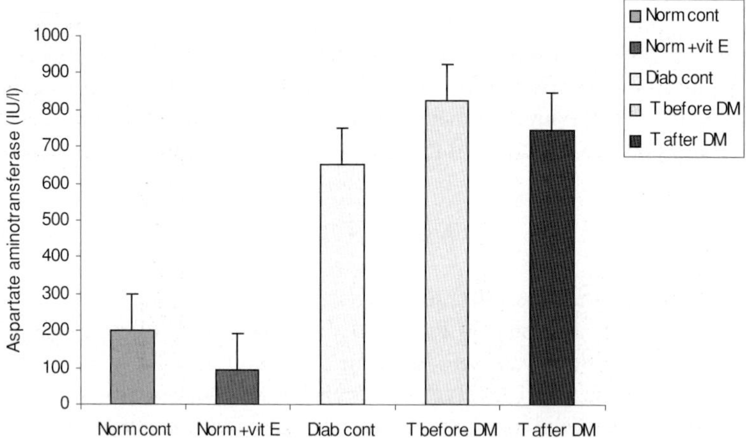

FIGURE 3. (**A**) Histograms showing the effect of 0.2 mg of vitamin E on plasma AST level of normal and diabetic rats. Vitamin E (0.2 mg) induced a significant decrease in the plasma AST level in rats treated after the onset of diabetes mellitus. $^*P < 0.05$ (diabetes cont versus treated after onset of DM). (Data are mean $\pm$ SD, $n = 6$.) DM = diabetes mellitus. (**B**) Histograms showing the effect of 0.4 mg of vitamin E on plasma AST level of normal and diabetic rats. (Data are mean $\pm$ SD, $n = 6$.) DM = diabetes mellitus.

of diabetic rats before and after the onset of diabetes with low dose of vitamin E reduced the level of BUN without any statistical significance. Treatment with moderate dose (0.4 mg) of vitamin E resulted in an increase in the level of BUN of normal and diabetic rats without any statistical significance (FIG. 6).

(A)

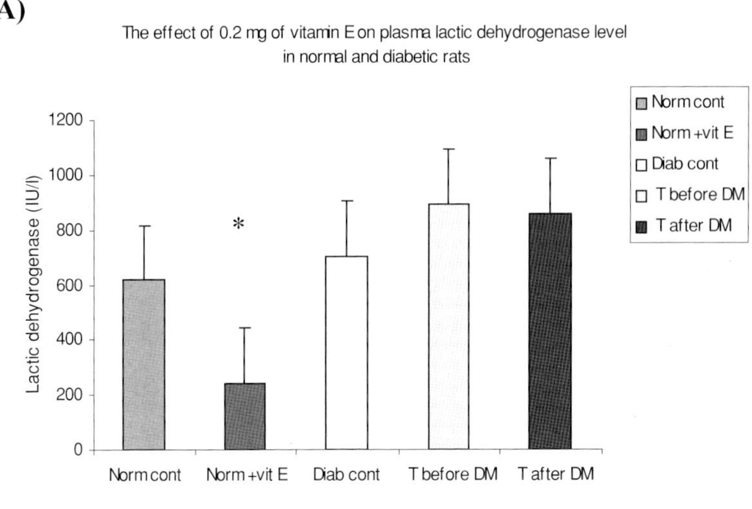

(B)

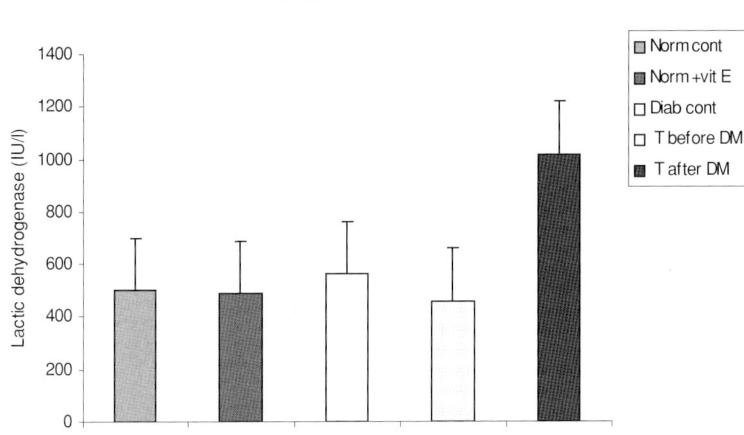

FIGURE 4. (**A**) Histograms showing the effect of 0.2 mg of vitamin E on plasma LDH level of normal and diabetic rats. Vitamin E (0.2 mg) induced a significant decrease in the plasma LDH level in normal nondiabetic rats. $^*P < 0.05$ (norm cont versus norm cont + vitamin E). (Data are mean ± SD, $n = 6$.) DM = diabetes mellitus. (**B**) Histograms showing the effect of 0.4 mg of vitamin E on plasma LDH level of normal and diabetic rats. (Data are mean ± SD, $n = 6$.) DM = diabetes mellitus.

The oral administration of high dose (0.8 mg) of vitamin E significantly ($P <$ 0.03) increased the BUN level of rats treated before the onset of diabetes. Also, high dose of vitamin E increased BUN level of normal-treated rats without any statistical significance (data not shown).

(A)

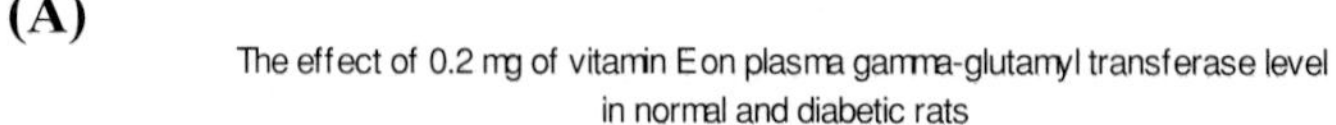

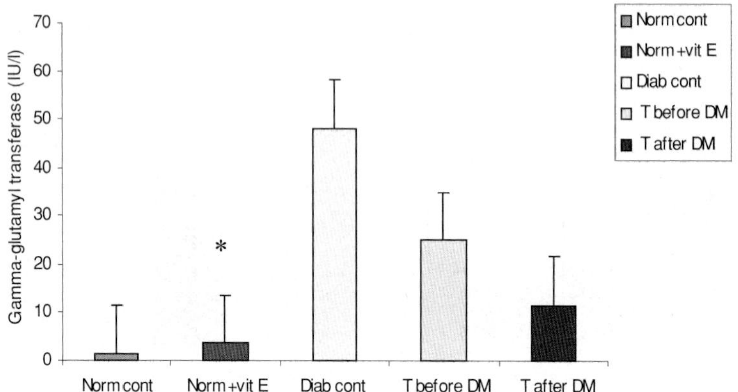

(B)

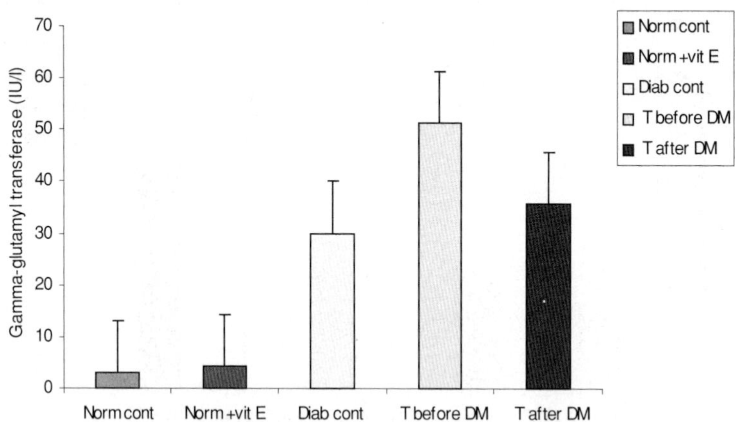

FIGURE 5. (**A**) Histograms showing the effect of 0.2 mg of vitamin E on plasma γ-GT level of normal and diabetic rats. Vitamin E (0.2 mg) induced a significant increase in the plasma γ-GT level in normal nondiabetic rats. $^{*}P < 0.05$ (norm cont versus norm + vitamin E). (Data are mean ± SD, $n = 6$.) DM = diabetes mellitus. (**B**) Histograms showing the effect of 0.4 mg of vitamin E on plasma γ-GT level of normal and diabetic rats. (Data are mean ± SD, $n = 6$.) DM = diabetes mellitus.

Plasma CRE Level

No significant changes in CRE level were observed in rats treated before and after the onset of diabetes. No change was observed in the plasma CRE level of normal and diabetic rats after oral administration of moderate dose of

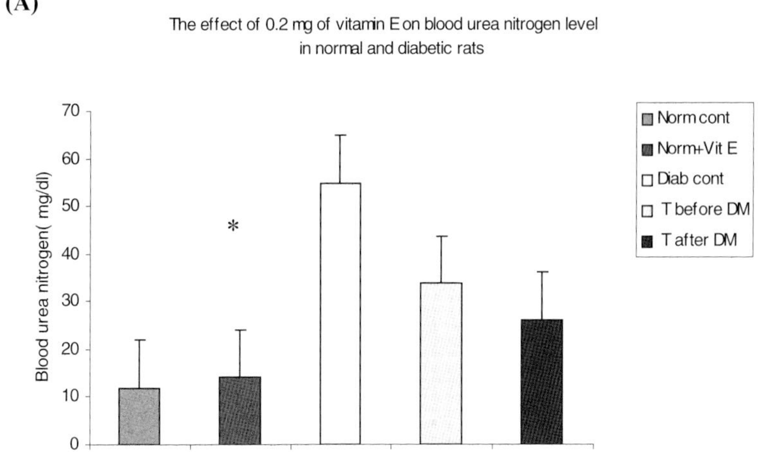

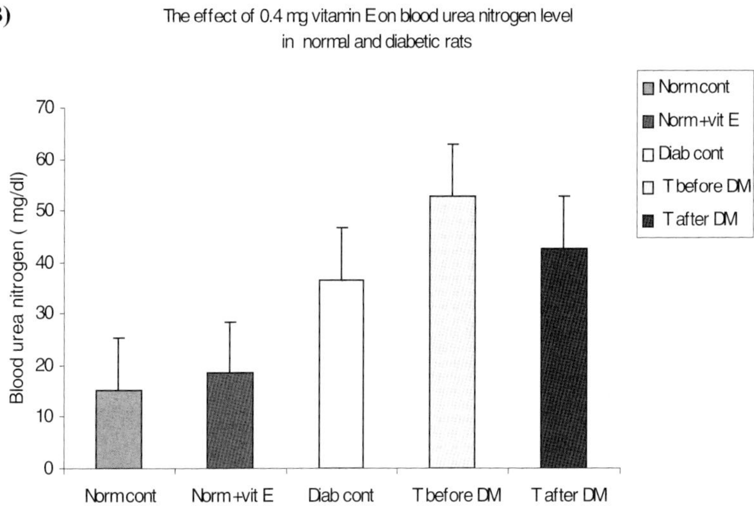

FIGURE 6. (**A**) Histograms showing the effect of 0.2 mg of vitamin E on BUN level of normal and diabetic rats. Vitamin E (0.2 mg) induced a significant increase in the BUN level of normal nondiabetic rats. $^{*}P < 0.05$ (norm cont versus norm + vitamin E). (Data are mean ± SD, $n = 6$.) DM = diabetes mellitus. (**B**) Histograms showing the effect of 0.4 mg of vitamin E on BUN level of normal and diabetic rats. (Data are mean ± SD, $n = 6$.) DM = diabetes mellitus.

vitamin E (FIG. 7). Also, after oral administration of high dose of vitamin E no significant change was observed in the plasma CRE level of normal rats. There was a decrease in the plasma CRE level of rats treated before and after the onset of diabetes. However, this decrease was not statistically significant (data not shown).

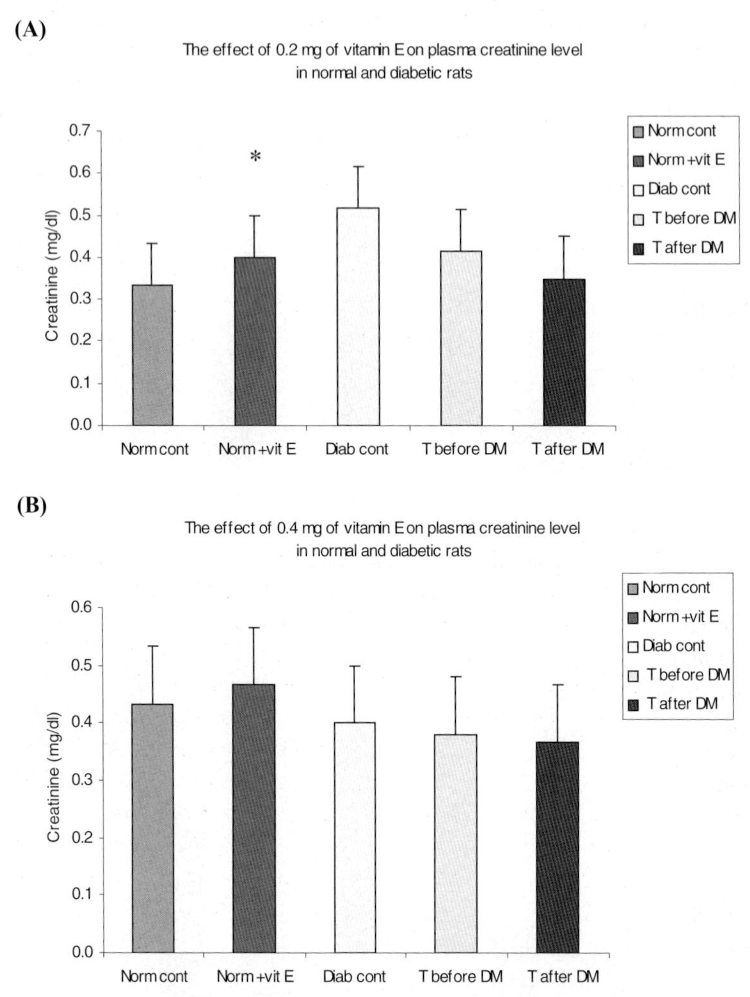

FIGURE 7. (**A**) Histograms showing the effect of 0.2 mg of vitamin E on plasma CRE level of normal and diabetic rats. Vitamin E (0.2 mg) induced a significant increase in the plasma CRE level of normal nondiabetic rats. $^*P < 0.05$ (norm cont versus norm + vitamin E). (Data are mean $\pm$ SD, $n = 6$.) DM = diabetes mellitus. (**B**) Histograms showing the effect of 0.4 mg of vitamin E on plasma CRE level of normal and diabetic rats. (Data are mean $\pm$ SD, $n = 6$.) DM = diabetes mellitus.

Effect of Vitamin E on the Electrolytes Level of Normal and Diabetic Rats

Plasma Calcium Level

STZ-induced diabetes caused large and significant increases in the plasma level of calcium. Low dose of vitamin E had no significant effect on plasma calcium level of normal rats. In contrast, low dose caused a significant ($P < 0.05$) increase in the plasma calcium level of rats treated for 10 days before the onset of diabetes. It also increased the plasma calcium level of rats treated after the onset of diabetes but without any statistical significance (FIG. 8). Moderate dose of vitamin E induced significant increases ($P < 0.002$) in plasma calcium level in normal rats when compared to normal untreated rats. On the other hand, the moderate dose reduced the plasma calcium level of rats treated before and after the onset of diabetes but without any statistical significance. The oral administration of high dose of vitamin E given 10 days before and after the onset of diabetes brought a small but not significant decrease in plasma calcium level. Also, the high dose failed to affect the plasma calcium level in normal rats (data not shown).

Plasma Phosphorus Level

There was no significant change in the plasma level of phosphorus after the onset of STZ-induced diabetes. FIGURE 9 shows the effect of low dose of vitamin E on plasma phosphorus level of normal rats. The result indicates that low dose of vitamin E failed to change the plasma phosphorus level in normal and diabetic rats. The moderate dose of vitamin E did not have any effect on the plasma phosphorus level of normal and rats treated for 10 days before the onset of diabetes. However, the moderate dose caused a significant decrease in the plasma phosphorus level of rats treated after the onset of diabetes compared to diabetic control. The oral administration of high dose of vitamin E did not have any significant effect on the plasma phosphorus level of normal rats and rats treated 10 days before the onset of diabetes. However, the high dose of vitamin E caused a significant increase in the plasma phosphorus level of rats treated after the onset of diabetes compared to diabetic control (data not shown).

Plasma Sodium Level

The plasma level of sodium decreased after the onset diabetes. Low dose of vitamin E affected the plasma sodium level in normal rats. In diabetic rats, the low dose of vitamin E caused significant increases in the plasma sodium level in rats treated before ($P < 0.02$) and after ($P < 0.005$) the onset of diabetes. The moderate dose of vitamin E also caused significant ($P < 0.003$) reduction in the plasma sodium level of rats treated 10 days after the onset of diabetes. There was an increase in the plasma sodium level of normal rats without any statistical significance (FIG. 10). In rats treated with high dose of vitamin E before and after the onset of diabetes the level of sodium was slightly increased when compared to control (data not shown).

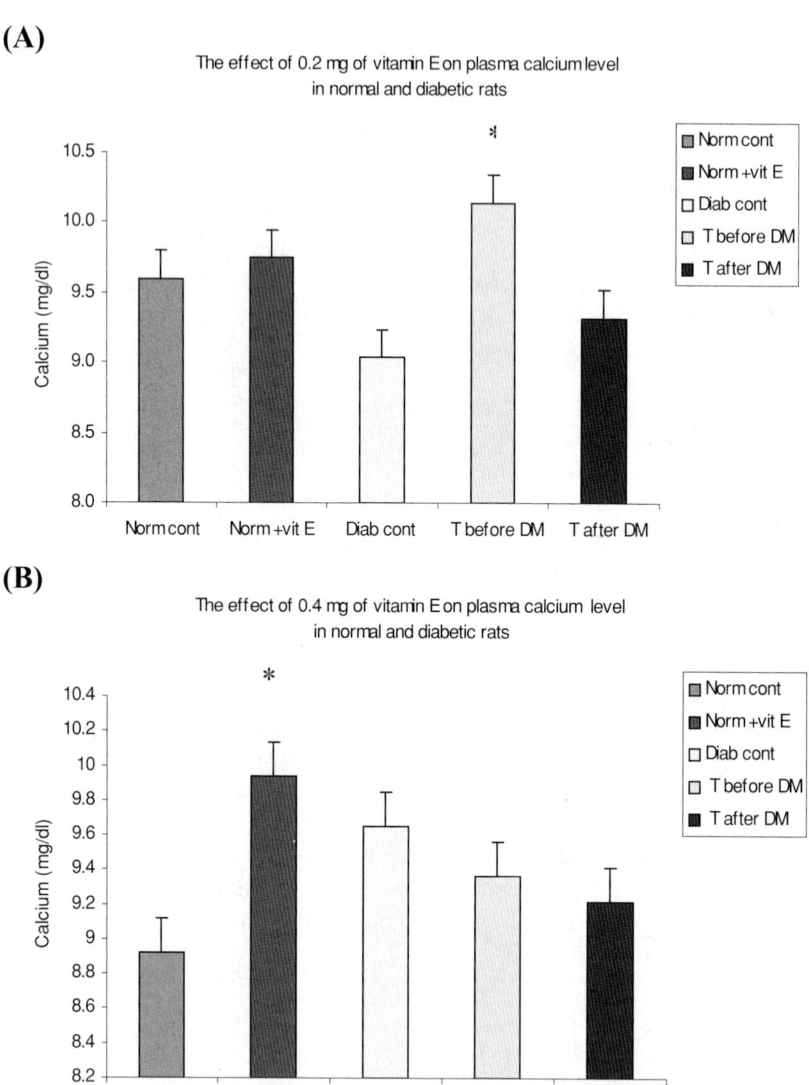

FIGURE 8. (**A**) Histograms showing the effect of 0.2 mg of vitamin E on plasma calcium level of normal and diabetic rats. Vitamin E (0.2 mg) induced a significant increase on the plasma calcium level in rats treated before the onset of diabetes mellitus. $^*P < 0.05$ (diabetes cont versus treated before DM). (Data are mean $\pm$ SD, $n = 6$.) DM = diabetes mellitus. (**B**) Histograms showing the effect of 0.4 mg of vitamin E on plasma calcium level of normal and diabetic rats. Vitamin E (0.4 mg) induced a significant increase in the plasma calcium level of normal nondiabetic rats. $^*P < 0.05$ (norm cont versus norm + vitamin E). (Data are mean $\pm$ SD, $n = 6$.) DM = diabetes mellitus.

(A)

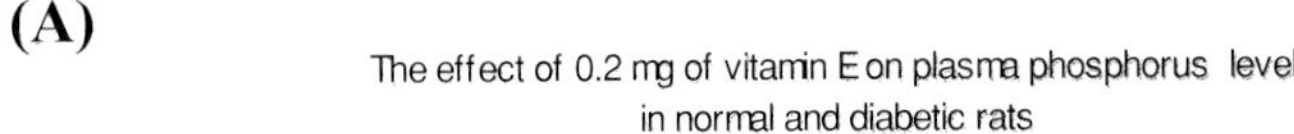

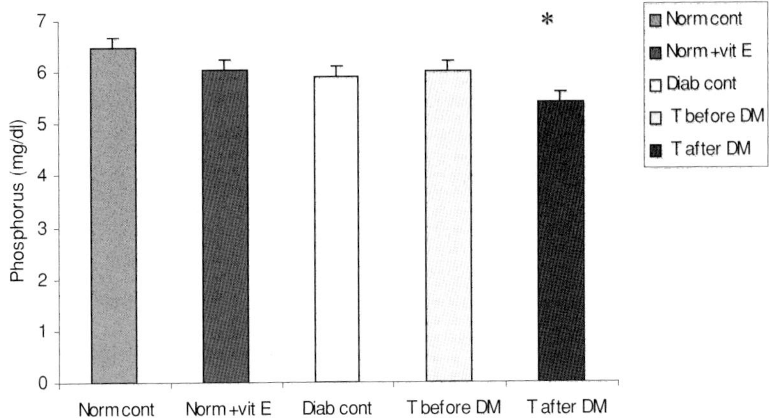

(B)

The effect of 0.4 mg/kg of vitamin E on plasma phosphorus level in normal and diabetic rats

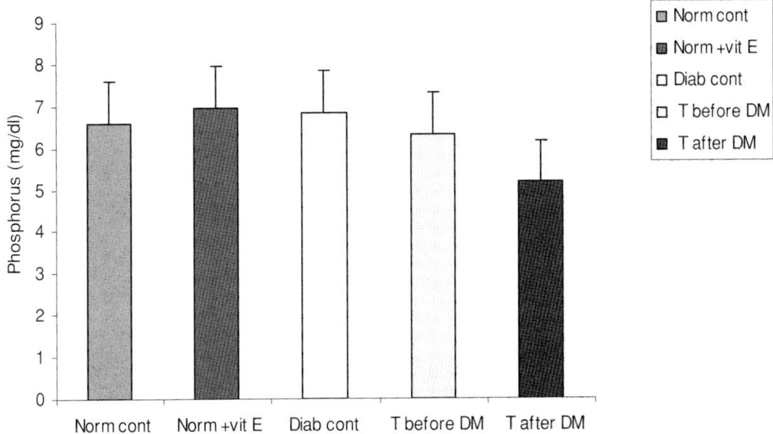

FIGURE 9. (**A**) Histograms showing the effect of 0.2 mg of vitamin E on plasma phosphorus level of normal and diabetic rats. Vitamin E (0.2 mg) induced a significant decrease in the plasma phorphorus level of rats treated after the onset of DM. $^*P < 0.05$ (diab cont versus treated after DM). (Data are mean ± SD, $n = 6$.) DM = diabetes mellitus. (**B**) Histograms showing the effect of 0.4 mg of vitamin E on plasma phosphorus level of normal and diabetic rats. (Data are mean ± SD, $n = 6$.) DM = diabetes mellitus.

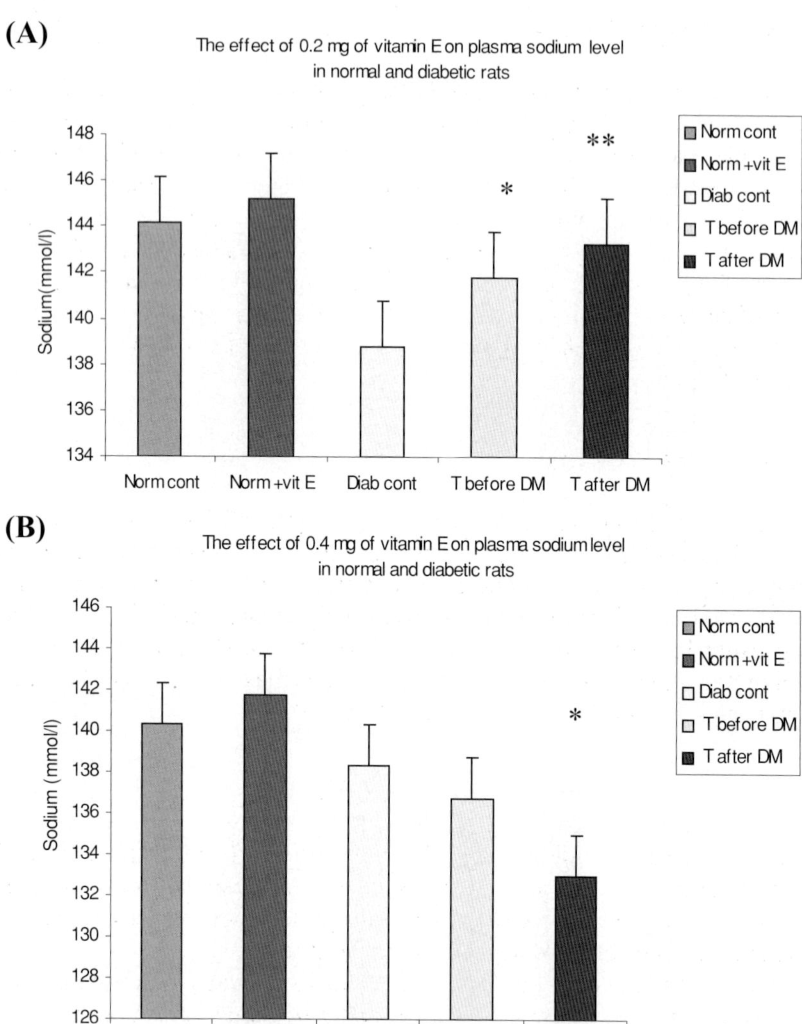

FIGURE 10. (**A**) Histograms showing the effect of 0.2 mg of vitamin E on plasma sodium level of normal and diabetic rats. Vitamin E (0.2 mg) induced a significant increase in the plasma sodium level in rats treated before and after the onset of diabetes mellitus. $^{*}P < 0.05$ (diabetes cont versus treated before DM); $^{**}P < 0.05$ (diabetes cont versus treated after DM). (Data are mean $\pm$ SD, $n = 6$.) DM = diabetes mellitus. (**B**) Histograms showing the effect of 0.4 mg of vitamin E on plasma sodium level of normal and diabetic rats. Vitamin E (0.4 mg) induced a significant decrease in the plasma sodium level in rats treated after the onset of DM. $^{*}P < 0.05$ (diabetes cont versus treated after DM). (Data are mean $\pm$ SD, $n = 6$.) DM = diabetes.

Plasma Potassium Level

There was no significant change in the plasma level of potassium after the onset of diabetes. The result shows that low dose of vitamin E has no effect on the plasma potassium level of normal rats and rats treated after the onset of diabetes. However, the low dose of vitamin E increased plasma potassium level of rats treated before the onset of diabetes. This increase did not reach statistical significance. The oral administration of moderate doses of vitamin E increased the plasma potassium level of normal and rats treated before the onset of diabetes (FIG. 11). High doses of vitamin E significantly increased the level of potassium in rats treated before and after the onset of diabetes without statistical significance (data not shown).

Plasma Magnesium Level

The plasma level of magnesium increased slightly after the induction of diabetes. The result indicates that low dose of vitamin E had no effect on plasma magnesium level of normal and diabetic rats. Moreover, the oral administration of moderate dose of vitamin E has no significant effect on the plasma magnesium level of normal and diabetic rats (FIG. 12). The oral administration of high dose of vitamin E had no effect on the plasma magnesium level of both normal and diabetic treated rats (data not shown).

DISCUSSION

Liver enzymes including ALT, AST, ALP, and γ-GT reflect different functions of the liver, such as excretion of anions, hepatocellular integration, formation, and subsequent free flow of bile and protein synthesis. ALT and AST are important indicators of hepatocellular damage.[14]

AST is found in several organs, such as the liver, brain, kidney, lungs, and pancreas, and it is present in cytosolic and mitochondrial enzymes. In this study the plasma level of AST increased after the onset of diabetes mellitus. Only treatment with low dose of vitamin E significantly reduced the AST level in rats treated 10 days after the onset of diabetes. The reason for the inability of other doses to significantly increase or decrease the level of AST in normal and diabetic rats is not clear.

ALT is more specific to liver and it is present in cytosolic enzyme. It is found in large quantities in the liver. The plasma level of ALT increased after the onset of diabetes mellitus. In contrast, the oral administration of low dose of vitamin E significantly decreased ALT in the plasma in rats treated 10 days before and after the onset of diabetes.

The hepatocellular injury is the trigger for the release of these enzymes into the circulation. The increase in the plasma level of these liver enzymes

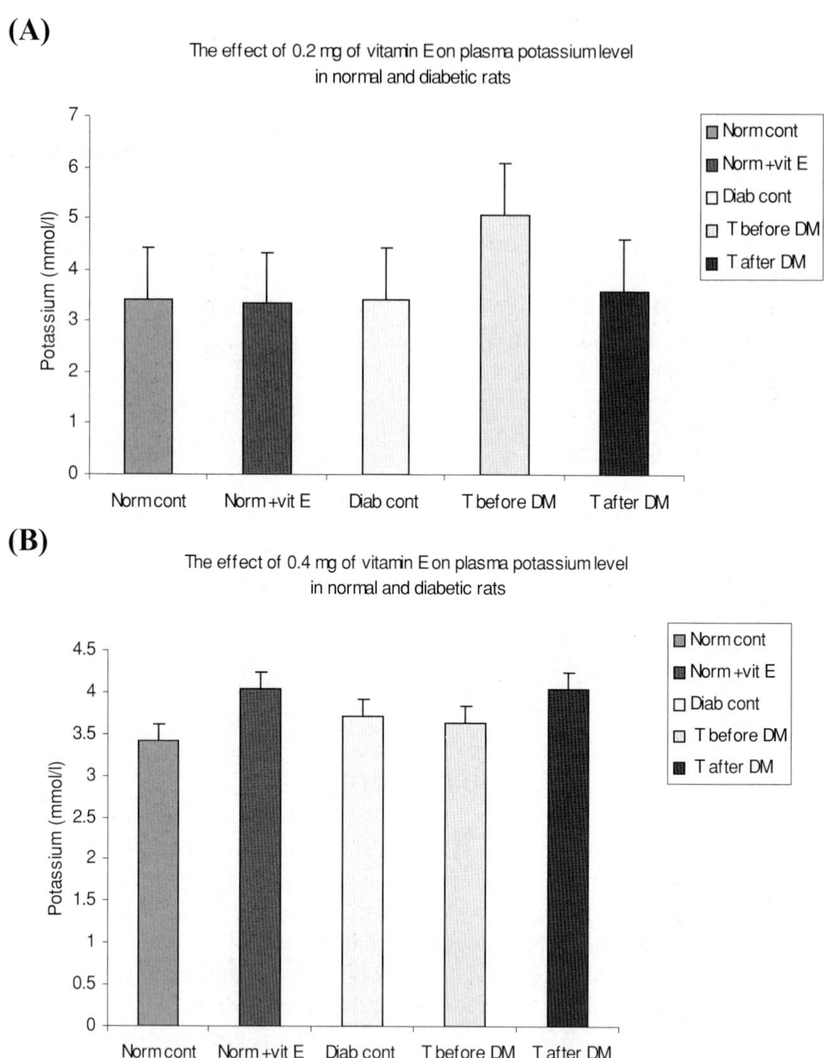

FIGURE 11. (**A**) Histograms showing the effect of 0.2 mg of vitamin E on plasma potassium level of normal and diabetic rats. (Data are mean ± SD, $n = 6$.) DM= diabetes mellitus. (**B**) Histograms showing the effect of 0.4 mg of vitamin E on plasma potassium level of normal and diabetic rats. (Data are mean ± SD, $n = 6$.) DM = diabetes mellitus.

shows that STZ had a toxic effect on the liver. Treatment with low dose of vitamin E reduced this toxic effect on the liver of diabetic rats. Moreover, this result indicated that low dose of vitamin E is more effective than moderate and high doses on plasma AST and ALT, and this may be due to what was reported previously, that the use of high single doses of micronutrient antioxidant

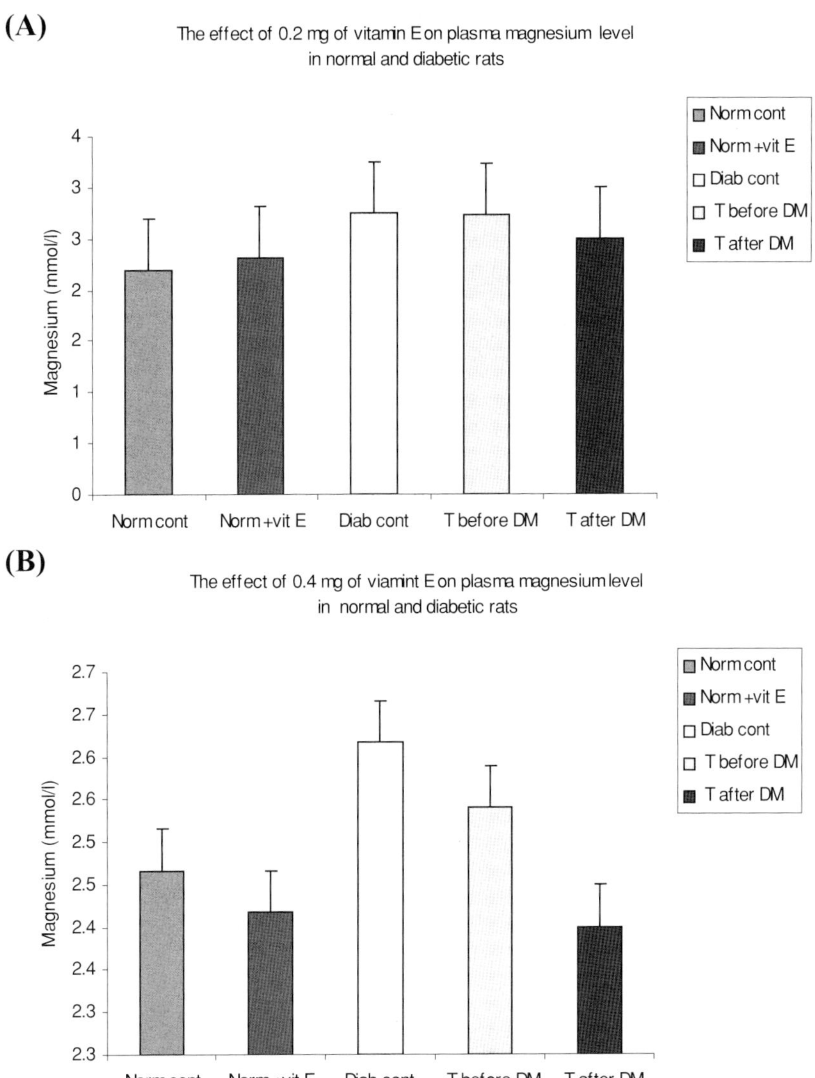

FIGURE 12. (**A**) Histograms showing the effect of 0.2 mg of vitamin E on plasma magnesium level of normal and diabetic rats. (Data are mean ± SD, $n = 6$.) DM = diabetes mellitus. (**B**) Histograms showing the effect of 0.4 mg of vitamin E on plasma magnesium level of normal and diabetic rats. (Data are mean ± SD, $n = 6$.) DM = diabetes mellitus.

supplements, such as vitamin E, poses potential risks because it could perturb the antioxidant–proxidant balance. It has been recommended that high doses of micronutrient antioxidant vitamins should be administered in combination rather than in single supplements.[15]

The plasma ALP level also increased after the onset of diabetes. ALP originates mainly from two sources, the liver and bone, and it may be present in many other tissues, such as the intestine, kidney, placenta, and blood. Hepatic ALP is present in the canalicular and luminal domain of bile duct epithelium and its level rises as a result of increased synthesis. The level of ALP may not rise until 2 days after biliary obstruction.[14] The oral administration of low doses of vitamin E caused a slight but not significant decrease in the ALP level in rats treated 10 days after the onset of diabetes. The plasma level of ALP increased significantly after the administration of low dose of vitamin E in normal nondiabetic rats.

The data obtained from this study show that low doses of vitamin E had a significant lowering effect on LDH level in normal rats. On the other hand, the LDH level in rats treated 10 days after the onset of diabetes is slightly similar to the level in normal rats. The oral administration of high dose of vitamin E significantly increased LDH level.

γ-GT is found in hepatocytes and biliary epithelial cells. Its level is raised in pancreatic disease, renal failure, and diabetes.[14] There was a significant increase in the γ-GT level in diabetic rats. After the oral administration of vitamin E there was a slight but not significant reduction in γ-GT level in rats treated either before or after the onset of diabetes. This means that treatment with vitamin E did have some beneficial effect on decreasing γ-GT level in diabetic rats.

Diabetes increased the BUN and plasma CRE level in rats. Elevated levels of BUN and CRE have been documented in experimental[16] and human[17] diabetes. Low dose of vitamin E caused a slight but not significant reduction in BUN and CRE level.

CONCLUSION

This study showed that liver enzymes, kidney parameters, and electrolytes are elevated during STZ-induced diabetes. The administration of vitamin E reduced the level of some of these enzymes. The results obtained from this study have provided insight into some of the hypoglycemic effects of vitamin E. Vitamin E may thus be a useful adjuvant therapy in the management of diabetes mellitus.

REFERENCES

1. Adeghate, E. 2001. Diabetes mellitus-multifactorial in aetiology and global in prevalence. Arch. Physiol. Biochem. **109:** 197–199.
2. Ishii, H.M., R. Jirousek, D. Koya, *et al*. 1996. Amelioration of vascular dysfunctions in diabetic rats by an oral PKC an inhibitor. Science **272:** 728–731.

3. Brownlee, M., A. Cerami & H. Vlassara. 1988. Advanced glycosylation end products in tissue and the biochemical basis of diabetic complications. N. Engl. J. Med. **318:** 1315–1321.
4. Nishio, Y., A. Kashiwagi, H. Taki, *et al.* 1998. Altered activities of transcription factors and their related gene expression in cardiac tissues of diabetic rats. Diabetes **47:** 1318–1325.
5. Ceriello, A. 2003. New insights on oxidative stress and diabetic complications may lead to a "causal" antioxidant therapy. Diabetes Care **26:** 1589–1596.
6. Young, A.J. & G.M. Lowe. 2001. Antioxidant and prooxidant properties of carotenoids. Arch. Biochem. Biophys. **385:** 20–27.
7. Betteridge, D.J. 2000. What is oxidative stress? Metabolism **49:** 3–8.
8. McGee, S.A., S.A. Wiggins & J.D. Pierce. 2003. What advanced practice nurses need to know about free radicals. J. Adv. Nurs. Pract. **6:** 210–217.
9. Drew, K.L., P.M. Tøien, M.A. Rivera, *et al.* 2002. Role of the antioxidant ascorbate in hibernation and warming from hibernation. Comp. Biochem. Phys. **133:** 483–492.
10. Shapiro, S.S. & C. Saliou. 2001. Role of vitamins in skin care. Nutrition **17:** 839–844.
11. Wang, X. & P.J. Quinn. 2000. The location and function of vitamin E in membranes. Mol. Membr. Biol. **17:** 143–156.
12. Eitenmiller, R. & W.O. Laneden Jr. 1998. Vitamin Analysis for the Health and Food Sciences. CRC Press. Boca Raton, FL.
13. Adeghate, E. 1999. Effect of subcutaneous pancreatic tissue transplants on streptozotocin-induced diabetes in rats. Tissue Cell **31:** 73–83.
14. Limidi, J.K. & G.M. Hyde. 2003. Evaluation of abnormal liver function tests. Postgrad. Med. J. **79:** 307–312.
15. Opara, E.C. 2002. Oxidative stress, micronutrients, diabetes mellitus and its complications. J. Roy. Soc. Health **122:** 28–34.
16. Yousef, W.M., A.H. Omar, N.M. Ghanayem, *et al.* 2006. Effect of some calcium channel blockers in experimentally induced diabetic nephropathy in rats. Int. J. Diabetes Metab. **14:** 39–49.
17. Aviles-Santa, L., R. Alpern & P. Raskin. 2002. Reversible acute renal failure and nephrotic syndrome in a type 1 diabetic patient. J. Diabetes Complications **16:** 249–254.

Vitamin E Decreases the Hyperglucagonemia of Diabetic Rats

MARIAM AL SHAMSI,[a] AMR AMIN,[b] AND ERNEST ADEGHATE[a]

[a]*Department of Anatomy, Faculty of Medicine and Health Sciences, UAE University, Al Ain, United Arab Emirates*

[b]*Department of Biology, Faculty of Science, UAE University, Al Ain, United Arab Emirates*

ABSTRACT: Vitamin E has the ability to scavenge a wide spectrum of free radicals, including singlet oxygen, superoxide, and hydroxyl radicals. It has beneficial effects against several other disorders, such as atherosclerosis and ischemic heart disease, because it acts as a transcriptional regulator for gene expression via a transcription factor TAP. The beneficial effect of vitamin E on plasma insulin and glucagon levels was examined using radioimmunoassay technique. Diabetes was induced in rats by a single intraperitoneal injection of streptozotocin at a dose of 60 mg/kg body weight. Vitamin E was given at a dose of either 0.2 mg, 0.4 mg, or 0.8 mg per animal 10 days before and after the onset of diabetes. Vitamin E significantly ($P < 0.05$) increased plasma insulin levels in normal rats but failed to increase the plasma insulin level in diabetic rats. In contrast, vitamin E caused a significant ($P < 0.05$) reduction in plasma glucagon level in rats treated before and after the onset of diabetes. Vitamin E may ameliorate some diabetic complication via reduction in the level of circulating glucagon.

KEYWORDS: radioimmunoassay; diabetes; insulin; hyperglucagonemia, rat

INTRODUCTION

Vitamin E is a lipid-soluble radical scavenger that rapidly oxidizes in atmospheric oxygen.[1] These properties of α-tocopherol limit its therapeutic application. Vitamin E has the ability to scavenge a wide spectrum of free radicals, including singlet oxygen, superoxide, and hydroxyl radicals.[2] Vitamin E does

Address for correspondence: Ernest Adeghate, M.D., M.F.M., Ph.D., Department of Anatomy, Faculty of Medicine and Health Sciences, UAE University, P.O. Box 17666, Al Ain, United Arab Emirates. Voice: 971-3-7137496; fax: 971-3-7672033.
e-mail: eadeghate@uaeu.ac.ae

Ann. N.Y. Acad. Sci. 1084: 432–441 (2006). © 2006 New York Academy of Sciences.
doi: 10.1196/annals.1372.032

not function as an antioxidant only, it has a great benefit against several disorders, such as atherosclerosis, ischemic heart disease, and tumors,[3,4] because it acts as a transcriptional regulator for gene expression via a transcription factor TAP.[5] Diabetes mellitus is associated with increase in the number of glucagon immunoreactive cells in pancreatic islet cells[6] with a concomitant hyperglucagonemia, a contributory factor in the development of short- and long-term complications of diabetes,[7] and it is a regular factor of the metabolic derangement.[8] Hyperglucagonemia has also been implicated in insulin resistance.[9] The streptozotocin (STZ)-induced diabetes is a model of type I diabetes that is characterized by islet inflammation and subsequent destruction of β cells. Moreover, free radicals have been implicated in the pathogenesis of type I diabetes. The aim of this article was to investigate the effect of vitamin E on the plasma level of insulin and glucagon before and after the onset of diabetes.

MATERIALS AND METHODS

Male Wistar rats weighting 200–300 g were obtained from the Faculty of Medicine and Health Sciences, United Arab Emirates University. All rats were housed in a temperature- (25°C) and humidity-controlled room, with 12-h light–dark periods. The animals were fed standard rat chow and tap water *ad libitum*.

Induction of Experimental Diabetes

Diabetes was induced in rats by a single intraperitoneal injection of STZ in (Sigma, St. Louis, MO) at a dose of 60 mg/kg body weight.[10]

Experimental Design

Rats were randomly divided into three groups according to three different doses of vitamin E (low, 0.2 mg; moderate, 0.4 mg; and high, 0.8 mg). Each of these groups were divided into five subgroups of six animals each: Group I served as normal untreated group, where the rats had not been treated either with STZ or with vitamin E. Group II served as diabetic control, that is, STZ-induced diabetic rats that were not treated with vitamin E. Group III served as diabetic treated group, where the rats were treated with three different doses (low, moderate, and high) of vitamin E for 10 days prior to the STZ induction of diabetes. Group IV also served as a diabetic treated group. This group was given STZ to induce diabetes, and 10 days after induction of diabetes it was treated with the three different doses—low, moderate, and high—of vitamin E.

Group V served as normal nondiabetic treated group. This group was treated with the three different doses of vitamin E only. Rats were treated orally by intubation tube.

Radioimmunoassay

Insulin Assay

All test samples and controls were assayed in duplicates. Insulin measurement was performed using LINCO Research Inc. (St. Charles, MO) radioimmunoassay kits. The procedure was conducted as described in the kit manual. Briefly, a volume of 200 μL of either calibrator controls or test samples were pipetted to previously labeled tubes. After this, 100 μL of hydrated ^{125}I-insulin was added to all tubes and then 100 μL of rat insulin antibody to all tubes was added except the total count and nonspecific binding (NSB) tubes and then vortexed. After vortexing, the tubes were covered with parafilm and incubated for 24 h at 4°C. On the following day, a volume of 1 mL of cold (4°C) precipitating reagent was added to all tubes except the total count tubes. Then the tubes were vortexed and incubated for 20 min at 4°C. After incubation all tubes except the total count tube were centrifuged for 20 min at 2000*g* at 4°C. The tubes were decanted gently and radioactivity was counted for 1 min using a gamma counter (Beckman, Fullerton, CA). Results were analyzed by using Beckman Immunofit EIA/RIA analysis software, version 2.00 and values were expressed in ng/mL.

Glucagon Assay

All test samples and controls were assayed in duplicates. Glass tubes were used for this assay because it has been shown that glucagon adheres onto plastic surfaces. Glucagon measurement was performed using LINCO Research Inc. radioimmunoassay kits. The procedure was conducted as described in the kit manual. Briefly, a volume of 200 μL of calibrator, control, or sample was pipetted into previously labeled tubes. After this, 100 μL of glucagon antiserum was added to all tubes except the NSB and total count tubes and vortexed. After vortexing, the tubes were covered with parafilm and incubated for 24 h at 4°C. After the first incubation, 100 μL of ^{125}I-glucagon was added to all tubes and vortexed. The samples were incubated for 24 h at 4°C. On the following day, a volume of 1 mL of cold (4°C) precipitating reagent was added to all tubes except the total count and centrifuged for 15 min at 1500*g* at 4°C. The tubes were decanted gently and radioactivity was counted for 1 min using a gamma counter (Beckman). Results were analyzed by using Beckman Immunofit EIA/RIA analysis software, version 2.00 and values were expressed in pg/mL.

Statistical Analyses

Data are expressed as the mean ± SD. Student's *t*-test was used to analyze the significance of differences between mean values, and different groups were analyzed by analysis of variance using Duncan's multiple range tests. A *P* value of less than 0.05 was considered statistically significant.

RESULTS

Plasma Insulin Level

FIGURE 1 shows the plasma insulin level in treated and untreated normal, and treated and untreated diabetic rats. Untreated diabetes is associated with low plasma levels of insulin. Low dose (0.2 mg) of vitamin E failed to increase the plasma insulin level when given to normal rats. Similarly, there was no significant difference in the insulin level of rats given 0.2 mg of vitamin E before the onset of diabetes. The level of insulin was further reduced in diabetic rats treated after the onset of diabetes when compared with untreated diabetic rats.

As shown in FIGURE 2, the plasma insulin level increased in normal rats treated with a moderate dose (0.4 mg) of vitamin E when compared to normal

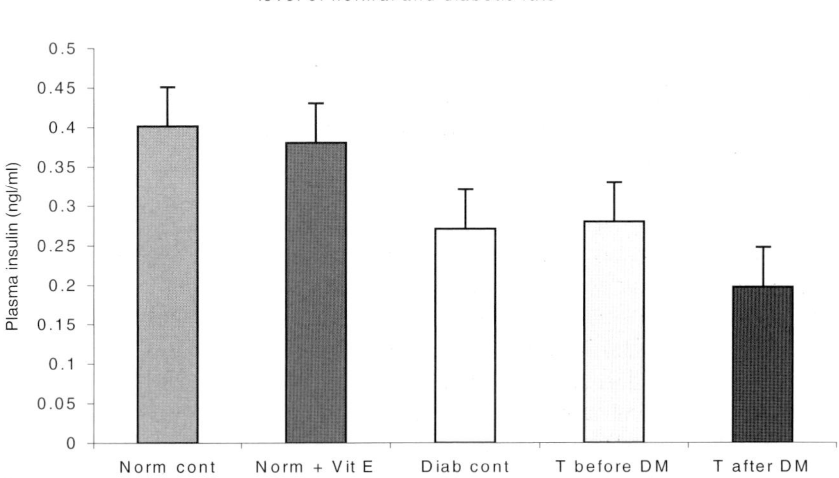

FIGURE 1. Histograms showing the effect of 0.2 mg of vitamin E on plasma insulin level of normal and diabetic rats. Vitamin E did not improve the plasma insulin level compared to control. (Data are mean ± SD, $n = 6$.) DM = diabetes mellitus.

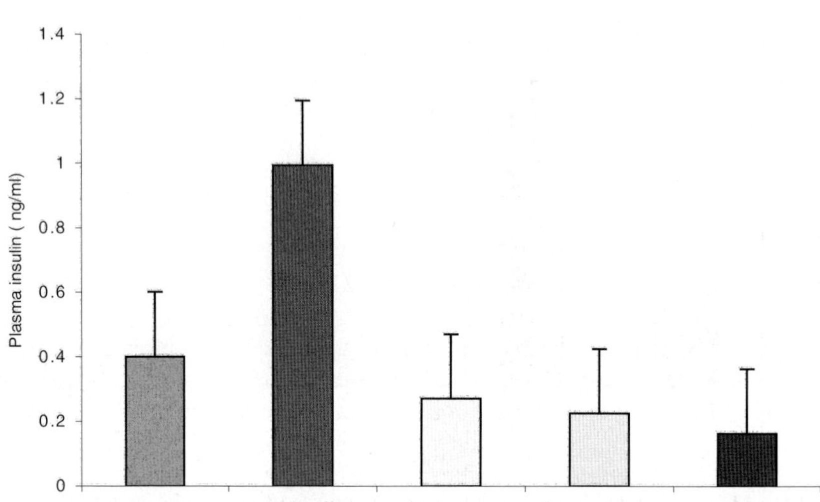

FIGURE 2. Histograms showing the effect of 0.4 mg of vitamin E on plasma insulin level of normal and diabetic rats. Vitamin E increased plasma insulin level in normal but not in diabetic rats. (Data are mean ± SD, $n = 6$.) DM = diabetes mellitus.

control. However, the increase in the plasma insulin level was not statistically significant. The level of plasma insulin was significantly reduced after the onset of diabetes. Moderate dose (0.4 mg) of vitamin E failed to increase the plasma insulin level when given to rats before and after the onset of diabetes. High dose (0.8 mg) of vitamin E also induced an increase in the plasma insulin level in normal nondiabetic rats. However, this increase was not statistically different compared to control (FIG. 3). In diabetic rats, the administration of a high dose of vitamin E did not improve plasma insulin level.

Plasma Glucagon Level

FIGURE 4 shows the effect of the low dose of 0.2 mg of vitamin E on plasma glucagon level of normal and diabetic rats. There was no difference between the plasma glucagon level of normal untreated rats and normal treated rats. The plasma glucagon level of untreated diabetic rats was significantly higher compared to normal. Low dose of vitamin E reduced the plasma glucagon level in rats treated before and after onset of diabetes rats but without statistical significance.

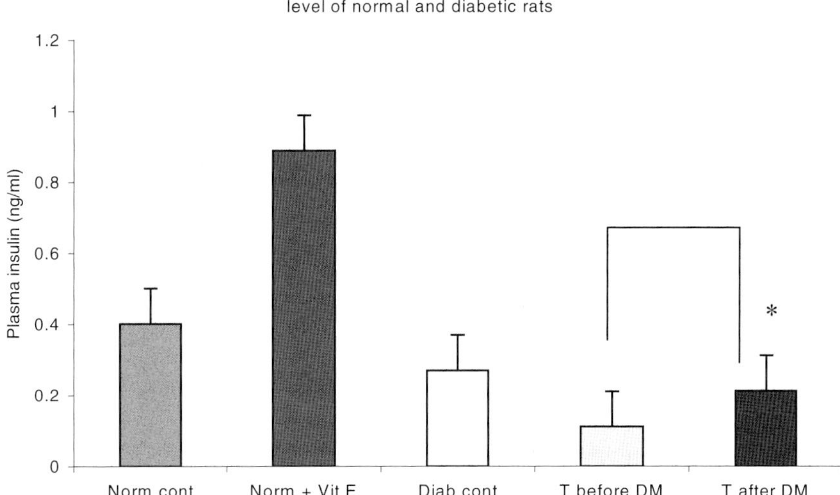

FIGURE 3. Histograms showing the effect of 0.8 mg of vitamin E on plasma insulin level of normal and diabetic rats. Vitamin E increased plasma insulin level in normal but not in diabetic rats.*$P < 0.05$ treated before DM versus treated after DM. (Data are mean $\pm$ SD, $n = 6$.) DM= diabetes mellitus.

As shown in FIGURE 5, the moderate dose (0.4 mg) of vitamin E increased the plasma glucagon level in normal rats. In contrast, moderate dose of vitamin E significantly ($P < 0.0073$) reduce the plasma glucagon level in rats treated before and after the onset of diabetes. The administration of a high dose (0.8 mg) of vitamin E caused a slight but not significant increase in plasma glucagon level in normal rats. In contrast, the high dose of vitamin E induced a significant ($P < 0.02$) reduction in the plasma level of glucagon when given before or after the onset of diabetes (FIG. 6).

DISCUSSION

Plasma Insulin Level

Hyperglycemia is widely known to be a cause of increased free radical concentration in diabetic subjects.[11] Antioxidants, such as vitamin E, have been shown to improve insulin action in healthy, elderly, and non–insulin-dependent diabetes.[11] Our study showed that vitamin E can cause increases in the plasma level of insulin in normal rats. Moreover, vitamin E can induce an increase in the number of insulin-immunoreactive cells in the pancreas

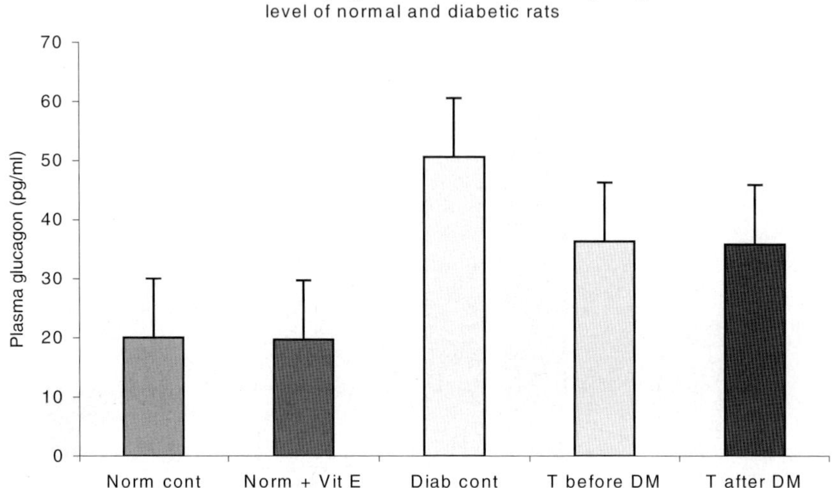

FIGURE 4. Histograms showing the effect of 0.2 mg of vitamin E on plasma glucagon level of normal and diabetic rats. Vitamin E at 0.2 mg caused a slight but not significant reduction in plasma glucagon level compared to control. (Data are mean ± SD, $n = 6$.) DM = diabetes mellitus.

of diabetic rats (personal observation). However, vitamin E failed to increase plasma insulin level when given to diabetic rats before or after the onset of diabetes. Reports by Gokkusu *et al.*[12] showed that vitamin E improved β cell function and increased plasma insulin level in type II diabetic patients. Our observation on type I diabetes and that of Gokkusu *et al.*[12] on type II diabetes indicate that vitamin E is most effective on intact or nearly intact pancreatic β cells. In addition, other reports show that vitamin E has a protective effect on β cell.[13] Others have shown that vitamin E deficiency causes glucose intolerance via disturbance in insulin sensitivity and secretion.[14] In this study, the reason for the lack of improvement in the plasma insulin level of diabetic rats after the administration of vitamin E may be due to the fact that most of the β cells have been lost after the induction of type I diabetes. It is widely known that type I diabetes is associate with more β cell destruction compared to type II. Thus, vitamin E has fewer β cells upon which to act compared to that of type II. Another reason for the failure of vitamin E to increase plasma insulin level is the dosage. The dosage used in this experiment may be inadequate. The moderate and high doses of vitamin E have the beneficial effects of increasing the number of insulin-positive cells in diabetic rats (data not included). The mechanism by which vitamin E causes the increase in the number of insulin-positive cells is unknown. However, this increase in the number of insulin-positive cells may be due the ability of vitamin E to reduce the toxic effect of

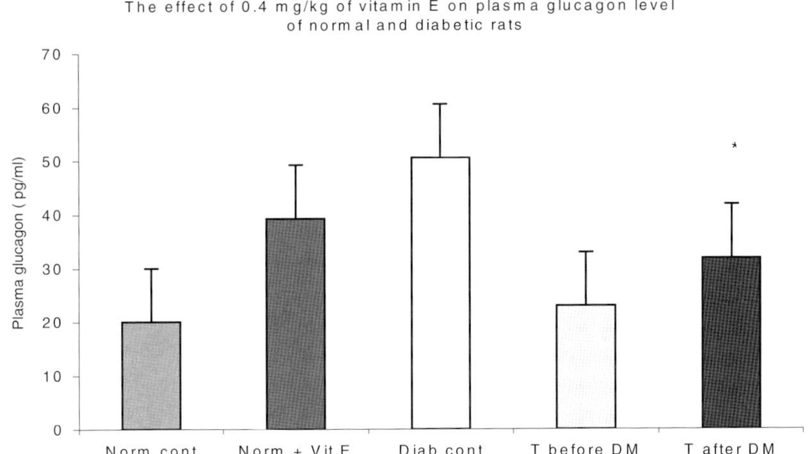

FIGURE 5. Histograms showing the effect of 0.4 mg of vitamin E on plasma glucagon level of normal and diabetic rats. Vitamin E caused a significant decrease in the plasma glucagon level of rats treated before and after the onset of DM rats, $^*P < 0.05$ (diab cont versus treated). (Data are mean $\pm$ SD, $n = 6$.) DM = diabetes mellitus.

STZ on β cell and it may also help in the regeneration of pancreatic β cells damaged by STZ.

Plasma Glucagon Level

The role of glucagon in the development of short- and long-term complications of diabetes has often been neglected. It is widely known that glucagon (hyperglucagonemia) increases glucose output via protein kinase that inhibits glycogen synthesis.[15] In addition, glucagon facilitates glycogenolysis and inhibits the conversion of phosphoenolpyruvate to pyruvate. It also decreases the level of fructose 2,6-diphosphate, which in turn inhibits the conversion of fructose 6-phosphate to fructose 1,6-diphosphate.[15] The resultant accumulation of glucose 6-phosphate leads to increased release of glucose into the bloodstream. The result of this study showed that vitamin E consistently reduced the hyperglucagonemia of diabetic rats treated before and after the onset of diabetes. The reduction was effective with all of the three (0.2 mg, 0.4 mg, 0.8 mg) doses of vitamin E used. The reduction was most significant with higher doses of vitamin E. It is not clear how and by what mechanism vitamin E reduces the plasma level of glucagon in diabetic rats. The reduction of plasma level of glucagon will thus have a beneficial effect on hyperglycemia and other complications that arise from it.

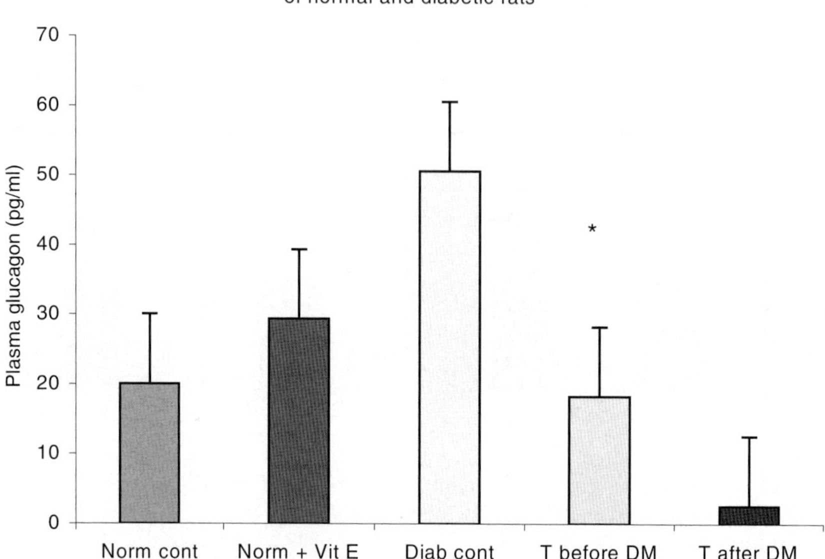

FIGURE 6. Histograms showing the effect of 0.8 mg of vitamin E on plasma glucagon level of normal and diabetic rats. Vitamin E caused a significant decrease in the plasma glucagon level of rats treated before and after the onset of DM rats, $^{*}P < 0.05$ (diab cont versus treated). (Data are mean ± SD, $n = 6$.) DM = diabetes mellitus.

REFERENCES

1. AZZI, A., R. GYSIN, P. KEMPNA, *et al.* 2004. Vitamin E mediates cell signaling and regulation of gene expression. Ann. N. Y. Acad. Sci. **1031:** 86–95.
2. SHAPIRO, S.S. & C. SALIOU. 2001. Role of vitamins in skin care. Nutrition **17:** 839–844.
3. AZZI, A., R. RICCIARELLI & J.M. ZINGG. 2002. Non-antioxidant molecular function of α-tocopherol (vitamin E). FEBS Lett. **519:** 8–10.
4. DRISKO, J.A., J. CHAPMAN & V.J. HUNTER. 2003. The use of antioxidant therapies during chemotherapy. Gynecol. Oncol. **88:** 434–439.
5. YAMAUCHI, J., T. IWAMOTO, S. KIDA, *et al.* 2001. Tocopherol-associated protein is a ligand dependent transcriptional activator. Biochem. Biophys. Res. Commun. **285:** 295–299.
6. ADEGHATE, E., A.S. PONERY, D.J. PALLOT & J. SINGH. 2000. Distribution of neurotransmitters and their effects on glucagon secretion from thc in vitro normal and diabetic pancreatic tissues. Tissue Cell **32:** 266–274.
7. ADEGHATE, E. 1999. Effect of subcutaneous pancreatic tissue transplants on streptozotocin-induced diabetes in rats, II: endocrine and metabolic functions. Tissue Cell **31:** 73–83.
8. YASUDA, H., Y. HARANO, K. KOSUGI *et al.* 1984. Development of early lesions of microangiopathy in chronically diabetic monkeys. Diabetes **33:** 415–420.

9. Raddatz, D., C. Rossbach, A. Buchwald, *et al.* 2005. Fasting hyperglucagonemia in patients with transjugular intrahepatic portosystemic shunts (TIPS). Exp. Clin. Endocrinol. Diabetes **113:** 268–274.
10. Ahmed, I., E. Adeghate, A.K. Sharma, *et al.* 1998. Effects of *Momordica charantia* fruit juice on islet morphology in the pancreas of streptozotocin-induced diabetic rats. Diabetes Res. Clin. Pract. **40:** 145–151.
11. Ceriello, A. 2000. Oxidative stress and glycemic regulation. Metabolism **49:** 27–29.
12. Gokkusu, C., S. Palanduz, E. Ademoglu & S. Tamer 2001. Oxidant and antioxidant systems in NIDDM patients: influence of vitamin E supplementation. Endocr. Res. **27:** 377–386.
13. Crino, A., R. Schiaffini, S. Manfrini, *et al.* & IMDIAB group. 2004. A randomized trial of nicotinamide and vitamin E in children with recent onset type 1 diabetes (IMDIAB IX). Eur. J. Endocrinol. **150:** 719–724.
14. Tsujinaka, K., T. Nakamura, H. Maegawa, *et al.* 2005. Diet high in lipid hydroperoxide by vitamin E deficiency induces insulin resistance and impaired insulin secretion in normal rats. Diabetes Res. Clin. Pract. **67:** 99–109.
15. Ganong, W.F. 1989. Endocrine functions of the pancreas and the regulation of carbohydrate metabolism. *In* Review of Medical Physiology. W. F. Ganong, Ed.: 280–300. Appleton and Lange. Connecticut.

Contraction and Cation Contents of Skeletal Soleus and EDL Muscles in Age-Matched Control and Diabetic Rats

APURVA CHONKAR,[a] RICHARD HOPKIN,[a] ERNEST ADEGHATE,[b] AND JAIPAUL SINGH[a]

[a]*Department of Biological Sciences, University of Central Lancashire, Preston, Lancashire, PR1 2HE UK*

[b]*Department of Human Anatomy, FMHS, United Arab Emirates University, Al-Ain, UAE*

ABSTRACT: Skeletal muscle atrophy and neuropathy are two of the major long-term complications of diabetes mellitus (DM). This article investigates the effect of streptozotocin (STZ)-induced type 1 DM on contraction and cation contents in soleus and EDL muscles compared to age-matched control rats. Adult Wistar rats were humanely killed and the soleus and EDL muscles located and excised rapidly and placed in organ baths. The muscles were electrically stimulated (EFS, 50 V, 1 ms, 1–50 Hz) and isometric contraction monitored using a chart recorder. At the end of the experiments the muscles were blotted, weighed, and dissolved in concentrated nitric acid for the measurements of cation contents. Diabetic rats have significantly ($P < 0.05$) reduced body and muscle weights and significantly ($P < 0.05$) elevated blood glucose (29.65 ± 0.33 mM, $n = 10$) compared to control (6.06 ± 0.21 mM, $n = 10$). EFS evoked frequency dependent contraction in both soleus and EDL muscles of healthy control rats. The response was significantly ($P < 0.05$, $n = 8$) increased in EDL compared to soleus. In the diabetic soleus and EDL muscles the force of contraction was significantly ($P < 0.05$, $n = 8$) reduced in both muscle types compared to control. The levels of total sodium (Na^+), potassium (K^+), calcium (Ca^{2+}), magnesium (Mg^{2+}), zinc (Zn^{2+}), copper (Cu^{2+}), and iron (Fe^{2+}) were significantly ($P < 0.05$) reduced in diabetic soleus and EDL muscles compared to control. The results indicate that STZ-induced skeletal muscle atrophy is associated with marked reductions in both the force of contraction and cation contents in EDL and soleus muscles of the rat.

KEYWORDS: diabetes mellitus; soleus; EDL muscle; rats; contraction; cations

Address for corresspondence: Prof. Jaipaul Singh, Department of Biological and Forensic Sciences, University of Central Lancashire, Preston, Lancashire, PR1 2HE UK. Voice: 0044-1772-893515; fax: 0044-1772-892929.

e-mail: jsingh3@uclan.ac.uk

Ann. N.Y. Acad. Sci. 1084: 442–451 (2006). © 2006 New York Academy of Sciences.
doi: 10.1196/annals.1372.006

INTRODUCTION

Diabetes mellitus (DM) is a major global health problem currently affecting around 180 million people worldwide and this number is predicted to increase to 300 million by the year 2025.[1–3] DM is a major metabolic disorder resulting from a lack of insulin secretion, insulin action due to its resistance or both.[4,5] The pancreatic beta cells have the unique ability to express the insulin gene and to synthesize and release insulin exactly according to the demands of the organisms.[3–5] The maintenance of appropriate plasma insulin levels is the result of two major mechanisms, namely minute-to-minute regulation of insulin release from individual beta cells and long-term adaptations of beta cells to peripheral demand of insulin. A deficient insulin production in relation to the insulin requirements of the body is a common denominator in all kinds of diabetes.[6] On basis of etiology, DM is divided into two main types, type 1 diabetes or insulin-dependent diabetes mellitus (IDDM) and type 2 diabetes or noninsulin-dependent diabetes mellitus (NIDDM).[7–9]

Insulin deficiency leads to hyperglycemia and disturbances in the metabolism of carbohydrates, fats, and proteins.[10,11] Progression of diabetes subsequently leads to such long-term complications as retinopathy, neuropathy, nephropathy, cardiomyopathy, exocrine insufficiencies, and skeletal muscle atrophy.[4,12] There is a marked reduction in the size of the skeletal muscle fibers thus reducing the strength of contraction.[4] This, in turn, decreases the quality of life for the patient. This study investigates the effect of streptozotocin (STZ)-induced DM on soleus and EDL skeletal muscle contraction and cation contents compared to age-matched control rats in order to understand the mechanism of DM-induced muscle atrophy.

METHODS

Materials

We used Analar grade chemicals, STZ, and nitric acid, which are all general laboratory reagents (Sigma, Dorset, UK).

General Procedures

All experiments were performed on adult male Wistar rats weighing about 200–530 g and relevant ethical approvals were obtained from the Ethics Committees of the University of Central Lancashire for the use of animals in experimental research. Rats were rendered diabetic by using a single intraperitoneal (i.p.) injection of STZ (60 mg kg/body weight) dissolved in citrate buffer.[13,14]

Age-matched control animals received an equivalent volume of citrate buffer i.p. Both control and DM-induced rats were tested for diabetes 4–5 days following STZ injection and 6–8 weeks later on the day of the experiment using a One Touch II Glucometer (Johnson & Johnson, Skipton, England, UK). Blood glucose concentration in excess of 300 mg dL^{-1} or 7 mmol confirmed DM.

Measurement of Contraction

On each day of the experiment, rats were humanely killed by a blow to the head followed by cervical dislocation. The EDL and soleus muscles were located from both the right and left hind limbs by making an incision in the limbs. There after, the muscles were gently teased out and then cut at both upper and lower ends. Following isolation, the muscles were immediately placed into an organ bath and stretched to 60% of its original length. Contraction was measured with an isometric transducer connected to a chart recorder. Throughout the experiments the muscles were bathed in Krebs's solution that was constantly aerated with 95% oxygen and 5% carbon dioxide and kept at constant temperature of 25°C. The normal physiological saline had the following composition (mM) :NaCl, 118.5; KCl, 4.7; $CaCl_2$, 3.4; KH_2PO_4, 1.2; $MgSO_4.7H_2O$, 1.2; $NaHCO_3$, 25; mannitol 35; glucose 11; and serum bovine albumin 0.1%.

Effect of electrical field stimulation (EFS) was conducted at frequencies of 1, 3, 7, 10, 20, 30, 40, and 50 Hz employing 50 V with pulse width 1 ms, for 15–20 s for each frequency. Following stimulation the physiological salt solution in the bath was changed with fresh solution. The muscle was then allowed to rest for 10–15 min after each series of EFS before being stimulated again. At the end of each experiment the length, diameter, and weight of each muscle were registered and contraction was expressed as force (N/cm^2) per cross-sectional area of the muscle.

Measurements of Cations

Soleus and EDL muscles from the above experiments were dissolved separately in 0.5 mL concentrated nitric acid in a 10 mL glass vial overnight.. A volume of 0.5 mL deionized water was added to each vial to increase the volume to 1 mL. An aliquot sample of 0.2 mL was pipetted in a 10 mL plastic tube and 9.8 mL of distilled water was added to this. This diluted sample was used to measure the level of either Ca^{2+}, Mg^{2+}, Fe^{2+}, Cu^{2+}, or Zn^{2+} using an atomic absorbance spectrophotometer. A Corning flame photometer (Steuben County, NY) was used for the measurements Na^+ and K^+. Cation concentrations were expressed as mM $(100 \text{ mg tissue})^{-1}$

TABLE 1. General characteristics of control and diabetic rats

Parameters	Control	Diabetic
Weight of rats (g)	501.83 ± 25.91	$222.19 \pm 10.51^*$
Blood glucose (mM)	6.06 ± 0.21	$29.65 \pm 0.33^*$
Blood insulin (mg dL^{-1})	20.63 ± 7.52	$4.81 \pm 1.28^*$
Weight of EDL (mg)	21 ± 0.05	$17 \pm 0.02^*$
Weight of soleus (mg)	0.23 ± 0.02	$0.174 \pm 0.02^*$

Data are mean ±SEM, $^*P < 0.05$; $n = 10$ rats for each parameter.

Statistical Analysis

Data are presented as mean ± standard error of the mean. All values were compared using Student's unpaired *t*-test and a value of $P < 0.05$ was taken as significant.

RESULTS

The general characteristics of age-matched control and diabetic rats are shown in TABLE 1. The results show that the diabetic rats have significantly ($P < 0.05$) less body and muscle weights. Moreover, they also have significantly ($P < 0.05$) increased blood glucose and significantly ($P < 0.05$) less plasma insulin compared to control animals.

FIGURE 1 shows the effect of EFS (10–50 Hz) on the force of contraction in soleus (solid squares) and EDL (solid diamonds) of age-matched healthy control rats. The results show that EDL muscle produced significantly ($P < 0.05$) more force compared to soleus muscle at 40–50 Hz. In healthy

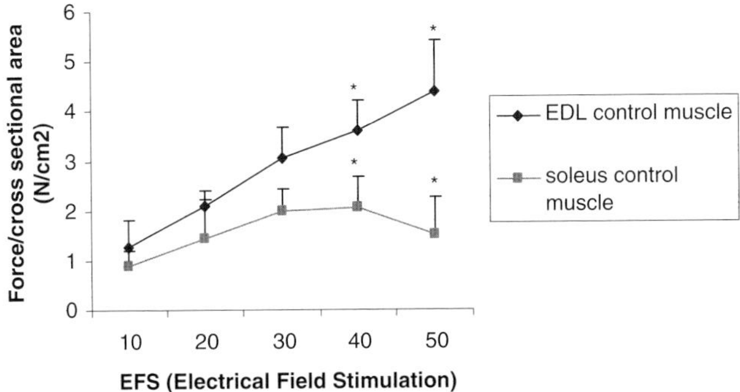

FIGURE 1. Effects of EFS (10–50 Hz, 50 V, 1 ms pulse width) on the force of contraction of EDL (diamonds) and soleus (squares) skeletal muscles of healthy age-matched control rats. Each point is ± SEM, $n = 8$. Note that EDL muscle produces significantly more force of contraction compared to soleus muscle. $^*P < 0.05$

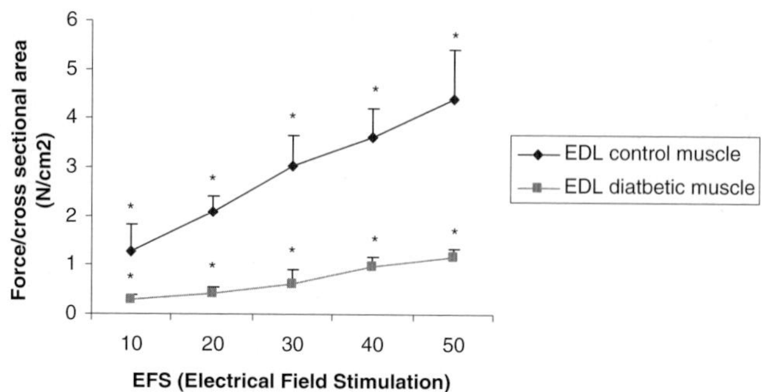

FIGURE 2. Effect of EFS (10–50 Hz, 50 V, 1 ms pulse width) on force of contraction of EDL muscle in age-matched control (diamonds) and STZ-induced diabetic (squares) rats. Each point is mean ± SEM, $n = 7$–8. Note that diabetic muscle produced significantly less force compared to control, * $P < 0.05$.

age-matched control rats, no difference in force was observed at frequencies of 1–10 Hz for the two muscles. FIGURE 2 shows the effect of EFS (10–50 Hz) on contraction in age-matched control (solid diamonds) and STZ-induced diabetic (solid squares) EDL muscle. The results clearly show that diabetic EDL muscle produced significantly ($P < 0.05$) less force of contraction at all frequencies tested in the study. FIGURE 3 shows the effect of EFS (10–50 Hz) on contraction in age-matched control and STZ-induced diabetic soleus muscle. Like EDL, the force of contraction in diabetic soleus muscle was also significantly ($P < 0.05$) reduced compared to control. FIGURE 4 shows the levels of sodium (panel A) and potassium (panel B) contents in control and diabetic EDL and soleus muscles. The results show that diabetic EDL and soleus muscles contain significantly ($P < 0.05$) less sodium and potassium contents compared to muscles for age-matched control muscles. FIGURE 5 shows the levels of Ca^{2+}, Mg^{2+}, Zn^{2+}, Fe^{2+}, and Cu^{2+} in EDL (panel A) and soleus (panel B) muscles of age-matched control and diabetic rats. The results show that both the diabetic EDL and soleus skeletal muscles contain significantly ($P < 0.05$) less cation contents (for all the ions tested) compared to age-matched control muscles. The results show further that the levels of Fe^{2+} and Cu^{2+} in EDL and Zn^{2+}, Fe^{2+}, and Cu^{2+} in soleus muscles fell to very low detection levels in the diabetic muscles.

DISCUSSION

The results of this study have demonstrated that 6-8-week old STZ-induced type 1 diabetic rats have significantly less body weights and EDL and soleus muscle weights, and significantly elevated blood glucose levels compared to age-matched control animals. Moreover, the diabetic animals have significantly less plasma insulin compared to control. These results are in

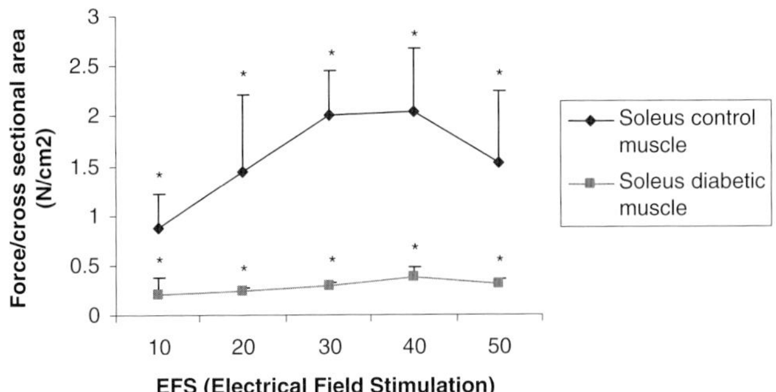

FIGURE 3. Effect of EFS (10–50 Hz, 50 V, 1 ms pulse width) on force of contraction of soleus muscle in age-matched control (diamonds) and STZ-induced diabetic (squares) rats. Each point is mean ± SEM, $n = 7$–8. Note that diabetic muscle produced significantly less force compared to control, $^*P < 0.05$.

complete agreement with findings from previous studies on the general characteristics of STZ-induced diabetic rats.[14–16] On close examination of the diabetic rats, both the body and the muscles contained a small amount of fatty tissues compared to control. In addition, both EDL and soleus muscles displayed signs of atrophy. The most likely reason for reduced body and muscle weights is that the diabetic rats either eat less, or they lose the weight directly because of diabetes, or both.[14–16]

The results have also shown that age-matched control EDL muscle produced significantly more force compared to age-matched healthy control soleus muscle. These effects were also frequency dependent with maximal response occurring at 50 Hz for EDL and 40 Hz for soleus muscles. Frequencies lower than 10 Hz did not affect the force of contraction significantly in both muscles.[17] Both EDL and soleus contain different types of fibers; soleus has slow twitch whereas EDL has fast twitch fibers. Soleus muscle is concerned with slow reaction for continuous support of the body against gravity and long continuing athletic events such as the marathon. Soleus muscle consists of small fibers, increased mitochondria to support increased levels of oxidative mechanism, and increased amount of blood vessels to supply high amounts of oxygen. The soleus muscle also contains large amounts of myoglobin. In contrast, EDL muscle is involved in rapid movement as in weight lifting. It is rich in glycogen and consists of few mitochondria. It depends on glycolysis for ATP production, fatigues easily, and has a low level of myoglobin.[17,18]

The present results have also shown that STZ-induced diabetes is associated with a marked reduction in the force of contraction in both EDL and soleus muscles compared to their respective age-matched controls. These effects were also frequency dependent with a larger reduction in force at 50 Hz for EDL and 40–50 Hz for soleus. These findings clearly demonstrate that DM is associated with reduced force. The question that now arises is: what is responsible for

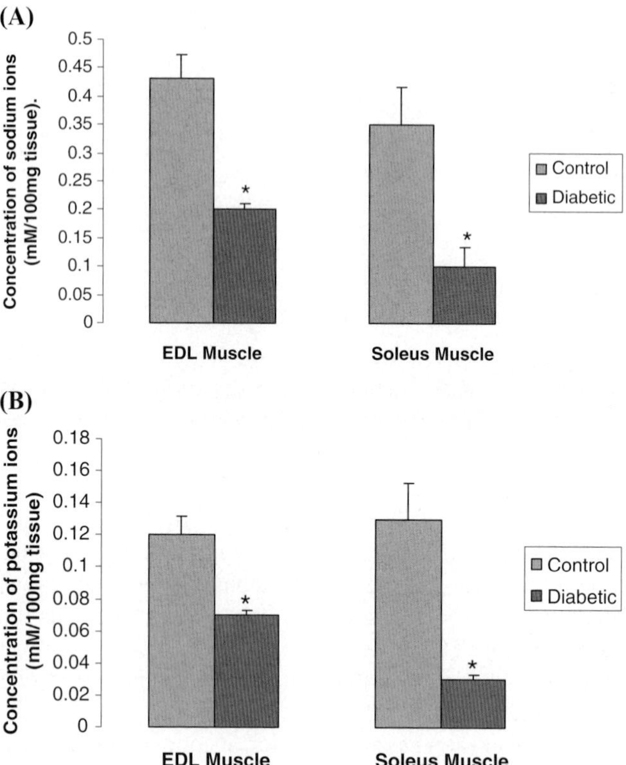

FIGURE 4. Concentrations of sodium (**A**) and potassium (**B**) contents in EDL and soleus skeletal muscles of age-matched control and STZ-induced diabetic rats. Each point is mean ± SEM, $n = 8$. Note that the diabetic EDL and soleus muscles have significantly less sodium and potassium contents compared to age-matched controls. ($^*P < 0.05$).

the reduced force in the diabetic muscle? One possible explanation is that the muscles are significantly smaller in the diabetic rats compared to control and as a result they generate less force. The decrease in size of the muscles and muscle fibers may be due to the neuropathy resulting from the diabetes.[4] Both atrophy and neuropathy are two major long-term complications of DM. In this situation, EFS will be an ineffective physiological tool to elicit contraction of the diabetic muscles because of reduced neurotransmitter release at the neuromuscular junction, compared to the responses obtained from age-matched healthy control muscles. Human diabetic neuropathy is a worrying complication of DM and it is responsible for severe disability.[5,19] Previous studies have shown that STZ-induced diabetes can result in a marked reduction in myelinated fiber size in rats.[20] It has also been demonstrated that myelinated fiber area, myelin thickness, and their axons are all significantly reduced in STZ-induced diabetic rats.[21] One of the most functional consequences of DM in the rodent model

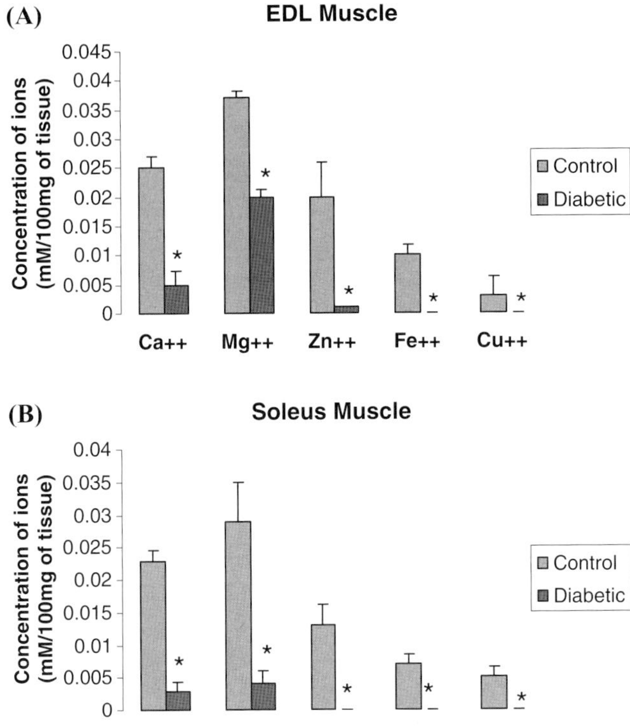

FIGURE 5. Concentrations of Ca^{2+}, Mg^{2+}, Zn^{2+}, Fe^{2+}, and Cu^{2+} in EDL (**A**) and soleus (**B**) skeletal muscles of age-matched control and STZ-induced diabetic rats. Each point is mean ± SEM, $n = 8$. Note that EDL and soleus skeletal muscles of diabetic rats have significantly less cation contents compared to age-matched controls in each muscle ($^*P < 0.05$).

is the marked reduction in strength of the fast twitch fibers, which is due to α-motor neurons in the muscle.[22]

The reduction in the force of contraction, which is seen in the STZ-induced diabetic rat EDL and soleus muscle is still not fully understood. One potential mechanism could be a disruption of the excitation–contraction coupling process. It is possible that the diabetic muscle is unable to utilize cellular Ca^{2+} efficiently, especially since Ca^{2+} is the trigger and mediator of muscle contraction.[23] Interestingly, the present results have also demonstrated that both diabetic EDL and soleus muscles contain significantly less total Na^+, K^+, Zn^{2+}, Cu^{2+}, Fe^{2+}, Mg^{2+}, and Ca^{2+} contents compared to age-matched healthy controls. The reduction in all these cations may be due to diabetes itself. This metabolic disorder is known to be associated with the reduction of many cations in tissues of the body.[4,19] Both Na^+ and K^+ are associated with depolarization and hyperpolarization of the muscle cell.[22] On the other hand, Ca^{2+} is associated with contraction and Mg^{2+} is the cofactor for a number of enzyme and transport systems during cellular regulation.[24] Moreover, diabetes is known to be associated with hypomagnesemia.[25] Zn^{2+}, Fe^{2+}, and Cu^{2+} are important cations in maintaining the integrity of muscles. As a result of diabetes, the muscles accumulate less cations.[26] Fe^{2+} is important in the metabolism of ATP for energy release whereas Zn^{2+} supports the functions of numerous metalloenzymes, which are involved in a multitude of metabolic processes including protein, DNA, and RNA synthesis.[26,27] On the other hand, Cu^{2+} is a cofactor for lysile oxidase that is an enzyme involved in collagen synthesis.[26]

In conclusion, the results of this study have shown that EFS can evoke marked frequency-dependent of contraction in EDL and soleus muscles with the maximal response obtained with EDL muscle. In the diabetic EDL and soleus muscles, the force of contraction was significantly reduced compared to age-matched controls. Moreover, the two muscle types contain significantly less Na^{+}, K^{+}, Ca^{2+}, Mg^{2+}, Zn^{2+}, Fe^{2+}, and Cu^{2+} in diabetic rats compared to control. The results indicate that STZ-induced diabetic muscle atrophy is associated with reduced force of contraction and this may be due to the reduction in the muscle cation contents.

ACKNOWLEDGMENTS

The authors would like to thank Roxy Afzal for typing the manuscript.

REFERENCES

1. AMOS, A., D. MCCARTY & P. ZIMMET. 1997. The rising global burned of diabetes and its complications, estimates and projections to the year 2010. Diabetic Med. **14:** S1–S85.
2. KING, H., R. AUBERT & W. HERMAN. 1998. Global burden of diabetes, 1995–2025. Prevalence, numerical estimates and projections. Diabetes Care **21:** 1414–1431.
3. ZIMMET, P. 2000. Globalization, cocoa-colonization and the chronic disease epidemic. Can the Doomsday scenario be averted? J. Med. **247:** 301–310.
4. KUMAR, P.J. & M. CLARK. 2002. Diabetes mellitus and other disorders of metabolism. Clinical Medicine. P.J. Kumar & M. Clark, Eds.: 1099–1121. WB Saunders. London.
5. EXPERT COMMITTEE ON THE DIAGNOSIS AND CLASSIFICATION OF DIABETES MELLITUS. 1997. Report of the Expert Committee on the diagnosis and classification of diabetes mellitus. Diabetes Care **20:** 1183–1197.
6. SILTIEL, A.R. & C.R. KHAN. 2001. Insulin signalling and the regulation of glucose and lipid metabolism. Nature **414:** 799–806.
7. WORLD HEALTH ORGANIZATION STUDY GROUP.1985. Diabetes Mellitus: WHO Technical Report, Series 727. Geneva: World Health Organization
8. WORLD HEALTH ORGANIZATION CONSULTATION.1999. Definition, diagnosis and classification of diabetes mellitus. Report of a WHO Consultation. Geneva: World Health Organization.

9. Zimmet, P., C. Cowie, J.M. Ekoe, *et al.* 2004. Classification of diabetes mellitus and other categories of glucose intolerance. *In* International Textbook of Diabetes Mellitus, 3rd ed. Chapter 1,3–14 John Wiley & Sons. UK.
10. Beverley, B. & E. Eschwege. 2003. The diagnosis and classification of diabetes and impaired glucose tolerance. *In* Textbook of Diabetes, 3rd ed. J.C. Pickup & G. Williams, Eds.: 2.1–2.11. Blackwell Sciences Ltd., UK.
11. Alterman, S.C. 1997. The insulin pump and oral drugs for diabetes. *In* How to Control Diabetes. 92–101, 121–126. Ballantine Pubs. Group. New York.
12. Singh, J., E. Adeghate, S. Aparico, *et al.* 2004. Exocrine pancreatic insufficiency in diabetes mellitus. Int. J. Diabetes Metab. **12:** 35–43.
13. Sharma, A.K., I.G.M. Duguid, D.S. Blanchard, *et al.* 1985. The effect of insulin-treatment on myelinated nerve-fibre maturation and integrity and on body growth on streptozotocin-diabetic rats. J. Neurol. Sci. **67:** 285–297.
14. Bracken, N.K., A.J. Woodall, F.C. Howarth, *et al.* 2004. Voltage-dependence of contraction in streptozotocin-induced diabetic myocytes. Mol. Cell. Biochem. **261:** 235–243.
15. Qureshi, M.A., N.K. Bracken, W. Winlow, *et al.* 2001. Time dependent effects of streptozotocin-induced diabetes on contraction in rat ventricular myocytes. Emirates Journal **19:** 35–41.
16. Bracken, N.K., F.C. Howarth, M. Qurechi, *et al.* 2002. Effects of diabetes on cation contents and contraction in the isolated heart. Adap. Biol. Med. **3:** 112–121.
17. Atherton, P.J., J.A. Babraf, K. Smith, *et al.* 2005. Selective activation of AMPK-PGC-1d on PKB-TSC2-mTOR signalling can explain specific adaptive responses to endurance or resistance training-like electrical muscle stimulation. FASED J. Express **Article 10.1096/Fj.04–2179 fjc:** 1–23.
18. Williamson, D.L., P.M. Gallagher, C.C. Carroll, *et al.* 2001. Reduction in hybrid single muscle fibre proportions with resistance training in humans. J. Appl. Physiol. **91:** 1955–1961.
19. Rajbhandari, S.M. & M.K. Piya. 2005. A brief review on the pathogenesis of human diabetic neuropathy: observations and postulations. Int. J. Diabetes Metab. **13:** 135–140.
20. Sharma, A.K., P.K. Thomas, G. Gabriel, *et al.* 1983. Peripheral nerve abnormalities in the diabetic mutant mouse. Diabetes **32:** 1152–1161.
21. Ahmed, I. 1999. Effect of Mornordica Charantia fruit juice on experimental diabetes and its complications. PhD thesis. University of Central Lancashire, UK
22. Lesniewski, L.A., T.A. Miller & R.B. Armstrong. 2003. Mechanism of force loss in diabetic mouse skeletal muscle. Muscle Nerve **28:** 493–500.
23. Vander, A., J. Sherman & D. Luciano. 2002. Human Physiology: Mechanism of Body Function, 5th ed. Chapter 11, 288–320. McGraw Hill. London.
24. Yago, M.D., M. Manas & J. Singh. 2000. Intracellular magnesium transport and regulation in epithelial secreting cells. Frontier Biosci. **5:** 602–618.
25. Chakrobourti, S., T. Chakrouborti, M. Mandal, *et al.* 2002. Protective role of magnesium in cardiovascular diseases: a review. Mol. Cell. Biochem. **238:** 163–179.
26. Whitney, C. & Rolfes. 1994. Understanding Normal Clinical Nutrition. West Publishing. New York.
27. Walter, R.M., J.Y. Uriu-Hare,O.K. Lewis, *et al.* 1991. Copper, zinc, manganese and magnesium status and complications of diabetes mellitus. Diabetes Care **14:** 1050–1056.

Calpains and Their Multiple Roles in Diabetes Mellitus

FREDERICK HARRIS,[a] SUMAN BISWAS,[b] JAIPAUL SINGH,[c] SARAH DENNISON,[d] AND DAVID A. PHOENIX[d]

[a]*Department of Forensic and Investigative Science, University of Central Lancashire, Preston, PR1 2HE, United Kingdom*

[b]*Department of Ophthalmology, Bristol Eye Hospital, Bristol, BS1 2LX, United Kingdom*

[c]*Department of Biology, University of Central Lancashire, Preston, PR1 2HE, United Kingdom*

[d]*Faculty of Science, University of Central Lancashire, Preston, PR1 2HE, United Kingdom*

ABSTRACT: Type 2 diabetes mellitus (T2DM) can lead to death without treatment and it has been predicted that the condition will affect 215 million people worldwide by 2010. T2DM is a multifactorial disorder whose precise genetic causes and biochemical defects have not been fully elucidated, but at both levels, calpains appear to play a role. Positional cloning studies mapped T2DM susceptibility to *CAPN10*, the gene encoding the intracellular cysteine protease, calpain 10. Further studies have shown a number of noncoding polymorphisms in *CAPN10* to be functionally associated with T2DM while the identification of coding polymorphisms, suggested that mutant calpain 10 proteins may also contribute to the disease. Here we review recent studies, which in addition to the latter enzyme, have linked calpain 5, calpain 3, and its splice variants, calpain 2 and calpain 1 to T2DM-related metabolic pathways along with T2DM-associated phenotypes, such as obesity and impaired insulin secretion, and T2DM-related complications, such as epithelial dysfunction and diabetic cataract.

KEYWORDS: diabetes; calpains; polymorphism; calcium; insulin; phenotype; epithelial dysfunction; cataract

INTRODUCTION

The occurrence of diabetes mellitus has reached epidemic levels and affects in excess of 170 million people globally. It has been estimated that by the year 2010 the incidence of the condition will have grown by 50%, with the highest increase in the developing nations of South America, Africa, and Asia.[1]

Address for correspondence: Prof. D.A. Phoenix, Dean, Faculty of Science, University of Central Lancashire, Preston, PR1 2HE, Lancashire, UK. Voice: +1772-893481; fax: +1772-894981.
e-mail: daphoenix@uclan.ac.uk

**Ann. N.Y. Acad. Sci. 1084: 452–480 (2006). © 2006 New York Academy of Sciences.
doi: 10.1196/annals.1372.011**

In more developed societies, the incidence of diabetes mellitus has reached approximately 6% of the population[2] and disturbingly, among the obese adolescents of these societies, 4% have the condition and 25% exhibit abnormal glucose tolerance.[3]

Diabetes mellitus represents a heterogeneous group of metabolic disorders whose development can involve both environmental and genetic contributions.[4–7] Type I diabetes mellitus (T1DM), or insulin-dependent diabetes, is caused by autoimmune destruction of the β cells of the pancreas, rendering the pancreas unable to synthesize and secrete insulin.[8–10] T1DM accounts for approximately 5–10% of all cases of diabetes with the major susceptibility gene mapping to the HLA region of chromosome 6.[11,12] However, type 2 diabetes mellitus (T2DM), or noninsulin dependent diabetes, is the major form of the disease and the most common worldwide, accounting for 90% or more of all cases of the condition.[7]

At the biochemical level, T2DM is characterized by defects in hepatic glucose production, insulin action, and insulin secretion. Insulin resistance is an early feature of T2DM, which is initially, at least partly, compensated for by hyperinsulinemia. This increased production of insulin by pancreatic β cells is such that normal glucose homeostasis is maintained or only mildly disturbed. The ability of insulin-resistant individuals to ward off T2DM depends largely upon the adaptive capacity of their pancreatic β cells to maintain increasing insulin concentrations. Those who cannot sustain sufficient hyperinsulinemia suffer deterioration in glucose homeostasis with an increasing disparity between escalating insulin resistance and inadequate compensatory hyperinsulinemia causing a progression into overt T2DM. By the time T2DM has developed, insulin resistance appears to be almost fully established. However, hyperglycemia continues to worsen due to increasingly compromised β cell function and as hyperglycemia becomes severe, β cell failure, due to exhaustion, is usually clearly evident. The combined effects of insulin resistance and impaired insulin secretion reduce insulin-mediated glucose uptake and utilization by skeletal muscle, and prevent insulin-mediated suppression of hepatic glucose output. Continuing deterioration of endocrine control exacerbates these metabolic disturbances and increases the hyperglycemia.[13–17] The combined forces of insulin resistance and hyperinsulinemia[18] have been implicated in the pathogenesis of polycystic ovary syndrome (PCOS)[19] and contribute either directly or indirectly to many other disorders, including: dyslipidemia,[20] hypertension,[21] atherosclerosis,[22] procoagulant states, cardiovascular disease,[23] end-stage renal disease,[24] retinopathy,[25] and reduced life expectancy.[26] The most devastating complications of T2DM are primarily microvascular and macrovascular diseases resulting from accelerated atherogenesis with cardiovascular morbidity in T2DM sufferers between two- and fourfold higher than in nondiabetic individuals.[1]

At the genetic level, there has been significant progress in elucidating factors that underlie T2DM over the last decade. Probably the best understood

TABLE 1. Varient genes and proteins that are associated with MODY

MODY	Gene	Function of protein
MODY1	*HNF-4-α*	Hepacyte nuclear factor (transcription factor)
MODY2	*GCK*	Glucokinase
MODY3	*HNF-1- α*	Hepacyte nuclear factor (transcription factor)
MODY4	*IPF1*	Insulin promotor factor
MODY5	*HNF-1β*	Hepacyte nuclear factor (transcription factor)
MODY6	*NEUROD1*	Neuro D1 transcription factor

Table 1 was adapted from Barroso *et al.*[27]

forms of T2DM are those that are monogenetic in origin and account for approximately 10% of all cases of the condition. Maturity-onset diabetes of the young (MODY) represents the most common of these forms of the condition and arises from mutations in a variety of genes that are expressed in pancreatic β cells, which are primarily manifested at the biochemical level as deficiencies in insulin secretion.[27,28] The first MODY gene was identified in the early 1990s as that encoding the glycolytic enzyme glucokinase.[29,30] A number of other MODY genes have been identified (TABLE 1). Other less common monogenetic forms of T2DM are known, which arise from mutations in maternally inherited mitochondrial genes, most frequently caused by a mutation in the mitochondrial gene encoding the transfer RNA for leucine. These forms of T2DM are associated with hearing loss, myopathy, and stroke-like episodes.[5,28] In a number of cases, recent studies have revealed misclassifications in relation to T2DM. Some forms of MODY have been misdiagnosed as T1DM and late-onset diabetes of the adult, which is often associated with T2DM, is strictly a late onset form of T1DM.[5,7]

Genetic factors that contribute to polygenic T2DM have been primarily sought using the candidate gene approach and the genome-wide scan approach. The first of these approaches examines specific genes with a plausible role in the disease process. To this aim, the statistical association of a given allele and a phenotype, such as insulin resistance and T2DM, is tested in unrelated individuals. Use of this approach has identified a number of candidate T2DM susceptibility genes[27] and those genes with the most significant associations are shown in TABLE 2. Currently, the candidate gene with the strongest statistical association is the widespread Pro12Ala variant of the peroxisome proliferator-activated receptor-γ (PPARγ), which putatively confers insulin resistance in liver, muscle, and fat.[7] In contrast to the latter methodology, the genome-wide scan or linkage approach is not based on assumptions regarding phenotypic linkage but locates genes through their genomic position and is based on the rationale that family members that share a specific phenotype will also share chromosomal regions surrounding the gene involved. Use of this approach has yielded several positive associations of genomic regions with T2DM[27] (TABLE 2). However, such findings are generally followed by positional cloning of the

TABLE 2. Varient genes and proteins that have been associated with T2DM via genomic searching

Gene	Encoded protein	Function of protein	Rare variant (allele/genotype)	Diabetes risk, odds ratio for rare allele (p)	Putative mechanism
PPARG	PPARγ	Nuclear receptor (transcription factor)	Ala12	0.79 ($P < 0.0001$)	Insulin resistance
GYS1	Glycogen synthase	Enzyme	A2 (XbaI)	0.60 ($P = 0.02$)	Alteration of glycogen storage
IRS1	Insulin receptor substrate 1	Docking protein (insulin signaling)	Arg972	1.27 ($P = 0.005$)	Probably β cell dysfunction
INS	Proinsulin	Hormone	class III VNTR	1.21 ($P = 0.01$)	β cell dysfunction
KCJN11	Potassium-inward rectifier 6.2	Potassium channel	Lys23	1.12 ($P = 0.002$)	β cell or α cell dysfunction
ABCC8	Sulfonylurea receptor 1	Potassium channel (subunit)	T761 (exon 18)	2.28 ($P < 0.05$)	Probably β cell dysfunction
SLC2A1	Glucose transporter 1	Facilitated transport	6.2 Kb allele (XbaI)	1.76 ($P < 0.05$)	Unclear
PPARGC1	PPARγ-coactivator-1	Transcriptional cofactor	Ser482	1.21 ($P < 0.001$)	Unclear, possibly pleiotropic
CAPN10	Calpain-10	Cystein protease	Intronic SNP43, G	1.15 ($P = 0.002$)	Unclear, possibly pleiotropic
			Intronic SNP44, C	1.17 ($P = 0.0003$)	Unclear, possibly pleiotropic

Table 2 was adapted from Stumvoll *et al.*[7]

causative gene and to date only *CAPN10* has been identified in this way in the NIDDM1 (noninsulin dependent diabetes mellitus 1) region of chromosome 2.[31] This gene encodes calpain 10, which is a member of a cysteine protease superfamily,[32,33] and it is becoming increasingly clear that other members of this family may also play roles in T2DM. Here, we give an overview of this enzyme family and review investigations into their contributions to T2DM.

Calpains

Calpains (EC 3.4.22.17) are a superfamily of 15 Ca^{2+}-dependent intracellular cysteine proteases, which can be either ubiquitous or tissue preferred.[34] These enzymes are believed to possess a domainal structure, which was recently confirmed for a number of Ca^{2+}-free forms of calpain 2 by high-resolution crystallography,[35,36] and for the majority of these proteins this structure is organized into domains I–IV.[34] On the basis of these crystallographic structures and the results of other studies, it has been shown that domain I forms an N-terminal extension of domain II and is autolytically processed upon calpain activation, thereby fulfilling a regulatory role.[37] Domain II houses the enzyme's active site, which is a papain-like cysteine protease domain and is divided into two subdomains, II a and II b.[38] Between them, these subdomains contain the amino acid residues necessary to form this site but in the absence of Ca^{2+}, interactions with other domains hold them apart, thus maintaining the active site in a disassembled state. Domain III is a Ca^{2+}-dependent lipid binding site[39] and also serves as a linker region[37] between the catalytic domain and domain IV, which contains a calmodulin-like Ca^{2+} binding domain with multiple EF-hands.[40,41] Calpains 1 and 2 also possess a smaller subunit, which possesses domains VI and V.[34] Domain VI possesses a calmodulin-like Ca^{2+} binding domain and associates with domain IV to facilitate dimerization with the large subunit[35,36] while domain V, which is largely cleaved from the small subunit during autolysis, interacts with lipid/membranes to lower the enzyme's Ca^{2+} requirement for activation.[42,43] It has been proposed that core events for the activation of calpain 2[35,36,44,45] involve Ca^{2+} binding to domains VI and VI,[40,41] which induces a series of both conformational and structural changes, including autolysis and subunit disassociation, leading to the realignment of domains II a and II b, assembly of the calpain 2 active site, and proteolytic activity.[35,36,44–46] Additionally, several studies have indicated the possibility that calpain activation could involve Ca^{2+} binding to domain II and domain III.[38,39,47–50]

Calpains with the structural organization described above are generally referred to as typical calpains and in addition to calpains 1 and 2,[34] include several major members of this enzyme family, such as calpain 3 and its splice variants.[51,52] A number of calpains, which have been designated as atypical, have been described where certain of the four domains associated with typical calpains have been either replaced or deleted with the most prominent

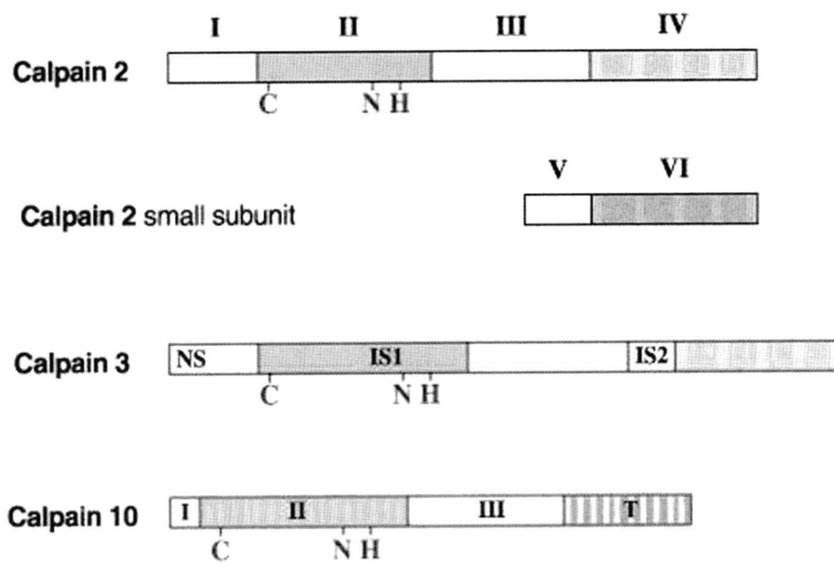

FIGURE 1. This figure shows the structural organization of representative calpains. Calpain 2 (and calpain 1) is dimeric, possessing a large (80 kDa) subunit comprising domains I–IV and a smaller (30 kDa) subunit comprising domains V–VI. Calpain 10 and calpain 3 are monomeric, possessing the structural organization of the calpain 2 larger subunit except that calpain 3 possesses a novel N terminus (NS) and the unique inserts, IS1 and IS2, in domains II and IV, respectively. *Lp82* (and *Lp85*) is a lens-specific variant of calpain 3, lacking IS1 and IS2, and possessing a modified N-terminal region (AX1). Also represented above, in domain IV of calpain 2 and calpain 3 are five EF-hand motifs that appear to be primarily responsible for the Ca^{2+} binding ability of these enzymes and other calpains. However, calpain 10 lacks domain IV and these EF-hands, instead possessing a divergent T (or III') domain. Annotated in domain II of the above calpains is the triad of amino acid residues, C, H, and N that forms the active site of these calpains. Essentially, the thiol group of this cysteine residue directly participates in covalent catalytic cleavage of the peptide bond of substrate. The histidine residue that is in close spatial proximity is also essential for the cysteine protease activity of calpains while other nearby residues provide groups for general acid-base catalysis.[32,34] (This figure was adapted from Biswas *et al.*[168])

member of this group being calpain 10.[32,53] The structural organization of representational calpains is shown in FIGURE 1.

In addition to humans and a wide variety of other mammals, calpains have been increasingly identified in a diverse range of lower eukaryotes.[54] This prevalence, clearly implies biological importance. Nonetheless, despite decades of intensive study, the physiological functions of calpains are still not fully understood[55] and roles for these enzymes in a variety of processes have been proposed,[34] ranging from signal transduction[56] and cell differentiation[57] to apoptosis and necrosis.[58,59] The biological importance of calpains is further reinforced by the fact that they have been implicated in a number of pathological conditions, thereby, giving calpains considerable medical relevance.[53,60,61] As examples: missense mutations in *CAPN3*, the gene encoding calpain 3, leads to loss of the enzyme's activity and the enzyme's resulting inability to proteolyse certain key substrates, appears to be responsible for the pathogeneisis of limb girdle muscular dystrophy 2A.[51,62] In contrast, changes in Ca^{2+} homeostasis leading to the overactivation of calpains has been linked to a range of disease states, such as degenerative conditions in the brain, including: cerebral ischemia, Alzheimer's disease, and Parkinson's disease.[63,64] In addition, there is accumulating evidence linking calpains to T2DM both at the genetic and biochemical level.[65]

Genetic Linking of Calpains to T2DM

Almost a decade ago, genome-wide scan studies on 330 sib pairs identified NIDDM1, the putative T2DM susceptibility locus, to the region D2S125–D2S140 on chromosome 2q37.3 of Mexican Americans.[66] Four years later, positional cloning studies revealed that NIDDM1 was a single gene, *CAPN10*, and that genetic variation in this gene accounted for 14% of the population-attributable risk to T2DM in this ethnic group.[31] An intronic single nucleotide polymorphism (SNP) in *CAPN10* (UCSNP43, G→A, FIG. 2) was significantly increased in affected individuals but the highest overall risk for T2DM was determined by a heterozygous combination of two haplotypes, which were defined by UCSNP43 and two further intronic SNPs: UCSNP19 (an insertion–deletion polymorphism with either two or three repeats, FIG. 1) and UCSNP63 (C→T, FIG. 2). These high-risk haplotypes are generally referred to as "112" (UCSNP43, allele 1; UCSNP19, allele 1; UCSNP63, allele 2, FIG. 2) and "121" (UCSNP43, allele 1; UCSNP19, allele 2; UCSNP63, allele 1, FIG. 2). This haplotype combination was found to confer an overall increased risk of T2DM in Mexican Americans of 2.8-fold, in Botnian Finns

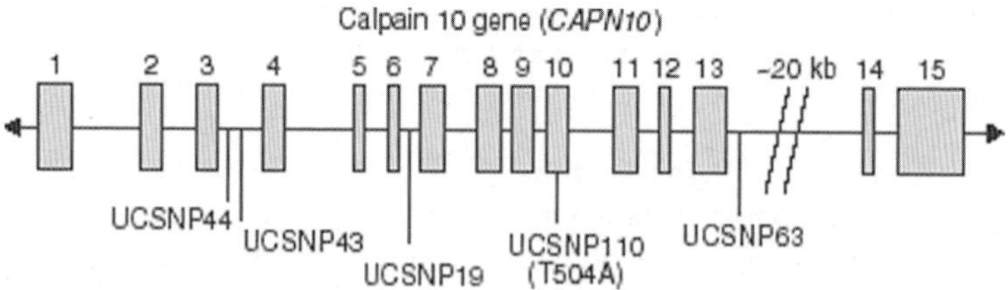

FIGURE 2. This figure shows the structure of *CAPN10*, the gene encoding human calpain 10 along with associated SNPs. The gene is located on chromosome and 2q37.3 comprises spans 31 Kb of genomic sequence. The gene contains 15 exons and encodes a protease with a full length of 672 amino acid residues. Annotated are UCSNP19, UCSNP43, and UCSNP63, which are the SNPs that form the risk haplotypes for T2DM. Along with UCSNP44, which is in almost perfect linkage disequilibrium with the missense coding mutation UCSNP110, these SNPs have also been associated with a variety of T2DM-associated phenotypes and disorders. (This figure was adapted from Turner *et al.*[33])

of 2.5-fold, and in Germans of almost 5-fold.[31] Since this initial work, there have been a number of follow-up studies on a diverse range of ethnic populations, which either confirmed or extended the associations of *CAPN10* with T2DM[67–76] or disputed the original findings.[77–86] A number of factors both statistical and genetic have been proposed to underlie this variation in results,[33,87,88] and to overcome problems of reproducibility in these studies, a series of meta-analyses of published *CAPN10* data have been performed. The first of these analyses found no evidence to support an association of either UCSNP43 or the 112/121 haplotype combination under either dominant or additive models with susceptibility to T2DM. Additionally, no evidence was found for associations between the UCSNP43 G homozygous genotype, or the 112/121 haplotype combination, and metabolic phenotypes. However, under a recessive model, subjects who were G homozygous for UCSNP43 had a 19% higher risk of T2DM.[89] In contrast to these latter studies, a second meta-analysis found no overtransmission of the G allele of UCSNP43 but revealed a significant overtransmission of the C allele of the rare T→C polymorphism at UCSNP44 from heterozygous parents to offspring affected with T2DM.[74] Similar observations were previously reported in a study on Britons[79] and the meta-analyses of Weedon[74]confirmed that the C allele of UCSNP44 is associated with T2DM. UCSNP44 is in perfect linkage disequilibrium with a missense mutation (UCSNP110) in a coding region of *CAPN10* that causes a T504A substitution in the calpain 10 amino acid sequence.[74,79] This substitution occurs in domain T (or domain III′), a region of calpain 10 whose function is poorly understood[32] (Fig. 1). UCSNP44 is also in perfect linkage disequilibrium with two polymorphisms in the 50-untranslated region of *CAPN10* (UCSNP-134 and UCSNP-135), providing alternatives as possible causal variants.[31,74,79] Other meta-analyses have suggested that increased risk of T2DM is associated with both UCSNP43 and UCSNP44[90] and that these polymorphisms may form the basis of an approach to predict the condition.[91] Compounding the issue, a recent statistical re-analysis of data in the original paper linking *CAPN10* to T2DM[31] has suggested that as yet unidentified variations in the gene may also be functionally associated with the disorder.[92] Moreover, *CAPN3*, the gene for calpain 3, appears to be functionally associated with *CAPN10*,[93] which led to the speculation that this enzyme may play a role in T2DM.[31] Possibly supporting this speculation, a recent study showed that reduced expression of *CAPN3* in skeletal muscle was associated with obesity and insulin resistance, often linked with T2DM, in both nondiabetic humans and Psammomys obesus, a polygenic animal model of obesity and T2DM.[94]

Genetic Linking of Calpains to T2DM-Related Phenotypes

In addition to T2DM, a number of studies have investigated links between *CAPN10* polymorphisms and phenotypes associated with the condition. Genetic polymorphisms associated with the enzyme have been found to correlate with several aspects of insulin action. Studies on nondiabetic British subjects with high risk haplotype (112/121) had increased plasma glucose levels both at fasting and after a 2-h oral glucose tolerance test concomitant with a decrease in the insulin secretory response.[69] Consistent with these data, polymorphism at SNP44 was found to modify the plasma glucose curve obtained from an oral glucose tolerance test in a manner that was indicative of T2DM association.[95] Surprisingly, nondiabetic German subjects that were homozygous for the G allele of SNP43 showed higher rates of insulin secretion and proinsulin processing.[96] However, it was suggested that these findings may be indicative of primary hypersecretion, which in its own right has been shown to predict T2DM, independent of insulin resistance.[97] *CAPN10* polymorphisms have been linked to both insulin resistance[71] and parameters of this resistance. Recent studies on nondiabetic Britons demonstrated associations between the G allele of UCSNP43 and abnormal microvascular function, which has been proposed to play a key role in insulin resistance.[98] Pima Indians possess a high prevalence of T2DM[99] and individuals of this ethnic group with homozygosity for the UCSNP43 G allele were associated with decreased rates of peripheral glucose turnover/insulin resistance.[72] Moreover, this investigation also found that nondiabetic Pima Indians possessing this polymorphism exhibited reduced skeletal muscle *CAPN10* mRNA, which led to the suggestion that it was linked to T2DM susceptibility.[72] Generally supporting this suggestion, it was recently shown that Danish individuals that were homozygous for the UCSNP43 G allele exhibited reduced levels of *CAPN10* mRNA in skeletal muscle and that in this case, transcription was under genetic control.[100] Further support for the suggestion of Baier *et al.*[72] came from the demonstration that intronic fragments of UCSNP43 and UCSNP44 variants showed different binding affinities with nuclear proteins.[31] These latter studies showed that alternative splicing of human *CAPN10* mRNA, produced at least eight different isoforms of the enzyme (calpains 10 a to 10 h), five of which were recognized in rat lens retina by an antibody specific for calpain 10 domain II.[101] An indepth analysis of human skeletal muscle mRNA showed that in this tissue the most abundant isoforms were calpain 10 a and 10 f and concluded that the likely cause of the reduced mRNA was reduced transcriptional initiation and/or pre-mRNA stability, and not altered mRNA splicing.[102] Nonetheless, other authors have disputed this conclusion and have argued that *CAPN10* polymorphisms contribute to T2DM susceptibility via altered transcriptional regulation.[65,103]

Obesity is a major factor in the development of T2DM with the elevated levels of lipolysis resulting from increased fat cell mass leading to skeletal muscle insulin resistance[104] and a number of authors have investigated associations between *CAPN10* polymorphisms and the condition. Investigations on an ethnically diverse range of populations have shown that there are associations between UCSNP19, UCSNP43, and UCSNP63 and anthropometric measures indicative of obesity, such as body mass index and waist–hip ratio.[72,73,105,106] Genetic variations in the *CAPN10* gene at UCSNP43, UCSNP-63, and haplotype combinations involving these polymorphism along with those at UCSNP19 and UCSNP63 have been shown to be associated with elevated free fatty acid levels.[71] Studies on a Chinese population found that the haplotype combination 112/121 was a potential risk factor for increased plasma cholesterol while studies on a Japanese population found that the UCSNP43 G allele was associated with increased levels of plasma cholesterol[77] and increased free fatty acid levels[80] and dyslipidemia.[107] Studies on a Swedish population found that individuals homozygous for the G allele of this latter polymorphism exhibited both elevated levels of triglyceride and reduced levels of *CAPN10* mRNA in adipose tissue although no association between UCSNP43 and obesity was detected.[108] Similarly, a study on German families with extremely obese offspring found no evidence for an association between the 112/121 haplotype combination and early onset obesity.[109] However, further support for a link between *CAPN10*, obesity, and T2DM was provided by studies on Otsuka Long–Evans Tokushima Fatty (OLEFT) polygenic type 2 diabetic rats. These obese rats spontaneously develop T2DM at the age of 18 weeks and were found to exhibit decreased *CAPN10* mRNA in white blood cells.[56] Moreover, genomic analysis showed that a quantitative trait locus involved in this diabetes contained *CAPN10*. A G$\rightarrow$A polymorphism in this gene was found to lead to a nonconservative S195G substitution in the protease domain of calpain 10, which it was suggested could be important to protein function and T2DM susceptibility in these rats.[110]

PCOS is associated with insulin resistance and a two- to sevenfold risk of T2DM. Previous studies have shown that PCOS and T2DM may share genetic susceptibility factors and on these observations, a number of studies have suggested that genes related to T2DM may play a role in POCS.[111] It has been demonstrated that the high-risk haplotype combination at *CAPN10* shows an association with PCOS and a predisposition to T2DM within POCS patients.[112] Moreover, later studies reported that specific *CAPN10* variations were associated with both PCOS[113] and hirsutism, a common clinical feature of POCS.[114] However, other studies have detected no association of *CAPN10* polymorphisms with PCOS[115] but interestingly, an association between specific haplotypes of the calpain 5 gene, *CAPN5*, and POCS have been reported.[113] These studies also showed that there were associations between *CAPN5* haplotypes and phenotypic differences between POCS patients including the presence of T2DM.

Calpains and T2DM Pathways

A number of earlier studies have suggested that calpains may be involved in T2DM-related pathways. In the late 1990s, it was demonstrated that calpains participate in adipocyte pathways[116] and mediate the insulin-induced downregulation of adipoyte insulin receptor substrate-1 (IRS-1), a key mediator of insulin action.[117] More recent studies strongly supported these latter findings when it was found that calpain-mediated downregulation of IRS-1 may involve direct interaction between the receptor and these enzymes.[118] Moreover, this IRS-1 downregulation was prevented by the presence of calpain inhibitors but enhanced by drug-induced overload of intracellular Ca^{2+} levels, an effect strongly associated with the overactivation of calpains.[34] Studies on calpain 10 found that UCSNP19 shows a strong association with the function of the lipolytic β3-adrenoreceptor in subcutaneous fat cells in obese individuals.[119] This polymorphism induced a 30-fold decrease in the lipolytic sensitivity of these receptors, leading the authors to conclude that calpain 10 could play a role in regulating thermogenesis. However, analogous studies of UCSNP63, UCSNP43, and UCSNP19 found that there was no association between these polymorphisms and either lipolysis or lipogenesis in adipocytes of nonobese subjects.[120] The link between calpain10 and β-3-adrenoreceptor function has, as yet, not been fully elucidated.

As described above, genetic analyses at the turn of the century have suggested that calpains may modulate insulin secretion and a number of studies have investigated this suggestion at the molecular level. In β cells, the regulated secretory pathway involves a complex series of events, which includes glycolysis, altered ion channel activity in the plasma membrane, and Ca^{2+}-dependent mechanisms that facilitate the relocation of insulin granules and their release from the cell.[121] In a recent study, the long-term exposure of murine pancreatic islets to a variety of calpain inhibitors was found to result in a large reversible decrease in glucose-induced insulin secretion. On the basis of these data, it was suggested that calpains may play an important role in intracellular trafficking either in glucose transport or in the movement of insulin granules.[122] The use of these inhibitors also attenuated the insulin secretory response to the mitochondrial substrate α-ketoisocaproate and suppressed both glucose metabolism and downstream intracellular Ca^{2+} responses to α-ketoisocaproate. These results led to the proposal that calpains play a role in glucose metabolism and that inhibition of these enzymes leads to the acute suppression of insulin secretion by limiting the rate of glucose metabolism through the regulation of mitochondrial function and metabolism. Interestingly, the short-term exposure of mouse pancreatic islets to the calpain inhibitors used by the latter authors[122] was found to enhance rather than decrease glucose-induced insulin secretion.[123] This temporal relationship of calpain inhibition has since been reproduced but as yet, the calpain(s) responsible for these effects and the mechanisms underlying this relationship still remain to be elucidated.[124] However, it has been suggested that this temporal relationship may reflect the existence of alternative signaling pathways or the fact that calpains may play different in different tissues or compartments within a given tissue.[88]

The extracellular matrix (ECM) is an important component of the pancreatic islet microenvironment, constituting a dynamic complex of different molecules that serve as a cellular scaffold regulating both differentiation and survival. It was recently reported that the laminin-5-rich ECM secreted by

804G cells induced increased spreading and improved insulin secretion in response to glucose in purified pancreatic β cells. Most recently, this ECM was used to investigate the role of calpains in the process of Ca^{2+}-induced insulin secretion and spreading of rat pancreatic β cells. Based on the use of calpain inhibitors, it was suggested by these latter authors that calpain could be a mediator of spreading on an ECM and the Ca^{2+}-induced insulin secretion of primary pancreatic β cells.[125] Consistent with this suggestion, a recent key study suggested that calpain 10 may be a major determinant of insulin exocytosis. Soluble *N*-ethyl maleimide-sensitive fusion protein attachment receptor (SNARE) proteins are key molecules that participate in the late stages of the secretory pathway[126–128] and play a role in the membrane targeting and membrane fusion of vesicles/granules.[129] In β cells, granule exocytosis is mediated by a complex that includes the vesicle-associated membrane protein, VAMP2, and the SNARE proteins, syntaxin 1 and SNAP-25[130] and calpain 10 was recently shown to bind these latter SNARE proteins.[131] Moreover, SNAP-25 was found to undergo Ca^{2+}-dependent partial proteolysis during stimulated secretion, which, along with insulin secretion, was inhibited by calpain inhibitors. This latter investigation also found that increasing levels of *CAPN10* overexpression correlated with increasing insulin secretion. On the basis these combined data, it was suggested that calpain 10 may function as a Ca^{2+} sensor to trigger SNARE rearrangement, granule fusion, and the exocytosis of insulin from β cells.[131]

Studies on the role of ryanodine receptor (RyR) Ca^{2+} release channels in the secretion of insulin from human pancreatic β cells led to the proposal that the endosomal system participated in Ca^{2+} influx-independent insulin secretion via RyR-mediated Ca^{2+} signaling.[132] Moreover, it was suggested that the reduced RyR activity associated with T2DM might contribute to hyperinsulinemia via these endosomal effects. There are two RyRs expressed in β cells and in a major study, it was recently shown that the inhibition of type 2 RyR Ca^{2+} flux in these cells, both human and murine, led to significantly increased levels of apoptosis.[124] This effect was strongly retarded by calpain inhibitors and correlated with increased levels of calpain10 mRNA. Moreover, the overexpression of *CAPN10* in mice increased apoptosis while mice lacking *CAPN10* did not exhibit RyR-stimulated apoptosis. This calpain 10-dependent apoptotic pathway was initiated by palmitate and was not associated with a hyperglycemic environment; indeed, its effects were enhanced by high glucose levels,[124] contrasting strongly with the classical caspase 3-dependent apoptosis pathway, which is induced by hyperglycemia.[133,134] In an effort to interpret these data, it has been suggested that hyperlipidemia, using the former apoptosis pathway, is a signal to β cells to induce apoptosis.[88] Thus, individuals who possess T2DM susceptibility will express calpian 10 at reduced levels and will be unable to express the higher levels of the protein needed to induce this pathway with unordered cell lysis and its consequences otherwise occurring. Support for this view comes from the recent demonstration that individuals with impaired glucose tolerance lack the ability of normal glucose tolerant individuals to increase their expression of *CAPN10* in skeletal muscle in response to insulin after long-term exposure to free fatty acids.[100]

The exposure of skeletal muscle strips and adipocytes to calpain inhibitors led to decreased levels of insulin-mediated glucose transport and glycogen synthesis.[123] These results clearly suggested that calpains may play a role in glucose transport, which is the major rate-limiting step in the metabolism of glucose in both muscle and fat tissue, and impaired glucose uptake by glucose transporter 4 (GLUT4) in these tissues is an important feature of insulin resistance.[135–138] Calpastatin is the endogenous inhibitor of calpains 1 and 2[139] and when overexpressed in the skeletal muscle of transgenic mice, this led to the intracellular accumulation of GLUT4 but with no concomitant increase in levels of the transporter protein at the plasma membrane or upregulation of glucose metabolism.[140] It was found by these latter authors that GLUT4 was degraded by calpain 2, which led to the suggestion that the enzyme was involved in the control of GLUT4 and the physiological effects were observed in these transgenic mice. Nonetheless, some controversy surrounds the participation of calpains in GLUT4-mediated glucose transport. It has been suggested[33] that the data of Otani *et al.*[140] would also be explained if the overexpression of calpastatin inhibited calpain 10 and thereby the ability of the enzyme to mediate the translocation of GLUT4-containing vesicle to the plasma membrane, which was recently demonstrated in intact 3T3-L1 adipocytes.[141] However, more recent studies reported that GLUT4 expression in 3T3-L1 adipocytes is not repressed by calpain inhibition but by proteasome inhibition.[142] As yet, neither the role of calpains in glucose transport nor the members of this enzyme family involved in these processes have been definitively defined and these remain questions to be answered. Nonetheless, several tentative models have been presented to describe the putative role(s) of calpain 10 in T2DM pathways[33,88] and that of the latter authors is summarized in FIGURE 3.

Calpains and T2DM Complications

Epithelial Dysfunction

T2DM is associated with a significantly increased risk of cardiovascular disease, which is the leading cause of morbidity and mortality in diabetic patients.[143] Hyperglycemia plays a key pathogenic role in the development of diabetic cardiovascular disease and a major result of the associated high blood glucose levels is endothelial dysfunction.[144] Using hyperglycemic rat models, it was recently shown that calpain activity in the microvasculature of these animals was increased in response to elevated blood glucose levels, resulting in endothelial dysfunction that could be attenuated by the presence of calpain inhibitors.[145] Increased calpain activity has also reported in several other diabetic tissues[146,147] and in combination, these results led Stalker *et al.*[148] to

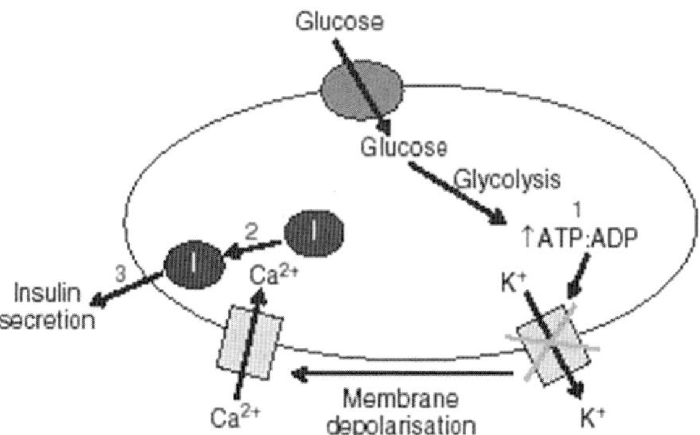

FIGURE 3. This figure shows proposed sites of action for calpain 10 in T2DM-related pathways: (1) The internalization of glucose leads to glycolysis and elevated ATP:ADP ratios through the action of mitochondria. This action is strongly diminished by calpain inhibition and calpain 10 is suggested to act as a regulator of mitochondrial fuel sensing. (2) The secretory stimulus is accompanied by cytoskeletal rearrangement, which leads to the transport of secretory granules containing insulin to active sites of exocytosis at the plasma membrane. In the case of adipocytes and skeletal muscle, this process proceeds via the translocation of vesicles containing GLUT4. This process is highly sensitive to calpin inhibition, either through the use of inhibitors or specific *CAPN10* antisense nucleotides, and roles for calpain 10 and calpain 1 have been suggested. (3) Exocytosis is mediated by a SNARE protein complex and a specific issoform of calpain 10 has been shown to associate with this complex. Based on a number of lines of evidence, it has been proposed that the enzyme functions as a pivotal Ca^{2+}-sensor in exocytosis in β cells.[33] (This figure was adapted from Turner *et al.*[33])

study Zucker diabetic fatty (ZDF) rats, a genetic model of type T2DM, for calpain-mediated endothelial dysfunction. These latter authors found that the microcirculation of these rats exhibited vascular inflammation, accompanied by increases in both the expression of cell adhesion molecules and levels of leukocyte trafficking. These effects, which are well-established characteristics of diabetes-mediated epithelial dysfunction[149] were accompanied by elevated calpain activity. However, it was also found by Stalker *et al.*[148] that the presence of calpain inhibitors strongly influenced these effects, suppressing the expression of cell adhesion molecules in the vasculature endothelium of these rats, and attenuating the interactions of leukocyte with the endothelium. Another major characteristic of diabetes-mediated endothelial dysfunction is the impaired release of nitric oxide (NO),[150] a molecule that exerts potent anti-inflammatory activity in the cardiovascular system.[151] Stalker *et al.*[148] measured the *in vivo* endothelial availability of NO in the microcirculation of ZDF rats and demonstrated large decreases in NO levels, which, however, was prevented by the presence of calpain inhibitors. This study also found that the microcirculation of ZDF rats exhibited strong decreases in the association of NO synthase with the molecular chaperone, heat shock protein 90 (hsp 90) that appears to play a major role in activating the enzyme.[152] The levels of this association were restored by the inhibition of calpain activity and interestingly, it has previously been shown that calpains degrades hsp 90 in several cell systems.[153,154] Most recently, it was shown that calpain-mediated degradation of hsp 90 decreases NO production in pulmonary artery endothelial cells.[155] Stalker *et al.*[148] attempted to identify the calpain(s) involved in the endothelial dysfunction of the ZDF rats studied and showed that there was increased proteolytic activity of calpain 1 but not calpain 2 in the vasculature of these rats. It was suggested that the difference in this isoform activation may be related to the selective activation of calpains according to pathological conditions. Consistent with this suggestion, previous studies have suggested that calpain 2 may be activated in response to large Ca^{2+} fluxes, such as in apoptosis whereas calpain 1 activation may be more important in the scenario of cell signaling,[34] a role previously suggested for calpains in the pathophysiology of diabetic vascular disease.[145] It was concluded by Stalker *et al.*,[148] that calpain 1, and possibly other calpains, may represent a novel molecular target for the prevention and treatment of diabetic vascular complications.

Eye Disorders

Six major calpains are known to be expressed in the eye: calpain 2,[156] the calpain 3 splice variants, *Lp82*[157,158] and *Lp85*,[159,160] and calpain 10[101] have been identified in the lens. In addition, the calpain 3 splice variants *Rt88* and *Cn94* are present in the retina[161] and in the cornea,[162] respectively.

Diabetic retinopathy is a major cause of blindness worldwide[163] and recently, there have been several investigations into the putative role of calpains in the disorder. Wistar Bonn/Kobari (WBN/Kob) rats serve as models for human retinal degeneration and recent studies on these rats showed that over their first 48 weeks of life, calpain 10, and *Rt88* played roles in the eye condition. It was also found by these latter authors that increased levels of retinal Ca^{2+} and the overactivation of calpains 1 and 2 were temporally associated with retinal degeneration.[164] Interestingly, male WBN/Kob rats spontaneously develop diabetes after approximately 52 weeks of life[165] and recent studies on the retinal tissues of rats have suggested that calpains may play a role in diabetic retinopathy.[166] However, the major investigations into calpains and T2DM-related eye disorders have been focused on diabetic cataract, which is another major cause of blindness.[167] In cataract, opacification of all or part of the lens prevents visible light from reaching the retina (FIG. 4), which reduces optical performance and is most commonly manifested by decreased visual acuity, glare, and contrast sensitivity.[168] Catarcatogenesis is known to be mediated by a number of lens insults[169,170] and there is accumulating evidence that associated pathological elevations in lenticular Ca^{2+} lead to the overactivation of calpains, thereby contributing to the condition (FIG. 5). Currently, calpain 2, calpain 10, *Lp82*, and *Lp85* have been linked to this eye condition both in diabetic and nondiabetic studies.

Calpain 10 and Cataract

Studies on male WBN/Kob rats, which exhibit spontaneous diabetic cataract at about the age of 1 year, showed calpain 10 to be localized in the lens cortex of these male rats and coincident with the onset of cataract, these lenses showed large rises in intracellular Ca^{2+}, which correlated with the overactivation of the enzyme.[171] Similar results were found in the studies on calpain 10 using a selenite model of rodent cataract,[101] which in contrast to WBN/Kob male rats, specifically exhibits opacification in the lens nucleus.[172] Consistent with this latter study, it was shown that calpain 10 possesses a putative nuclear localization signal and to localize to the nucleus of αTN4-1 mouse cells with levels of this localization enhanced by elevated Ca^{2+}.[101] It was suggested by these latter authors, that the normal function of calpain 10 may be in the differentiation of epithelial cells but in the presence of pathologically elevated Ca^{2+}, increased uptake of the enzyme into the nuclei of lens epithelial cells may occur, thereby facilitating its participation in selenite cataract. Possibly supporting this suggestion, it was found that lenses of healthy mice, the highest levels of calpain 10 expression were in regions that were associated with the differentiation of epithelial cells.[173]

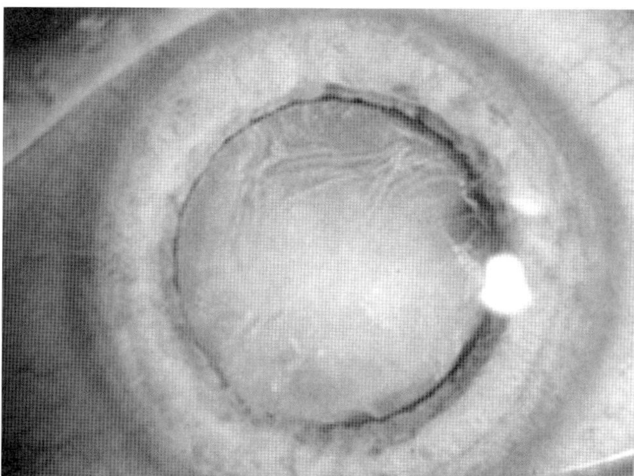

FIGURE 4. This figure shows an advanced cortical cataract in a 48-year-old female with a 12-year history of T2DM. Due to the dense opacity of the cataract, it is difficult to visualize and therefore determine, if there is nuclear opacity as well. (This figure was adapted from Biswas *et al.*[168])

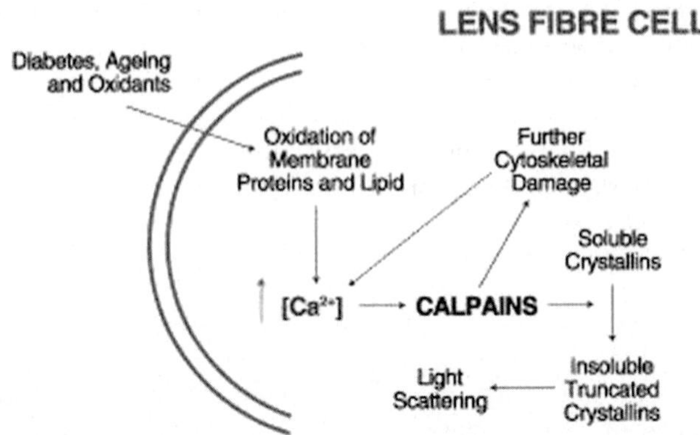

FIGURE 5. This figure shows biochemical pathways that can induce light scattering and cataract. The aging process and lens insults, such as oxidation and diabetes, can lead to impaired membrane function, which results in pathologically elevated levels of lenticular Ca^{2+}. Under these Ca^{2+} conditions, calpains are overactivated and the resulting deregulated proteolysis of soluble crystallins leads to their insolubilization and aggregation, thereby compromising their function(s) in maintaining lens transparency and producing the reduced lens performance associated with cataract. Overactivated calpains also proteolyse lens cytoskeletal proteins, such as vimentin, which, can further elevate lenticular Ca^{2+}, thus excavating calpain overactivation and cataract formation.[168] Calpains have been implicated in a number of cellular processes but for clarity, these biochemical pathways are not shown. (This figure was adapted from Biswas *et al.*[192])

Lp82 and Cataract

Lp82 has been localized to the nuclear and cortical regions of lens from new-born mice[174] and has been shown to co-localize in the fibers of embryonic and postnatal mouse lenses with crystallins.[173] The highly ordered packing of these soluble proteins is primarily responsible for lens transparency with their insolubilization leading to aggregation and the reduced lens performance associated with cataract.[168] The normal function of *Lp82* appears to be in the posttranslational processing of crystallins with low levels of the enzyme required in adult mouse lenses to maintain crystallin structure.[173,175] However, in maturing mouse lenses, mouse cataracts,[176] and mouse lenses with congenital nuclear cataract, the presence of elevated Ca^{2+} levels leads to increased crystallin proteolysis by *Lp82.*[177] Most recently, *in vitro* light scattering studies showed that the Ca^{2+}-mediated overactivation of endogenous mouse lens calpains led to the production of high levels of insoluble α-A-crystallin that were C terminally truncated.[178] *Lp82* showed the highest levels of these effects and taken with the results of other studies[177] it was proposed that the enzyme is the major calpain involved in mouse cataract formation.[178]

Lp82 from rat lenses was found to localize to the nuclear regions of the lens[160] and exogenous *Lp82* was shown to cleave endogenous rat lens α-A-crystallins, producing insoluble C-terminally truncated forms of the protein with levels enhanced by increasing Ca^{2+} levels.[179] A specific cleavage fragment α-A, residues 1–168, produced by this proteolysis has been implicated in cataract formation[180,181] and has also been identified as a product in the *Lp82* proteolysis of mouse α-A-crystallin.[178] Using this cleavage fragment as a biomarker of *Lp82* proteolysis of α-A-crystallin, several studies have suggested that *Lp82* may be the major calpain involved in selenite cataract formation in rats.[175,179] The crystalline cleavage fragment, α-A, residues 1–168, has been identified in various other mammalian lenses and most recently, in bovine lenses, which led to the proposal that the enzyme may also be the major calpain in these lenses.[182] While *Lp82* is currently believed to be absent in humans,[183] it is interesting to note that C terminally truncated crystallins, cleaved at sites identical to those associated with the *Lp82*-mediated proteolysis of these proteins, have been identified in human lenses[184–186] and some human cataracts.[177] Moreover, the novel AX1 N terminus of *Lp82*, which appears to play an important role in the ocular tissues of rodents, appears to be possessed by calpain 3 isoforms present in human ocular tissue.[162]

Calpain 2 and Cataract

There is an abundance of evidence suggesting that calpain 2 is involved in animal cataract. Earlier studies established that the enzyme cleaved crystallins and that calpain inhibitors could prevent rodent cataract, induced by the Ca^{2+}-mediated activation of calpain 2.[156,187,188] Taken with more recent studies,[189] it is now generally accepted that calpain 2 plays a major role in rodent lens opacification while several studies have shown the enzyme to be the major calpain activated in murine diabetic cataractogenesis.[171,190] Most recently, calpain 2 has been shown to induce cataractogenesis, and to cleave crystallins, in the lenses of a variety of other mammalian species including: mice and guineapigs,[175,182,191] monkeys and rabbits,[162] and calves[182] and pigs.[192] The presence of calpain 2 in human lenses is generally accepted and was shown to be the major calpain in the epithelial cells of human lenses exhibiting age-related cortical cataract.[193] Human lenses with cortical cataract are known to have increased levels of intracellular Ca^{2+}, while treating healthy human lenses with extracellular Ca^{2+} leads to discrete cortical cataracts.[156] The activity of calpain 2 has previously been demonstrated in the cortex of human lenses but it was only recently that the Ca^{2+}-induced activation of calpain 2 in this type of human cataract was demonstrated under physiologically relevant conditions.[194] Using cultured human lenses, it was shown that when Ca^{2+} in these lenses was elevated within physiological limits, cortical opacification resulted, accompanied by a significant loss of crystallins from the soluble fraction of these lenses. Moreover, analysis of the insoluble fraction from these lenses revealed high levels of proteolyzed vimentin, a lens substrate of calpain 2 whose proteolysis is indicative of the enzyme's activation.[156] There is some evidence to support a role for calpain 2 in human diabetic cataract[190,195] and taken overall, these results strongly suggest that the enzyme may play a role in at least some forms of human cataract, although clearly, further definitive evidence is required.

CONCLUDING REMARKS

This review has shown that there is strong statistical evidence for a functional association between genetic variations in *CAPN10* and T2DM. This statistical evidence is robustly supported by experimental results, which have shown calpain 10, to play a role in the control of glucose metabolism, insulin action, and β cell function. Clearly, a better knowledge of the genetic risk factors underlying T2DM will enhance understanding of the primary physiology of the disorder, which should be accompanied by the development of more specific and cost-effective therapies. Moreover, the methodologies developed and lessons learnt from the positional cloning studies on *CAPN10* have laid the foundations for investigations into other complex genetic disorders, such as Crohn's disease and asthma.[87]

In addition to calpain 10, a variety of other calpians have also been shown to participate in T2DM-related pathways, phenotypes, and complications through the use of calpain inhibitors. On the basis of such studies, the therapeutic potential of calpain inhibitors is now being investigated and a recent focus of these studies has been the development of these inhibitors as anticataract agents. The successful development of these compounds would be invaluable for use in cases where surgery is not an option, and in the treatment of diabetic cataract as a complement to conventional diabetes therapy.[168]

There are a variety of therapies available for treating T2DM and its complications, but these are not accessible to many poorer populations of the world. While there are many questions yet to be answered about the role(s) of calpain 10, and other calpains, in T2DM, progress over the last 5 years has provided a number of breakthroughs. It is hoped that this will catalyze the development of innovative new therapeutic interventions in the treatment of T2DM and thereby provide benefit to mankind on a global scale.

REFERENCES

1. ZIMMET, P., K.G. ALBERTI & J. SHAW. 2001. Global and societal implications of the diabetes epidemic. Nature **414:** 782–787.
2. KING, H., R.E. AUBERT & W.H. HERMAN. 1998. Global burden of diabetes, 1995–2025: prevalence, numerical estimates, and projections. Diabetes Care **21:** 1414–1431.

3. SINHA, R. *et al.* 2002. Prevalence of impaired glucose tolerance among children and adolescents with marked obesity. N. Engl. J. Med. **346:** 802–810.
4. GORODEZKY, C. *et al.* 2006. HLA and autoimmune diseases: type 1 diabetes (T1D) as an example. Autoimmun. Rev. **5:** 187–194.
5. HANSEN, L. & O. PEDERSEN. 2005. Genetics of type 2 diabetes mellitus: status and perspectives. Diabetes Obes. Metab. **7:** 122–135.
6. REDONDO, M.J. & G.S. EISENBARTH. 2002. Genetic control of autoimmunity in type I diabetes and associated disorders. Diabetologia **45:** 605–622.
7. STUMVOLL, M., B.J. GOLDSTEIN & T.W. VAN HAEFTEN. 2005. Type 2 diabetes: principles of pathogenesis and therapy. Lancet **365:** 1333–1346.
8. ADORINI, L., S. GREGORI & L.C. HARRISON. 2002. Understanding autoimmune diabetes: insights from mouse models. Trends Mol. Med. **8:** 31–38.
9. CASTANO, L. & G.S. EISENBARTH. 1990. Type-I diabetes: a chronic autoimmune disease of human, mouse, and rat. Annu. Rev. Immunol. **8:** 647–679.
10. BACH, J.F. 1994. Insulin-dependent diabetes mellitus as an autoimmune disease. Endocr. Rev. **15:** 516–542.
11. CONCANNON, P. *et al.* 1998. A second-generation screen of the human genome for susceptibility to insulin-dependent diabetes mellitus. Nat. Genet. **19:** 292–296.
12. HERR, M. *et al.* 2000. Evaluation of fine mapping strategies for a multifactorial disease locus: systematic linkage and association analysis of IDDM1 in the HLA region on chromosome 6p21. Hum. Mol. Genet. **9:** 1291–1301.
13. ARNER, P. 2003. The adipocyte in insulin resistance: key molecules and the impact of the thiazolidinediones. Trends Endocrinol. Metab. **14:** 137–145.
14. BAILEY, C.J. 1999. Insulin resistance and antidiabetic drugs. Biochem. Pharmacol. **58:** 1511–1520.
15. BAILEY, C.J. 2000. Potential new treatments for type 2 diabetes. Trends Pharmacol. Sci. **21:** 259–265.
16. PETERSEN, K.F. & G.I. SHULMAN. 2002. Pathogenesis of skeletal muscle insulin resistance in type 2 diabetes mellitus. Am. J. Cardiol. **90:** 11G–18G.
17. SACKS, D.B. & J.M. MCDONALD. 1996. The pathogenesis of type II diabetes mellitus. A polygenic disease. Am. J. Clin. Pathol. **105:** 149–156.
18. SCHEEN, A.J. & F.H. LUYCKX. 2002. Obesity and liver disease. Best Pract. Res. Clin. Endocrinol. Metab. **16:** 703–716.
19. BALEN, A. & M. RAJKOWHA. 2003. Polycystic ovary syndrome—a systemic disorder? Best Pract. Res. Clin. Obstet. Gynaecol. **17:** 263–274.
20. NAOUMOVA, R.P. & D.J. BETTERIDGE. 2002. A new drug target for treatment of dyslipidaemia associated with type 2 diabetes and the metabolic syndrome? Lancet **359:** 2215–2216.
21. CONLIN, P.R. 2001. Efficacy and safety of angiotensin receptor blockers: a review of losartan in essential hypertension. Curr. Ther. Res. **62:** 79–91.
22. PLUTZKY, J., G. VIBERTI & S. HAFFNER. 2002. Atherosclerosis in type 2 diabetes mellitus and insulin resistance: mechanistic links and therapeutic targets. J. Diabetes Complicat. **16:** 401–415.
23. ALI RAZA, J. & A. MOVAHED. 2003. Current concepts of cardiovascular diseases in diabetes mellitus. Int. J. Cardiol. **89:** 123–134.
24. ZANELLA, M.T. & A.B. RIBEIRO. 2002. The role of angiotensin II antagonism in type 2 diabetes mellitus: a review of renoprotection studies. Clin. Ther. **24:** 1019–1034.
25. GARDNER, T.W. *et al.* 2002. Diabetic retinopathy: more than meets the eye. Surv. Ophthalmol. **47**(Suppl 2): S253–S262.

26. Coppini, D.V. *et al.* 2000. Showing neuropathy is related to increased mortality in diabetic patients—a survival analysis using an accelerated failure time model. J. Clin. Epidemiol. **53:** 519–523.
27. Barroso, I. 2005. Genetics of type 2 diabetes. Diabet. Med. **22:** 517–535.
28. Gloyn, A.L. 2003. The search for type 2 diabetes genes. Ageing Res. Rev. **2:** 111–127.
29. Froguel, P. *et al.* 1992. Close linkage of glucokinase locus on chromosome 7p to early-onset non-insulin-dependent diabetes mellitus. Nature **356:** 162–164.
30. Hattersley, A.T. *et al.* 1992. Linkage of type 2 diabetes to the glucokinase gene. Lancet **339:** 1307–1310.
31. Horikawa, Y. *et al.* 2000. Genetic variation in the gene encoding calpain-10 is associated with type 2 diabetes mellitus. Nat. Genet. **26:** 163–175.
32. Suzuki, K. *et al.* 2004. Structure, activation, and biology of calpain. Diabetes **53:** S12–S18.
33. Turner, M.D., P.G. Cassell & G.A. Hitman. 2005. Calpain-10: from genome search to function. Diabetes Metab. Res. Rev. **21:** 505–514.
34. Goll, D.E. *et al.* 2003. The calpain system. Physiol. Rev. **83:** 731–801.
35. Hosfield, C.M. *et al.* 1999. Crystal structure of calpain reveals the structural basis for Ca(2+)-dependent protease activity and a novel mode of enzyme activation. EMBO J. **18:** 6880–6889.
36. Strobl, S. *et al.* 2000. The crystal structure of calcium-free human m-calpain suggests an electrostatic switch mechanism for activation by calcium. Proc. Natl. Acad. Sci. USA **97:** 588–592.
37. Hosfield, C.M., J.S. Elce & Z. Jia. 2004. Activation of calpain by Ca2+: roles of the large subunit N-terminal and domain III–IV linker peptides. J. Mol. Biol. **343:** 1049–1053.
38. Hata, S. *et al.* 2001. Domain II of m-calpain is a Ca(2+)-dependent cysteine protease. FEBS Lett. **501:** 111–114.
39. Tompa, P. *et al.* 2001. Domain III of calpain is a Ca2+-regulated phospholipid-binding domain. Biochem. Biophys. Res. Commun. **280:** 1333–1339.
40. Dutt, P. *et al.* 2000. Roles of individual EF-hands in the activation of m-calpain by calcium. Biochem. J. **348**(Pt 1): 37–43.
41. Kretsinger, R.H. 1997. EF-hands embrace. Nat. Struct. Biol. **4:** 514–516.
42. Arthur, J.S. & C. Crawford. 1996. Investigation of the interaction of m-calpain with phospholipids: calpain-phospholipid interactions. Biochim. Biophys. Acta **1293:** 201–206.
43. Dennison, S.R. *et al.* 2005. Investigations into the membrane interactions of m-calpain domain V. Biophys. J. **88:** 3008–3017.
44. Reverter, D., H. Sorimachi & W. Bode. 2001. The structure of calcium-free human m-calpain: implications for calcium activation and function. Trends Cardiovasc. Med. **11:** 222–229.
45. Reverter, D. *et al.* 2001. Structural basis for possible calcium-induced activation mechanisms of calpains. Biol. Chem. **382:** 753–766.
46. Reverter, D. *et al.* 2002. Flexibility analysis and structure comparison of two crystal forms of calcium-free human m-calpain. Biol. Chem. **383:** 1415–1422.
47. Alexa, A. *et al.* 2004. Contribution of distinct structural elements to activation of calpain by Ca2+ ions. J. Biol. Chem. **279:** 20118–20126.
48. Bozoky, Z. *et al.* 2005. Multiple interactions of the 'transducer' govern its function in calpain activation by Ca2+. Biochem. J. **388:** 741–744.

49. HOSFIELD, C.M. *et al.* 2001. Calpain mutants with increased Ca2+ sensitivity and implications for the role of the C(2)-like domain. J. Biol. Chem. **276:** 7404–7407.
50. MOLDOVEANU, T. *et al.* 2001. Ca(2+)-induced structural changes in rat m-calpain revealed by partial proteolysis. Biochim. Biophys. Acta. **1545:** 245–254.
51. BRANCA, D. 2004. Calpain-related diseases. Biochem. Biophys. Res. Commun. **322:** 1098–1104.
52. GARCIADIAZ, B.E., S. GAUTHIER & P.L. DAVIES. 2006. Ca^{2+} Dependency of calpain 3 (p94) activation. Biochemistry **45:** 3714–3722.
53. HUANG, Y. & K.K. WANG. 2001. The calpain family and human disease. Trends Mol. Med. **7:** 355–362.
54. SORIMACHI, H. & K. SUZUKI. 2001. The structure of calpain. J. Biochem. (Tokyo) **129:** 653–664.
55. CARAFOLI, E. & M. MOLINARI. 1998. Calpain: a protease in search of a function? Biochem. Biophys. Res. Commun. **247:** 193–203.
56. SATO, K. & S. KAWASHIMA. 2001. Calpain function in the modulation of signal transduction molecules. Biol. Chem. **382:** 743–751.
57. YAJIMA, Y. & S. KAWASHIMA. 2002. Calpain function in the differentiation of mesenchymal stem cells. Biol. Chem. **383:** 757–764.
58. RAMI, A. 2003. Ischemic neuronal death in the rat hippocampus: the calpain-calpastatin-caspase hypothesis. Neurobiol. Dis. **13:** 75–88.
59. YAMASHIMA, T. 2000. Implication of cysteine proteases calpain, cathepsin and caspase in ischemic neuronal death of primates. Prog. Neurobiol. **62:** 273–295.
60. CARRAGHER, N.O. 2006. Calpain inhibition: a therapeutic strategy targeting multiple disease states. Curr. Pharm. Des. **12:** 615–638.
61. SAZONTOVA, T.G., A.A. MATSKEVICH & Y.V. ARKHIPENKO. 1999. Calpains: physiological and pathophysiological significance. Pathophysiology **6:** 91–102.
62. BARTOLI, M. & I. RICHARD. 2005. Calpains in muscle wasting. Int. J. Biochem. Cell. Biol. **37:** 2115–2133.
63. NIXON, R.A. 2000. A "protease activation cascade" in the pathogenesis of Alzheimer's disease. Ann. N. Y. Acad. Sci. **924:** 117–131.
64. VANDERKLISH, P.W. & B.A. BAHR. 2000. The pathogenic activation of calpain: a marker and mediator of cellular toxicity and disease states. Int. J. Exp. Pathol. **81:** 323–339.
65. HARRIS, F. *et al.* 2004. Role of calpains in diabetes mellitus: a mini review. Mol. Cell. Biochem. **261:** 161–167.
66. HANIS, C.L. *et al.* 1996. A genome-wide search for human non-insulin-dependent (type 2) diabetes genes reveals a major susceptibility locus on chromosome 2. Nat. Genet. **13:** 161–166.
67. GARANT, M.J. *et al.* 2002. SNP43 of CAPN10 and the risk of type 2 diabetes in African Americans: the Atherosclerosis Risk in Communities Study. Diabetes **51:** 231–237.
68. LEIPOLD, H. *et al.* 2004. Calpain-10 haplotype combination and association with gestational diabetes mellitus. Obstet. Gynecol. **103:** 1235–1240.
69. LYNN, S. *et al.* 2002. Variation in the calpain-10 gene affects blood glucose levels in the British population. Diabetes **51:** 247–250.
70. MALECKI, M.T. *et al.* 2002. Homozygous combination of calpain 10 gene haplotypes is associated with type 2 diabetes mellitus in a Polish population. Eur. J. Endocrinol. **146:** 695–699.

71. ORHO-MELANDER, M. *et al.* 2002. Variants in the calpain-10 gene predispose to insulin resistance and elevated free fatty acid levels. Diabetes **51:** 2658–2664.
72. BAIER, L.J. *et al.* 2000. A calpain-10 gene polymorphism is associated with reduced muscle mRNA levels and insulin resistance. J. Clin. Invest. **106:** 69–73.
73. CASSELL, P.G. *et al.* 2002. Haplotype combinations of calpain 10 gene polymorphisms associate with increased risk of impaired glucose tolerance and type 2 diabetes in South Indians. Diabetes **51:** 1622–1628.
74. WEEDON, M.N. *et al.* 2003. Meta-analysis and a large association study confirm a role for calpain-10 variation in type 2 diabetes susceptibility. Am. J. Hum. Genet. **73:** 1208–1212.
75. NG, M.C.Y. *et al.* 2001. Association of calpain 10 genetic polymorphisms with type 2 diabetes and insulin response in non-diabetic Chinese. Diabetes **50:** A234.
76. FURUTA, M., H. FURUTA & K. UEDA. 2001. Relationship between genetic variation in the calpain 10 gene and insulin sensitivity in Japanese. Diabetes **50:** A490.
77. DAIMON, M. *et al.* 2002. Calpain 10 gene polymorphisms are related, not to type 2 diabetes, but to increased serum cholesterol in Japanese. Diabetes Res. Clin. Pract. **56:** 147–152.
78. ELBEIN, S.C. *et al.* 2002. Role of calpain-10 gene variants in familial type 2 diabetes in Caucasians. J. Clin. Endocrinol. Metab. **87:** 650–654.
79. EVANS, J.C. *et al.* 2001. Studies of association between the gene for calpain-10 and type 2 diabetes mellitus in the United Kingdom. Am. J. Hum. Genet. **69:** 544–552.
80. FINGERLIN, T.E. *et al.* 2002. Variation in three single nucleotide polymorphisms in the calpain-10 gene not associated with type 2 diabetes in a large Finnish cohort. Diabetes **51:** 1644–1648.
81. HEGELE, R.A. *et al.* 2001. Absence of association of type 2 diabetes with CAPN10 and PC-1 polymorphisms in Oji-Cree. Diabetes Care **24:** 1498–1499.
82. HORIKAWA, Y. *et al.* 2003. Genetic variations in calpain-10 gene are not a major factor in the occurrence of type 2 diabetes in Japanese. J. Clin. Endocrinol. Metab. **88:** 244–247.
83. RASMUSSEN, S.K. *et al.* 2002. Variants within the calpain-10 gene on chromosome 2q37 (NIDDM1) and relationships to type 2 diabetes, insulin resistance, and impaired acute insulin secretion among Scandinavian Caucasians. Diabetes **51:** 3561–3567.
84. SUN, H.X. *et al.* 2002. Single nucleotide polymorphisms in CAPN10 gene of Chinese people and its correlation with type 2 diabetes mellitus in Han people of northern China. Biomed. Environ. Sci. **15:** 75–82.
85. TSAI, H.J. *et al.* 2001. Type 2 diabetes and three calpain-10 gene polymorphisms in Samoans: no evidence of association. Am. J. Hum. Genet. **69:** 1236–1244.
86. XIANG, K. *et al.* 2001. The impact of calpain-10 gene combined-SNP variation on type 2 diabetes mellitus and its related metabolic traits. Zhonghua Yi Xue Yi Chuan Xue Za Zhi. **18:** 426–430.
87. COX, N.J. *et al.* 2004. Linkage of calpain 10 to type 2 diabetes: the biological rationale. Diabetes **53**(Suppl 1): 19–25.
88. RIDDERSTRALE, M., H. PARIKH & L. GROOP. 2005. Calpain 10 and type 2 diabetes: are we getting closer to an explanation? Curr. Opin. Clin. Nutr. Metab. Care **8:** 361–366.

89. Song, Y. *et al.* 2004. Are variants in the CAPN10 gene related to risk of type 2 diabetes? A quantitative assessment of population and family-based association studies. Am. J. Hum. Genet. **74:** 208–222.
90. Parikh, H. & L. Groop. 2004. Candidate genes for type 2 diabetes. Rev. Endocr. Metab. Disord. **5:** 151–176.
91. Lyssenko, V. *et al.* 2005. Genetic prediction of future type 2 diabetes. PLoS Med. **2:** 1299–1308.
92. Sun, L., N.J. Cox & M.S. McPeek. 2002. A statistical method for identification of polymorphisms that explain a linkage result. Am. J. Hum. Genet. **70:** 399–411.
93. Cox, N.J. *et al.* 1999. Loci on chromosomes 2 (NIDDM1) and 15 interact to increase susceptibility to diabetes in Mexican Americans. Nat. Genet. **21:** 213–215.
94. Walder, K. *et al.* 2002. Calpain 3 gene expression in skeletal muscle is associated with body fat content and measures of insulin resistance. Int. J. Obes. Relat. Metab. Disord. **26:** 442–449.
95. Tschritter, O. *et al.* 2003. Assessing the shape of the glucose curve during an oral glucose tolerance test. Diabetes Care **26:** 1026–1033.
96. Stumvoll, M. *et al.* 2001. Functional significance of the UCSNP-43 polymorphism in the CAPN10 gene for proinsulin processing and insulin secretion in nondiabetic Germans. Diabetes **50:** 2161–2163.
97. Weyer, C. *et al.* 2000. A high fasting plasma insulin concentration predicts type 2 diabetes independent of insulin resistance: evidence for a pathogenic role of relative hyperinsulinemia. Diabetes **49:** 2094–2101.
98. Shore, A.C. *et al.* 2002. Association of calpain-10 gene with microvascular function. Diabetologia **45:** 899–904.
99. Knowler, W.C. *et al.* 1978. Diabetes incidence and prevalence in Pima Indians: a 19-fold greater incidence than in Rochester, Minnesota. Am. J. Epidemiol. **108:** 497–505.
100. Carlsson, E. *et al.* 2005. Genetic and nongenetic regulation of CAPN10 mRNA expression in skeletal muscle. Diabetes **54:** 3015–3020.
101. Ma, H. *et al.* 2001. Characterization and expression of calpain 10. A novel ubiquitous calpain with nuclear localization. J. Biol. Chem. **276:** 28525–28531.
102. Yang, X. *et al.* 2001. Reduced skeletal muscle calpain-10 transcript level is due to a cumulative decrease in major isoforms. Mol. Genet. Metab. **73:** 111–113.
103. Cox, N.J. 2001. Challenges in identifying genetic variation affecting susceptibility to type 2 diabetes: examples from studies of the calpain-10 gene. Hum. Mol. Genet. **10:** 2301–2305.
104. Leahy, J.L. 2005. Pathogenesis of type 2 diabetes mellitus. Arch. Med. Res. **36:** 197–209.
105. Shima, Y. *et al.* 2003. Association of the SNP-19 genotype 22 in the calpain-10 gene with elevated body mass index and hemoglobin A1c levels in Japanese. Clin. Chim. Acta **336:** 89–96.
106. Ji, L., L. Chen & X. Han. 2001. The role of calpain10 gene polymorphisms in genetic susceptibility to type 2 diabetes in a Chinese population. Diabetes **50:** A206–A207.
107. Sugimoto, K. *et al.* 2003. UCSNP-43 G/A polymorphism of calpain-10 gene is associated with hypertension and dyslipidemia in Japanese population. Am. J. Hypertens. **16:** A82.
108. Carlsson, E. *et al.* 2004. Variation in the calpain-10 gene is associated with elevated triglyceride levels and reduced adipose tissue messenger ribonucleic

acid expression in obese Swedish subjects. J. Clin. Endocrinol. Metab. **89:** 3601–3605.
109. HINNEY, A. *et al.* 2002. No evidence for involvement of the calpain-10 gene 'high-risk' haplotype combination for non-insulin-dependent diabetes mellitus in early onset obesity. Mol. Genet. Metab. **76:** 152–156.
110. MURAMATSU, Y. *et al.* 2003. Capn10, a candidate gene responsible for type 2 diabetes mellitus in the OLETF rat. IUBMB Life **55:** 533–537.
111. OVALLE, F. & R. AZZIZ. 2002. Insulin resistance, polycystic ovary syndrome, and type 2 diabetes mellitus. Fertil. Steril. **77:** 1095–1105.
112. EHRMANN, D.A. *et al.* 2002. Relationship of calpain-10 genotype to phenotypic features of polycystic ovary syndrome. J. Clin. Endocrinol. Metab. **87:** 1669–1673.
113. GONZALEZ, A. *et al.* 2002. Comment: CAPN10 alleles are associated with polycystic ovary syndrome. J. Clin. Endocrinol. Metab. **87:** 3971–3976.
114. ESCOBAR-MORREALE, H.F. *et al.* 2002. Common single nucleotide polymorphisms in intron 3 of the calpain-10 gene influence hirsutism. Fertil. Steril. **77:** 581–587.
115. HADDAD, L. *et al.* 2002. Variation within the type 2 diabetes susceptibility gene calpain-10 and polycystic ovary syndrome. J. Clin. Endocrinol. Metab. **87:** 2606–2610.
116. PATEL, Y.M. & M.D. LANE. 1999. Role of calpain in adipocyte differentiation. Proc. Natl. Acad. Sci. USA **96:** 1279–1284.
117. SMITH, L.K., K.M. RICE & C.W. GARNER. 1996. The insulin-induced downregulation of IRS-1 in 3T3-L1 adipocytes is mediated by a calcium-dependent thiol protease. Mol. Cell. Endocrinol. **122:** 81–92.
118. ZHANG, H., H. HOFF & C. SELL. 2003. Downregulation of IRS-1 protein in thapsigargin-treated human prostate epithelial cells. Exp. Cell. Res. **289:** 352–358.
119. HOFFSTEDT, J., E. NASLUND & P. ARNER. 2002. Calpain-10 gene polymorphism is associated with reduced beta(3)-adrenoceptor function in human fat cells. J. Clin. Endocrinol. Metab. **87:** 3362–3367.
120. HOFFSTEDT, J. *et al.* 2002. Polymorphism in the calpain 10 gene influences glucose metabolism in human fat cells. Diabetologia **45:** 276–282.
121. RORSMAN, P. & E. RENSTROM. 2003. Insulin granule dynamics in pancreatic beta cells. Diabetologia **46:** 1029–1045.
122. ZHOU, Y.P. *et al.* 2003. A 48-hour exposure of pancreatic islets to calpain inhibitors impairs mitochondrial fuel metabolism and the exocytosis of insulin. Metabolism **52:** 528–534.
123. SREENAN, S.K. *et al.* 2001. Calpains play a role in insulin secretion and action. Diabetes **50:** 2013–2020.
124. JOHNSON, J.D. *et al.* 2004. RyR2 and calpain-10 delineate a novel apoptosis pathway in pancreatic islets. J. Biol. Chem. **279:** 24794–24802.
125. PARNAUD, G. *et al.* 2005. Inhibition of calpain blocks pancreatic beta-cell spreading and insulin secretion. Am. J. Physiol. Endocrinol. Metab. **289:** 313–321.
126. PELHAM, H.R. 2001. SNAREs and the specificity of membrane fusion. Trends Cell. Biol. **11:** 99–101.
127. HAY, J.C. 2001. SNARE complex structure and function. Exp. Cell. Res. **271:** 10–21.
128. CHEN, Y.A. & R.H. SCHELLER. 2001. SNARE-mediated membrane fusion. Nat. Rev. Mol. Cell. Biol. **2:** 98–106.

129. ROTHMAN, J.E. 1994. Mechanisms of intracellular protein transport. Nature **372:** 55–63.
130. OHARA-IMAIZUMI, M. *et al.* 2004. Correlation of syntaxin-1 and SNAP-25 clusters with docking and fusion of insulin granules analysed by total internal reflection fluorescence microscopy. Diabetologia **47:** 2200–2207.
131. MARSHALL, C. *et al.* 2005. Evidence that an isoform of calpain-10 is a regulator of exocytosis in pancreatic beta-cells. Mol. Endocrinol. **19:** 213–224.
132. JOHNSON, J.D. *et al.* 2004. Ryanodine receptors in human pancreatic β cells: localization and effects on insulin secretion. FASEB J. **10:** 878–880.
133. MAEDLER, K. *et al.* 2002. Glucose-induced beta cell production of IL-1beta contributes to glucotoxicity in human pancreatic islets. J. Clin. Invest. **110:** 851–860.
134. ZHOU, Y.P. *et al.* 1998. Apoptosis in insulin-secreting cells. Evidence for the role of intracellular Ca2+ stores and arachidonic acid metabolism. J. Clin. Invest. **101:** 1623–1632.
135. CUSHMAN, S.W. & L.J. WARDZALA. 1980. Potential mechanism of insulin action on glucose transport in the isolated rat adipose cell. Apparent translocation of intracellular transport systems to the plasma membrane. J. Biol. Chem. **255:** 4758–4762.
136. BUTLER, P.C. *et al.* 1990. Effect of insulin on oxidation of intracellularly and extracellularly derived glucose in patients with NIDDM. Evidence for primary defect in glucose transport and/or phosphorylation but not oxidation. Diabetes **39:** 1373–1380.
137. CLINE, G.W. *et al.* 1999. Impaired glucose transport as a cause of decreased insulin-stimulated muscle glycogen synthesis in type 2 diabetes. N. Engl. J. Med. **341:** 240–246.
138. ROTHMAN, D.L., R.G. SHULMAN & G.I. SHULMAN. 1992. 31P nuclear magnetic resonance measurements of muscle glucose-6-phosphate. Evidence for reduced insulin-dependent muscle glucose transport or phosphorylation activity in non-insulin-dependent diabetes mellitus. J. Clin. Invest. **89:** 1069–1075.
139. WENDT, A., V.F. THOMPSON & D.E. GOLL. 2004. Interaction of calpastatin with calpain: a review. Biol. Chem. **385:** 465–472.
140. OTANI, K. *et al.* 2004. Calpain system regulates muscle mass and glucose transporter GLUT4 turnover. J. Biol. Chem. **279:** 20915–20920.
141. PAUL, D.S. *et al.* 2003. Calpain facilitates GLUT4 vesicle translocation during insulin-stimulated glucose uptake in adipocytes. Biochem. J. **376:** 625–632.
142. COOKE, D.W. & Y.M. PATEL. 2005. GLUT4 expression in 3T3-L1 adipocytes is repressed by proteasome inhibition, but not by inhibition of calpains. Mol. Cell. Endocrinol. **232:** 37–45.
143. VARUGHESE, G.I., J. TOMSON & G.Y.H. LIP. 2005. Type 2 diabetes mellitus: a cardiovascular perspective. Int. J. Clin. Pract. **59:** 798–816.
144. AVOGARO, A. *et al.* 2006. Endothelial dysfunction in type 2 diabetes mellitus. Nutr. Metab. Cardiovasc. Dis. **16:** 39–45.
145. STALKER, T.J., C.B. SKVARKA & R. SCALIA. 2003. A novel role for calpains in the endothelial dysfunction of hyperglycemia. FASEB J. **17:** 1511–1513.
146. KOBAYASHI, S., T. NAITOH & M. KIMURA. 1989. Diabetic state-induced regulation of glucose uptake to skeletal muscle by insulin: a possible mechanism of its enhancement and autoinhibition. Diabetes Res. Clin. Pract. **7**(Suppl 1): S11–S13.

147. SRIVASTAVA, K. & D. DASH. 2002. Changes in membrane microenvironment and signal transduction in platelets from NIDDM patients—a pilot study. Clin. Chim. Acta **317:** 213–220.
148. STALKER, T.J., Y. GONG & R. SCALIA. 2005. The calcium-dependent protease calpain causes endothelial dysfunction in type 2 diabetes. Diabetes **54:** 1132–1140.
149. DANDONA, P. *et al.* 2004. Endothelial dysfunction, inflammation and diabetes. Rev. Endocr. Metab. Disord. **5:** 189–197.
150. COSENTINO, F. & G.E. ASSENZA. 2004. Diabetes and inflammation. Herz **29:** 749–759.
151. LEFER, A.M. & R. SCALIA. 2001. Nitric oxide in inflammation. *In* Physiology of Inflammation. K. Ley, Ed.: 447–472 Oxford University Press. Oxford, UK.
152. FONTANA, J. *et al.* 2002. Domain mapping studies reveal that the M domain of hsp90 serves as a molecular scaffold to regulate Akt-dependent phosphorylation of endothelial nitric oxide synthase and NO release. Circ. Res. **90:** 866–873.
153. BELLOCQ, A. *et al.* 1999. Somatostatin increases glucocorticoid binding and signaling in macrophages by blocking the calpain-specific cleavage of Hsp 90. J. Biol. Chem. **274:** 36891–36896.
154. MINAMI, Y. *et al.* 1994. The carboxy-terminal region of mammalian HSP90 is required for its dimerization and function *in vivo*. Mol. Cell. Biol. **14:** 1459–1464.
155. SU, Y.C. & E.R. BLOCK. 2000. Role of calpain in hypoxic inhibition of nitric oxide synthase activity in pulmonary endothelial cells. Am. J. Physiol.—Lung Cell. Mol. Physiol. **278:** L1204–L1212.
156. SHEARER, T.R. *et al.* 2000. Calpains in the lens and cataractogenesis. Methods Mol. Biol. **144:** 277–285.
157. MA, H. *et al.* 1998. Cloning and expression of mRNA for calpain Lp82 from rat lens: splice variant of p94. Invest. Ophthalmol. Vis. Sci. **39:** 454–461.
158. MA, H. *et al.* 1998. Protein for Lp82 calpain is expressed and enzymatically active in young rat lens. Exp. Eye Res. **67:** 221–229.
159. SHIH, M. *et al.* 2006. Biochemical properties of lens-specific calpain Lp85. Exp. Eye Res. **82:** 146–152.
160. MA, H. *et al.* 2000. Lp85 calpain is an enzymatically active rodent-specific isozyme of lens Lp82. Curr. Eye Res. **20:** 183–189.
161. AZUMA, M. *et al.* 2000. Identification and characterization of a retina-specific calpain (Rt88) from rat. Curr. Eye Res. **21:** 710–720.
162. NAKAJIMA, T. *et al.* 2001. Different expression patterns for ubiquitous calpains and Capn3 splice variants in monkey ocular tissues. Biochim. Biophys. Acta **1519:** 55–64.
163. CIULLA, T.A., A.G. AMADOR & B. ZINMAN. 2003. Diabetic retinopathy and diabetic macular edema: pathophysiology, screening, and novel therapies. Diabetes Care **26:** 2653–2664.
164. AZUMA, M. *et al.* 2004. Involvement of calpain isoforms in retinal degeneration in WBN/Kob rats. Comp. Med. **54:** 533–542.
165. NAKAMA, K. *et al.* 1985. Spontaneous diabetes-like syndrome in WBN/KOB rats. Acta Diabetol. Lat. **22:** 335–342.
166. ROY, K. *et al.* 2005. Effects of streptozotocin-induced type 1 diabetes mellitus on protein and ion concentrations in ocular tissues of the rat. Int. J. Diabetes Metab. **13:** 154–158.

167. KYSELOVA, Z., M. STEFEK & V. BAUER. 2004. Pharmacological prevention of diabetic cataract. J. Diabetes Complicat **18:** 129–140.

168. BISWAS, S. *et al.* 2005. Calpains: enzymes of vision? Med. Sci. Monit. **11:** RA301–RA310.

169. LOU, M.F. 2003. Redox regulation in the lens. Prog. Retin. Eye Res. **22:** 657–682.

170. STITT, A.W. 2001. Advanced glycation: an important pathological event in diabetic and age related ocular disease. Br. J. Ophthalmol. **85:** 746–753.

171. SAKAMOTO-MIZUTANI, K. *et al.* 2002. Contribution of ubiquitous calpains to cataractogenesis in the spontaneous diabetic WBN/Kob rat. Exp. Eye Res. **75:** 611–617.

172. SHEARER, T.R. *et al.* 1997. Selenite nuclear cataract: review of the model. Mol. Vis. **3:** 8.

173. REED, N.A. *et al.* 2003. Protein expression patterns for ubiquitous and tissue specific calpains in the developing mouse lens. Exp. Eye Res. **76:** 433–443.

174. MA, H. *et al.* 2000. Influence of specific regions in Lp82 calpain on protein stability, activity, and localization within lens. Invest. Ophthalmol. Vis. Sci. **41:** 4232–4239.

175. UEDA, Y., M.K. DUNCAN & L.L. DAVID. 2002. Lens proteomics: the accumulation of crystallin modifications in the mouse lens with age. Invest. Ophthalmol. Vis. Sci. **43:** 205–215.

176. MA, H. *et al.* 1999. Lp82 is the dominant form of calpain in young mouse lens. Exp. Eye Res. **68:** 447–456.

177. BARUCH, A. *et al.* 2001. Defining a link between gap junction communication, proteolysis, and cataract formation. J. Biol. Chem. **276:** 28999–29006.

178. AZUMA, M. *et al.* 2003. Differential influence of proteolysis by calpain 2 and Lp82 on in vitro precipitation of mouse lens crystallins. Biochem. Biophys. Res. Commun. **307:** 558–563.

179. UEDA, Y. *et al.* 2002. Mass measurements of C-terminally truncated alpha-crystallins from two-dimensional gels identify Lp82 as a major endopeptidase in rat lens. Mol. Cell. Proteom. **1:** 357–365.

180. SHARMA, K.K., K. KESTER & N. ELSER. 1996. Identification of new lens protease(s) using peptide substrates having in vivo cleavage sites. Biochem. Biophys. Res. Commun. **218:** 365–370.

181. TAKEMOTO, L. 1994. Release of [alpha]-A sequence 158–173 correlates with a decrease in the molecular chaperone properties of native [alpha]-crystallin. Exp. Eye Res. **59:** 239–242.

182. UEDA, Y. *et al.* 2001. Purification and characterization of lens specific calpain (Lp82) from bovine lens. Exp. Eye Res. **73:** 625–637.

183. FOUGEROUSSE, F. *et al.* 2000. Human-mouse differences in the embryonic expression patterns of developmental control genes and disease genes. Hum. Mol. Genet. **9:** 165–173.

184. COLVIS, C.M. *et al.* 2000. Tracking pathology with proteomics: identification of in vivo degradation products of alphaB-crystallin. Electrophoresis **21:** 2219–2227.

185. LUND, A.L., J.B. SMITH & D.L. SMITH. 1996. Modifications of the water-insoluble human lens alpha-crystallins. Exp. Eye Res. **63:** 661–672.

186. TAKEMOTO, L.J. 1995. Identification of the *in vivo* truncation sites at the C-terminal region of alpha-A crystallin from aged bovine and human lens. Curr. Eye Res. **14:** 837–841.

187. ANDERSSON, M., J. SJOSTRAND & J.O. KARLSSON. 1996. Calpains in the human lens: relations to membranes and possible role in cataract formation. Ophthalmic Res. **28**(Suppl 1): 51–54.
188. AZUMA, M. *et al.* 1997. Activation of calpain in lens: a review and proposed mechanism. Exp. Eye Res. **64:** 529–538.
189. INOMATA, M. *et al.* 2000. Aminoguanidine-treatment results in the inhibition of lens opacification and calpain-mediated proteolysis in Shumiya cataract rats (SCR). J. Biochem. (Tokyo) **128:** 771–776.
190. THAMPI, P. *et al.* 2002. Enhanced C-terminal truncation of alphaA- and alphaB-crystallins in diabetic lenses. Invest. Ophthalmol. Vis. Sci. **43:** 3265–3272.
191. FUKIAGE, C. *et al.* 1997. SJA6017, a newly synthesized peptide aldehyde inhibitor of calpain: amelioration of cataract in cultured rat lenses. Biochim. Biophys. Acta **1361:** 304–312.
192. BISWAS, S. *et al.* 2004. The in vitro retardation of porcine cataractogenesis by the calpain inhibitor, SJA6017. Mol. Cell. Biochem. **261:** 169–173.
193. ANDERSSON, M. *et al.* 1994. Calpains in lens epithelium from patients with cataract. Exp. Eye Res. **59:** 359–364.
194. SANDERSON, J., J.M. MARCANTONIO & G. DUNCAN. 2000. A human lens model of cortical cataract: Ca2+-induced protein loss, vimentin cleavage and opacification. Invest. Ophthalmol. Vis. Sci. **41:** 2255–2261.
195. THAMPI, P., S. ZARINA & E.C. ABRAHAM. 2002. Alpha-crystallin chaperone function in diabetic rat and human lenses. Mol. Cell. Biochem. **229:** 113–118.

Lipid Peroxidation and Serum Antioxidant Enzymes in Patients with Type 2 Diabetes Mellitus

FEROZA N. AHMED, FARZANA N. NAQVI, AND FAKHRA SHAFIQ

Department of Genetics, University of Karachi, Karachi-75270, Pakistan

ABSTRACT: Diabetes mellitus is characterized by fasting hyperglycemia, with both type 1 and type 2 diabetes. Persons are also known to be prone to develop complications related to elevated blood glucose concentrations, including atherosclerosis, retinal damage, cataract, and neuropathy. Hyperglycemia may also result in increased production of the reactive oxygen species within numerous biochemical pathways that have the potential to initiate changes in endothelial function. This article demonstrates the presence of lipid peroxidation products in the red cell membranes of type 2 diabetic patients compared to the normal subjects. These membranes are more susceptible to exogenous oxidative stress than those of normal healthy individuals. Significantly higher activities of antioxidant enzymes, namely, serum peroxidase, superoxide dismutase (SOD), and catalase (CAT) were found in type 2 diabetic patients as compared to control. This study led us to conclude that elevated levels of glucose induce oxidative stress that is ultimately reflected by the increased malondialdehyde (MDA) levels in erythrocyte ghost membranes of diabetic patients. Hyperglycemia also induced an increase in antioxidant enzymes and a relationship seems to exist between diabetic complications and elevated levels of these enzymes. It is suggested that these antioxidant enzymes may be considered as markers for vascular injury.

KEYWORDS: NIDDM; lipid peroxidation; antioxidant enzymes

INTRODUCTION

Hyperglycemia is an important determinant in the pathogenesis of the long-term complications in both insulin-dependent diabetes mellitus (type 1, IDDM) and non insulin-dependent diabetes mellitus (type 2, NIDDM).[1] Hyperglycemia may also result in increased production of the reactive oxygen species (ROS) within numerous biochemical pathways that have potential to initiate changes in endothelial functions.

Address for corespondence: Farzana N. Naqvi, Department of Genetics, University of Karachi, Karachi-752 70, Pakistan.Voice: 92-21-9243030, 92-21-8201674, 0333-2183710.
e-mail: naqvi.farzana@gmail.com

Ann. N.Y. Acad. Sci. 1084: 481–489 (2006). © 2006 New York Academy of Sciences.
doi: 10.1196/annals.1372.022

Free radicals are physiologically useful and necessary for life but can be harmful if present in excess amounts.[2] The attack by free radicals, collectively known as oxidative stress, is capable of causing cells to lose their structure and function and eventually destroy them.[3] Oxidative stress plays an important role in the pathogenesis of the long-term complications of diabetes.[4] Oxygen-free radicals could therefore be responsible for most of the erythrocyte abnormalities associated with noninsulin-dependent diabetes and could indeed be intimately involved in the mechanism of tissue damage in diabetic complications.[5] Lipid peroxidation is indicative of cell damage. Studies have shown increased level of plasma lipid in diabetic individuals as compared to their control.[6,7]

It is well known that a number of enzymatic systems protect cells from the damage caused by excessive production of ROS. These systems include superoxide dismutase (SOD) in the cytosol that convert superoxide into hydrogen peroxide, together with the glutathione peroxidase (GPX) and catalase (CAT) enzymes in the cytosol and peroxisomes that convert hydrogen peroxide to water.[8] High blood glucose can induce an overexpression of CuZn-SOD, CAT, and GPX in human endothelial cells from umbilical vein and immortalized human endothelial cells.[9]

The aim of the present article is to determine the effect of hyperglycemia (oxidative stress) on the biochemical parameters of diabetic patients compared to control. Lipid peroxidation product of thiobarbituric acid compound (malondialdehyde [MDA]) was used as an indicator of membrane damage while levels of antioxidant enzymes were considered as markers for vascular injury.

MATERIALS AND METHODS

This study was conducted on 71 subjects. Informed consent was obtained from each person who agreed to participate in this study, while the survey was based on standardized interviews and questionnaire. Subjects were grouped as diabetics, diabetic control (who had family history of diabetes but they are not affected), and healthy control (who had no diabetes status of their parents as well as themselves). Blood pressure, glucose levels, hypertension, and other related complications were recorded. The information gathered was used for the construction of pedigrees, two of the representative pedigrees of healthy control and diabetic subjects are shown (FIGS. 1 and 2).

Isolation of Erythrocyte Ghost Membranes

For the isolation of erythrocyte ghost membranes (EGMs), blood sample was collected into anticoagulant tubes from all subjects. After separation of plasma, RBCs were suspended in 10 volumes of cold isotonic phosphate buffer pH 7.4[6] and centrifuged at 3000 rpm for 10 min. This was repeated again and

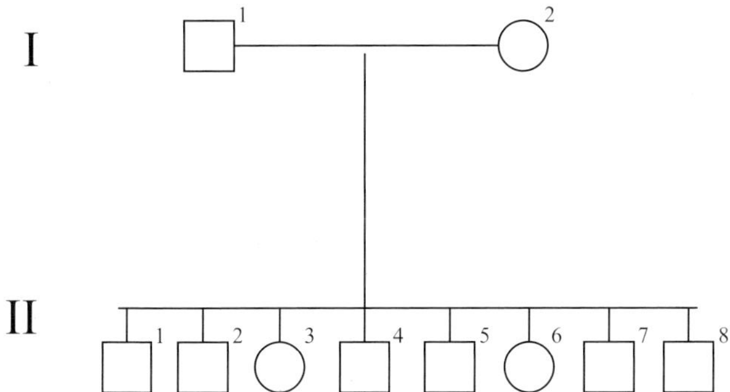

FIGURE 1. Pedigree of healthy control.

any buffy coat was carefully aspirated. The packed cells were then resuspended in 10 volumes of cold hypotonic 5 mM phosphate buffer pH 7.4 and allowed to stand on ice for 30 min after vortexing for 1–2 min. Centrifugation was later carried out at 16,000 rpm for 10 min at 4°C. The supernatant as well as the dense pellet at the bottom of the tubes was carefully aspirated. The membranes obtained were washed four times in 10 volumes of the same buffer and later resealed by resuspension in 10 volumes of the isotonic phosphate buffer pH 7.4 followed by centrifugation at 16,000 rpm for 10 min. The membrane samples were stored in the same buffer at 4°C and used within 12 h for measuring MDA content.

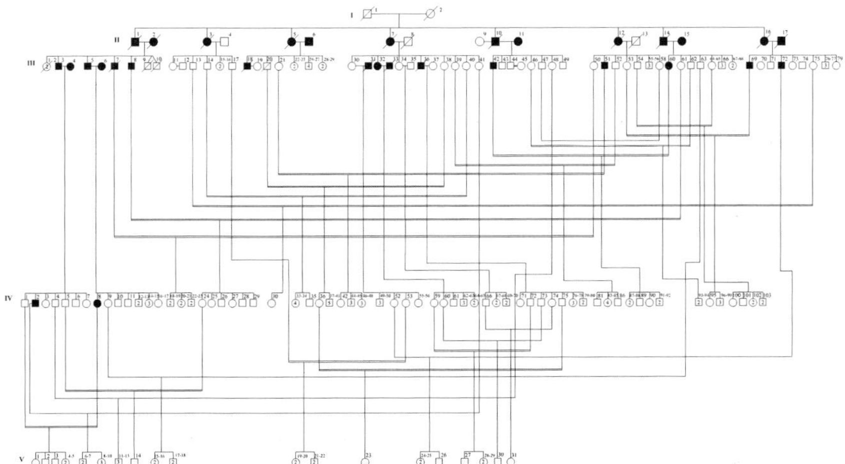

FIGURE 2. Pedigree of diabetic subjects. Male □ Female ○ Affected ■ • Consanguineous marriage □—○.

Estimation of Lipid Peroxidation in EGMs

Protein concentration in EGM was assayed[10] using BSA as standard followed by assessment of lipid peroxidation[11] as follows. Membranes were incubated in an isotonic phosphate buffer pH 7.4 containing iron sulphate (100 μM), ascorbic acid (1 mM), and hydrogen peroxide (200 μM). Membranes with and without exogenous stress were suspended in isotonic phosphate buffer at a final concentration of 1 mg/mL and incubated at 37°C in a shaking water bath for 5 h. A 0.5 mL of 0.75% thiobarbituric acid (TBA) in 0.1M HCl was later added to 0.5 mL of the incubation mixture already quenched with 0.5 mL of 10% acetic acid. The mixture was heated at 90–95°C for 20 min and after cooling centrifuged for 10 min at 16,000 rpm. The pink color of MDA was assayed spectrophotometrically at 532 nm. Lipid peroxidation was expressed as (A 532 nm/mg protein) against reagent blank.

Estimation of Antioxidant Enzymes

Plasma was used for the quantitative estimation of antioxidant enzymes, including SOD, CAT, and peroxidase (POD). The method used for the quantitative estimation of SOD is described.[12] Pipetted into a series of tubes were 200 μL EDTA cyanide, 100 μL NBT, 150 μL plasma, and 3000 μL phosphate buffer (pH 7.8). Two tubes with no enzyme were used as control. The tubes were placed in a light box providing uniform light intensity and incubated for 5–8 min to achieve a standard temperature. At zero time and at intervals 50 μL riboflavin was added and all tubes were again incubated in the light box for 12 min. Absorbance was recorded at 560 nm against reagent blank. Specific activity was reported as O.D/mg protein/12 min. The method[13] was used for the quantitative estimation of CAT. UV spectrophotometer (Hitachi Model: U-3200; Hitachi, Japan) was set with strip chart recorder and temperature control at 240 nm and 25°C. In quartz cuvette 2.99 mL of diluted hydrogen peroxide solution (substrate) and 10 μL plasma was pipetted. After mixing, initial absorbance was noted at 0 min, after 1-min observation was repeated. Reagent blank with no enzyme was used as a standard. Specific activity was expressed as (O.D at 240 nm/mg protein). Decline in absorbance is usually observed during 0-1-min interval.

The method[14] was followed for quantitative estimation of POD. Fifty microliters of plasma was transferred into a tube containing 3.75 mL of 0.15 M phosphate buffer and 100 μL of 176 mM H_2O_2. At zero time, 100 μL of 0.1 M guaicol was added as a substrate. The reaction was allowed to proceed for 8 min. The reaction mixture was then shaken after adjusting total volume up to 5 mL with distilled water. Absorbance of solution was recorded at 470 nm against reagent blank and one unit of enzyme is considered to be change in the optical density/8 min, whereas specific activity is expressed as the OD at 470 nm/mg protein/8 min.

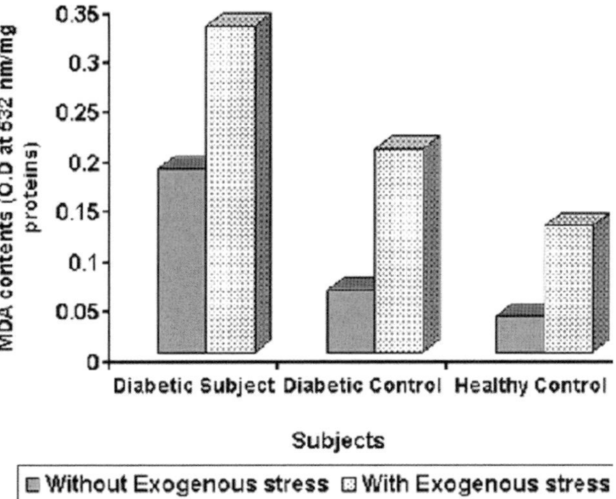

FIGURE 3. Lipid peroxidation with and without oxidative stress among diabetic subjects, diabetic controls, and healthy controls. Without oxidative stress■ With oxidative stress□.

The data obtained were analyzed statistically using SPSS version 10 (SPASS Inc., Chicago, IL). One-way analysis of variance (ANOVA) and Duncan's multiple range test was performed for mean comparisons among the three groups studied.

RESULTS

The results obtained are consistent, with elevated significant increase in MDA levels without exogenous oxidative stress in EGMs of NIDDM subjects as compared to diabetic controls and healthy controls (FIG. 3, TABLE 1). MDA contents were further enhanced in EGMs of diabetic patients subjected

TABLE 1. Analysis of variance for lipid peroxidation with and without oxidative stress MDA, SOD, CAT, and POD

		Mean squares (A 532 nm/mg protein)				
Sources of variation	*d.f*	MDA levels without oxidative stress	MDA levels with oxidative stress	SOD	CAT	POD
Between groups	2	0.0969**	0.1938**	0.1857**	0.2095**	0.0044**
Within groups	69	0.0115	0.2800	0.0161	0.0562	0.0004
Total	71					

**Significant at 0.01 level probability.

TABLE 2. Duncan multiple range test for mean MDA, SOD, CAT, and POD contents among diabetics, diabetic controls, and healthy controls

Subjects	Mean MDA levels: Without oxidative stress	Mean MDA levels: With oxidative stress	Mean SOD (nm/mg protein/10 min)	Mean CAT (nm/mg protein/60 s)	Mean POD (nm/mg protein/8 min)
Diabetic subjects	0.0354[a]	0.1270[a]	0.0356[a]	0.4441[a]	0.0096[a]
Diabetic controls	0.0668[a]	0.2089[a]	0.0346[a]	0.4972[a]	0.0245[b]
Healthy controls	0.1683[b]	0.3287[b]	0.1890[b]	0.6374[b]	0.0400[c]

Homogenous means are indicated by similar alphabets.

to exogenous oxidative stress as compared to their respective controls. Furthermore, diabetic controls also showed a significant increase in MDA levels as compared to healthy control (TABLE 2).

Comparison of SOD and CAT activities indicated that diabetic subjects have significantly higher levels of these enzymes as compared to diabetic control and healthy control. Both enzymes, however, are nonsignificantly different between healthy controls and diabetic controls. Diabetic subjects and diabetic controls also have significantly elevated levels of POD as compared to healthy controls (TABLE 2).

DISCUSSION

Hyperglycemia is a major factor in the development of diabetic complications, although the mechanisms of how increased glucose levels contribute to these changes have not been fully elucidated. Adverse biochemical changes associated with hyperglycemia include increased flux of glucose through the polyol pathway, enhanced nonenzymatic glycation, and activation of the diacylglycerol–protein kinase C pathway. Hyperglycemia may also result in increased production of the ROS within numerous biochemical pathways that have the potential to initiate adverse changes in endothelial function.[15]

Oxygen-free radicals had been suggested to be a contributory factor in complications of diabetes mellitus. There are many reports that indicate that the changes in biochemical parameters are due to diabetes-induced oxidative stress. The data of acute symptoms among diabetic subjects show high prevalence of cardiovascular disease, blood pressure, and accelerated atherosclerotic macrovascular disease.[16]

In these studies, mean glucose levels of the diabetic subjects were higher compared to diabetic controls and healthy control. This may be due to the fact that insulin stimulates glycogen accumulation through a coordinated increase in glucose transport and glycogen synthesis.[17]

The results indicate the presence of higher levels of MDA in EGMs of type 2 patients as compared to diabetic and healthy controls. Further increase was found in membranes of all three groups when exposed to exogenous oxidative stress. The amount of MDA was significantly more in diabetic subjects compared to diabetic controls and healthy controls. Results indicate that EGMs of NIDDM subjects were more prone toward lipid peroxidation compared to their respective controls. Increased levels of MDA in diabetic subjects are indication of lipid peroxidation. The EGM's of type 2 diabetic subjects were shown to be more susceptible to exogenously generated oxidative stress than those of normal healthy individuals. The detection of significant amounts of lipid breakdown products in a membrane after oxidative stress induced by incubation gives the impression that ROS capable of initiating peroxidation of membrane phospholipids are being generated in the membrane.[6]

Increased production of MDA has also been demonstrated in the erythrocyte membranes of diabetic patients[18,19] and high-lipid peroxides levels are also observed in diabetic rats.[20] It is suggested that increased MDA levels leading to damage in erythrocyte cells membrane is important not only for the progress of diabetes but also in the development of diabetic complications.[21]

When quantitative estimation of SOD is assessed, significant differences were observed among the three groups studied. Diabetic patients have higher activity of SOD whereas a lower enzyme activity is noted in control subjects. It has been reported that high glucose concentration induces an increase in mRNA levels and biological activity of Cu-Zn SOD, CAT, and GPX in fibroblast from diabetic subjects with nephropathy as compared to normal subjects.[22] In diabetic rats, high SOD activity in the liver, heart, and pancreas is also reported along with increased levels of thiobarbituric acid reactive substances (TBARS), GPX, and CAT in tissues and blood compared to control.[23] Similar to SOD, CAT activity is also significantly higher in diabetic subjects as compared to diabetic controls and healthy controls. Increase in CAT activity has been reported in fibroblasts from control subjects, nephropathic nondiabetic subjects, and diabetic subjects without nephropathy.[22]

The enzyme activity of POD was significantly higher in diabetic subjects compared to healthy controls. The possible reason for this increase is that the excessive amount of glucose in the blood of diabetic patients increased the production of hydrogen peroxide and this toxic molecule increases as a result of the activity of CAT and POD in order to convert it into water and molecular oxygen. Levels of POD were higher in diabetic patients compared to healthy controls. This work is an addition to the confirmation of earlier reports that have demonstrated that serum concentration of free radical scavenging enzymes in response to hyperglycemia are significantly higher in type 2 diabetic patients compared to healthy control subjects. A relationship thus seems to exist between diabetic complications and elevated levels of these enzymes. It is suggested that these enzymes may be considered as biomarkers for vascular injury.

REFERENCES

1. Accili, D., Y. Kido, J. Nakae, *et al.* 2001. Genetics of type 2 diabetes: insight from targeted mouse mutants. Curr. Mol. Med. **1:** 9–23.
2. Palanduz, S., E. Ademoglu & C. Gokkusu. 2001. Plasma antioxidants and type 2 diabetes mellitus. Res. Commun. Mol. Pathol. Pharmacol. **109:** 309–318.
3. Martim, A.C., R.A. Sanders & J.B. Watkins. 2003. Oxidative stress and antioxidants. A review. J. Biochem. Mol. Toxicol. **17:** 24–38.
4. Dhalla, N.S., R.M. Temsah & T. Netticadan. 2000. Role of oxidative stress in cardiovascular disease. J. Hypertens. **18:** 655–673.
5. Sailaja, Y.R., R. Baskar & D. Saralakumari. 2003. The antioxidant status during maturation of reticulocytes to erythrocytes in type 2 diabetes. Free Radic. Biol. Med. **35:** 24–38.
6. Okunade, G.W., O.O. Odunuga & O.O. Olorunsogo. 1999. Iron-induced oxidative stress in erythrocyte ghost membrane of non-insulin dependent diabetic Nigerians. Biosci. Reports **19:** 1–9.
7. Sajid, M. & F.N. Naqvi. 2005. Familial clustering and analysis of some biochemical parameters among control and diabetic subjects. Paper presented at 8th Biennial National Conference of Pakistan Society for Biochemistry and Molecular Biology. Abstract 59.
8. Kesavulu, M.M., R. Giri, R.B. Kameswara & C. Apparao. 2000. Lipid peroxidation and antioxidant enzymes levels in type 2 diabetic with macrovascular complications. Diabetes. Metab. **26:** 387–392.
9. Ceriello, A., P. Russo, P. Amstad & P. Cerutti. 1996. High glucose induces antioxidant enzymes in human endothelial cells in culture: evidence linking hyperglycemia and oxidative stress. Diabetes. **45:** 471–477.
10. Lowry, O.H.N., N.J. Rosebrough, A.D. Farr & A.J. Randall. 1951. Protein measurement with folin reagent. J. Biol. Chem. **193:** 265–275.
11. Rice Evans, C., S.C. Omorphos & E. Baysal. 1986. Biochem. J. **237:** 265–269. Cited in Okunade GW, Odunuga OO & Olorunsogo O O. 1999. Iron induced oxidative stress in erythrocyte ghost membrane of non-insulin dependent diabetic Nigerians. Biosci. Reports **19:**1–9.
12. Winterbourn, C., R. Hawkins, M. Brain & R. Carrell. 1975. The estimation of red cell superoxide dismutase activity. J. Lab. Clin. Med. **85:** 337–341.
13. Scebba, F., L. Sebastiani & C. Vitagliano. 1999. Protective enzymes against activated oxygen species in wheat (Triticum aestivum L) seedlings: response to cold acclimation. J. Plant Physiol. **155:** 762–768.
14. Evers, J., C.J. Maria & A.M. Mario. 1994. Peroxidative activities of hemoglobin and hemoglobin derivatives. *In* Methods in Enzymology. J. Evers, K.M. Vandegriff, R.M. Winslow, Eds.: 547–561 Academic Press. New York.
15. Giugliano, D., A. Ceriello & G. Paolisso. 1996. Oxidative stress and diabetic vascular complications. Diabetes Care **19:** 257–267.
16. Brownlee, M. 2001. Biochemistry and molecular cell biology of diabetic complications. Nature **414:** 813–820.
17. Saltiel, A.R. & K. Ronald. 2001. Insulin signaling and the regulation of glucose and lipid metabolism. Nature **414:** 799–805.
18. Mahboob, M., M.F. Rahman & P. Grover. 2005. Serum lipid peroxidation and antioxidant enzymes levels in male and female diabetic patients. Singapore Med. J. **46:** 322–324.

19. MARITIM, A.C., R.A. SANDERS & J.B. WATKINS. 2003. Oxidative stress and antioxidants a review. J. Biochem. Mol. Toxicol. **17:** 24–38.
20. UNLUCERCI, Y., S. BEKPINAR & H. KOCAK. 2000. Testis glutathione peroxidase activities in amino guanidine treated diabetic rats. Arch. Biochem. Biophys. **379:** 217–220.
21. DEVARAJ, S. 2000. Increased oxidative stress in type 2 diabetic subjects with macro vascular complications: effect of alpha tocopherol supplementation. www.ideallibrary.com.
22. CERIELLO, A. 2000. Intracellular antioxidant enzyme production in type 1 diabetic patients with nephropathy. Am. Diabetes Assoc. www.Find articles.com.
23. CEYLAN, A., C. KARASU, F. AKTAN, *et al.* 2003. Effects of simvastation treatment on oxidant/antioxidant state and ultrastructure of diabetic rat myocardium. Gen. Physiol. Biophys. **22:** 535–547.

Signaling Proteins Associated with Diabetic-Induced Exocrine Pancreatic Insufficiency in Rats

REKHA PATEL,[a] PHILIP ATHERTON,[a] HENNING WACKERHAGE,[b] AND JAIPAUL SINGH[a]

[a]*Department of Biological Sciences, University of Central Lancashire, Preston, Lancashire, PR1 2HE United Kingdom*

[b]*Department of Biomedical Sciences, University of Aberdeen, Aberdeen, AB24 3FX Scotland, United Kingdom*

ABSTRACT: **Diabetes mellitus (DM) is associated with pancreatic atrophy and compromised digestion of carbohydrates as a result of exocrine pancreatic insufficiency and lower alpha-amylase synthesis and secretion. The reduced production of digestive enzymes is likely to be caused by deregulated protein metabolism. The relative concentrations and phosphorylation of signaling proteins associated with protein translation, such as PKB, p70S6K1, 4E-BP1, ERK1/2, and also some of those implicated in protein breakdown, such as ubiquitin and NF-κB, in the pancreas of streptozotocin (STZ)-induced type I diabetic pancreas were measured using Western blotting. There were significant decreases in the levels of total PKB, p70S6K, 4E-BP1, ERK1/2, and NF-κB in the diabetic pancreas compared to control. In contrast, the phosphorylation of p70S6K1, 4E-BP1, ERK1/2, and protein ubiquitination increased significantly compared to controls. Together, these results indicate that STZ-induced DM leads to reduced levels of enzymes mediating protein synthesis while their phosphorylation is actually increased, perhaps in an attempt to maintain protein homeostasis, which is further compromised by heightened ubiquitin-dependent protein breakdown. It is likely that these factors are responsible for pancreatic atrophy, enzyme synthesis, and net protein loss in DM.**

KEYWORDS: **diabetes mellitus; rat; pancreas; signaling proteins**

INTRODUCTION

The pancreas contains both endocrine and exocrine portions, and it is sometimes regarded as two separate organs.[1] The endocrine pancreas secretes a

Address for corresspondence: Prof. Jaipaul Singh, Department of Biological and Forensic Sciences, University of Central Lancashire, Preston, Lancashire, PR1 2HE UK. Voice: 0044-1772-893515; fax: 0044-1772-892929.
e-mail: jsingh3@uclan.ac.uk

**Ann. N.Y. Acad. Sci. 1084: 490–502 (2006). © 2006 New York Academy of Sciences.
doi: 10.1196/annals.1372.026**

number of regulatory hormones, including insulin, glucagon, somatostatin, and pancreatic polypeptide.[2] By contrast, the exocrine pancreas secretes a number of digestive enzymes, fluids, and bicarbonate that help in the efficient digestion of food stuffs.[3] There are also marked interactions between the metabolic hormones of the endocrine pancreas and the digestive hormones and endogenous neurotransmitters, which control exocrine pancreatic secretion that produce sustained and voluminous secretion.[4–6] In diabetes mellitus (DM), the exocrine pancreas is unable to secrete an adequate amount of alpha-amylase, which is responsible for the digestion of carbohydrates. This dysfunction of the pancreas is referred to as exocrine pancreatic insufficiency and it can lead to weight loss and other long-term complications.[7] Several factors have been proposed for the development of exocrine pancreatic insufficiency. These include a derangement in calcium and magnesium homeostasis,[8] insensitivity of CCK receptors on acinar cells,[9] a decrease in gene expression for alpha-amylase,[10] and reduced activity of Na^+-K^+-ATPase and glucose uptake into pancreatic acinar cells.[11]

The exocrine pancreas is a highly active gland that is responsible for enhanced synthesis of a number of digestive enzymes.[12] In DM, the pancreas is unable to synthesize sufficient alpha-amylase resulting in reduced secretion of the enzyme.[11] This defect is believed to be due to a reduction in either gene expression for alpha-amylase or a deficit of the pancreas in the diabetic state to translate mRNA.[13] In fact, a global decrease in protein synthesis in DM is probably responsible for atrophy and reduced weight of both the subject and the pancreas. The signaling mechanism(s) responsible for reduced pancreatic weight and protein output in DM has not yet been previously investigated. Thus, this study measured marker proteins of protein synthesis, such as protein kinase B (PKB), p70 S6 kinase (p70 S6K), and 4E binding protein 1 (4E-BP1), regulators of ribosomal integrity, and initiation of translation; and also protein breakdown, measured as ubiquitination-mediated degradation through the 26S proteasome as well as nuclear factor kappa B (NF-κB; activated during inflammation). Furthermore, the transcriptional controlling mitogen-activated protein kinase (MAPK), extracellular regulated kinase 1/2 (ERK1/2) was examined. This approach revealed disturbed cellular signaling that controls both transcription and protein metabolism in the pancreas of streptozotocin (STZ)-induced type 1 DM and provided mechanistic insights into the causes of pancreatic insufficiency.

METHODS

General Procedure

Adult male Wistar rats weighing between 250–275 g were used in this study. They were supplied by the Animal Service of the University of

Central Lancashire. Type I diabetes was induced in male Wistar rats by a single intraperitoneal injection (i.p.) of STZ (60 mg kg^{-1}; Sigma [Dorset, England, UK], S-0130).[14] STZ was dissolved in a citrate acid buffer solution (0.1 M citric acid; Sigma, C-0759, and 0.1 M sodium citrate; Sigma, S-4641 pH 4.5). Age-matched control rats received an equivalent volume of citrate acid buffer solution alone. Diabetes was confirmed 4 days following STZ injection (>7.1 mM blood glucose concentration to indicate DM) and immediately prior to humanely killing of the animal 7–8 weeks following STZ injection prior to experimentation. Glucose was measured using a Glucometer (Accu Chek; Roche Diagnostic, East Sussex, UK). This study had the relevant ethical clearance from the Ethics Committee of the University of Central Lancashire to undertake the experiments.

Protein Extraction

Both age-matched healthy control and STZ-induced diabetic rats were humanely killed by a blow on the head followed by cervical dislocation. An incision was made in the abdomen and the pancreas excised rapidly and snap frozen. Proteins were extracted from 8 control and 8 STZ-induced diabetic pancreas. Approximately 30 mg of tissue was homogenized on ice in 0.6 mL of homogenization buffer (50 mM Tris-HCL; 0.1% Triton-X; 1 mM EDTA; 1 mM EGTA; 50 mM NaF; 10 mM β-glycerophosphate; 5 mM Na pyrophosphate; 0.1% 2-mercaptoethanol; 100 nM okadaic acid; 50 μM sodium orthovanadate; 1 tablet of a protease inhibitor cocktail). Samples were rotated for 60 min at 4°C, before being centrifuged at 13,000 *g* for 10 min. Protein concentration of the supernatant was measured using the Bradford assay and adjusted to 2 mg mL^{-1} by diluting in SDS sample buffer (3.55 mL deionized water, 1.25 mL 0.5 M Tris-HCl, pH 6.8; 2.5 mL glycerol; 2 mL 10% (w/v) SDS; 0.2 mL 0.5% (w/v) bromophenol blue).

Electrophoresis and Western Blotting

Samples (20 μg) were electrophoresed in running buffer (1% SDS; 192 mM glycine; 25 mM Tris-base; pH 8.3) on a 10% SDS-PAGE (13.5% high-bis gel for 4E-BP1) gel at 100 V for 30 min through the stacking layer and then 200 V until the dye marker reached the bottom of the gel. Precisely, 10 μL of a kaleidoscope molecular size marker was loaded into the final lane in order to later confirm detection of the correct protein size. Following conclusion of electrophoresis, the polyvinylidene difluoride (PVDF) membrane was permeabilized in 100% methanol for 1 min before both the gel and prewetted membrane were equilibrated in transfer buffer (192 mM glycine; 25 mM Tris-base; 20% w/v methanol; pH 8.3) for 30 min. The transfer was run for 2 h at a constant

100 V. Upon completion of transfer, the uniformity of loading was checked with Ponceau S before the membrane was incubated in 30 mL of blocking buffer (TBS with 0.1% Tween-20; 5% w/v nonfat milk powder) for 2 h. Following incubation with the blocking buffer, the membrane was washed three times for 5 min with wash buffer (TBS with 0.1% Tween-20) in 30 mL with gentle agitation. Samples were exposed to the following total antibodies: anti-NF-κB (NEB3034; 1:2000); anti-PKB/AKT (Courtesy of Sir P. Cohen; 1:2000); anti-p70S6K (NEB9202; 1:2000); anti-ERK1/2, anti-4E-BP1 (courtesy of Prof. C.G. Proud; 1:1,000), and anti-ubiquitin (NEB3936; 1:1,000) overnight at 4°C. Phosphorylation status was measured using: phospho-PKB (NEB9271; Ser473; 1:2000); phospho-p70S6K (NEB9205; Thr389; 1:2000); phospho-ERK1/2 (p44/p42) (NEB9101; Thr202/Tyr204; 1:2000); and phospho-4E-BP1 (NEB9459; Ser37/46; 1:2000) also overnight at 4°C. The following morning, the membrane was rinsed in wash buffer three times for 5 min each time in 30 mL. The membrane was then incubated for 1 h at ambient temperature with gentle agitation in 30 mL of blocking buffer containing the appropriate secondary antibody, either: HRP-linked anti-mouse IgG (NEB 7072; 1:2000); anti-rabbit IgG (NEB7074; 1:2000); or anti-sheep IgG (courtesy of Prof. Chris Proud; 1:5000). The membrane was cleared in wash buffer three times for 5 min in 30 mL wash buffer. Membranes were exposed to ECL chemiluminescent detection reagents mixed 1:1 in 10 mL for 1 min. Membranes were partially dried, wrapped in saran, and exposed to X-ray film. X-ray films were scanned using a Bio-Rad Imaging densitometer (Model GS-670; Hertfordshire, England, UK) to detect the relative band intensity. Each band was identified and the optical density volume adjusted by subtraction of the background.

Statistical Analysis

Since two mini gels were used (containing $n = 4$ each) and only relative differences in density on the same gel can be used, all control values obtained from each blot were normalized so that the average resting control band intensity was set to 100 thus allowing comparison between gels. Statistical significance was assessed by the use of a two-tailed t-test. All data were expressed as means ± standard errors of the means (SEM). Only values with $P < 0.05$ were accepted as significant.

RESULTS

In this study, diabetic rats and pancreas weighed significantly ($P < 0.05$) less than their age-matched controls. Typically, the body weight and pancreas of diabetic animals were 190.12 ± 5.41 g ($n = 20$) and 1.02 ± 0.05 g

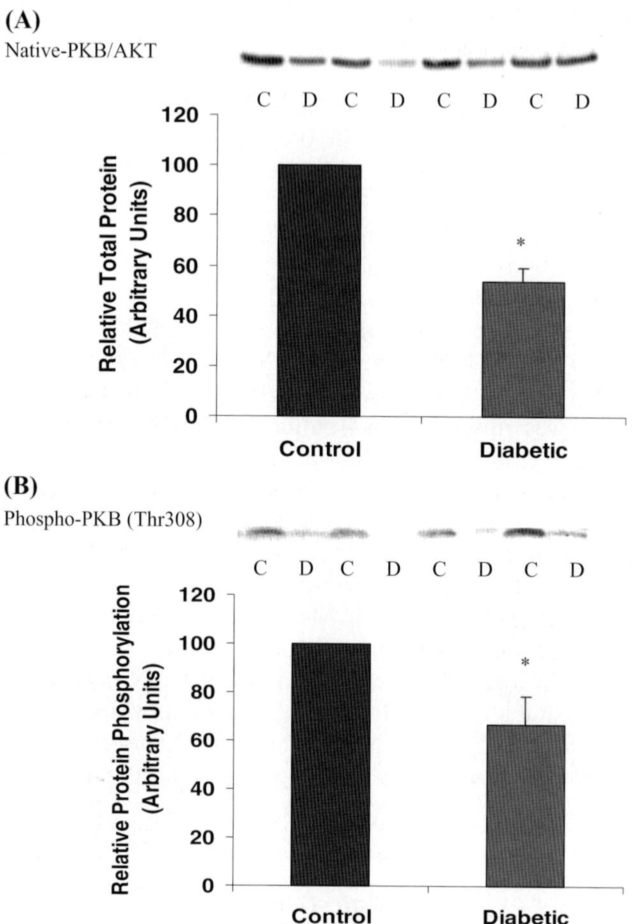

FIGURE 1. Representative immunoblots showing and bar charts the effect of STZ-induced diabetes upon the relative protein levels of both total (**A**) and phosphorylation (**B**) of PKB at Thr308. All values were normalized to the relative intensity of the control bands. Immunoblots represent $n = 4$ healthy control (C) and 4 STZ-induced diabetic (D) rats. Data are displayed as means $\pm$ SEM $n = 8$, $^*P < 0.05$.

($n = 20$) compared to weight and pancreas of control rats 391.83 ± 37.91 ($n = 20$) and 1.30 ± 0.07 g ($n = 20$), respectively. In contrast, the blood of diabetic rat contained significantly ($P < 0.05$) elevated glucose (>500 mg dL^{-1}, $n = 27$) compared to control (92.40 ± 2.42 mg dL^{-1}, $n = 27$).

FIGURE 1 shows the relative total protein level (arbitrary units) for total PKB/Akt and the phospho-PKB-(Thr308) in control and diabetic rat pancreas. The figure also shows the respective original immunoblots for comparison.

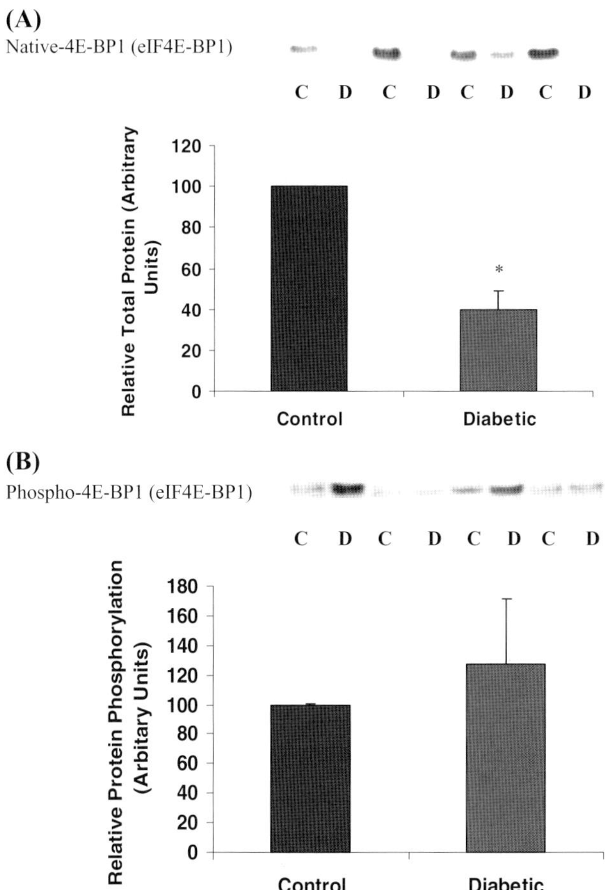

FIGURE 2. Representative immunoblots and bar charts showing the effect of STZ-induced diabetes upon the relative protein levels of both total (**A**) and phosphorylation (**B**) of 4E-BP1 at Thr37/46. All values were normalized to the relative intensity of the control bands. Immunoblots represent $n = 4$ healthy control (C) and STZ-induced diabetic (D) rats. Data are displayed as means ± SEM $n = 8$, $^*P < 0.05$.

The results show that there was a significant ($P < 0.05$) decrease in both the total and the phosphorylated form of PKB in diabetic rat pancreas compared to control. FIGURE 2 shows original immunoblots and histograms of total 4E-BP1 (eIF4E-BP1) (panel A) and its phosphorylated form (panel B). The results show that the diabetic pancreas contained significantly ($P < 0.05$) less total 4E-BPI compared to age-matched control pancreas. In contrast, the diabetic pancreas contained significantly ($P < 0.05$) more phosphorylated form of the 4E-BP1 protein compared to control. FIGURE 3 shows original immunoblots

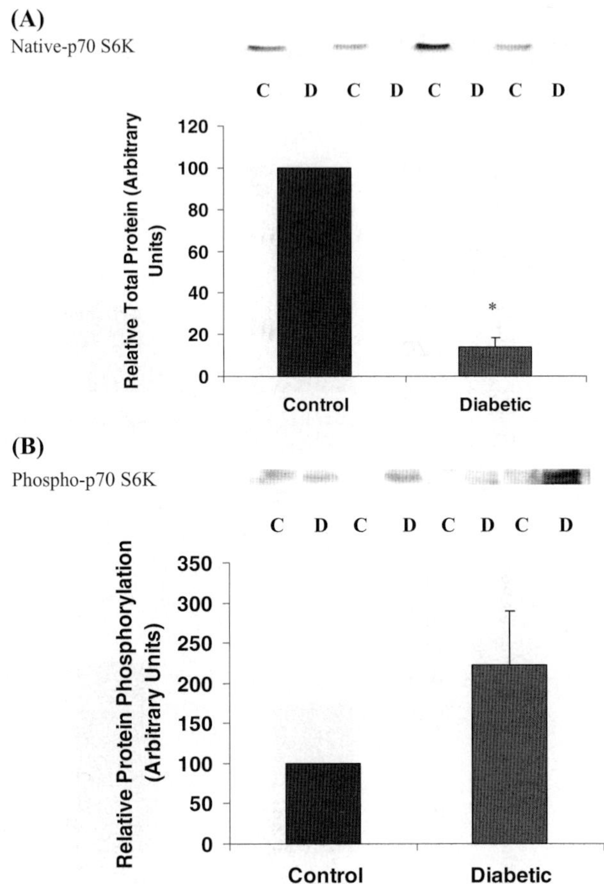

FIGURE 3. Representative immunoblots and bar charts showing the effect of STZ-induced diabetes upon the relative protein levels of both total (**A**) and phosphorylation (**B**) of p70 S6K at Thr389. All values were normalized to the relative intensity of the control bands. Immunoblots represent $n = 4$ healthy control (C) and STZ-induced diabetic (D) rats. Data are displayed as means ± SEM $n = 8$, $^*P < 0.05$.

and bar charts of total p70S6K (panel A) and its phosphorylated form (panel B). The data revealed that the level of the total p70S6K decreased significantly ($P < 0.05$) in the diabetic pancreas compared to age-matched control tissues. In contrast, the level of the phosphorylated form of the signaling protein increased significantly ($P < 0.05$) in the diabetic pancreas compared to control. FIGURE 4 shows original immunoblots and bar charts of the relative total level of ERK1/2 (p44/p42) (panel A) and phosphorylated form (panel B) in control and diabetic pancreas. The data show that the diabetic pancreas contains significantly

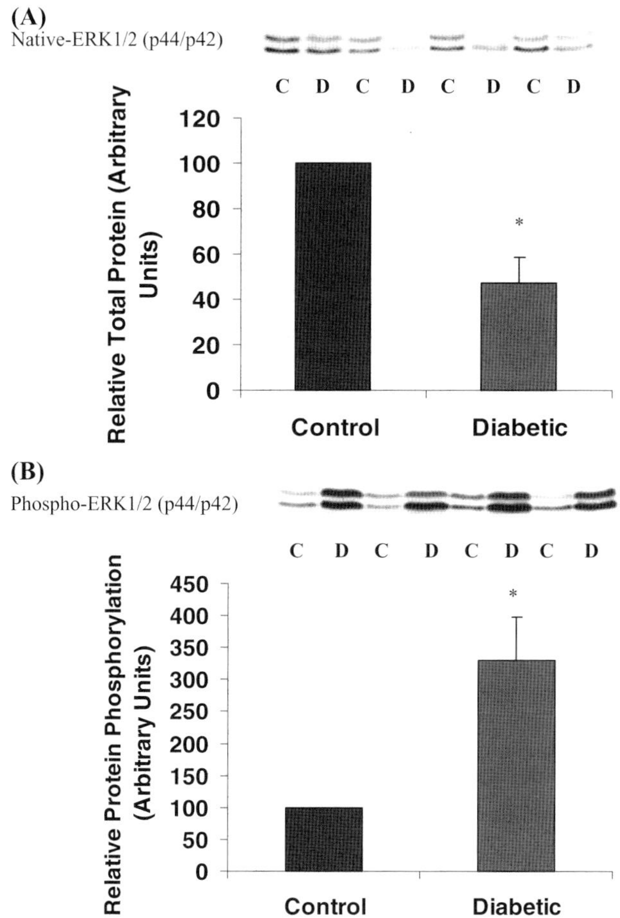

FIGURE 4. Representative immunoblots and bar charts showing the effect of STZ-induced diabetes upon the relative protein levels of both total (**A**) and phosphorylation (**B**) of ERK1/2 at Thr202/Tyr204. All values were normalized to the relative intensity of the control bands. Immunoblots represent $n = 4$ healthy control (C) and STZ-induced diabetic (D) rats. Data are displayed as means ± SEM $n = 8$, $^*P < 0.05$.

($P < 0.05$) less total protein and significantly ($P < 0.05$) more phosphorylated protein compared to control. FIGURE 5 shows the original immunoblots for NF-κB (p65) (panel A) and ubiquitinated protein (panel B). In addition, FIGURE 5 shows the molecular weight markers of the ubiquitinated protein. The results show that diabetic pancreas contains significantly ($P < 0.05$) less total NF-κB compared to age-matched control, and displays heightened ubiquitination (indicated by darker intensity of diabetic animals).

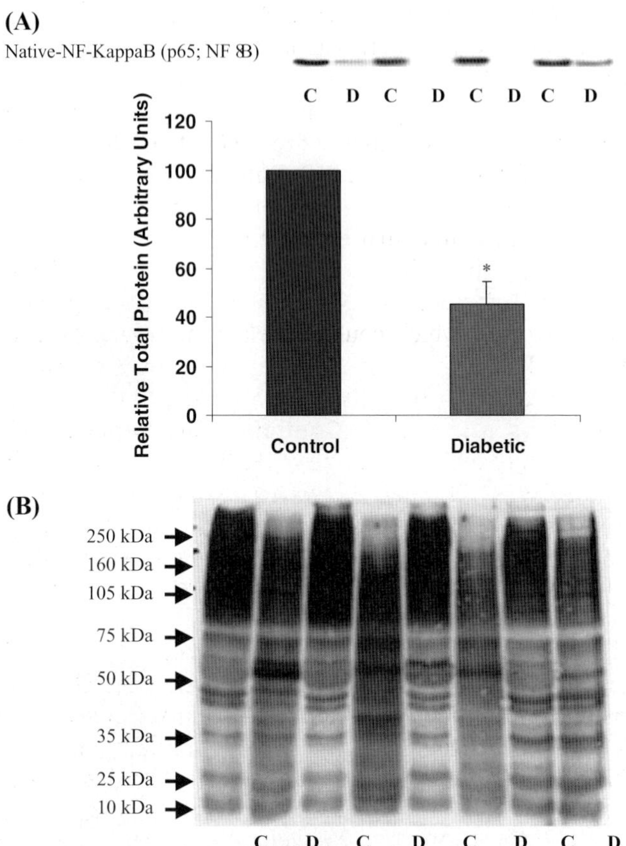

FIGURE 5. Western blots of NF-κB (**A**) and ubiquitinated protein (**B**) in the healthy control (C) and STZ-induced diabetic (D) rat pancreas ($n = 4$ for control and diabetic rats). Each lane represents one animal. The molecular weight markers show the approximate molecular weights of the ubiquitinated proteins.

DISCUSSION

The results of this study have demonstrated that the STZ-induced diabetic rats and their pancreas weigh significantly ($P < 0.05$) less than respective age-matched control. In contrast, the blood of diabetic rats contains significantly ($P < 0.05$) elevated glucose compared to control. These data are in agreement with results from other studies.[8,15] The weight loss may be due to the fact that the diabetic animals eat less, have protein loss in skeletal muscles (the animals are indeed wasted), and the inability to digest foodstuffs and to use sufficient glucose. Indeed, exocrine pancreatic insufficiency is a major long-term complication of DM in which the subject is unable to digest carbohydrates efficiently, which in turn leads to weight loss.[7] Several mechanisms have been proposed to contribute to the development of exocrine pancreatic insufficiency. These include derangements in calcium and magnesium homeostasis and a decrease in gene expression of amylase,[11] reduced enzyme synthesis and secretion,[8] insensitivity of receptors to CCK that usually act to stimulate amylase release,[9] and reduced amino acid and glucose uptakes and Na^+/K^+ ATPase activities in pancreas acinar cells.[16] The results of this study for the first time, demonstrate that exocrine pancreatic insufficiency may be due to changes in signaling, which controls protein turnover and transcription.

The results show a decrease in PKB concentration (FIG. 1), both total and phospho-specific forms, which could be related to a lack of insulin in the diabetic pancreas. It should be stated that since the PKB kinase performs so many cellular functions an explanation for this is speculative. However, since PKB is activated by insulin to promote GLUT translocation and is downstream of the insulin receptor (IR), perhaps, the lack of circulating insulin leads to a downregulation of PKB expression since there is no longer the requirement for insulin to signal through this intermediate. This would be independent to the reduced levels of p70S6K and 4E-BP1 since these are also activated in a PKB-independent manner, such as by nutrients through mTOR.[17]

The total concentration of translational regulators 4E-BP1 and p70S6K (FIGS. 2, 3, respectively) were significantly reduced in the STZ-induced pancreas compared to control. The output of a signal transduction pathway is dependent on both the activity and total protein concentration as proposed by the metabolic control theory.[18] Therefore, it is likely that this reduction in key signaling proteins may reflect a reduced translation signaling capacity that in turn could mediate the pancreatic atrophy and reduced protein available for secretion. In contrast to this, the phosphorylation of p70, 4E-BP1 was actually higher in diabetic pancreas. This at first seems unexpected since reduced total protein levels as shown here would presumably have been concomitant with blunted phosphorylation. One possible explanation for this increase in protein phosphorylation is to compensate for reduced total protein levels (secretory enzymes, ribosomal proteins, etc.) in the pancreas. This in turn could act as a defense mechanism to maintain protein mass, the cellular activity of these proteins actually increases in an attempt to maximize the output from remaining protein levels. This pattern has been previously shown to be evident in aged rats, which actually reveal upregulation of p70S6K activity despite the state of sarcopenia.[19]

The MAPK protein ERK1/2 also showed an increased phosphorylation in tandem with a reduced total protein level (FIG. 4). ERK1/2 is in part responsible for mediating translation through phosphorylating p90 RSK, which in turn activates eukaryotic elongation factor 2 kinase (EF2K).[20] Activation of eEF2K regulates peptide elongation by phosphorylation of eEF2 enabling translocation of charged tRNA to the ribosome. Therefore, the increase in ERK1/2 phosphorylation could lead to the enhanced phosphorylation of p90 RSK and thus eEF2K and promote peptide elongation in order to counter the decrease in ERK1/2 total protein levels in an attempt to maintain pancreatic protein translation. In addition, the phosphorylation of ERK1/2 controls many transcription factors, which regulate the genes involved in response to stress and growth factors.[21] Therefore, increased ERK1/2 phosphorylation suggests heightened transcriptional activity.

The role of NF-κB in pancreas is controversial since NF-κB activation has been shown to both induce cell death while in contrast to this, a protective role of NF-κB activation against cell death has been observed in some tumor cell lines.[22] NF-κB has been implicated in cytokine-mediated TNF-α-induced tissue wasting, and has also been shown to be elevated in type I diabetes.[23] Furthermore, TNF-α levels have been shown to be increased in STZ diabetic rats.[24] This study showed a reduction in NF-κB protein in chronic STZ-induced diabetes (FIG. 5), which may attenuate increased TNF-α signaling in an attempt to maximize maintenance of cell mass and viability. Furthermore, NF-κB has a role in glucose-stimulated insulin secretion[25] and since this process is attenuated in experimental diabetes, then the downregulation could be due to the fact that the acinar cells no longer need NF-κB to assist insulin secretion. To make more specific conclusions, the specific activity or DNA binding of NF-κB would need to be assessed. Interestingly, it has been shown that the STZ requires NF-κB to destroy islet cells since its inhibition abrogates the effects of STZ; therefore STZ-induction of diabetes perhaps alters NF-κB, rather than the diabetes itself. Clearly, the role of this protein in STZ-induced diabetes warrants further investigation.

The ubiquitination of total cellular proteins was higher in the diabetic state. Since ubiquitin is the tag, which marks proteins for proteolytic degradation by the 26S proteasome, this suggests that there is elevated protein breakdown in the chronic STZ state. This would provide some explanation for the reduced protein levels of PKB, p70S6K, 4E-BP1, and ERK1/2 in this advanced stage of the type I metabolic disease state, as well as the pancreatic and skeletal atrophy.

In conclusion, the results of this study have highlighted possible explanations for pancreatic insufficiency indicated by alteration in the regulation of key signaling proteins controlling transcription and translation in STZ-induced diabetes. While total protein levels involved in mediating protein synthesis have been downregulated, the phosphorylation of these proteins is actually elevated. It is therefore, suggested that this increase in phosphorylation is a cellular defense mechanism in an attempt to maintain protein synthesis to counteract gross loss of protein as indicated by reduced levels of translation proteins and enhanced ubiquitination; both markers for increased global protein breakdown. These defects in translation-mediating proteins and altered ERK1/2 activity may affect translation and transcription of secretory enzymes and also contribute to the considerable atrophy of the STZ-induced pancreas by altering the protein breakdown:synthesis ratio in favor of the breakdown.

REFERENCES

1. WILLIAMS, J.A. & I.D. GOLDFINE. 1993. The insulin acinar relationship. *In* The Exocrine Pancreas: Biology, Pathobiology, and Disease, 2nd. ed. V.L.M. Go, E.P. DiMagno, J.D. Gardner, *et al.*, Eds.: 789–802. Raven Press. N.Y.
2. YAGO, M.D., M. MANAS & J. SINGH. 2000. Intracellular magnesium: transport and regulation in epithelial secretory cells. Front. Biosci. **5:** D602–D618.
3. PETERSEN, O.H. 1992. Stimulus-secretion coupling: cytoplasmic calcium signals and the control of ion channels in exocrine acinar cells. J. Physiol. **448:** 1–51.
4. JUMA, L.M., J. SINGH, D.J. PALLOT, *et al.* 1997. Interactions of islet hormones with acetylcholine in the isolated rat pancreas. Peptides **18:** 1415–1422.
5. SINGH, J., M.D. YAGO & E. ADEGHATE. 2001. Involvement of cellular calcium in exocrine pancreatic insufficiency during streptozotocin-induced diabetes mellitus. Arch. Physiol. Biochem. **109:** 252–259.
6. YAGO, M.D., E. ADEGHATE & J. SINGH. 1999. Interactions between the endocrine and exocrine pancreas. Effects of islet hormones, secretagogues, and nerve stimulation. *In* Neural Regulation in the Vertebrate Endocrine System: Neuroendocrine Regulation. R.A. Prasada Rao, R. Peters, Eds.: 197–217. Kluwer Academic/ Plenum, N.Y.
7. KUMAR, P.J. & M.L. CLARK. 2002. Diabetes mellitus and other disorders of meabolism. *In* Clinical Medicine P. Kumar & M. Clark, Eds.: 1069–1121. WB Saunders. London.
8. PATEL, R., M.D. YAGO, M. MANAS, *et al.* 2004. Mechanism of exocrine pancreatic insufficiency in streptozotocin-induced diabetes mellitus in rat: effect of cholecystokinin-octapeptide. Mol. Cell. Biochem. **261:** 83–89.
9. OTSUKI, M., T. AKIYAMA, H. SHIROHARA, *et al.* 1995. Loss of sensitivity to cholecystokinin stimulation of isolated pancreatic acini from genetically diabetic rats. Am. J. Physiol. **268:** E531–E536.
10. KIM, S.K., L.M. CUZZORT & E.D. ALLEN. 1991. Effects of age on diabetes- and insulin-induced changes in pancreatic levels of alpha-amylase and its mRNA. Mech. Ageing Dev. **58:** 151–161.
11. SINGH, J., E. ADEGHATE, S. APARICO, *et al.* 2004. Exocrine pancreatic insufficiency in diabetes mellitus. Int. J. Diabetes Metab. **12:** 35–43.
12. SINGH, J. 1983. Effects of amino acids, glucagon, insulin and acetylcholine on cyclic nucleotide metabolism and amylase secretion in isolated mouse pancreatic fragments. Biochem. Pharmacol. **32:** 2017–2023.
13. PATEL, R. 2005. Cellular mechanism of exocrine pancreatic insufficiency in diabetes mellitus. Ph.D Thesis,The British Library England, UK.
14. SHARMA, A.K., I.G. DUGUID, D.S. BLANCHARD, *et al.* 1985. The effect of insulin treatment on myelinated nerve fibre maturation and integrity and on body growth in streptozotocin-diabetic rats. J. Neurol. Sci. **67:** 285–297.
15. OKABAYASHI, Y., M. OTSUKI, A. OHKI, *et al.* 1988. Effect of diabetes mellitus on pancreatic exocrine secretion from isolated perfused pancreas in rats. Dig. Dis. Sci. **33:** 711–717.

16. HOOTMAN, S.R., J.E. JONES, R. KAPOOR, *et al.* 1998. Sodium, potassium-activated triphophatase activity is impaired in the guinea pig pancreatic duct system in streptozotocin-induced diabetes. Biochem. Biophys. Res. Commun. **24:** 869–873.
17. HARA, K., K. YONEZAWA, Q.P. WENG, *et al.* 1998. Amino acid sufficiency and mTOR regulate p70 S6 kinase and eIF-4E BP1 through a common effector mechanism. J. Biol. Chem. **273:** 14484–14494.
18. DE VIENNE, D., B. BOST, J. FIEVET, *et al.* 2001. Optimisation of enzyme concentrations for unbranched reaction chains: the concept of combined response coefficient. Acta Biotheor. **49:** 341–350.
19. PARKINGTON, J.D., N.K. LEBRASSEUR, A.P. SIEBERT, *et al.* 2004. Contraction-mediated mTOR, p70S6k, and ERK1/2 phosphorylation in aged skeletal muscle. J. Appl. Physiol. **97:** 243–248.
20. WANG, X., W. LI, M. WILLIAMS, *et al.* 2001. Regulation of elongation factor 2 kinase by p90(RSK1) and p70 S6 kinase. EMBO J. **20:** 4370–4379.
21. WILLIAMS, J.A., M.D. SANS, M. TASHIRO, *et al.* 2002. Cholecystokinin activates a variety of intracellular signal transduction mechanisms in rodent pancreatic acinar cells. Pharmacol. Toxicol. **91:** 297–303.
22. SCHOTT-OHLY, P., A. LGSSIAR, H.J., H.J. PARTKE, *et al.* 2004. Prevention of spontaneous and experimentally induced diabetes in mice with zinc sulphate-enriched drinking water is associated with activation and reduction of NF-kappa B and AP-1 in islets, respectively. Exp. Biol. Med. (Maywood) **229:** 1177-1185.
23. TANTI, J.F., P. GUAL, T. GREMEAUX, *et al.* 2004. Alteration in insulin action: role of IRS-1 serine phosphorylation in the retroregulation of insulin signalling. Ann. Endocrinol. (Paris) **65:** 43–48.
24. EL SEWEIDY, M.M., S.E. EL SWEFY, R.S. AMEEN, *et al.* 2002. Effect of age receptor blocker and/or anti-inflammatory coadministration in relation to glycation, oxidative stress and cytokine production in stz diabetic rats. Pharmacol. Res. **45:** 391–398.
25. HAMMAR, E.B., J.C. IRMINGER, K. RICKENBACH, *et al.* 2005. Activation of NF-kappa B by extracellular matrix is involved in spreading and glucose-stimulated insulin secretion of pancreatic beta cells. J. Biol. Chem. **34:** 30630–30637.

Effects of Streptozotocin-Induced Type 1 Diabetes Mellitus on Total Protein Concentrations and Cation Contents in the Isolated Pancreas, Parotid, Submandibular, and Lacrimal Glands of Rats

NAVIN R. CHANGRANI,[a] APURVA CHONKAR,[a] ERNEST ADEGHATE,[b] AND JAIPAUL SINGH[a]

[a]*Department of Biological Sciences, University of Central Lancashire, Preston, Lancashire, PR1 2HE UK*

[b]*Department of Anatomy, Faculty of Medicine and Health Sciences, United Arab Emirates University, Al-Ain, UAE*

ABSTRACT: This study investigated the effect of streptozotocin (STZ)-induced type 1 diabetes mellitus (DM) on total protein concentration and levels of sodium (Na^{+}), potassium (K^{+}), magnesium (Mg^{2+}), zinc (Zn^{2+}), copper (Cu^{2+}), calcium (Ca^{2+}), and iron (Fe^{2+}) in the pancreas, parotid, submandibular, and lacrimal glands of the rat, compared to age-matched control animals. Protein concentrations were measured by the Bradford Assay, whereas levels of Na^{+}, K^{+}, Mg^{2+}, Zn^{2+}, Cu^{2+}, Ca^{2+}, and Fe^{2+} were measured by flame photometry and atomic absorbance spectrophotometry. The results show marked changes in the characteristics of diabetic and control animals. Diabetic rats and their different glands weighed significantly ($P < 0.05$) less compared to age-matched controls. Diabetic rats also have significantly elevated blood glucose and significantly reduced plasma insulin, compared to controls. The results also show that the concentrations of proteins and levels of cations were significantly ($P < 0.05$) reduced in the pancreas, parotid, submandibular and lacrimal glands of diabetic rats, compared to glands from age-matched animals. These differences in the cation contents and protein levels in STZ-induced DM in this study, along with supporting evidences from previous studies, may provide evidence for the development of long-term complications of DM including exocrine gland deficiencies.

Address for corresspondence: Prof. Jaipaul Singh, Department of Biological and Forensic Sciences, University of Central Lancashire, Preston, Lancashire, PR1 2HE UK. Voice: 0044-1772-893515; fax: 0044-1772-892929.

e-mail: jsingh3@uclan.ac.uk

Ann. N.Y. Acad. Sci. 1084: 503–519 (2006).
doi: 10.1196/annals.1372.019

Keywords: streptozotocin; diabetes; total protein; rat; pancreas; parotid; submandibular; lacrimal; cations

INTRODUCTION

Diabetes mellitus (DM) is one of the oldest conditions characterized in humans, having been recognized since antiquity. It is a major health problem at present affecting about 180 million people worldwide.[1] DM is a generalized chronic disorder characterized by certain abnormalities in carbohydrate, fat, electrolyte, and protein metabolism.[2] The occurrence of DM is either due to a lack of insulin or the presence of factors that oppose the action of insulin.[3] This in turn results in an increase in blood glucose concentration (hyperglycemia) that ultimately leads to several acute and chronic complications including neuropathy, nephropathy, retinopathy, cardiomyopathy, microangiopathy, atherosclerosis, and foot ulcers.[2,4] In the UK alone, about 2 million people are diagnosed as diabetic and an estimated 1 million remain undiagnosed. The National Health Service bears a cost of about £5.5 billion annually for the diagnosis, treatment, and care for diabetic patients.[3]

The basic structure of all exocrine glands, including the pancreas, parotid, lacrimal, and the submandibular glands is the same except for the pancreas, which has endocrine cells. The bulk of the exocrine glands is composed of exocrine cells and their associated ducts.[5] In the pancreas, embedded within this exocrine tissue are roughly 1 million small clusters of cells called the islets of Langerhans, which are the endocrine cells of the pancreas and secrete insulin, glucagon, and several other hormones. The exocrine cells are arranged in grape-like clusters called acini. These cells secrete a fluid that contains water, electrolytes, mucus, proteins, and specific enzymes, all of which flow out of the acinus into collecting ducts.[6] The exocrine cells themselves are packed with membrane-bound secretory granules, which contain digestive enzymes that are exocytosed into the lumen of the acinus. From there these secretions flow into larger and larger, intralobular ducts, which eventually collect into the main pancreatic duct that drains directly into the duodenum.[7]

The lumen of an acinus communicates directly with intralobular ducts, which coalesce into interlobular ducts and then into the major exocrine duct. Epithelial cells of the intralobular ducts actually project "back" into the lumen of the acinus, where they are called centroacinar cells.[8] The anatomy of the main exocrine duct varies among species. In some animals, two ducts of the pancreas enter the duodenum rather than a single duct. In some species, the main exocrine duct fuses with the common bile duct just before its entry into the duodenum.[9]

There is much evidence that in DM, exocrine glands including the pancreas and the parotid are unable to secrete adequate amount of α-amylase for the effective digestion of carbohydrates, leading to indigestion and weight loss.[10] Both the lacrimal and submandibular glands are also exocrine glands and it is possible that they secrete less protein in DM.[11] In addition to reduction in amylase secretion, it is also possible that the exocrine glands secrete less fluid, which is associated with ion output in the secretions.[12] This is a comparative study, which employs the pancreas, parotid, submandibular and lacrimal glands of age-matched control and diabetic rats to investigate the levels of total proteins and cation contents. The rationale is to ascertain whether there are any differences in the protein and cation concentrations of the four glands during DM compared to normal conditions.

METHODS

Induction of DM

Adult male Wistar rats weighing about 150–500 g were employed in this study and were supplied by the Animal Service of the University of Central Lancashire. Type 1 DM was induced in male Wistar rats by a single intraperitoneal injection (i.p.) of streptozotocin (STZ)[10,13] (60 mg/kg; Sigma [Dorset, UK], S-0130). STZ was dissolved in a citrate acid buffer solution (0.1 M citric acid; Sigma, C-0759 and 0.1 M sodium citrate; Sigma, S-4641 pH 4.5). Age-matched control rats received an equivalent volume of citrate acid buffer solution alone. Diabetes was confirmed 4–5 days following STZ injection and immediately prior to humanely killing of the animal 7–8 weeks following STZ injection prior to experimentation.[14] Glucose was measured using a Glucometer (Accu Chek; Roche Diagnostic, East Sussex, UK). This study had the relevant ethical clearance from the Ethics Committee of the University of Central Lancashire, to undertake the experiments.

Experimental Procedure

Adult age-matched control and STZ-induced diabetic male rats were humanely killed by a blow on the head followed by cervical dislocation. An incision was made in the abdomen and the thoracic region of the rat and the pancreas, parotid, and submandibular glands were located and removed swiftly from the animal. Incisions were made on either side of the eye and the lacrimal glands were located and swiftly removed. The tissues were placed in a modified Krebs–Henseleit (K–H) solution of the following composition (mM): NaCl, 103; KCl, 4.7; $CaCl_2$, 2.6; $MgCl_2$,, 1.1; $NaHCO_3$, 25; NaH_2PO_4, 1.1; D-glucose, 2.8; sodium pyruvate, 4.9; sodium fumarate, 2.7; and sodium glutamate, 4.9. The solution was kept at pH 7.4 while being continuously gassed with a mixture of 95% O_2–5% CO_2 and maintained at 37°C. The tissue was subsequently removed from the solution, blotted, and any connective or fatty tissues were dissected away from the gland and discarded. All the glands were quickly weighed, placed into a 5 mL vial, and frozen at –80°C until used for experimentation. On the day of the measurements, the glands and tissues were thawed out and one group (right parotid, submandibular, and lacrimal glands, and a part of the pancreas) was dissolved in 1 mL concentrated nitric acid in a 10 mL glass vial overnight. These samples were used for the determination of the concentration of ions in them. The other glands (left parotid, submandibular and lacrimal glands) and pancreatic tissues were sonicated (MSE Soniprep 150; TCP Inc., Jersey City, New Jersey) for 15 s separated by 4-min intervals on ice, in 1 mL deionized water, until the sample was fully digested, for the measurement of total protein.[14]

Measurement of Total Protein Using the Bradford Method

The Bradford protein assay is a dye-binding assay based on the differential color change of a dye in response to various concentrations of protein.[15] This technique is based on the observation that the absorbance maximum for an acidic solution of Coomassie Brilliant Blue G-250 shifts from 465 nm to 595 nm when binding to protein occurs.

The Bradford reagent was prepared by adding 0.1 g Coomassie Brilliant Blue G-250 in 50 mL 95% ethanol. One hundred milliliters of 85% orthophosphoric acid was added and diluted to 1 L. The solution was filtered and stored in a brown glass bottle in a dark environment at 4°C.

Protein standard solutions ranging from 0.25–4 mg mL^{-1} bovine serum albumin (BSA) were prepared from a 4 mg mL^{-1} stock BSA solution. When required, aliquoted samples were allowed to defrost at room temperature. A volume of 50 μL of the standards and diluted samples were pipetted into dry test tubes. A volume of 50 μL of deionized water was also added in a test tube as "blank." To all tubes, 2.5 mL of dye reagent (Bradford's reagent) was added, vortexed, and incubated for about 20 min at room temperature. The absorbance of each protein standard was measured versus the reagent blank at 595 nm in a spectrophotometer (Novaspec II; Pharmacia Biotech, Cambridge, UK). Similarly, a volume of 50 μL of either control or diabetic protein samples were added to a dry test tube and 2.5 mL of Bradford reagent was added. Each sample was tested in duplicate. The total protein concentration on each sample was determined against a protein standard curve and results expressed as μg mL^{-1} (100 mg of tissue)$^{-1}$.

Sample Preparation for the Measurement of Ions

A volume of 0.2 mL of the tissue sample was dissolved in 1 mL concentrated nitric acid, diluted 50 times by the addition of 9.8 mL deionized water. This solution was vortex mixed and was used for the measurements of Na^+ and K^+ using flame photometry and for measurements of Ca^{2+}, Mg^{2+}, Cu^{2+}, Zn^{2+}, and Fe^{2+}, using flame atomic absorption spectrophotometry (FAAS).

Measurement of Ions Using FAAS

Appropriate standard ion solutions were made ranging from 5–20 mg mL^{-1} from a standard stock concentration of 20 mg mL^{-1} of either Ca^{2+}, Fe^{2+}, Mg^{2+}, Cu^{2+}, or Zn $^{2+}$. The concentrations of these ions were determined in the samples by the use of FAAS (Unicam 929 AA spectrometer; Unicam Ltd., Cambridge, UK).

The flame atomic absorption spectrophotometric method detects metals and metalloids and is based on the fact that ground state metals absorb light at specific wavelengths. During combustion, metal ions in a solution were reduced to free, unexcited ground state atoms by means of a flame whose temperature ranges from 2100 to 2800°C. A light beam from a lamp whose cathode was made of the element being determined was passed through the flame. A device such as a photomultiplier detected the amount of reduction of the light intensity due to absorption by the analyte, and this was directly related to the amount of the element in the sample.[10,13,14] The amount of light absorbed was measured against a standard curve and ion contents were expressed as µg mL^{-1} (100 mg of tissue)$^{-1}$.

Measurement of Ions Using Flame Photometry

Levels of Na^+ and K^+ were measured by the flame photometry method (Corning, Model 420 Flame Photometer; Sherwood Scientific, Steubin County, NY). Sample preparation was performed in exactly the same way as for FASS. Standards ranging from 5 to 20 mg mL^{-1} were made from a stock concentration of 20 mg mL^{-1} of either potassium or sodium. The absorbance of these standards was measured by using the flame photometer and the results were plotted to give a standard curve of each of the ions. Deionized water was used in this entire process, as a blank. The concentrations of potassium and sodium were determined using exactly the same technique as employed for determining the standard graph values. These results were plotted on the standard graph to determine the concentrations of each of the samples. All values were expressed as mg mL^{-1} (100 mg of tissue)$^{-1}$.

Statistical Analysis

The concentrations of either proteins or cations in each sample were obtained from the standard curve and the values were analyzed as mean ± standard error of the mean (SEM). Age-matched control and diabetic tissue values were compared by using the Student's unpaired *t*-test and the one-way analysis of variance (ANOVA) test. The SPSS software was used in all cases (SPSS for Windows, Version 13.0.1, 2004; London, UK). Only values with $P < 0.05$ were accepted as significant.

RESULTS

General Characteristics

TABLE 1 shows the general characteristics of control and diabetic rats. The results show that diabetic rats and their glands weigh significantly ($P < 0.05$) less and they have significantly ($P < 0.05$) elevated plasma glucose and significantly ($P < 0.05$) reduced plasma insulin compared to age-matched control rats. Similarly, the glands of diabetic rats weigh significantly ($P < 0.05$) less as compared to those of age-matched control rats.

Measurement of Total Protein

FIGURE 1 shows bar charts for protein concentrations in the parotid, lacrimal, pancreas, and submandibular glands of control and diabetic rats as determined by the Bradford assay. The results show that STZ-induced DM had significant ($P < 0.05$) effects on protein concentrations in the diabetic tissues as compared to the age-matched control tissues. Analysis of the results showed that there was a significant ($P < 0.05$) decrease in the protein content in all four diabetic glands as compared to those of age-matched control rats.

Measurement of Cation Contents

Sodium (Na^+)

FIGURE 2 shows bar charts of sodium concentrations in the pancreas, parotid, submandibular, and lacrimal glands of control and diabetic rats. The results indicate that the sodium concentrations in diabetic rats were notably lower in all the four diabetic glands as compared to the glands of age-matched control animals.

TABLE 1. General characteristics of age-matched control and diabetic rats and their glands

Parameters	Control	Diabetic
Weight of rats (g)	501.83 ± 25.91	222.19 ± 10.51*
Blood glucose (mM)	6.06 ± 0.21	29.65 ± 0.33*
Blood insulin (mg dL^{-1})	20.63 ± 7.52	4.81 ± 1.28*
Weight of pancreas (mg)	331.68 ± 18.03	291.32 ± 25.50*
Weight of parotid glands (mg)	254.13 ± 14.27	198.90 ± 19.88*
Weight of submandibular glands (mg)	186.19 ± 23.98	84.33 ± 20.15*
Weight of lacrimal glands (mg)	96.97 ± 7.42	53.68 ± 5.38*

Data are mean ± SEM, $^*P < 0.05$; $n = 18$ rats for each parameter.

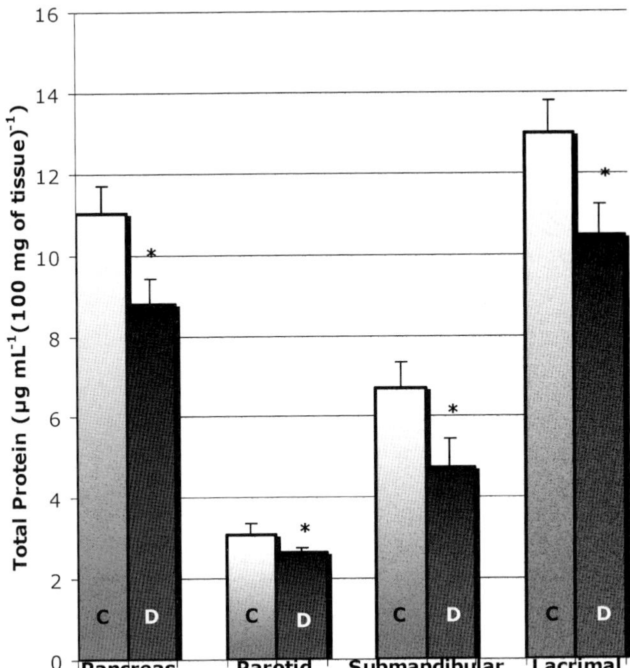

FIGURE 1. Bar charts showing total protein in the pancreas, parotid, submandibular, and lacrimal glands of diabetic (D) and age-matched control (C) rats. Data are mean ± SEM, $n = 36$, taken from 18 rats. $^{*}P < 0.05$. Note that the results show a significant ($P < 0.05$) decrease in protein content in the glands of diabetic rats compared with those of age-matched control rats.

Potassium (K^+)

FIGURE 3 shows bar charts of potassium concentrations in the pancreas, parotid, submandibular, and lacrimal glands of control and diabetic rats. The results show that the potassium concentration in diabetic rats was seen to be lower than the concentration in the glands of age-matched control rats. The potassium concentrations in the parotid and submandibular glands were lowered by a very low value in the diabetic animals, and were not significant as they fell in the range of the standard error of mean, but the potassium concentration in the pancreas and lacrimal glands of diabetic rats was significantly ($P < 0.05$) reduced as compared to the concentrations in these glands of the age-matched control rats.

Iron (Fe^{2+})

FIGURE 4 shows bar charts of the iron concentration of the four glands of diabetic and control rats. The results indicate that there was a significant ($P <$

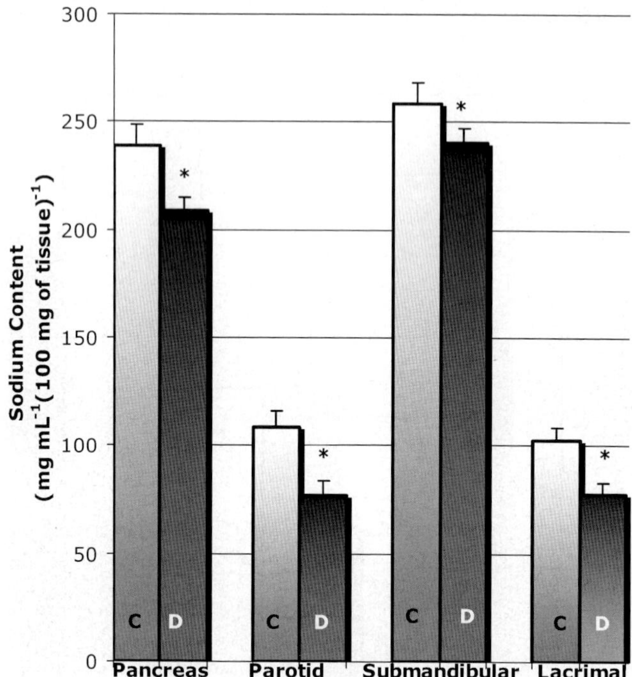

FIGURE 2. Bar charts showing sodium contents in the pancreas, parotid, submandibular, and lacrimal glands of diabetic (D) and age-matched control (C) rats. Data are mean ± SEM, $n = 36$, taken from 18 rats. $^*P < 0.05$. Note that there was a significant ($P < 0.05$) reduction in the concentration of sodium in all four glands of diabetic rats, as compared to those of age-matched control rats.

0.05) increase in the iron content in the diabetic pancreas as compared to the age-matched controls, but the parotid, submandibular, and lacrimal glands showed a decrease in the iron content of diabetic glands, but the decrement falls in the range of the standard error of mean and can thus be ignored.

Magnesium (Mg^{2+})

The results shown in FIGURE 5 indicate that the magnesium content in the pancreas, parotid, submandibular, and lacrimal glands of the diabetic rats was significantly ($P < 0.05$) reduced as compared to that of age-matched control rats.

Zinc (Zn^{2+})

FIGURE 6 shows bar charts of the concentration of zinc in the four glands of diabetic and control rats. The results show a significant ($P < 0.05$) decrease

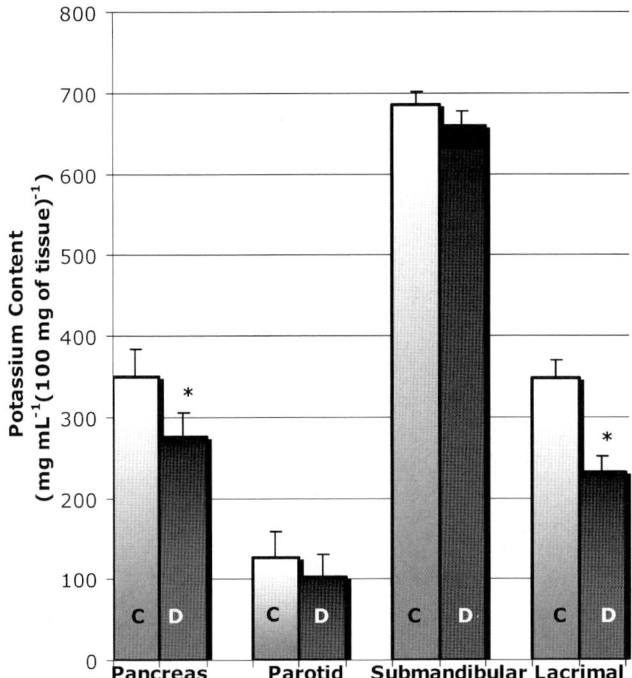

FIGURE 3. Bar charts showing potassium content in the pancreas, parotid, submandibular, and lacrimal glands of diabetic (D) and age-matched control (C) rats. Data are mean ± SEM, $n = 36$, taken from 18 rats. $^*P < 0.05$. Note that there was a significant ($P < 0.05$) decrease in the potassium concentration in the pancreas and lacrimal glands of diabetic rats compared to those of control rats. A decrease in the potassium concentration was also seen in the parotid and submandibular glands of diabetic rats, but this deviation was not significant as the values fell in the range of the SEM.

in concentration of zinc in the pancreas, parotid and submandibular glands of diabetic rats as compared with age-matched controls. The concentration of zinc in the lacrimal glands was significantly ($P < 0.05$) increased in diabetic rats, compared to the age-matched control rats.

Copper (Cu^{2+})

FIGURE 7 shows bar charts of the copper content in the four glands of control and diabetic animals. The results are conclusive in the pancreas and parotid gland and indicate a clear and significant ($P < 0.05$) reduction in the concentration of copper in the diabetic rats as compared to age-matched control rats. The results for the lacrimal and submandibular glands were also reduced for the diabetic glands, but proved to be insignificant as they fell within the range of the standard error of mean.

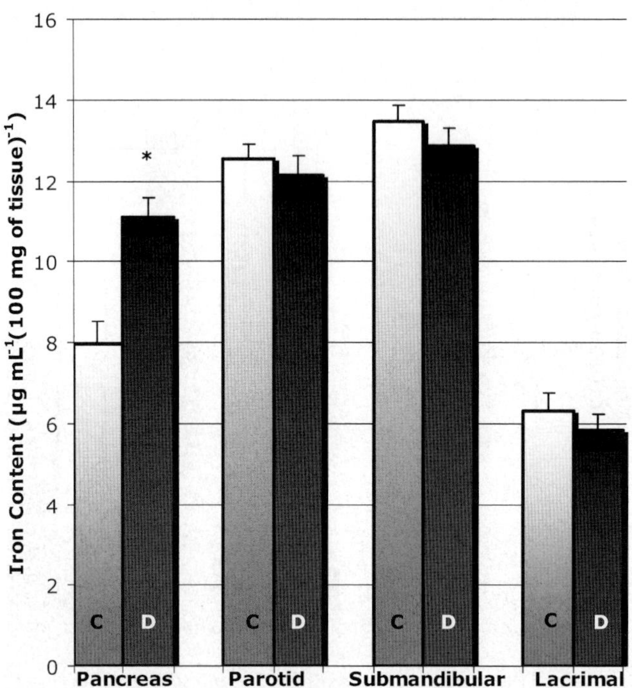

FIGURE 4. Bar charts showing iron content in the pancreas, parotid, submandibular, and lacrimal glands of diabetic (D) and age-matched control (C) rats, determined by the use of flame atomic absorption spectrophotometry. Data are mean ± SEM, $n = 36$, taken from 18 rats. $^*P < 0.05$. Note that the iron concentration in the diabetic pancreases was significantly ($P < 0.05$) increased, while the iron concentrations in the parotid, submandibular, and lacrimal glands were reduced slightly, but were not significant.

Calcium (Ca^{2+})

FIGURE 8 shows bar charts of the calcium content in the four glands of the control and diabetic rats. Analysis of the results indicate that the concentration of calcium was seen to be significantly ($P < 0.05$) decreased in the pancreas and parotid glands, while it was significantly ($P < 0.05$) increased in the submandibular and lacrimal glands of diabetic animals, as compared to the glands of the respective age-matched control animals.

DISCUSSION

The results of this investigation have shown marked differences in the characteristics of the diabetic rats compared to healthy age-matched control animals. STZ is a diabetogenic agent that elevated blood glucose, causing a condition

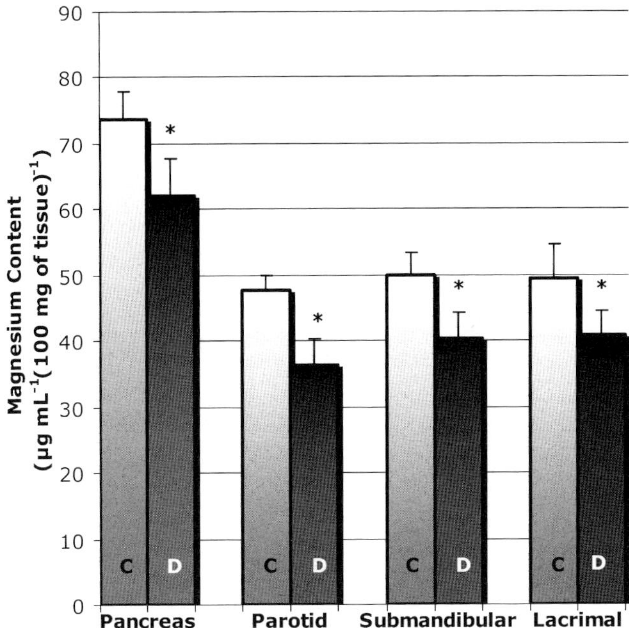

FIGURE 5. Bar charts showing magnesium content in the pancreas, parotid, submandibular, and lacrimal glands of diabetic (D) and age-matched control (C) rats, determined by the use of FAAS. Data are mean ± SEM, $n = 36$, taken from 18 rats. $^*P < 0.05$. Note that the concentration of magnesium in all the four glands of diabetic rats is reduced significantly ($P < 0.05$) compared to glands of age-matched control rats.

known as hyperglycemia, within 4–5 days following its injection.[16] Hyperglycemia was caused due to partial destruction of β cells of the endocrine pancreas.[14] Levels of blood glucose, monitored throughout the time course of the diabetes, remained elevated at all times, and this was associated with a significant decrease in the plasma insulin levels.[13] Diabetic rats gained significantly less weight compared to control. The weights of the glands employed in this study; namely, the pancreas, parotid, submandibular, and the lacrimal glands; had a significant variation between diabetic and control animals. The glands of diabetic rats weighed considerably less than the glands of age-matched control animals. The reason for the reduced weight of the animals and their glands may be due to the fact that diabetic animals eat less, and this in turn may lead to reduced body and gland weights.[2]

In addition to understanding the general characteristics of control and diabetic rats, this study was mainly designed to investigate the effect of STZ-induced type 1 DM on total protein concentration and levels of Na^+, K^+, Mg^{2+}, Zn^{2+}, Cu^{2+}, Ca^{2+}, and Fe^{2+} in the pancreas, parotid, submandibular, and lacrimal glands of the rat, compared to age-matched control animals. The

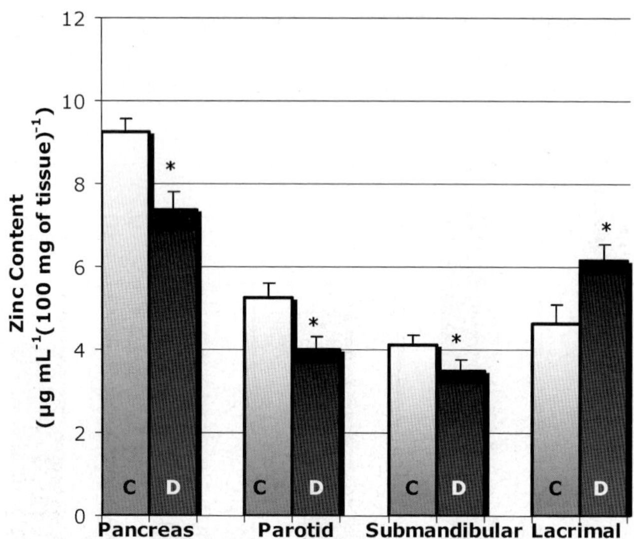

FIGURE 6. Bar charts showing zinc content in the pancreas, parotid, submandibular, and lacrimal glands of diabetic (D) and age-matched control (C) rats, determined by the use of FAAS. Data are mean ± SEM, $n = 36$, taken from 18 rats. $^{*}P < 0.05$. Note that the zinc contents of the diabetic pancreas, parotid, and submandibular glands were significantly ($P < 0.05$) elevated. In contrast, the zinc concentration in the lacrimal glands was reduced ($P < 0.05$) significantly.

results have demonstrated that STZ-induced diabetes produced marked reductions in the total protein concentration in the pancreas, parotid, submandibular and lacrimal glands of diabetic rats compared to age-matched control animals. Furthermore, the present investigation also gave a clear indication of the concentration of different cations in each of the four glands and provided new insights into the role of each of the ions in the different glands that were studied. This discussion is focused on the effects of STZ-induced diabetes on the rat pancreas, parotid, submandibular, and lacrimal glands and aims at providing further knowledge and understanding about the possible reasons for the variations in the concentrations of proteins and ions within the diabetic and control glands, as well as between each of the four diabetic glands.

This study has shown that the diabetic glands contained significantly less proteins compared to age-matched control glands. In previous studies, it was also shown that either the diabetic parotid glands[17,18] or the diabetic pancreas[13,14] secrete significantly less proteins and amylase compared to control. The reduction in either protein content or its secretion may be due to several mechanisms including a disturbance in the $[Ca^{2+}]_i$ and $[Mg^{2+}]_i$ homeostasis, parotid and pancreatic atrophy, altered intracellular signaling and gene regulation, deranged protein synthesis release and breakdown, and a derangement in gene expression for protein synthesis.[10,19–21] Not much work has

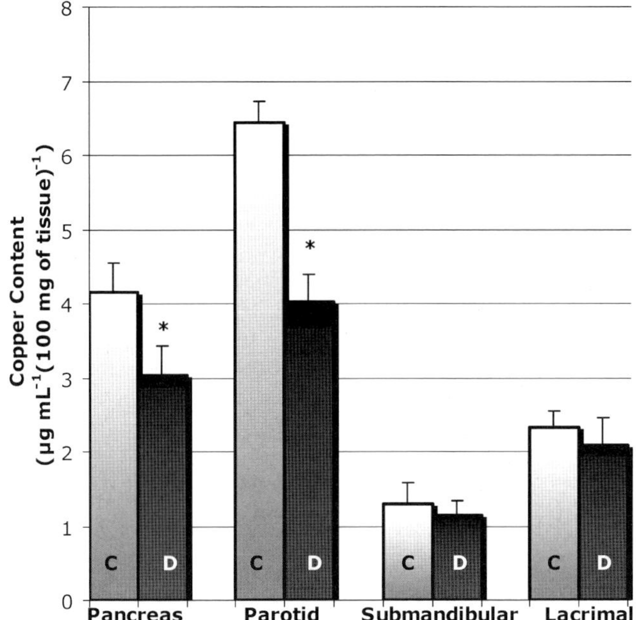

FIGURE 7. Bar charts showing copper content in the pancreas, parotid, submandibular and lacrimal glands of diabetic (D) and age-matched control (C) rats, determined by the use of FAAS. Data are mean ± SEM, $n = 36$, taken from 18 rats. $^{*}P < 0.05$. Note that the concentration of copper was significantly ($P < 0.05$) reduced in the diabetic pancreas and parotid glands as compared with glands of age-matched control rats, while the decrease in the concentration of copper in the submandibular and lacrimal glands was not significant enough to be conclusive of an interrelationship of reduction in copper content with diabetes.

been done on diabetic lacrimal and submandibular glands, but since these are exocrine glands like the pancreas and the parotid glands, it is possible to speculate that diabetes may be related with reduction in protein synthesis and/or its release from these glands as well.

This study also measured the levels of cations, such as Na^{+}, K^{+}, Fe^{2+}, Cu^{2+}, Ca^{2+}, Zn^{2+}, and Mg^{2+} which coregulate many processes in the pancreas, salivary glands, and the lacrimal gland. These cations are involved in intracellular regulation and thus, it is important to understand their homeostasis in control and diabetic conditions.

The content of Zn^{2+} in the pancreas, parotid, and submandibular glands of STZ-induced diabetic rats was significantly reduced. Since it has been shown that Zn^{2+} deficiency impairs both insulin secretion and production,[22] this may be a factor contributing to the inability to produce insulin in type 1 DM as well as islet cell destruction. Zn^{2+} and arachidonic acid have been found to lower glucose via improvement in insulin sensitivity in genetically diabetic rats.[23] Decrease in Zn^{2+} content of diabetic tissues, as seen from the results of this

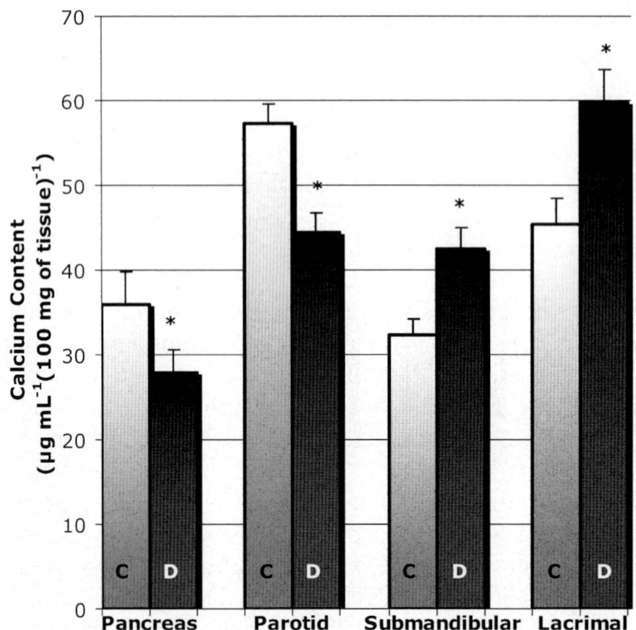

FIGURE 8. Bar charts showing calcium content in the pancreas, parotid, submandibular and lacrimal glands of diabetic (D) and age-matched control (C) rats, determined by the use of FAAS. Data are mean ± SEM, $n = 36$, taken from 18 rats. $^{*}P < 0.05$. Note that the concentration of calcium was significantly ($P < 0.05$) reduced in the diabetic pancreas and parotid glands as compared with glands of age-matched control rats, while there was a significant ($P < 0.05$) increase in the concentration of calcium in the submandibular and lacrimal glands of diabetic rats.

investigation, may thus provide additional proof to this role of low levels of zinc in causing diabetes.[24] The results also show that Zn^{2+} levels increase in the diabetic lacrimal glands compared to the control lacrimal glands. The reason for this elevation is still not clear. It is possible that zinc behaves differently in the tear glands. Diabetic rats develop cataract and the high levels of Zn^{2+} in the lacrimal glands of the diabetic rats could indicate that low levels of zinc may play a protective role in the prevention of cataract at least in the control animals.[23,25] Zinc also supports the functions of numerous metalloenzymes involved in a multitude of metabolic processes.[26]

Two cations that have been studied extensively in many previous investigations employing these glands are the concentrations of Ca^{2+} and Mg^{2+}.[13,14,17,18,27] The results from such investigations performed on both pancreatic, parotid, and submandibular acinar cell suspensions and on single acini cells demonstrate decreased intracellular levels of both $[Ca^{2+}]_i$ and $[Mg^{2+}]_i$, in CCK-8 and ACh-evoked STZ-induced diabetic rats compared to controls. The results in this study on the Mg^{2+} content in the different glands are in agreement with the results for such previous experiments.[13,21] In the pancreas and the parotid glands of diabetic animals compared to glands from control animals, both $[Ca^{2+}]_i$ and $[Mg^{2+}]_i$ decreased during basal and following secretagogue stimulation.[27] Cellular-free calcium is an important physiological mediator in the stimulus-secretion coupling process[5,28] and is closely linked to $[Mg^{2+}]_i$.[19,29] Therefore, it may be concluded that significant decreases in the Mg^{2+} content in tissues may be directly linked to the deactivation of the different enzyme systems responsible for calcium-dependent amylase secretion,[13] thereby reducing the Ca^{2+} content of tissues. Magnesium has also been found to improve insulin sensitivity and metabolic control in diabetic patients and is associated with metabolism of a number of ions and enzymes.[5]

The results also show the Na^+ and K^+ contents of all four of the glands were seen to be reduced in diabetic rats, compared to the healthy control rats. The findings are in accordance with previous studies that have shown that Ca^{2+}, Mg^{2+}, Na^+, as well as K^+ to be inversely related to diabetes.[30] This can be further reinforced by the fact that high serum concentrations of cortisol cause greater excretions of Na^+ and K^+. It is also possible that low serum concentrations of insulin could be the factor causing greater release of Na^+, K^+, and Mg^{2+} in the diabetic state, because it affects the energy furnished to their cell wall pumps. Potassium cannot be absorbed efficiently in the presence of a magnesium deficiency and magnesium tends to be correlated with potassium intake.[31]

The concentration of Fe^{2+} was highly elevated in the diabetic pancreas, as compared to age-matched controls. It is suggested that an excessive absorption and storage of dietary iron might contribute in the pathogenesis of DM and its complications.[2] During normal conditions, iron acts as a vital element by which cells generate energy.

The concentration of Cu^{2+} was lowered in the glands of diabetic animals, compared to control. A significant decrease seen in concentration of Cu^{2+} in the pancreas and the parotid gland could indicate its role in pancreatic and parotid insufficiency. It has been proved that Cu^{2+} depletion doubled glucose levels in blood of diabetic rats that were fed glucose. Also, the level of sucrose was seen to be about 50% higher in cases of low levels of Cu^{2+}.[32] Along with supporting evidence from such studies, the results indicate a definite role of copper catalyzed enzymes somewhere in the process. Adequate copper has been shown to help prevent insulin-dependent diabetes in STZ-poisoned mice and it can thereby be concluded that there could be similar effects of adequate content of Cu^{2+} on humans. A possible mechanism by which copper produces its effects may be through super oxidase dismutase, because previous studies have shown that the antioxidant metalloporphyrin-based superoxide dismutase (SOD) can prevent or delay the onset of the autoimmune cascade in diabetes in mice.[30]

In conclusion, the results of this study have demonstrated marked changes in control and diabetic rats regarding body and tissue weights, and blood glucose and insulin levels. The data clearly show marked decreases in total proteins and the majority of cations in diabetic glands as compared to controls. It is possible that these changes are due to DM itself and they can lead to the long-term complications of DM.

REFERENCES

1. DANIELSSON, A. 1974. Effects of glucose, insulin and glucagons on amylase secretion from incubated mouse pancreas. Pflugers Arch. **348:** 333–342.
2. KUMAR P. & M. CLARK. 2002. Diabetes mellitis and other disorders of metabolism. *In* Clinical Medicine. P. Kumar & M. Clark, Eds.: 1069–1121. WB Saunders.
3. ZIMMET, P., K.G. ALBERTI & J. SHAW. 2001. Global and societal implications of the diabetes epidemic. Nature **414:** 782–787.
4. WILLIAMS, J.C. & G. PICKUP. 1998. Complications of diabetes mellitis. *In* Handbook of Diabetes. 14–18 Cambridge University Press. Blackwell Science. Livingston, UK.
5. YAGO, M.D., E. ADEGHATE & J. SINGH. 1999. Interactions between the endocrine and exocrine pancreas. Effects of islet hormones, secretagogues, and nerve stimulation. *In* Neural Regulation in the Vertebrate Endocrine System: Neuroendocrine Regulation. R.A. Prasada Rao & R. Peters. Eds.: 197–217. Kluwer Academic/Plenum. New York.
6. MARTINI, F.H. & K. WELCH. 2004. The digestive system. *In* Applications Manual to Accompany Fundamentals of Anatomy & Physiology, 6th ed. 136–147. Pearson Education. Cambridge, UK.
7. BASTIAN, J.F. 1994. Structures and functions of the pancreas. *In* An Illustrated Review of Anatomy & Physiology. 40–41. Harper Collins College Publishers. New York.
8. WIDMAIER, E.P., H. RAFF & K.T. STRANG. 2006. Digestive system. *In* Vander's Human Physiology—The Mechanisms of Body Function. 575–601 McGraw-Hill London, UK.
9. TORTORA, G.J. & S.R. GRABOWSKI. 2003. A detailed review of digestive system. *In* Principles of Anatomy & Physiology, 10th ed. 531–534, 858–864, 874–888. John Wiley & Sons. London, UK.
10. SINGH, J., E. ADEGHATE, S. APARICO & R. HOPKIN. 2004. Exocrine pancreatic insufficiency in diabetes mellitus. Int. J. Diabetes Metab. **12:** 35–43.
11. BERNE, R.M., M.N. LEVY, B.M. KOEPPEN & B.A. STANTON. 1998. A detailed review of the digestive system. *In* Physiology, 4th ed. 632–637. New York. Mosby.
12. PEARSON, G.T., J. SINGH & O.H. PETERSEN. 1984. Adrenergic nervous control of cAMP-mediated amylase secretion in the rat pancreas. Am. J. Physiol. **246:** G563–G573.
13. PATEL, R., M.D. YAGO, M. MANAS, *et al.* 2004. Mechanism of exocrine pancreatic insufficiency in streptozotocin-induced diabetes mellitus in rat: effect of cholecystokinin-octapeptide. Mol. Cell. Biochem. **261:** 105–110.
14. PATEL, R. 2005. Cellular mechanism of exocrine pancreatic insufficiency in diabetes mellitus. PhD thesis, University of Central Lancashire.
15. BRADFORD, M.M. 1976. A rapid and sensitive method for the quantitation of microgram quantities of protein utilizing the principle of protein-dye binding. Anal. Biochem. **72:** 248–254.

16. BOUREY, R.E., L. KORANYI, D.E. JAMES, *et al.* 1990. Effects of altered glucose homeostasis on glucose transporter expression in skeletal muscle of the rat. J. Clin. Invest. **86:** 542–547.
17. MAHAY, S., W. WINLOW, J. SINGH, *et al.* 2002. Effects of ageing on morphology and α-amylase release in the isolated rat parotid gland. J. Physiol. **543P:** 15P.
18. MAHAY, S.K. 2005. The effects of aging and streptozotocin (STZ)–induced diabetes mellitus on the rodent parotid gland. PhD thesis, University of Central Lancashire.
19. WISDOM, D., J. SINGH, P.J. CAMELLO, *et al.* 1993. Effect of secretion on vagal stimulation-evoked exocrine pancreatic secretion in the rat. Rev. Esp. Fisiol. **49:** 31–35.
20. BURNHAM, D.B., P. MUNOWITZ, S.R. HOOTMAN & J.A. WILLIAMS. 1986. Regulation of protein phosphorylation in pancreatic acini. Distinct effects of Ca^{2+} ionophore A23187 and 12-O-tetradecanoylphorbol 13-acetate. Biochem. J. **235:** 125–131.
21. WISDOM, D.M., G.M. SALIDO, L.M. BALDWIN & J. SINGH. 1996. The role of magnesium in regulating CCK-8-evoked secretory responses in the exocrine rat pancreas. Mol. Cell. Biochem. **154:** 123–132.
22. CHAUSMER, A. 1998. Zinc, insulin and diabetes. J. Am. Coll. Nutr. **17:** 109–115.
23. HONNORAT, J., M. ACCOMINOTTI, C. BROUSSOLLE, *et al.* 1992. Effects of diabetes type and treatment on zinc status in diabetes mellitus. Biol. Trace Elem. Res. **32:** 311–316.
24. SATO, T.P. & K. MIKAMI. 2002. Recovery of a patient with a recurrent dysgeusia monitored by salivary variables and serum zinc content. Pathophysiology **8:** 275–281.
25. JONES, L.T. 1966. The lacrimal system and its treatment. Am. J. Ophthalmol. **62:** 503–523.
26. ANDERSON, R.A., A.M. ROUSSEL, N. ZOUARI, *et al.* 2001. Potential antioxidant effects of zinc and chromium supplementation in people with type 2 diabetes mellitus. J. Am. Coll. Nutr. **20:** 212–218.
27. MATA, A.D., D. MARQUES, M.F. MESQUITA & J. SINGH. 2002. Effect of extracellular magnesium on secretagogue-evoked amylase secretion in the isolated rat parotid gland segments. Mag. Res. **15:** 161–165.
28. PETERSEN, O.H. 1992. Stimulus-secretion coupling: cytoplasmic Ca^{2+} signals and control of ion channels in exocrine acinar cells. J. Physiol. **448:** 1–51.
29. WOODS, N.M., K.S. CUTHBERTSON & P.H. COBBOLD. 1986. Repetitive transient rises in cytoplasmic free calcium in hormone-stimulated hepatocytes. Nature **319:** 600–602.
30. ISBIR, T., L. TAMER, A. TAYLOR & M. ISBIR. 1994. Zinc, copper and magnesium status in insulin-dependent diabetes. Diabetes Res. **26:** 41–45.
31. MATHER, H.M. & G.E. LEVIN. 1979. Magnesium status in diabetes. Lancet **1:** 924.
32. FAILLA, M.L. & C.Y. GARDELL. 1985. Influence of spontaneous diabetes on tissue status of zinc, copper, and magnesium in the BB Wistar rat. Proc. Soc. Exp. Biol. Med. **180:** 317–322.

Mucormycosis Mimicks Sinusitis in a Diabetic Adult

GYÖRGY SZALAI,[a] VERONIKA FELLEGI,[a] ZSUZSANNA SZABÓ,[b] AND LAJOS CSOKONAI VITÉZ[a]

[a]*National Medical Center, Department of ENT, 1135-Budapest, Szabolcs u.35, Hungary*

[b]*St. László Hospital, Department of Pathology, H-1097 Budapest, Hungary*

ABSTRACT: Fungal sinusitis caused by invasive fungal infections, such as *Mucormycosis*, occurs predominantly in an immunocompromised patient. However, invasive cranial bone mycoses are rare and are usually associated with host immunodeficiency. They are difficult to diagnose, and in many cases are fatal. Treatment consists of antifungal chemotherapy, radical surgical debridement, and control of the underlying immunological condition. We report a case of *Mucormycosis* in a patient with type 1 diabetes mellitus. The patient had a history of dental pathology and associated renal dysfunction. The patient was managed by extensive surgical debridement followed by amphotericin B lipid complex injection (Abelcet 5 mg/bw kg/day) as an antifungal agent. Our patient's ocular function was affected. The radical treatment and follow-up by a multidisciplinary team eliminated the mucor-related consequences, however, the patient died because of end-stage renal failure. In conclusion, type 1 diabetes may be associated with invasive fungal sinusitis.

KEYWORDS: cranial bone mucormycosis; surgical debridement; immunosuppression

INTRODUCTION

Mucormycosis is considered to be the most invasive and rapidly progressive fungal infection in humans. However, early detection and treatment are the key elements for survival.[1] The wildly spread mucor rarely appears clinically in an otherwise immunocompetent person.[2] Mucormycosis commonly occurs in diabetic, immunocompromised hosts, patients with leukemia, lymphoma, multiple myeloma, septicemia, hepatitis, cirrhosis, renal failure, and patients of chemotherapy or on steroids. Intravenous drug abusers are also at risk.[3]

Address for correspondence: György Szalai, M.D., Ph.D., National Medical Center, ENT Department, Szabolcs utca 35. 1135-Budapest, Hungary. Voice/fax: +36-1-350-4731.
e-mail: szalaigy@ogyik.hu

Ann. N.Y. Acad. Sci. 1084: 520–530 (2006).
doi: 10.1196/annals.1372.010

Rhinocerebral mucormycosis is the most common form of mucormycosis and is seen particularly in cases of uncontrolled diabetes mellitus.[4]

Rhinocerebral mucormycosis is an invasive, opportunistic fungal infection usually seen in immunocompromised patients, and particularly in the setting of diabetes or immune deficiency. It is assumed that the port of entry is colonization of the nasal mucosa, allowing the fungus to spread via the paranasal sinuses into the orbit. Involvement of the brain and sometimes that of the cavernous sinus occurs by way of the orbital apex; therefore sphenoethmoidectomy with or without maxillectomy seems to be the definitive method to eradicate this infection.[5,6]

Rhinocerebral mucormycosis can be clinically diagnosed in patients, upon histological confirmation. Diabetes is the most common underlying disorder seen in these patients. In this study, the patient was assessed for predisposing factors, presenting signs and symptoms, the number and sites of surgical debridement, as well as the outcome. Ocular, sinonasal, and facial soft tissue involvement and involvement of the pterygopalatine fossa at the time of debridement were evident. No invasion through the lamina papiracea or the walls of the maxillary sinus was identified. The patient's death was caused by hypokalemia, cardiac arrhythmia, and end-stage renal failure. The pterygopalatine fossa is considered to be the main reservoir for rhinocerebral mucormycosis, and extension into the orbit and facial soft tissues usually follows.[7,8]

MATERIALS AND METHODS

Diagnosis

A 29-year-old male with type 1 diabetes was presented to our department complaining of unilateral headache, nasal congestion, nasal discharge, nausea, vomiting, and blurred vision in the right eye that rapidly progressed to near total blindness within 2 days. The patient had a dental intervention 5 days prior to the onset of his symptoms. He was not sure when he took his insulin regimen. Diabetic ketoacidosis was present upon admission.

The physical examination was remarkable for signs of florid inflammation of the right nasal turbinate and the right side of the palatal mucosa that appeared gray. Computed tomography (CT) scan of the head with contrast blood-stain revealed right nasal mucosal thickening, opacification of the right maxillary and ethmoid sinuses, and normal lateral flow in the cavernous sinuses and periorbital indurations. The patient presented the symptoms of subcomplete ophthalmoplegia with some light seeing. There was an almost total blindness with pupillary difference and fixation on the right side. Ophthalmoscopy revealed a grayish-white retina, a hazy optic disc, and a flat, dark macula. The left eye was normal in all respects.

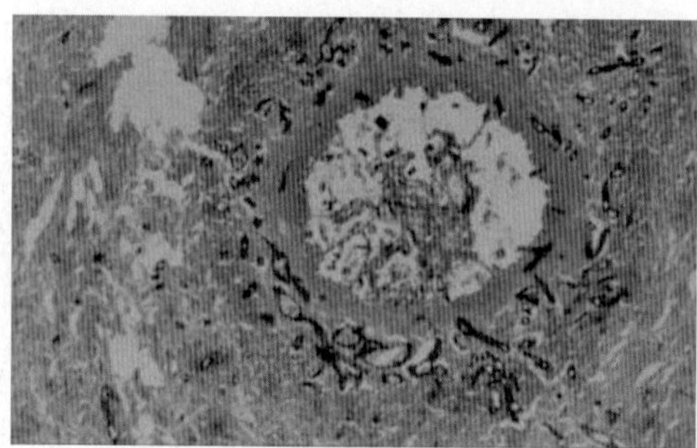

FIGURE 1. Nonseparate hyphae branching at right angles consistent with *Mucor* species HE and Grocot stain.

Treatment

A preliminary evaluation and diagnosis of rhinocerebral infection were made without excluding the possibility of zygomycosis. The drug of choice for most invasive mycoses is amphotericin B, but its use is limited by both frequent nephrotoxicity and the noticeable pharmacokinetic differences among the lipid-based formulations. Upon admission, amphotericin B (1.5 mg/kg of bw/day) was administered with wide spectrum antibiotics parentally.

The first operative plan was a right Winkler–Jansen transmaxillary–ethmoidectomy and a request for frozen tissue section and a periodic acid Schiff (PAS) stain from the tissue samples. Access was gained to the maxillary antrum by a Caldwell–Luc approach. The ethmoid complex was opened and diseased mucosa was cleared completely. Histopathologic evaluation revealed nonseparate hyphae branching at right angles consistent with *Mucor* species (FIG. 1).

CT of the brain was performed on the sixth day post surgery and revealed a relevant enhancement with inflammatory changes in the frontal lobe (FIG. 2). CT obtained on the first and seventh days after the initial surgery showed marked enhancement of the right temporal lobe compatible with inflammatory changes. Laboratory studies of the serum showed 0.33–0.24 red blood cells/mL; nucleated cells 22.4–4.6 × G/L. In addition there was an increase in serum creatinine levels (FIG. 3). Due to the decline in the patent's renal function and lack of response to treatment with conventional amphotericin B therapy, the patient was switched to amphotericin B lipid complex (ABELCET®) at a dose of 3 mg/bw kg/day (150 mg a day). G-CSF was administered to improve presumed minimal neutrophil function.[9]

Follow-up CT on days 7 and 21 showed a slowly diminished abnormal enhancement at the right frontal lobe of the brain (FIG. 4).

Second surgery was taken on day 8 in hospital. Right total maxillectomy, sphenoidectomy, and orbital exenteration were performed.

(A)

(B)

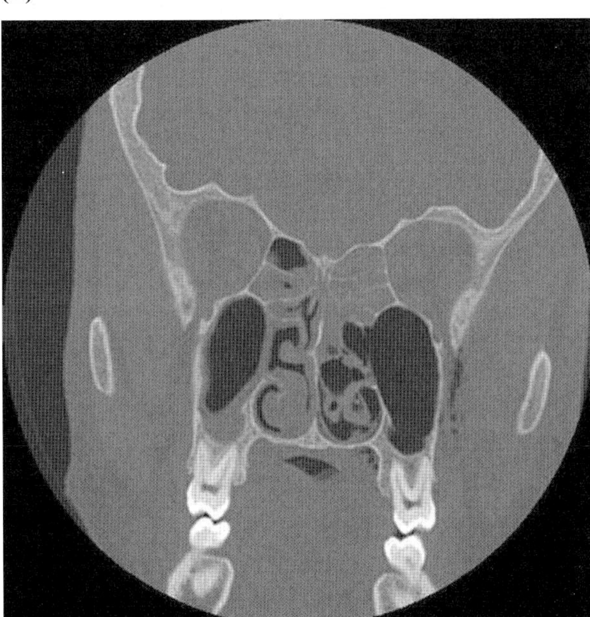

FIGURE 2. CT obtained first (**A**) and seventh (**B**) days after the initial surgery shows marked enhancement of the right temporal lobe compatible with inflammatory changes and periosteal bubble formation.

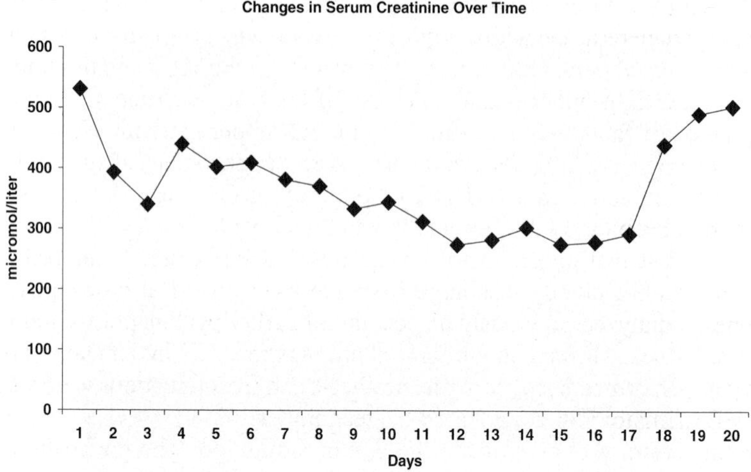

FIGURE 3. A curve demonstrating the difficulty in keeping serum creatinine level to a lower range specially from day 19 in the hospital.

Oral morphine 15 mg every 6–8 h as needed was also administered from admission to day 7.

Patients Outcome

Eight days prior to being admitted to hospital he was presented with facial pain after the right upper incisivus was treated twice by a dentist and

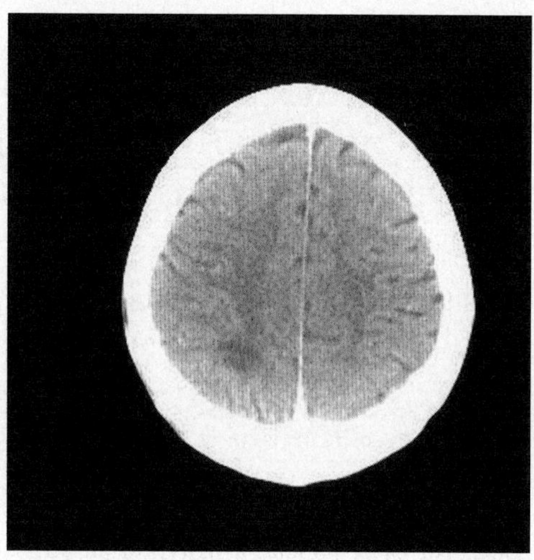

FIGURE 4. CT of the brain at day 7 presents some intracranial lesion at the right frontal lobe of the brain.

supplemented with clindamycin. Approximately 5 days following the initial visit, the patient returned with complaints of worsening symptoms that included right-sided facial pain with right eye involvement, numbness and tingling sensation in the right upper palate, and loss of taste on the same side. He also complained of fatigue and weakness in the left upper extremity. The patient denied having fevers, chills, rhinorrhea, sore throat, or visual disturbances. There were no complaints of nausea, vomiting, or diarrhea. The patient was admitted to hospital for further workup and treatment.

On the first day of admission to the hospital he became subfebrile and presented with a bloody discharge from the right nostril at blowing. In the anamnesis: dialyzed previously on account of earlier pyelonephritis and renal abscess. CT scan showed no intraorbital propagation. A Winkler–Jansen operation was performed under general anesthesia and frozen sections were stained with HE (hematoxylin-eosin) and PAS techniques.

Amphotericin was given from the day of admission. The medication was switched to amphotericin B lipid complex (Abelcet, 150 mg per day) on day 4 after histology confirmed the diagnosis. Empirical therapy with oral itraconazole at 200 mg bid and oral amoxicillin-clavulanate at 875 mg bid and 2 × 0.3 mL nadropain, 3 × 1 g meropenem, later 20 mg famotidine, alprazolam, and sertraline was administered, with some clinical improvement. Gram stain of the sinus aspirate revealed heavy red blood cells, rare leukocytes, and no microorganisms.

The patient was treated with 14U-12U-13U-8U-4U of recombinant human insulin with a daily 150 g carbohydrate diet under continuous serum glucose control adjustment (FIG. 5).

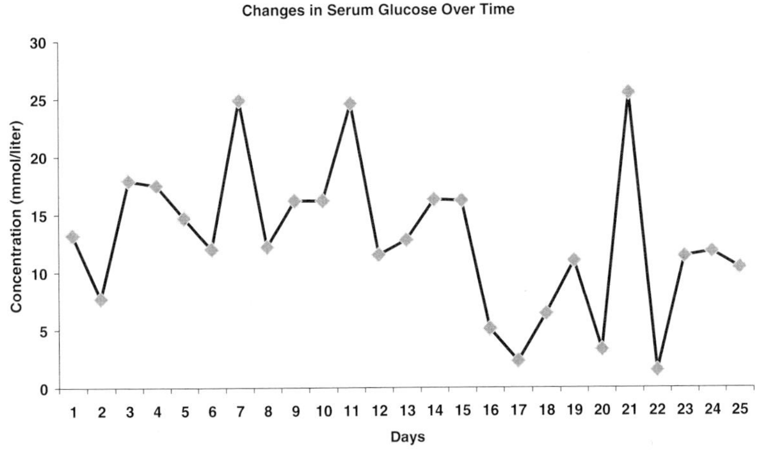

FIGURE 5. Serum glucose over time with the recombinant insulin treatment and repeated control at bedside. The *curve* presents a sign of major difficulty to adjust serum glucose level to the acceptable range.

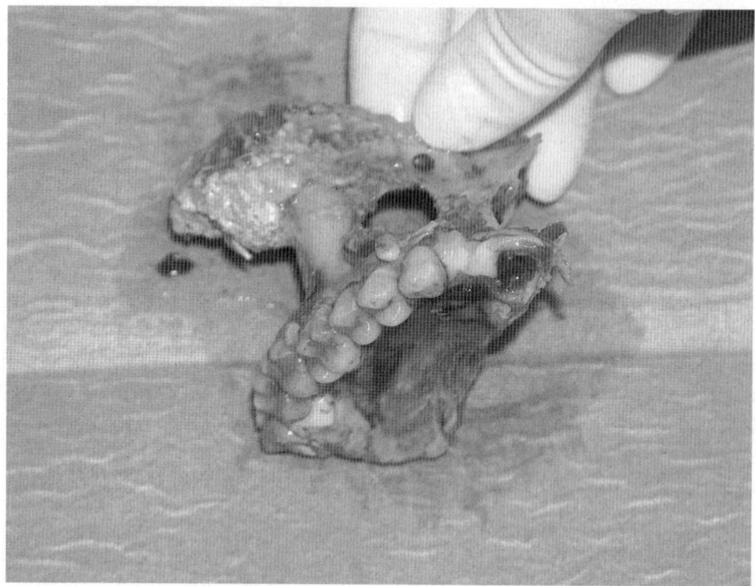

FIGURE 6. Resected right maxilla.

At day 6, control CT presented a niveau in the right sphenoid sinus, orbital propagation of the inflammation till orbital apex with the sign of gas formation in tissues. CT showed hypodensity in right parietal lobe, a sign of possible septic embolization. Right radical maxillectomy was performed with orbital exenteration under general anesthesia (FIG. 6).

At day 21, TIVA (total intravenous anesthesia) and PEG (percutaneous gastrostomy) were performed.

During hospital treatment daily debridement was made. Because of left upper arm weakness, physiotherapy was performed daily. On day 29, a bulla was found over the right elbow. Surgical incision and drainage was performed and showed methicillin-resistant staphylococcus aureus (MRSA) infection after microbiological examination. At the beginning of the treatment, renal function improved slowly with intravenous hydration and low-dose dopamine.

Vancomycin treatment was initiated. On day 30, hemoculture showed a rapidly progressing metabolic acidosis, which resulted in the death of the patient.

Grocot stain showed wide and nonseptate mycelia with rhizoids coming off directly from the stolon and sporangiophore. The sporangium was round and filled with spores. Identification of the subtype of mucor species had not been performed. Following isolation of the mold, sinus debridement was performed and Grocot staining of a maxillary sinus tissue showed broad, nonseptate

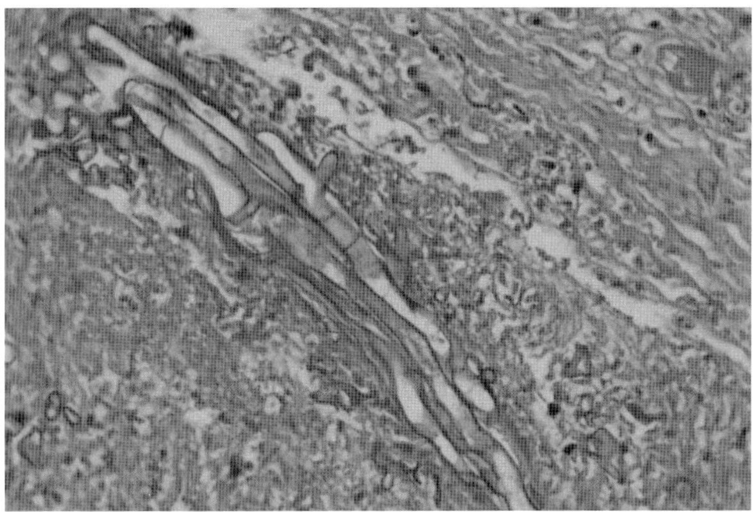

FIGURE 7. Tissue sample stained with HE: hyphae are present in the wall and lumen of necrotic blood vessels highly suggestive of angioinvasion.

hyphae consistent with a zygomycete. Hyphae present in the walls and lumen of necrotic blood vessels were highly suggestive of angioinvasion (FIG. 7).

Radiological investigations included magnetic resonance imaging scans of the brain and sinuses and showed extensive sinus disease and an unusually aerated right sphenoid wing. CT imaging of the cervical spine found no evidence of lesions or other abnormalities.

Treatment over 1 month with maximally tolerated doses of amphotericin halted intracranial extension but rapid metabolic complications resulted in the death of the patient. During pathological dissection there were no detectable mucor around resection lines and within 1 month after the surgery, all the clinical signs were resolved. Serial biopsies that included histopathologic investigation confirmed eradication of the invasive mucor.

Full reassessment at the time failed to demonstrate any residual fungus.

Following confirmation of infection with a zygomycete, liposomal amphotericin B was initiated at a dose of 3–5 mg/kg/day for approximately 4 weeks (total dose of 5500 mg) with concurrent, often daily, surgical debridement of the sinuses and nasal washes with amphotericin solution (1 mg/5 mL bid). In addition, very aggressive management of his diabetes mellitus was undertaken. He was initially placed on insulin.

CONCLUSION

Mucormycosis is an uncommon infection caused by fungi of the *Zygomycetes* class that comprised the orders *Mucorales* and *Entomophthorales*.

The members of the order *Mucorales* have most often been implicated as pathogens in human disease and include the genera *Rhizopus, Mucor, Rhizomucor, Absidia, Apophysomyces, Saksenaea, Cunninghamella, Syncephalastrum,* and *Cokeromyces*.[10–12] The zygomycetes are hyaline fungi found in air, soil, and food and produce wide, ribbon-like, nonseptate, or sparsely septate hyphae in human tissue. The primary route of transmission is inhalation of spores from the environment; however, cutaneous or percutaneous routes of exposure have also been implicated in the disease.[2,13] Demonstration of invasive disease due to these organisms generally requires growth from a specimen obtained from a normally sterile site or identification of fungal elements within tissue, as colonization and laboratory contamination have been reported.[10]

Several studies show that zygomycosis represent approximately 5–12% of all fungal infections in high-risk patient groups and are considered opportunistic pathogens.[10] Similar to *Aspergillus* spp., zygomycetes cause a spectrum of clinical diseases that affect a variety of systems, including the sinonasal, rhinocerebral, pulmonary, cardiac, gastrointestinal, and cutaneous systems.[14–16] Rhinocerebral or craniofacial zygomycosis is the most frequently encountered form and is usually fulminant and rapidly fatal. *Rhizopus* spp. are the most commonly implicated organisms causing craniofacial zygomycosis, accounting for about 90% of all infections with the Zygomycetes.[10,15] The host is typically immunocompromised, with granulocytopenic and acidotic patients being at highest risk. Diabetes mellitus is the single most common predisposing illness associated with the development of this infection.[10] In this report, we present a case of rhinocerebral mucormycosis in a patient with diabetes mellitus and end-stage renal disease that responded to surgical treatment and therapy with high-dose liposomal amphotericin B.

Identification of the mucor was important in terms of clinical management. Histopathologic examination of biopsied-debrided-exentered sinus tissue revealed characteristic aseptate branching hyphae with invasion of the blood vessels consistent with zygomycosis.

This case highlights the difficulty and importance of early diagnosis of zygomycosis as the patient was initially thought to have a dental infection and later a bacterial sinusitis.[17] This 5- to 8-day delay could translate into complications and treatment failures at first.[18,19] Hospital evaluation and prompt administration of antifungal treatment was efficient but IDDM and the rapid progression to the end-stage renal status resulted in the death of the patient.

Although zygomycosis is a rare fungal infection in immunocompetent hosts, it most frequently develops in patients with diabetes mellitus or hematologic malignancies, and is characterized by a mortality rate of approximately 70%.[18] Cases of zygomycosis reported in the literature include patients with acute leukemia or lymphoma and other hematologic malignancies, as well as organ or stem cell transplant recipients with their associated immunosuppressive treatments.[10,18,20] Clinical practice experience suggests that successful treatment of zygomycosis requires (*a*) early and aggressive surgical excision of necrotic lesions, (*b*) recovery of immune function or control of underlying disease, and (*c*) intensive antifungal therapy.[12,14,21,22] To date, the literature supports the use of intravenous amphotericin B as the primary antifungal treatment for all forms of zygomycosis.[11,13]

In this case, cranial nerve abnormalities on presentation, combined with the patient's history of IDDM, and renal disease-related immunosuppression, placed zygomycosis at the top of the differential diagnosis. Considering that special stains of samples from the paranasal sinuses revealed a Rhizopus species being the offending organism, the drug of choice was liposomal amphotericin B, which enabled aggressive and continuous antifungal therapy. Treatment was both appropriate and effective against craniofacial zygomycosis in this patient.

REFERENCES

1. HENDRICKSON, R.G., J. OLSHAKER & O. DUCKETT. 1999. Rhinocerebral mucormycosis: a case of a rare, but deadly disease. J. Emerg. Med. **17:** 641–645.
2. PRABHU, R.M. & R. PATEL. 2004. Mucormycosis and entomophthoramycosis: a review of the clinical manifestations, diagnosis and treatment. Clin. Microbiol. Infect. **10**(Suppl 1): 31–47.
3. TUGSEL, Z., B. SEZER & T. AKALIN. 2004. Facial swelling and palatal ulceration in a diabetic patient. Oral Surg. Oral Med. Oral Pathol. Oral Radiol. Endod. **98:** 630–636.
4. LEHRER, R.I., T. GANZ, M.E. SELSTED, *et al.* 1988. Neutrophils and host defense. Ann. Intern. Med. **109:** 127–142.
5. HOSSEINI, S.M. & P. BORGHEI. 2005. Rhinocerebral mucormycosis: pathways of spread. Eur. Arch. Otorhinolaryngol. **262:** 932–938.
6. FEELEY, M.A., P.D. RIGHI, T.E. DAVIS & A. GREIST. 1999. Mucormycosis of the paranasal sinuses and septum. Otolaryngol. Head Neck Surg. **120:** 750.
7. KHOR, B.S., M.H. LEE, H.S. LEU & J.W. LIU. 2003. Rhinocerebral mucormycosis in Taiwan. J. Microbiol. Immunol. Infect. **36:** 266–269.
8. VERMA, A., B. BROZMAN & C.K. PETITO. 2006. Isolated cerebral mucormycosis: report of a case and review of the literature. J. Neurol. Sci. **240:** 65–69.
9. ALEXANDER, B.D. & J.R. WINGARD. 2005. Study of renal safety in amphotericin B lipid complex-treated patients. Clin. Infect. Dis. **40:** S414–S421.
10. SPELLBERG, B., J. EDWARDS, Jr., & A. IBRAHIM. 2005. Novel perspectives on mucormycosis: pathophysiology, presentation, and management. Clin. Microbiol. Rev. **18:** 556–569.
11. GROLL, A.H. & T.J. WALSH. 2001. Uncommon opportunistic fungi: new nosocomial threats. Clin. Microbiol. Infect. **7**(Suppl. 2): 8–24.
12. RIBES, J.A., C.L. VANOVER-SAMS & D.J. BAKER. 2000. Zygomycetes in human disease. Clin. Microbiol. Rev. **13:** 236–301.
13. HANDZEL, O., Z. LANDAU & D. HALPERIN. 2003. Liposomal amphotericin B treatment for rhinocerebral mucormycosis: how much is enough? Rhinology **41:** 184–186.
14. STEINBACH, W.J. & J.R. PERFECT. 2003. Newer antifungal therapy for emerging fungal pathogens. Int. J. Infect. Dis. **7:** 5–20.

15. O'Neill, B.M., A.S. Alessi, E.B. George & J. Piro. 2006. Disseminated rhinocerebral mucormycosis: a case report and review of the literature. J. Oral Maxillofacial Surg. **64:** 326–333.
16. Weber, A.L., L.V. Romo & N.R. Sabates. 1999. Pseudotumor of the orbit: clinical, pathologic, and radiologic evaluation. Radiol. Clin. North Am. **37:** 151–168.
17. Kim, J., J.K. Fortson & H.E. Cook. 2001. A fatal outcome from rhinocerebral mucormycosis after dental extractions: a case report. J. Oral Maxillofacial Surg. **59:** 693–697.
18. Pagano, L., M. Offidani, L. Fianchi, *et al.* 2004. Mucormycosis in hematologic patients. Haematologica **89:** 207–214.
19. Wirth, F., R. Perry, A. Eskenazi, *et al.* 1997. Cutaneous mucormycosis with subsequent visceral dissemination in a child with neutropenia: a case report and review of the pediatric literature. J. Am. Acad. Dermatol. **36:** 336–341.
20. Procop, G.W. & G.D. Roberts. 2004. Emerging fungal diseases: the importance of the host [review]. Clin. Lab. Med. **24:** 691–719.
21. Talmi, Y.P., A. Goldschmied-Reouven, M. Bakon, *et al.* 2002. Rhino-orbital and rhino-orbito-cerebral mucormycosis. Otolaryngol. Head Neck Surg. **127:** 22–31.
22. Hochman, I.I., H. Elran, G. Zucker, *et al.* 2000. Surgical management of aggressive fungal infection involving the anterior skull base. Oper. Tech. Otolaryngol. Head Neck Surg. **11:** 268–270.

Index of Contributors

Adeghate, E., xiii–xiv, 1–29, 71–88, 178–190, 223–234, 296–303, 361–370, 371–390, 391–401, 402–410, 411–431, 432–441, 442–451, 503–519
Adem, A., xiii–xiv, 155–165, 223–234, 402–410
Adili, F., 329–349
Afandi, B., 319–324
Agarwal, S.C., 191–207
Ahmad, S., 319–324
Ahmed, F.N., 481–489
Al Haj Ali, M., 402–410
Al Hakim, A., 49–57
Al Mazrouei, M., 155–165
Al Qaydi, M., 155–165
Al Shamisi, M., 49–57
Al Shamsi, N., 155–165
Al Shamsi, M., 371–390, 411–431, 432–441
Alaveras, A., 89–117, 166–177
Alexandraki, K., 89–117
Amin, A., 371–390, 391–401, 411–431, 432–441
Assaf, H., 319–324
Atherton, P., 490–502
Atkins, S., 350–360
Azim Mabrouk, A., 325–328

Batbayar, B., 280–295
Benedict, S., 223–234
Bin-Othman, S., 325–328
Biswas, S., 452–480
Bracken, N., 178–190, 208–222
Bradley-Watson, P., 132–140

Chandranath, S.I., 155–165, 223–234, 402–410
Changrani, N.R., 503–519
Chonkar, A., 178–190, 442–451, 503–519
Corban, R., 350–360

Dashora, U.K., 191–207
Dennison, S., 452–480
Dhalla, N.S., 141–154
Dhanasekaran, S., 267–279
Dunn, E., 1–29

Eapen, V., 325–328
Elkhumaidi, S., 319–324
Ezimokhai, M., 132–140

Fahim, M., 223–234
Fehér, E., 280–295
Fellegi, V., 520–530
Frampton, C.M., 267–279

Gbewonyo, A., 361–370
Gebbie, J., 191–207, 304–318

Haghighatpanahb, M., 329–349
Harris, F., 166–177, 452–480
Herder, C., 30–48
Home, P., 191–207, 304–318
Hopkin, R., 442–451
Howarth, F.C., 155–165, 208–222, 361–370
Hsu, D.K., 49–57
Hussain, M., 178–190

Joseph, A., 132–140

Kalofoutis, A., 89–117, 166–177
Kalofoutis, C., 89–117, 166–177
Kamiya, H., 235–249
Karkoukli, M.A., 319–324
Kazzam, E., 155–165
Kelly, B., 319–324
Kempf, K., 30–48
Kleophas, U., 30–48
Kolb, H., 30–48

Larijani, B., 329–349
Latt, Z., 178–190
Law, H.N., 191–207, 304–318
Liu, X., 141–154
Lotfy, M., 391–401
Lukic, M.L., 49–57

Martin, S., 30–48
Martinez, M.A., 58–70
Martinez-Burgos, M.A., 71–88
Martinus, R., 350–360
Matear, D., 319–324
Mensah-Brown, E., 49–57, 267–279
Mohamed, S., 118–131
Morrison, J.F.B., 267–279

Naqvi, F.N., 481–489
Nyberg, F., 402–410

Obineche, E., xiii–xiv, 223–234

Padmanabhan, R., 118–131
Parekh, K., 49–57
Pariente, J.A., 58–70, 71–88
Patel, R., 58–70, 71–88, 490–502
Phoenix, D.A., 166–177, 452–480
Piperi, C., 89–117, 166–177
Ponery, A.S., 402–410

Qureshi, A., 155–165

Rajbandari, S., 296–303
Rashed, H., 296–303, 361–370
Rose, B., 30–48

Saadi, H., xiii–xiv, 319–324
Sabri, S., 325–328
Saeed, T., 361–370
Salido, G.M., 58–70, 71–88
Schattner, P., 1–29
Sethi, R., 141–154
Shafiq, F., 481–489
Shafiullah, M., 391–401
Shahin, A., 49–57
Sheen, R., 267–279
Shervington, A., 71–88
Sibal, L., 191–207, 304–318
Sima, A.A.F., 235–249
Singh, J., 58–70, 71–88, 89–117, 166–177, 178–190, 208–222, 296–303, 350–360, 442–451, 452–480, 490–502, 503–519
Singh, S., 118–131
Suzuki, H., 141–154
Szabó, Z., 520–530
Szalai, G., 520–530

Takeda, N., 141–154
Tappia, P.S., 141–154

Vér, Á., 280–295
Vitéz, L.C., 520–530

Wackerhage, H., 350–360, 490–502

Zelles, T., 280–295
Ziegler, D., 250–266
Zisaki, A., 166–177